Learning Disabilities

For Churchill Livingstone

Senior Commissioning Editor: Susan Young
Project Development Manager: Karen Gilmour
Project Manager: Derek Robertson
Design Direction: Judith Wright

Learning Disabilities

Edited by

Bob Gates MSc BEd(Hons) DipN RNMH RMN CertEd RNT

Head of Learning Disability, Faculty of Health and Human Sciences,
Thames Valley University, Berkshire, UK

FOURTH EDITION

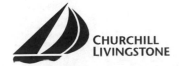
CHURCHILL
LIVINGSTONE

CHURCHILL LIVINGSTONE
An imprint of Elsevier Science Limited

ISBN 0443 071357

British Library Cataloguing in Publication Data
A catalogue record for this book is available from the British Library

Library of Congress Cataloguing in Publication Data
A catalog record for this book is available from the Library of Congress

Note
Medical knowledge is constantly changing. As new information becomes available, changes in treatment, procedures, equipment and the use of drugs become necessary. The editors, contributors and the publishers have taken care to ensure that the information given in this text is accurate and up to date. However, readers are strongly advised to confirm that the information, especially with regard to drug usage, complies with the latest legislation and standards of practice.

Cover photos from www.JohnBirdsall.co.uk

The
Publisher's
policy is to use
**paper manufactured
from sustainable forests**

Printed in China by RDC Limited

Contents

Contributors

Maggie Anderson
Director of Clinical Services, London Early Autism Project, Leap House, London, UK
Chapter 11 – Autistic spectrum disorder

Helen Atherton
Lecturer in Learning Disability Nursing, Department of Learning Disabilities, Faculty of Health, University of Hull, Hull, UK
Chapter 3 – A history of learning disabilities

Owen Barr
Lecturer in Learning Disability Nursing, School of Health Sciences, University of Ulster, Coleraine, Northern Ireland
Chapter 24 – Working effectively with families of people with learning disabilities

Ms Barbro Blomberg
University Lecturer, Department of Health Sciences and Social Work, Vaxjo University, Vaxjo, Sweden
Chapter 27 – Sweden

Tom Bush
Principal Lecturer, Faculty of Human Sciences, Institute of Health Studies, University of Plymouth, Exeter, UK
Chapter 9 – Employment, leisure and learning disabilities

Elaine Chaplin
Consultant Art Therapist, Independent Community Living Ltd, Caerphilly, Swansea, UK
Chapter 21 – Art, drama and music therapies

David Dickinson
Principal Educational Psychologist, Lincoln, UK
Chapter 7 – Compulsory school education

Linda Dickinson
Learning Support Teacher, Lincoln, UK
Chapter 7 – Compulsory school education

Rita Ferris-Taylor
Lecturer, Kensington and Chelsea College; Tutor, Makaton Vocabulary Development Project; Freelance Trainer, Advocate, Willesden, London UK
Chapter 15 – Communication

Bob Gates
Head of Learning Disability, Faculty of Health and Human Sciences, Thames Valley University, Berkshire, UK
Chapter 1 – The nature of learning disabilities
Chapter 5 – Residential alternatives for people with learning disabilities
Chapter 13 – Self-injurious behaviour

Sue Hart
Lecturer (Clinical) in Learning Disability, EIHMS, Duke of Kent Building, University of Surrey, Guildford, UK
Chapter 16 – Health and health promotion

Robert Jenkins
Senior Lecturer, School of Care Science, University of Glamorgan, Pontypridd, UK
Chapter 18 – Specialist learning disability services in the UK

Mark Jukes
Senior Lecturer (Learning Disabilities), Faculty of Health and Community Care, School of Continuing Care and Community Nursing, University of Central England in Birmingham, Birmingham, UK
Chapter 30 – Management and leadership in learning disability

Odete Lopes
Oxfordshire Learning Disability NHS Trust, Oxford, UK
Chapter 14 – People with learning disabilities who have offended in law

Steve McNally
Lecturer/Practitioner, School of Health Care Studies, Oxford Brookes University, Isis Education Centre, Oxford, UK
Chapter 25 – Helping to empower people

Richard Manners
Consultant Art Therapist, Independent Community Living Ltd, Caerphilly, Swansea, UK
Chapter 21 – Art, drama and music therapies

Ian Mansell
Senior Lecturer, School of Care Sciences, University of Glamorgan, Pontypridd, UK
Chapter 18 – Specialist learning disability services in the UK

Jill Manthorpe
Reader, Department of Social Work, University of Hull, Hull, UK
Chapter 4 – Accessing services and support

David Marsland
Project Manager, QUEST, East Yorkshire Learning Disability Institute, Faculty of Health, University of Hull, Hull, UK
Chapter 6 – Evaluating the quality of support services for people with learning disabilities

Ruth Northway
Professor of Learning Disability Nursing, School of Care Sciences, University of Glamorgan, Pontypridd, UK
Chapter 18 – Specialist learning disability services in the UK

Peter Oakes
Consultant Clinical Psychologist and Lecturer, Department of Clinical Psychology, Faculty of Health, University of Hull, Hull, UK
Chapter 23 – Sexual and personal relationships

Chris Parkin
Lecturer, Hull College, Hull, UK
Chapter 8 – Post-compulsory education

Rob Parry
Teaching Dean, School of Nursing and Midwifery, University of Dundee, Dundee, UK
Chapter 29 – Education and training

Karen Paton
Clinical Specialist Aromatherapist, Berkshire Healthcare NHS Trust; Lecturer/Practitioner, Thames Valley University, Berkshire, UK
Chapter 20 – Complementary therapies

Cathy Renouf
Formerly Education Officer, English National Board for Nursing, Midwifery and Health Visiting, York, UK
Chapter 29 – Education and training

Sabine Rothe
Professor of Social Psychology, University of Applied Sciences, Frankfurt am Main, Germany
Chapter 28 – Germany

Dermot Rowe
Consultant Psychiatrist, Waddiloves Health Centre, Bradford District Care Trust, Bradford, UK
Chapter 14 – People with learning disabilities who have offended in law

Helen Sanderson
Regional Advisor, North West Training and Development Team, Manchester, UK
Chapter 19 – Person-centred planning

Truce Soeter
Senior Lecturer, Hogeschool Van Arnhem Em Nijmegen, Faculty of Health Nursing, Nijmegen, The Netherlands
Chapter 26 – The Netherlands

Gillian Stevens
Senior Music Therapist, Arts Therapies Department, Alders House, Cwmbran Torfaen, UK
Chapter 21 – Art, drama and music therapies

Ibrahim Turkistani
Consultant and Assistant Professor in Psychiatry and Epilepsy, Faculty of Medicine and Medical Sciences, University Hospital, Um-Al-Qura-University, Makkah, Saudi-Arabia
Chapter 12 – Mental ill health in learning disabilities

Eileen Wake
Lecturer in Paediatrics, University of Hull, Hull, UK
Chapter 17 – Profound and multiple disability

Angie Walker
Lecturer, Hull College, Hull, UK
Chapter 8 – Post-compulsory education

Deborah Watson
Tutor, School of Nursing, Faculty of Health, University of Hull, Hull, UK
Chapter 2 – Causes and manifestations of learning disabilities
Chapter 17 – Profound and multiple disability

David Wilberforce
Lecturer/Practitioner, Faculty of Health, University of Hull, Hull, UK
Chapter 1 – The nature of learning disabilities
Chapter 22 – Psychological approaches

Mick Wolverson
Lecturer/Practitioner, Faculty of Health, University of Hull and Rotherham Priority Health Trust, Hull, UK
Chapter 10 – Challenging behaviour

Jane Wray
Research Associate, East Yorkshire Learning Disability Institute, University of Hull, Hull, UK
Chapter 20 – Complementary therapies

Preface

In the foreword to the recent, and long awaited White Paper for people with learning disabilities (DOH 2001), the current Prime Minister of the UK, Tony Blair stated:

People with a learning disability can lead full and rewarding lives as many already do. But others find themselves pushed to the margins of our society. And almost all encounter prejudice, bullying, insensitive treatment and discrimination at some time in their lives.

Whereas the White Paper is intended to provide central government direction for England only, it is likely that the other constituent countries of the UK will adopt similar themes and directions. Given the enormous importance of this piece of legislation it would seem opportune to briefly outline its main features in the preface to this new edition of *Learning Disabilities*. It is 30 years since the last publication of the now famous, historically at least, White Paper (DHSS 1971) that sought to provide central and strategic policy on the future direction of services for people with learning disabilities. This White Paper has stood as a landmark in the development of more appropriate and informed services for people with learning disabilities and their families. Similarly, the new White Paper articulates the potentially exciting nature of future service configurations for people with learning disabilities in England.

The new vision for people with learning disabilities is based upon four fundamental principles: rights, independence, choice and inclusion. In addition, new national objectives and targets are set to assist local agencies to benchmark their progress toward obtaining them. The main body of the White Paper (Chapters 2 to 10) is concerned with promoting better life chances for people with learning disabilities. Having outlined the problems and challenges in learning disabilities in Chapter 1 – including, amongst other things, epidemiology; services and expenditure, and developments since 1971 – Chapter 2 moves on to present the underlying value base of the White Paper. Chapter 3 explores many of the issues currently facing disabled children and young people. The Paper, quite rightly, identifies the many barriers that such children and their families' face in fully participating in their communities. The Paper promotes the benefits to be obtained by children with learning disabilities by educational opportunities, good health and social care whilst living with their families, or in other settings. To assist in this, it is proposed that children with learning disabilities and their families will benefit from improved funding to special schools, assistance in accessing mainstream schools and the new Connexions Service. Chapter 4 outlines the need for more choice and for the control of lifestyle to be located with people with learning disabilities themselves. Perhaps not surprisingly, the need to accelerate the use made of direct payments by people with learning disabilities and advocacy services are promoted. Central to this is person-centred planning – and the Government commits itself to issuing guidance from the Department of Health. Supporting carers has long been an issue in the research literature, therefore a specific chapter that outlines how the government will achieve this is provided. Recognition that a significant number of people with learning disabilities are cared for by older carers and that the government has committed itself to identifying that a percentage of these people will have an agreed plan is to be particularly welcomed. Similarly to be welcomed is Chapter 6, which identifies a range of specific issues concerning the health of people with learning disabilities; this issue has been repeatedly reported in the research literature for at least two decades. Attention to issues around consent to treatment, specialist learning disability services, the identification of Health Facilitators (by 2003) and a Health Action Plan (by 2005), will impact upon the way we work with people with learning disabilities for many years to come. Chapter 7 focuses upon housing, fulfilling lives and employment. Given recent research in England concerning the quality and costs of different types of residential accommodation (see Chapter 5 of this book) the White Paper says 'No housing solution should be routinely disregarded as a matter of deliberate policy' (DOH 2001; 7.5.). Equally important is recognition that the issue of where they live is not the only determinant of quality issues in people's lives. The White Paper acknowledges the importance of management style and staff training; this is explored in considerable detail in Chapter 8. It is to be hoped that the Partnership Boards proposed in the White Paper bring about a genuine choice of housing options for people with learning disabilities. Research literature from the field of learning disabilities has told us for some time that of those able to express a view, many people with learning disabilities wish to live within their communities leading full and productive lives supported by friends. In addition, people with learning disabilities expect to be able to access recreation and employment without discrimination. To this end, the key actions and objectives around these issues are encouraging. However, some concern ought to be raised at the perception of people with learning disabilities as a homogenous group (Aylot 2001). The extent of user involvement, whilst to be applauded, might not necessarily represent

the pluralistic views of people with profound and/or complex needs. Let us hope that those people with profound learning disabilities and complex needs are not paradoxically marginalised by the very policy that seeks to bring about their inclusion. Chapter 8 explores issues of quality, training and some detail is given to exploring people with additional and complex needs. Of enormous importance are the key actions surrounding quality that include setting minimum national standards for residential care, local quality assurance frameworks, guidance on user surveys and physical intervention, collation of data of abuse and assistance of vulnerable witnesses to give evidence in a court of law. Concerning training there are to be Health and Social Care strategies to provide new opportunities for learning disability staff, the arrival of the Learning Disability Awards Framework, development of leadership initiatives and local work force planning. Chapter 9 outlines the need to establish new learning disability Partnership Boards and identifies how these Boards will implement Joint Investment Plans, that will secure 'inter-agency planning and commissioning of comprehensive, integrated and inclusive services'. This chapter also identifies that future guidance on the work of community learning disability teams is to be forthcoming. Finally, in Chapter 10, the White Paper identifies how the government intends to bring about this new vision of services for people with learning disabilities and their families. This includes the setting up of a Learning Disability Task Force, the creation of a Learning Disability Fund, setting up a national Implementation Support Team, and the creation of an information base on learning disability. Even as this preface is been written, national and regional directors have been appointed to an implementation support team. At the end of Chapter 10, a five-year delivery plan is outlined that identifies key milestones for implementation.

Let us hope that this White Paper does improve life chances of people with learning disabilities, and brings about their inclusion into the communities in which they live.

This book, now in its fourth edition, hopes to assist those who work with people with learning disabilities by making a small contribution to the enormous agenda for modernising health and social services. Hopefully, it will assist this by providing nurses, social workers, therapists – indeed any one with an interest in this area – by providing them with a sufficient knowledge base concerning people with learning disabilities. The fourth edition of *Learning Disabilities* has been completely rewritten. This has been done not only to take account of the recent White Paper, but also because of developments in the field of learning disabilities. Evidently there was need for a more substantive text book accessible enough to attract a wider readership than the last issue, yet substantial enough to support vocational programmes of study in learning disabilities from the Learning Disability Award Framework through to that of undergraduate programmes of study. It is also hoped that parents and interested others may also use this text.

In this edition, in addition to areas previously covered, there are new chapters on person-centred planning, people who have offended, management and leadership, education and training, self-injurious behaviour, monitoring and evaluation of services, psychological approaches, art and music, further education, autistic spectrum disorder, mental health, specialist services and services in three other European countries. The book is divided into eight sections and comprises 30 chapters in total. Each chapter is supported by contemporary research and other relevant literature. Extensive use of reader activities has been made throughout the book and nearly all chapters provide further resources.

Learning Disabilities has become a highly regarded text book in the field of learning disability and is currently used by many professionals and students from a wide range of different professional and academic backgrounds. Its success is due entirely to the excellent contributions of friends and colleagues from across the United Kingdom and other countries and I thank them for their trust in me as editor by contributing to this text book. As importantly, I hope you the reader find this textbook helpful and that in some small part it assists in bringing about the inclusion of people with learning disabilities into our communities.

BG, Ottringham 2003

REFERENCES

Aylott J 2001 The new learning disabilities White Paper: did it forget something? British Journal of Nursing. 10(8): 512

Department of Health and Social Security (DHSS) 1971 Better Services for the Mentally Handicapped. London: HMSO

DOH 2001 Valuing people: A new strategy for learning disability for the 21st Century. Cm 5806. SO, London.

1

Understanding learning disabilities

In this section three important areas are explored that provide a foundation of knowledge upon which the remaining content of the book is based. In Chapter 1, David Wilberforce and Bob Gates outline the nature of learning disabilities and provide some case illustrations that demonstrate the heterogeneous variation of a complex phenomena – learning disability. In Chapter 2, Debbie Watson identifies a range of causes and manifestations of learning disabilities, and in Chapter 3, Helen Atherton provides a comprehensive history of learning disabilities, focussing chiefly on the United Kingdom.

1

The nature of learning disabilities

Bob Gates, David Wilberforce

KEY ISSUES

- Defining learning disability is difficult because it means many things to many people.
- Generally it is agreed that learning disability comprises significant sub-average intellectual functioning that coexists with below average social functioning and that this manifests itself before the age of 18.
- Over time intellectual ability, legislative definitions and social competence have all been used for establishing whether someone has learning disabilities.
- Throughout history different academic disciplines have attempted to account for learning disabilities in different ways and this has often dictated how services for this group of people have been formulated.
- It is generally agreed that 3–4 persons per 1000 of the general population will have severe and 25–30 persons per 1000 of the general population will have mild learning disabilities.

INTRODUCTION TO LEARNING DISABILITY

The first part of this chapter explores how it is decided whether someone has learning disabilities and to this extent it enables us to define what learning disability means. Defining learning disability is much easier to talk about than it is to achieve. Understanding any concept, idea or phenomenon requires access to a prescribed language that expresses some common understanding amongst people as to what is being discussed, explored or studied. This is necessary for the development of knowledge and the study of learning disability is no exception. Herein lies a problem; this is because, as will be explained later in the chapter, the term 'learning disability' means many different things to many different people. This is discussed in the second part of the chapter where we explore a range of issues surrounding the terminology used in learning disability. We next move to present an overview, albeit very brief, of a number of theoretical ways in which we might try and understand learning disability. Following this we explore some of the important issues surrounding the incidence and prevalence of learning disabilities. The final part of the chapter provides the reader with four extended case illustrations concerning people with learning disabilities and their families. These case illustrations are included to bring to this introductory chapter a sense of authenticity about the lives of people with learning disabilities and the experiences of their families.

The new White Paper *Valuing People* (DOH 2001) is based upon the principles of rights, independence, choice and inclusion. The role of the professional and of the lay carer in assisting people with learning disabilities to move towards achieving these principles is, at least in part, dependent upon a knowledgeable and skilled work force. This first chapter lays a foundation for the remainder of this text which articulates a knowledge and value base that promotes people with learning disabilities as equal citizens. As specialist services for people with learning disabilities become more scarce, it will become increasingly important that people with learning disabilities do not become a forgotten people, as has been the case in the past (see Ch. 3). It is vitally important that those who work with this heterogeneous group of people truly understand the nature of learning disabilities.

HOW DO WE DECIDE WHETHER SOMEONE HAS LEARNING DISABILITIES?

Intellectual ability

Some would argue that intelligence is an obvious criterion upon which to judge whether someone

has a learning disability. An immediate problem with this is being able to decide just what intelligence is. This chapter does not have sufficient space to explore this issue in any great depth, but it is assumed that intelligence is something to do with the ability to solve problems and that this ability, or the absence of it, can be measured. One way of measuring intelligence is by using intelligence tests. These tests have been used since the turn of the century; they serve the purpose of enabling one to measure the intellectual ability of one individual to complete a range of standardised tests against a large representative sample of the general population of a similar chronological age. The score that an individual attains can then be converted into a percentile, in order that one may understand how this individual compares with others in the general population. Normally the percentile is converted to an intelligence quotient (IQ) and this has been, and still is, used as a means for identifying learning disability. The intelligence test seeks to compare the mental age of individuals against their chronological age. This is achieved by using the following formula:

$$\frac{\text{Mental age}}{\text{Chronological age}} \times 100 = IQ$$

In the above formula, chronological age refers to the actual age of an individual and mental age refers to the developmental stage that an individual has reached in comparison to others of a similar age. If the sum of the number reached by dividing mental age by chronological age is multiplied by 100 then one arrives at the IQ. Clearly, given the nature of this formula, if one were to continue using it throughout an individual's life then IQ would progressively diminish, therefore the formula is only of use until the chronological age of around 18 years. For the student who wishes to study both the concept and the history of IQ, Gross (1991) is recommended. Given that intelligence is present in the population, and is evenly distributed, it is possible to measure how far an individual moves away from what constitutes 'normal'.

The World Health Organisation has characterised the degree of disability ('retardation') according to how far an individual moves away from the normal distribution of IQ for the general population (see Fig. 1.1). Using this system, an individual who consistently scores below 2 standard deviations of an IQ test, i.e. a measured IQ of less than 70, would be said to have learning disabilities. Those individuals whose IQ is in the range 50–69 are generally identified as having mild learning disability (F70), and those with an IQ of between 71 and 84 are said to be on the borderline of intellectual functioning. Moderate learning disability (F71) is identified when the IQ is in the range of 35–49; the term severe mental retardation (F72) is reserved for people whose IQ is in the range of 20–34, and finally the term profound mental retardation (F73) is reserved for those whose complex additional disabilities, for example sensory, physical or behavioural, make the measurement of IQ difficult. Of course, the use of all these labels, with the exception of F78, relies on the use of standardised tests that offer high validity and reliability.

Intelligence tests were used extensively during the 1960s and 1970s; however, recognition by psychologists and others of the many limitations of their use has made them less popular today. These limitations include cultural bias, poor predictive ability, and an incomprehensive relevance for the identification of learning disability. Despite the range of criticisms constructed against the use of intelligence tests, if they are used appropriately and by properly trained technicians then they do provide a relatively objective measure of the intellectual ability of an individual. In addition, if such a measure is used in conjunction with other criteria, such as social competence, this may be helpful in identifying whether or not an individual has learning disabilities.

Legislative definitions

Legislators, both within the UK and in other countries, have for centuries attempted to use the law to define learning disability. This may in part be explained by the conflation of learning disability with mental illness; this 'clumping' together of two states of being has resulted in people with learning disabilities being the subject of much unnecessary legislation. This brief exploration only considers legislation this century, and in particular focuses upon mental health legislation; the historical passage of legislation focused on people with learning disabilities is to be found in Chapter 3.

The Mental Deficiency Act of 1913 said: 'Mental defectiveness means a condition of arrested or incomplete development of mind existing before the age of eighteen years, whether arising from inherent causes or induced by disease or injury'. This Act followed the Radnor Commission of 1908, and introduced the compulsory certification of 'defectives'. In a sense, this Act reflected the strong eugenics movement of the time; not surprisingly the Act required that 'defectives' be identified and then segregated from the rest of society. By 1959 terminology, and perhaps attitudes, had changed and the Mental Health Act of 1959 introduced the terms listed in Box 1.1.

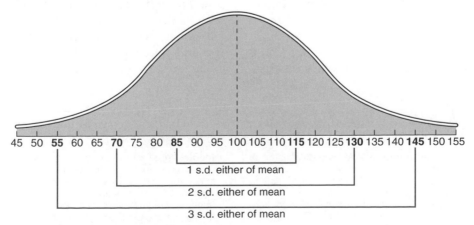

Figure 1.1 The normal distribution curve of intelligence.

Box 1.1   Classifications of the 1959 Mental Health Act

- **Subnormality** – A state of arrested or incomplete development of mind, not amounting to severe subnormality, which includes subnormality of intelligence, and is of a nature or degree which requires, or is susceptible to, medical treatment or other special care or training of the patient.
- **Severe subnormality** – A state of arrested or incomplete development of mind which includes subnormality of intelligence and is of such a nature or degree that the

patient is incapable of living an independent life or guarding himself/herself against serious exploitation, or will be so incapable when of an age to do so.
- **Psychopathic disorder** – A persistent disorder or disability of mind, whether or not including subnormality of intelligence, which results in abnormally aggressive or seriously irresponsible conduct on the part of the patient and requires, or is susceptible to, medical treatment.

This Act required local authorities to make day service and residential provision for people with a 'mental subnormality' and placed a new emphasis on the reintegration of this group of people into the communities to which they belonged. However, this Act must be seen in context, and it should be remembered that it followed the implementation of the NHS Act (1948). The consequential medicalisation of 'mental subnormality' following the NHS Act is clearly reflected in the Mental Health Act of 1959, and therefore its definitions reflected this. Note the strong emphasis, in the definitions, that was placed on treatment. In addition, the Act made extensive reference to the Responsible Medical Officer. It is at this point in the history of mental health legislation that the influence of medicine in defining the nature of learning disability exerted its greatest impact. As a result of continued social reform and pressure from a range of lobby groups, mental health legislation was again reformed in 1983; the old Act of 1959 was replaced with the 1983 Mental Health Act. Once again old terminology was changed and replaced with the terms shown in Box 1.2.

It can be seen that the nature of these definitions excluded the large majority of people with learning disability; i.e. unless people's learning disability (mental or severe mental impairment) coexisted with aggressive or seriously irresponsible behaviour, then they were not subject to this new piece of legislation. This Act represented a major shift in how people with a learning disability were perceived in mental health legislation; for the first time learning disability and mental illness were separated by law.

Social competence

The final criterion used for identifying learning disability in this chapter is that of social competence. Mittler (1979) has suggested that most countries have used criteria based on social competence which include the ability of an individual to adapt to the changing demands made by the society in which that individual lives. Of course this sounds relatively straightforward; one simply identifies people who are socially incompetent, and who do not respond well to changing societal demands. Burton (1996) has said, 'Social competence concerns such areas as understanding and following social rules, adjusting social behaviour to the situation, social problem solving,

---

Box 1.2   Classifications of the 1983 Mental Health Act

- **Severe mental impairment** – A state of arrested or incomplete development of mind, which includes severe impairment of intelligence and social functioning and is associated with abnormally aggressive or seriously irresponsible conduct of the person concerned.
- **Mental impairment** – A state of arrested or incomplete development of mind (not amounting to severe mental impairment) which includes significant impairment of intelligence and social functioning and is associated with abnormally aggressive or seriously irresponsible conduct on the part of the person concerned.

and understanding others. These are the areas where people typically fail independent living' (Burton 1996, p. 40).

On the basis of individuals performing significantly below what might be considered as 'normal', one presumably may say that they might have a learning disability. However, there are a number of problematic issues to consider in relation to the criterion of social competence.

First, social incompetence is to be found in a wide cross-section of people, and not just those with a learning disability. Consider, for example, people with chronic mental health problems as well as nonconformists to societal norms. Alternatively, problems of communication, hearing and vision could also be the cause of social incompetence, and may not necessarily involve a learning disability.

Secondly, there is an issue here of expectation and the notion of a self-fulfilling prophecy. Assume, momentarily, that an individual is identified as having a learning disability, on the basis of measured social incompetence. Is it the case that this individual genuinely has a learning disability, or is the social incompetence merely an artefact of that person having spent his formative years in a hospital setting? Such a finding is not beyond the realms of credibility. It is only relatively recently that the large learning disability hospitals have been closing. In the past thousands of people with learning disabilities were segregated from society, and led very devalued lives. Opportunities for the development of social competence were few and far between; even when opportunities arose they were often perverted attempts to create some kind of social reality within an institutional setting. There have been numerous studies undertaken of the effects on people of being deprived of normal environments. Dennis (1973) found that institutionalised children were delayed in basic competencies such as sitting, standing and walking, and reported that they had no opportunity to practise these skills. It was also noted that with the additional lack of stimulation there was also significant delay in language acquisition, social skill development and emotional expression:

. . . as babies they lay on their backs in their cribs throughout the first year and often for much of the second year . . . Many objects available to most

children did not exist . . . There were no building blocks, no sandboxes, no scooters, no tricycles, no climbing apparatus, no swings. There were no pets or other animals of any sort . . . they had had no opportunities to learn what these objects were. They never saw persons who lived in the outside world, except for rather rare visitors. (Dennis 1973, pp 22–23)

In short, the expectations of people in these environments were low, and therefore it is not unreasonable to assume that their ability to develop social competence in such environments was reduced. Despite the criticisms made in this section, social competence as a means for the identification of a learning disability remains a globally used criterion.

DEFINITIONS OF LEARNING DISABILITY

Generally speaking in the UK the term learning disability is used, and this is accepted to mean:

- A significantly reduced ability to understand new or complex information, to learn new skills (impaired intelligence), with,
- A reduced ability to cope independently (impaired social functioning);
- Which started before adulthood, with a lasting effect on development. (DOH 2001, p. 14).

In the USA the American Association on Mental Retardation define what we would call learning disability as follows:

'Mental retardation refers to substantial limitations in present functioning. It is characterised by significantly sub-average intellectual functioning, existing concurrently with related limitations in two or more of the following applicable adaptive skill areas: communication, self-care, home living, social skills, community use, self direction, health and safety, functional academics, leisure, and work. Mental retardation manifests itself before age 18' (American Association on Mental Retardation 1997).

Both of these are discussed in more detail below along with an exploration of the problematic nature of all terms in the area of learning disabilities.

Terminology

It should be pointed out that the term 'learning disability' is relatively new. Emerson et al (2001) have suggested that its origin lies in a speech to Mencap by Stephen Dorrell, Minister for Health in England in 1991.

Its general usage in the UK is to describe a group of people with significant developmental delay that results in arrested or incomplete achievement of the 'normal' milestones of human development. These milestones relate to intellectual, emotional, spiritual and social aspects of development. Significant delays in a number of these areas may lead to a person being described, defined or categorised as having learning disabilities. Despite wide usage of this term in the UK it should be remembered that it is not one that is used internationally (see the AAMR definition of learning disability (mental retardation) above), nor is it a term that has been used for very long in this country. Until recently the term 'mental handicap' was much more frequently used but was replaced, because it was felt that it portrayed a negative image of people with disability. Interestingly, a relatively recent study by Nursey et al (1990) demonstrated that parents and doctors had preferences in the words that they chose to use when referring to people with learning disability. The study was conducted using a questionnaire and established that both parents and doctors preferred the term 'mental handicap' or 'learning difficulties'. However, doctors were more inclined to accept the words dull, backward and developmentally delayed. In the USA (see above) the term 'mental retardation' is widely used in the classification of learning disability. The USA system is based upon the ICD–10 classification of mental and behavioural disorders (WHO 1993). This uses the term 'mental retardation' to refer to: 'a condition of arrested or incomplete development of the mind, which is especially characterised by impairment skills manifested during the developmental period which contribute to the overall level of intelligence, i.e. cognitive, language, motor and social abilities' (WHO 1993).

Interestingly the USA is currently engaged in considerable debate about the use of the term mental retardation: 'as all of us have experienced, the term mental retardation has expanded from a diagnostic label embedded in both legislative and social norms to a pejorative, stigmatising term that is increasingly offensive to a large group of individuals' (Schalock 2001, p. 4).

Notwithstanding this, the American Association on Mental Retardation (AAMR) noted that after 2 years of exploration for an alternative term they had not found one that meant the same thing, and on this basis they recommended that the term should not be replaced.

In the field of learning disability, one of the problems in deciding which term to use is the possibility that the term may become used as a label that conjures up negative imagery. The use of labels for people with a learning disability has in the past served as a way of segregating this group from society at large. It is becoming increasingly common for professional carers not to use these categories (Emerson et al 2001). This is because they represent static measures that tell us nothing of the needs of each individual person; these needs will vary considerably between people, even if their measured IQs are an exact match. For further information concerning the history of labelling in learning disability the reader should refer to Williams (1978), Ryan & Thomas (1987) and Hastings & Remington (1993), and to Chapter 3 of this book.

 Reader activity 1.1

Box 1.3 lists labels in common usage for people with learning disabilities. Do you know any more? How do you think such labels assist in devaluing this group of people?

THEORETICAL APPROACHES TO UNDERSTANDING LEARNING DISABILITY

Clarke (1986) has said that 'Learning disability has been a source of speculation, fear, and scientific enquiry for hundreds of years. It has been regarded in turn as an administrative, medical, eugenic, educational and social problem.'

> **Box 1.3** Terms used to describe people with a learning disability
>
> - Learning disability
> - Learning difficulty
> - Mentally impaired
> - Imbecile
> - Moron
> - Cretin
> - Benny
> - Spastic
> - Idiot
> - Mentally subnormal
> - Mentally retarded
> - Intellectual disability
> - Morally defective
> - Educationally subnormal
> - Ineducable

The manner in which learning disability has been catered for throughout history has, to some extent, reflected the dominant theoretical perspective that has been used at any one time in order to understand it. This next section provides a brief overview of five different theoretical perspectives that are commonly associated with learning disabilities.

A sociological perspective

Sociology has been defined as 'the science or study of society' (Seymour-Smith 1986, p. 263). Sociology concerns itself with the study of the social phenomena of modern industrial societies, and employs methods of analysis and investigation to understand the component parts of society, and how these parts relate to one another. Sociological theory can be divided into two traditions: structuralist and interpretative approaches. Reid (1978) has said that *structuralist sociology* is concerned with understanding man as a manipulator and creator of society. Within this section an approach to understanding sociology from the structuralist viewpoint is explored. For further guidance and/or information in this area, refer to Bennett (1992).

Kurtz (1981) has provided a short, but none the less powerful, chapter on a sociological approach to understanding learning disability. He suggest-ed that individuals within any society are incumbents of the status that is attached to the role that they occupy in that society. He cited Guskin (1963) who had noted that people with a learning disability play a very generalised role. This role, it was suggested, emphasised the inability of a person with a learning disability to undertake functional activities adequately. The functional activities referred to were everyday experiences for most people, such as going to work, taking care of one's self, behaving in an acceptable way, or managing one's own finances. It was suggested that the person with a learning disability could not adequately perform these activities. Of particular interest to this approach was the question of whether one could identify the causation of such inability. Simply, was the inability caused by the learning disability, or was it a consequence of those with learning disabilities behaving in the ways that people expected them to? Guskin (1963) suggested that:

... one could hypothesise non achievement orientation, dependency behaviour, and rebelliousness as patterns of behaviour determined by previous and present interactions with people who have role concepts of the defective emphasising inability, helplessness, and lack of control, respectively.

Kurtz (1981) has argued that because of the ways in which learning disability had been perceived two important images emerged of such individuals in the USA. These images were:

- the person with learning disabilities as a sick person
- the person with learning disabilities as a developing person.

He suggested that the first of these images was chiefly held by medical personnel, whilst the second was held by educators, psychologists and, possibly, parents.

In conclusion, the sociological approach to learning disability focuses on the role of this group of people within society. It is suggested that because of the images that society holds of them, expectations for their role are limited. Dexter (1958) has argued that it is in this sense that learning disability is a construction of society.

A psychological perspective

Psychology is concerned with the study of human behaviour and as some human behaviour is deemed abnormal, a branch of study has developed known as abnormal psychology. This branch of psychology is concerned specifically with the study of abnormal behaviour. Paradoxically, like learning disability, abnormal behaviour is difficult to define, so there is a need to identify criteria in order to distinguish abnormal from normal behaviour (Atkinson et al 1990). In general, abnormal behaviour is identified by the following criteria:

- deviation from statistical norms
- deviation from social norms
- maladaptive behaviour
- personal distress.

This chapter has already outlined how IQ tests are used to establish whether people deviate from statistical norms, in relation to their measured intelligence.

Within the USA, a category system has been used for the identification of abnormality. This is known as the *Diagnostic and Statistical Manual of Mental Disorders*, and approximates to the international system of the World Health Organisation identified earlier in this chapter. The system comprises a number of diagnostic categories that are themselves comprised of subclassifications. Using this system, an individual is evaluated against a number of dimensions from which developmental disorders, such as learning disability, can be identified.

Within such a large academic discipline as psychology it is not surprising to find different theoretical explanations for learning disability. In behavioural psychology, for example, the major focus of interest is on the systematic observation of behaviour. The behavioural approach can be traced back to the work of Skinner (1974) and is concerned with what people do, rather than what they feel or think. In short, behavioural psychology is concerned with observable behaviour rather than with hypothetical constructs. It is concerned with individual problems and the identification of clear objectives for enhancing an individual's ability to perform behaviours that he or she is currently unable to do. It is thus an interventionist approach. Schwartz & Goldiamond (1975) have emphasised that it is not only observable behaviour that is important, but also environmental aspects, such as thought and feelings. Alternatively, Bijou (1992) has reviewed and evaluated a range of concepts in learning disability within the scientific discipline of psychology. His review concluded that the 'restricted developmental' approach to understanding learning disability was the most advanced and defensible. He also argued its superiority to other approaches because it was an integral component of empirically based behaviour theory of human development. Waitman & Conboy-Hill (1992) have provided an overview of psychotherapeutic themes related to learning disability; along with other theoretical approaches, this demonstrates that psychology offers varied and valuable insights into the nature of learning disability, and practical approaches which can enhance the lives of people with a learning disability.

A medical perspective

Brechin et al (1980) have provided a useful and comprehensive analysis of this approach to understanding learning disability. It is the case that cures, the alleviation and prevention of disease, and restoring and preserving health, are the central concerns of medicine. The practice of Western medicine rests upon the so-called positivistic paradigm; i.e. it is concerned with the establishment of hypotheses and the acceptance or refutation of their predictions. Therefore, the medical model uses a deductive approach that follows a diagnostic path in search of an explanation for disease, often referred to as the cause–effect relationship. The whole point of Western medicine is to identify diseases and disorders, and to determine their causes in order that the disease or disorder can be prevented and/or ameliorated. Illsley (1977) has identified four central assumptions of the medical model:

- illness is thought of as being the result of a physical cause
- physicians are seen as the key players in health care

- hospitals are seen as the repositories and treatment centres of the sick
- advances in health care are viewed as developing from improved medical technology.

It was noted earlier in this chapter that services for people with a learning disability transferred to the NHS following its genesis in the 1940s and that with the absorption of learning disability services by the NHS came the medicalisation of learning disability, which unfortunately carried the corollary of learning disability and mental illness being viewed as one and the same. Therefore, the tremendous advances made in mental health, especially pharmacological advances, were extrapolated to people with learning disabilities. For example, the phenothiazines, which were developed for use in the treatment of people with psychotic mental health problems, became 'treatments of choice' for people with learning disabilities who had behavioural problems. It is fair to say that the medical model in learning disability has been extremely influential since that time. Some have argued that this approach to understanding learning disability has been unhelpful. Hattersley et al (1987) have said:

The emergence of treatment for mental illness was seen in the 1950s, and of the developmental change that took place within the psychiatric services there is no doubt. The revolution that was brought about, particularly by the introduction of phenothiazines (major tranquillisers), changed the world of psychiatric institutions. Unfortunately, the same model of providing services was bestowed on mentally handicapped people as well – but drugs do not cure mental handicap (Hattersley et al 1987, p. 101).

It may be the case that the medical approach to understanding learning disability has not always served the best interests of this group of people. However, the medical approach has contributed to our understanding of some of the more biological dimensions of learning disability, and therefore the contribution of medicine to the lives of people with learning disabilities remains valid.

An anthropological perspective

Anthropology has been defined as 'the study of man and his work' (Pelto 1965, p. 1). Anthropology may be divided into two separate but related branches:

- **Physical anthropology**. Physical anthropology is concerned with the examination of evidence for the evolution of man from 'lower' forms of life. This branch of anthropology is also concerned with the study of the variations of the population *Homo sapiens* including, for example, Mongoloid, Negroid and Caucasoid. More recently, physical anthropology has become concerned with aspects of human growth and constitution, in particular body builds. This has brought anthropology closer to a number of other academic disciplines, for example the study of medicine and physiology.
- **Cultural (social) anthropology**. A distinguishing feature of the behaviour of man is that it is pervasively cultural (Pelto 1965). There are many different dimensions to human culture including, for example, history, social structures and language. One area of particular interest to anthropologists is that of ethnology – the study of peoples and/or races. Of particular interest is the study of the varieties of human behaviour that can be observed across a range of peoples in different cultures. Anthropologists live with a particular group of people in order to observe their patterns of behaviour, assuming the role of participant observers. Their study attempts to bring understanding and meaning to the different patterns of behaviour observed.

It is the second of these two branches of anthropology, which this section, on theoretical perspectives, concentrates upon.

Edgerton (1975) identified that learning disability was a culturally defined phenomenon. He provided fascinating insights as to how cultural differences make terms like 'learning disability' very deceptive. Consider the following:

Not only do games fail to interest them, they are almost completely unable to participate in most activities. They could not be taught to whistle, sing or even hum a simple tune. I wrote: 1111 2222 3_ _ _ _ _4_ _55_ on a sheet of paper and asked a number of eight year olds who had never been to school to fill in the missing numbers. They could not. Nor were they able to draw a circle, a square, raise their fingers, or spell their names (Gazaway 1969).

These children probably did not have learning disabilities at all; rather the children all lived in a very deprived area of the USA where such 'levels of attainment' were considered not unusual within that culture. Edgerton (1975) has said:

Most of us, myself included, are sometime guilty of writing (and perhaps believing) that the mentally retarded and their lives are simpler than they really are. Granted, writers about any aspect of human reality could be similarly accused, but the charge here may not be entirely gratuitous since the retarded are by definition 'simple' and our accounts of them cannot be praised for their efforts to discover complexity (Edgerton 1975, p. 139).

More recently new and sensitive life-history accounts of people with learning disabilities appear to be emerging within the literature. These accounts provide fascinating and in-depth accounts of the experience of living with a learning disability and are clearly contextualised within the cultural fabric of the communities and societies to which these people belong. An example of this approach is offered by Bogdan & Taylor (1994), based upon an earlier edition. In their book they have provided biographies of two people with learning disabilities – Patti and Ed. Another fascinating account that has offered an emotional insight into the nature of learning disability is the autobiography of Deacon (1974). More recently David Barron (1996) has written a moving account of his 35 years of life in long stay institutions; this is compulsory reading for those who really wish to begin to understand some of the temporal dimensions of learning disability. Such biographical and autobiographical accounts, along with other anthropological methods, have the potential to provide both professional carers and the general public with valuable insights into the nature of learning disability.

INCIDENCE AND PREVALENCE OF LEARNING DISABILITY

Calculating the incidence of learning disability is extremely problematic. This is because there is no way of detecting the vast majority of those infants who have learning disabilities at birth. It is only the obvious manifestations of learning disability that can be detected at birth; for example in Down syndrome the physical characteristics enable an early diagnosis and the ability to calculate incidence of this disorder. Where there is no obvious physical manifestation, one must wait for delay in development in order to ascertain whether a child has learning disabilities, therefore it is more common in learning disability to talk about the prevalence.

Prevalence is concerned with an estimation of the number of people with a condition, disorder or disease as a proportion of the general population. If one uses IQ as an indicator of learning disability then one is able to calculate that 2–3% of the population have an IQ below 70. This represents a large segment of society. Given that a large number of people with such an estimated IQ never come into contact with a caring agency, it is more common to refer to the 'administrative prevalence'. Administrative prevalence refers to the number of people provided with some form of service from caring agencies.

Historically, there has been a general consensus that the overall prevalence of moderate and severe learning disabilities was approximately 3–4 persons per 1000 of the general population (see, for example, Open University 1987, DOH 1992). Such prevalence would appear to be universally common; for example, Craft (1985) has suggested that international studies have identified prevalence for severe and moderate learning disability as 3.7 per 1000 population. The Department of Health has suggested that mild learning disability is actually quite common; prevalence has been estimated to be in the region of 20 persons per 1000 of the general population. In the UK it has been further calculated that of the 3–4 persons per 1000 population with a learning disability, approximately 30% will present with severe or profound learning disabilities. Within this group it is not uncommon to find multiple disability that includes physical and/or sensory impairments or disability as well as behavioural difficulties. This group of people require lifelong support in order for them to achieve and maintain a valued lifestyle. More recently Emerson et al (2001), drawing on more recent and extensive epidemiological data, have confirmed the above estimation of prevalence rate for severe learning disabilities. They state it to be somewhere in the region of 3–4 persons per 1000 of the general population. The prevalence rate given by Emerson et al for that section of the learning disabled population referred to as having mild learning disabilities is much more imprecise. It is estimated that this figure might lie between 25 and 30 people per 1000 of the general population. Based on these estimates it can be assumed that there are some 230 000–350 000 persons with severe learning disabilities, and possibly 580 000–1 750 0000 persons with mild learning disabilities. It is also known that there is a slight imbalance in ratio of males to females both in people with mild and those with severe learning disabilities, with males having slightly elevated prevalence rates. People with learning disabilities clearly represent a significant section of society who, like other citizens, are entitled to access the resource of skilled professionals who are able to meet their health and social care needs, when they are required.

Earlier in the chapter it was said that people use different criteria for determining learning disability. This differing use of terminology has implications for calculating incidence and prevalence, so it should be acknowledged that there is some controversy associated with being able to identify accurately the incidence and prevalence of learning disabilities. Some would argue that not being able to calculate prevalence accurately is unimportant, as the epidemiological study of learning disability creates labelling, which perpetuates inappropriate models of care that are developed outside the day-to-day services that are available for ordinary people. One problem, amongst many others, with this line of argument is that without careful epidemiological studies in this area, it is very difficult to know how best to target resources for those who may need them. It has oft and long been complained that people with a learning disability are not afforded the same rights as other citizens. Careful measurement of prevalence provides one way of ensuring that people with specialist needs are provided with specialist resources when they are required.

CASE ILLUSTRATIONS

The case illustrations that follow (Case illustrations 1.1–1.4) are based on real people, but all names have been changed. They are intended to illustrate four people's lives which explore various issues pertaining to learning disabilities. They do not contain the whole truth of an individual's life nor can they be regarded as representative of any group. Perhaps they begin to show the diversity of individuals described as being 'learning disabled'. Nothing more than this is intended.

Case illustration 1.1   Jack's story

Jack has mild learning disabilities, sufficient to impact upon his ability to live independently in that he needs some level of support with regard to various skills of daily living, for example budgeting, shopping and cooking. He possesses functional levels of literacy and numeracy and good communication skills in terms of both expressive and receptive language.

However, it is not for those characteristics that he is so very well known to the local learning disability services and indeed also to the police, the general hospital accident and emergency department and short stay ward and social services. His life becomes sporadically chaotic precipitating crisis interventions from those various agencies. He has a long history of what are regarded of para-suicide episodes – usually related to paracetamol or other drug overdoses. This is in addition to the presentation of various somatic complaints, threats of self-harm, threatened and actual physical aggression towards his family, particularly his mother and younger sister, damage to property (such as breaking windows), petty theft and fraudulent minor scams such as selling stolen raffle tickets. He has also on occasion chosen to stay out and sleep rough in local parks, even in freezing conditions.

Perhaps strangely, Jack is quite popular within the helping services and, in contrast to the image that such activity may conjure up, Jack actually presents in a very friendly, 'hail fellow well met', almost stereotypically jolly manner (his large 17 stone frame adds to this image). He always smiles at those he meets and he is an instant 'friend' of everyone, except his family during one of his 'episodes'.

Case illustration 1.1   Jack's story *(Cont'd)*

 ## Reader activity 1.2

Do you know of individuals who smile and appear happy yet who engage in self-destructive behaviour of some kind? See the work of Valerie Sinason (Sinason 1986, 1991, Sinason & Stokes 1992) on secondary handicap as a defence against trauma and 'the handicapped smile' for ideas around this process.

Jack was 1 month premature, a 'blue baby', and he spent 2 weeks of his prenatal period on an incubator. His mother had contracted TB and spent the first 6 months of Jack's life in quarantine whilst he was cared for by his maternal grandparents – he saw his mother only once during this period. Jack's father was a 'Deckie' on deep-sea trawlers and consequently also spent long periods away from home.

An unusually quiet baby with delayed milestones, Jack was diagnosed as having a mental handicap at age 4. Although he began his education in a mainstream school he was soon transferred to learning disability provision, where Jack began truanting and refusing meals. This was to become a familiar pattern along with his 'overdosing' on between 4 and 8 paracetamol, which began from the age of 11. Unfortunately as he grew older his behaviour became more intimidating and chaotic and although he still lived at home there began a series of repeated admissions to the local mental handicap hospital.

His younger sister and mother became regular victims of threatening behaviour and physical aggression. Paradoxically, his relationship with his mother became very clingy and dependent. Jack would insist on her physical proximity to him for much of the time and he would also want her to do things for him (for example, shaving) which he was actually capable of himself. This clingy and dependent relationship would continue for some years with both Jack and his family feeling somewhat stuck. The times when this status quo was challenged invariably evoked distress and rage in Jack and the predictable crisis would follow.

 ## Reader activity 1.3

What impact can early disruptive attachment experiences have upon an individual's adult relationships? See Bowlby (1988).

Eventually and inevitably there followed a repeated series of admissions to the nearest mental handicap hospital. Since the closure of the hospital, Jack has had a number of residential placements, which have rarely lasted for very long, ostensibly as a result of the residence being unable to safely manage Jack's distressed acting out.

Jack is now in his early 40s and, though his father has died, he still wishes to live with his mother. She, in turn, hopes that he could settle into living elsewhere. This tension continues to pervade their relationship, with Jack's distress periodically breaking through.

Perhaps when deeper emotional issues are not properly addressed they remain unresolved; unable to be forgotten they manifest, however, like the grief, guilt and rage we see in Jack. The general population has access to counselling and therapy services, but do people with learning disabilities have similar and sufficient opportunities to resolve their emotional and spiritual difficulties?

Meanwhile, whilst Jack's mother appears increasingly weighed down by the struggle, Jack keeps smiling, everybody's friend.

 Case illustration 1.2   Jenny's story

Jenny is 6 years old and has never spoken a word. It almost seems that she hardly needs to. Jenny has autism and, except when distressed, seems to exude an almost Zen-like calm, appearing self-contained and far away. This lends Jenny an air of mystery that is often apparent around people with autism.

Jenny's parents are still, to some extent, seeking answers, seeking to resolve some of the mystery. Unfortunately, whilst there are a number of speculative books on the causes of autism, there is no definitive explanation.

 ## Reader activity 1.4

How important for parents would it be to know *why* their children had autism? Would it be better to focus on and deal with autism's effects?

Case illustration 1.2   Jenny's story *(Cont'd)*

Sometimes Jenny would become very distressed, screaming and crying in such a pained way it seemed that nothing would calm or comfort her. More often than not her parents could not link her distress to any outside event or trigger. Her mother naturally wishes to hold her child but has learnt that until the storm has passed, trying to do so will only heighten Jenny's distress. Sometimes 'Jenny's Box', which contains her collection of small plastic discs, might distract and calm her. She would spend her time sorting and lining them up in rows. She always did this in the same way and her absorption in the task seemed to calm her. Other times, the box would be ignored or even thrown.

Throughout the house, Jenny would line up her 2p coins on the floor, long rows of coins, some going from one room to another. If a coin was out of place Jenny would put it back or begin to get anxious, pacing around, hand waving in her particular way, until her mother replaced it as it should be. This obsession began in only a small way with short lines of coins until over time, as with many of Jenny's obsessions, the family became a prisoner to the routine. To change or challenge it would now involve such a battle and such distress for Jenny that the path of least resistance seems preferable.

Jenny's diet also causes her parents considerable concern. Basically she will eat bread, cereal, rolls, milk and jam. Again the 'why' remains something of a mystery and thus their approaches to diet are somewhat hit and miss. Is this diet another type of obsession/routine or can she not tolerate other types of food? How do they balance her nutritional needs against her psychological needs? Her parents had received various advice, from 'this is a phase, don't worry' to 'Jenny is being awkward or attention seeking', none of which were particularly helpful.

Trips out were anxiety provoking. Familiar journeys would generally be fine as long as the same route was followed. Sometimes on the way there would be things that they must do, like sit on a particular seat or twirl around a particular lamp post, but they managed. However, new places and untoward events could seem to overwhelm Jenny and she would become distressed. Sometimes they would have to abandon their journey and return home.

Although Jenny and her parents seemed trapped in a series of routines and obsessions, to some extent many of these had become second nature to them. Only when the context changed did they become more of a challenge. Jenny could also, on her terms and when she chose, be extremely loving and even cuddly. Despite the mystery of the disorder, Jenny's parents feel they know her pretty well. They can predict how she will be in certain circumstances and how she will respond to certain stimuli. They also see her unique personality emerging, her playfulness and humour, her tender side – traits that would still be hers in the absence of autism.

Reader activity 1.5

Should such behaviour be defined as 'challenging'? How might such obsessive behaviour be managed and should the family seek to introduce an element of control? What might the impact be on Jenny in the short term and in the long term?

See Turner (1997) for a discussion on repetitive behaviours in autism.

Case illustration 1.3   Gordon's story

At 7.30 a.m. whether he was awake or not, Gordon would be lifted from his bed by his father, carried downstairs and placed upon his beanbag in the sitting room. His father would then make his own breakfast and go off to work.

At 8.00 a.m. Gordon's mother would prepare his breakfast and feed him, sometimes he would eat and sometimes not, depending on his mood. If he was in a good mood not only would he eat but he would more likely cooperate in the task of getting dressed. He might also speak a combination of familiar words, snatches of songs or old stories.

The task of getting Gordon ready for the day was not straightforward. Gordon was sometimes doubly incontinent and wore disposable nappies; he had pressure areas, which needed careful attention, and a skin condition, which required treatment with a cream. Gordon has hydrocephalus and his head is disproportionately large compared with his small and rather frail, wasted looking body. He has a severe scoliosis, which has left him permanently twisted. He is quadriplegic, his eyesight is failing and he has epilepsy too.

Although his occasional resistance makes getting dressed even more difficult, to his mother this show of

Case illustration 1.3 Gordon's story *(Cont'd)*

independence and assertion of will sometimes seems preferable to his more frequent passive, sleepy acquiescence.

His mother says Gordon once walked, ran and talked, a normal boy for a while. The thought of Gordon being normal would still sometimes bring tears but this mood would pass. Gordon was loved for who he was now, with all his imperfections, perfect in his own way.

Reader activity 1.6

How can parents be helped to explore their sometimes ambivalent feelings about disabled children? What might these feelings be?
See Meyer (1995) and Ditchfield (1992) for discussion on parental reactions and adjustment issues.

Gordon's parents were told when he was very young that he would be unlikely to live long into adulthood. He is now in his 30s. This constant expectation of loss, whilst somehow heightening their appreciation of their time together with Gordon, also keeps grief close by.

By 9.00 a.m. or so Gordon is ready for the local authority bus. He would now have his familiar objects around him, old colourful toys, now mostly ignored, remnants from a previous time. He is already beginning to doze. The bus driver lifts him into his made-to-measure wheelchair, and then onto the bus. He is taken to the centre, which caters for around thirty other individuals with severe or profound and multiple handicaps. Gordon has been attending the centre since he left school.

Much of the staff's work involves dealing with basic and everyday aspects of life for the people attending the centre, eating and drinking, continence, mobilisation,

hygiene, epilepsy and so on. Inevitably, Gordon is left to his own devices for periods of the day. Mostly he dozes.

Reader activity 1.7

In these circumstances what can staff do to create and maintain a stimulating environment? What part does boredom play in the culture of such settings? Is it inevitable? Can environment play some part which allows staff to stay somehow emotionally detached and do this work?
See Smith (1992) on 'emotional labour' for ideas on this final point.

Gordon returns home on the bus at around 4.15 p.m. His mother prepares his evening meal and feeds him around 5.00 p.m. Again, he may eat it or he may not. She then washes and prepares him for bed in the early evening.

Reader activity 1.8

See Chapter 3 on issues of social exclusion and isolation.

Mum, Dad and Gordon watch TV for a couple of hours. They rarely if ever go out and equally rarely have visitors.

His father carries him up to bed around 9.30 or 10.00 p.m. Gordon dozes and talks to himself for a while before sleeping.

Case illustration 1.4 Said's story

Said is 16 years old. He attends a special school and has just moved into the '16 plus' department where the focus will be on the development of social skills, independent living skills and so on. He can stay until he is 19, a rather prolonged sixth form perhaps, without an academic focus. Unfortunately, no place at university will follow.

He lives with his parents and younger brother. He has a mild hemiplegia on his left side, which gives him an awkward gait. Said is forever knocking things over and bumping into things; overt enthusiasm meets a lack of coordination and balance. His speech is very difficult to understand even when the listener is reasonably familiar

with him, and pretty much impossible for strangers. He uses a combination of Makaton, a sign language developed by Margaret Walker in the 70s for people with learning disabilities, and his own set of idiosyncratic and often very creative signs and gestures.

Said generally manages to show a remarkable level of persistence and patience with such 'stupid' others. He needs to, given that he loves to talk and fires incessant questions, being bright and endlessly curious about the world. He also has a sharp wit; unfortunately the necessary repetition takes the edge off his *bon mots*.

Case illustration 1.4   Said's story *(Cont'd)*

Said can also become frustrated, impatient and angry; because of his lack of coordination he sometimes does not seem to know how hard he pinches and grabs. This has caused much concern between school and home over the years, possibly more so now as he grows bigger and stronger. His parents have attended many 'something must be done' meetings and still dread the note home from school. Said is very familiar with the headmistress' office.

Like all teenagers, Said wants relationships, both platonic and romantic. However, his lack of social skills sometimes makes this difficult and frustrating for him. His humorous charm never-the-less often gains him favour and forgiveness. He, of course, rebels against parental authority in his own creative and unique ways. His parents struggle with whether they are dealing with a normal teenager or a disabled teenager. Said can go from charming and amusing to stubborn and back again very quickly. His wilfulness can make life very difficult, but his parents also know that given his disabilities, such a trait is probably necessary in order for him to get on in his life.

Said's brother Zaffar, whilst involved in taking care of his brother, has become somewhat emotionally distanced. At times there is conflict between the brothers, yet their relationship lacks the more intimate, emotional and competitive edge one might expect to find in siblings only 2 years apart in age. At times Zaffar has felt pushed out. He does not bring his friends home and although very intelligent, he is regarded as something of an underachiever at school. He sometimes expresses resentment at what he regards as the preferential treatment of his brother, particularly in relation to discipline.

Reader activity 1.10

What effects on siblings may the presence of a learning disabled person have? The effects may be positive and/or negative.
Consider in particular a younger sibling having to assume the role of 'older' sibling to the disabled individual.
See also Begun (1989) and Edgar & Crnic (1989) for discussion of sibling relationships.

Reader activity 1.9

How different are the parenting tasks between disabled and non-disabled teenagers? Should allowances be made for the disability in relation to, say, risk taking?
What dilemmas may arise and how might they manifest within the family?
See Hornby (1995), McCormack (1992) and Allan (1993) for ideas and for discussions of these and similar issues.

Said is approaching an age when the notion of independence is becoming more relevant. Whilst life within the family remains a struggle at times, thoughts about Said's future evoke mostly anxiety. How will he cope outside of the protection of his family? Whilst he is developing the skills necessary for an independent life, his understanding of the responsibilities that come with this remains limited.

CONCLUSION

In this chapter we have attempted to portray the very wide nature and different manifestations of learning disabilities. Many textbooks refer to 'people with learning disabilities' unproblematically as a homogeneous group. This is simplistic and unhelpful, both for people with learning disabilities and their families, and for professional carers. People with learning disabilities form a very diverse group. In the case illustrations above, both Gordon and Said might be said to have learning disabilities, but each is a very different, unique being with his own very personal needs and aspirations. Notwithstanding this, people with learn-

ing disabilities, regardless of the impact of those learning disabilities, share a common humanity with the general population. Most people desire love and a sense of connection with others; they wish to be safe, to learn, to lead a meaningful life, to be free from ridicule and harm, to be healthy and free from poverty; and in this respect people with learning disabilities are no different. It is in the spirit of this common humanity that the rest of this text is presented. It is hoped that it will in some small part help carers to bring about the inclusion of people with learning disabilities into their communities.

REFERENCES

Allan I 1993 View of the family. In: Shanley E, Starrs T (eds) Learning disabilities: a handbook of care, 2nd edn. Churchill Livingstone, Edinburgh

American Association on Mental Retardation 1997 Mental retardation: definition, classification, and systems of support, 9th edn. AAMR, Washington, p. 5

American Psychiatric Association 1994 Diagnostic and statistical manual of mental disorders, 4th edn. American Psychiatric Association, Washington DC

Atkinson R L, Atkinson R C, Smith E E, Bem D J, Hilgard E R 1990 Introduction to psychology, 10th edn. Harcourt Brace Jovanovich, London

Barron D 1996 A price to be born. Mencap Northern Division, Harrogate

Begun A 1989 Sibling relationships involving developmentally disabled people. American Journal of Mental Retardation 5: 566–574

Bennett K 1992 The sociological self. In: Kenworthy N, Snowley G, Gilling C (eds) Common foundation studies in nursing. Churchill Livingstone, Edinburgh, pp 59–74

Bicknell J, Conboy-Hill S 1992 The deviancy career and people with a mental handicap. In: Waitman A, Conboy-Hill S (eds) Psychotherapy and mental handicap. Sage Publications, London

Bijou S W 1992 Concepts of mental retardation. Psychological Record 42: 305–322

Bogdon R, Taylor S 1994 The social meaning of mental retardation. Teachers College Press, London

Bowlby J 1988 A secure base: parent-child attachment and healthy human development. Basic Books, Harper & Row, New York

Burton M 1996 Intellectual disability: developing a definition. Journal of Learning Disabilities for Nursing, Health and Social Care 1(1): 40

Clarke D 1986 Mentally handicapped people living and learning. Baillière Tindall, London

Craft M 1985 Classification criteria, epidemiology and causation. In: Craft M, Bicknell J, Hollins S (eds) Mental handicap: a multidisciplinary approach. Ballière Tindall, London

Deacon J J 1974 Tongue tied: fifty years of friendship in a subnormality hospital. Mencap, London

Dennis W 1973 Children of the creche. Appleton Century-Crofts, New York

Dexter L 1958 A social theory of mental deficiency. American Journal of Mental Deficiency 62: 920–928

Ditchfield H 1992 The birth of a child with a mental handicap: coping with loss? In: Waitman A, Conboy-Hill S (eds) Psychotherapy and mental handicap. Sage, London

DOH 1992 Social care for adults with learning disabilities. (Mental Handicap LAC(92)15). HMSO, London

DOH 2001 Valuing people: a new strategy for learning disability for the 21st century. Cm 5086, HMSO. London.

Edgar L, Crnic K 1989 Psychological predictors of adjustment by siblings of developmentally disabled children. American Journal of Mental Retardation 3: 292–302

Edgerton R 1975 Issues relating to the quality of life among mentally retarded persons. In: Begab M, Richardson S (eds) The mentally retarded and society: a social science perspective. University Park Press, Baltimore, pp 127–140

Emerson E, Hatton C, Felce D, Murphy G 2001 Learning disabilities: the fundamental facts. The Foundation for people with Learning Disabilities, London

Gazaway R 1969 The longest mile. Doubleday, Garden City, New York

Gross R D 1991 Psychology: the science of mind and behaviour. Hodder and Stoughton, London

Guskin S 1963 Social psychologies of mental deficiency. In: Ellis N (ed) Handbook of mental deficiency. McGraw-Hill, New York

Hastings R P, Remington S 1993 Connotations of label for mental handicap and challenging behaviour: a review and research evaluation. Mental Handicap Research 6(3): 237–249

Hattersley J, Hoskin G P, Morrow D, Myers M 1987 People with a mental handicap: perspectives on intellectual disability. Faber & Faber, London

Hornby G 1995 Working with parents of children with special needs. Cassell, London

Illsley R 1977 Health and social policy – priorities for research. SSRC report of Advisory Panel to Research Initiatives Board

Kurtz R 1981 The sociological approach to mental retardation. In: Brechin A, Liddiard P, Swain J (eds) Handicap in a social world. Hodder and Stoughton, Suffolk

Lobato D 1983 Siblings of handicapped children: a review. Journal of Autism and Developmental Disorders 13: 347–364

McCormack M 1992 Special children, special needs. Families talk about living with mental handicap. Thorsons, London

Meyer D (ed) 1995 Uncommon fathers: reflections on raising a child with a disability. Woodbine, USA

Mittler P 1979 People not patients: problems and policies in mental handicap. Methuen, London

Nursey N, Rhode J, Farmer R 1990 The words used to refer to people with mental handicaps. Mental Handicap 18(1): 30–32

Open University 1987 Mental handicap: patterns for living. Open University Press, Milton Keynes

Pelto P 1965 The study of anthropology. Charles E Merrill, Ohio

Reid I 1978 Sociological perspectives on school and education. Open Books, London

Ryan J, Thomas F 1987 The politics of mental handicap. Free Association Books, London

Schalock R 2001 Consortium on language presents phase one report. American Association on Mental Retardation. News and Notes. May–June 2001, 1–4

Schwartz A, Goldiamond I 1975 Social casework: a behavioural approach. Columbia University Press, New York

Seymour-Smith C 1986 Macmillan dictionary of anthropology. Macmillan, London

Sinason V 1986 Secondary mental handicap and its relationship to trauma. Psychoanalytic Psychotherapy 2(2): 131–154

Sinason V 1991 The sense in stupidity: psychotherapy and mental handicap. Free Association Books, London

Sinason V, Stokes J 1992 Secondary handicap as a defence. In: Waitman A, Conboy-Hill S (eds) Psychotherapy and mental handicap. Sage Publications, London

Skinner B F 1974 About behaviourism. Jonathan Cape, London

Smith P 1992 The emotional labour of nursing. How nurses care. Macmillan, London

Turner M 1997 Towards an executive dysfunction account of repetitive behaviour on autism. In: Russels J (ed) Autism as an executive disorder. Oxford University Press, New York

Waitman A, Conboy-Hill S (eds) 1992 Psychotherapy and mental handicap. Sage, London

WHO 1993 Describing developmental disability. Guidelines for a multiaxial scheme for mental retardation (learning disability), 10th revision. World Health Organisation, Geneva

Williams P 1978 Our mutual handicap: attitudes and perceptions of others by mentally handicapped people. Campaign for Mutually Handicapped People, New York

Williams P 1985 The nature and foundations of the concept of normalisation. In: Kracos E (ed) Current issues in clinical psychology. Clinical psychology 2. Plenum, New York

FURTHER READING

American Association on Mental Retardation 1997 Mental retardation, definition, classification, and systems of support, 9th edn. AAMR, Washington

Emerson E, Hatton C, Felce D, Murphy G 2001 Learning disabilities: the fundamental facts. The Foundation for people with Learning Disabilities, London

Malin N 1995 Services for people with learning disabilities. Routledge, London

Thompson T, Mathias P 1998 Standards and learning disability, 2nd edn. Baillière Tindall, London

USEFUL ADDRESSES

American Association on Mental Retardation
www.aamr.org/index.ns4.7.shtml

Association of Practitioners in Learning Disability (APLD)
APLD@apld.freeserve.co.uk

Association of Residential Care
www.arcuk.org.uk/

British Institute of Learning Disability
www.bild.org.uk

Innovation and Best Value
www.IBV.org.uk

Mencap
www.mencap.org.uk

The Tizard Centre
http://www.ukc.ac.uk/tizard

Values into Action (VIA)
www.demon.co.uk//via/

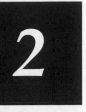

2

Causes and manifestations of learning disabilities

Debbie Watson

KEY ISSUES

- There are a number of known factors that contribute toward, or result in learning disabilities.
- There are four distinct periods when learning disabilities may occur, and these are preconceptual, prenatal, perinatal and postnatal.
- The causative factors operating during these periods can be roughly divided into two areas, those of heredity or environmental factors. Each area can then be further subdivided to concentrate on the more specific causal agents.
- The manifestations of the various conditions are identified, but it must be emphasised that clinical features and the prognosis of a

particular condition should only be used as an aid to planning person centred care that is flexible and individualistic in approach.

INTRODUCTION

What causes learning disabilities is a frequently asked question. However, only partial answers have been found since the first attempts to define the condition were made. Since the beginning of history, in even the simplest of societies, assumptions have been made about the causation of learning disabilities. 'Learning disabilities' can usefully be described as an umbrella term under which all affected individuals are described as having varying degrees of impairment of intellectual and social functioning. Learning disabilities are diverse and may be the result of a range of causative factors. Such conditions are manifested during different stages of the developmental process – preconceptual, prenatal, perinatal and postnatal – and can be described as being genetic or environmental in nature (Fig. 2.1).

It is difficult to state the precise number of people who have a learning disability, but it is estimated that currently, in England, there are 1.2 million people with a mild or moderate disability and about 210 000 people with severe learning disabilities (DOH 2001). Even if there were a more precise method of establishing these numbers, the actual number of known causes would still remain small because of the diverse and complex aetiologies of the various conditions.

An understanding of the potential causes and manifestations of learning disabilities is essential for professionals who wish to work holistically with people with learning disabilities. Arguably it allows carers to develop, in partnership with such people, appropriate person-centred care that takes into consideration any specific health-related issues that may impact upon the individual's daily and future life. However, it must be emphasised that labelling someone with a particular condition can have a negative effect. Simply slotting people into categories that inform treatment or aid prognosis should be avoided if we are truly to work with people in an individual and holistic manner. As human beings it is important that we should all

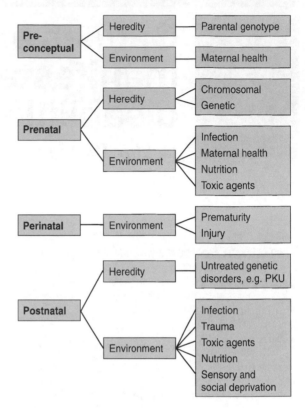

Figure 2.1   Causative factors of learning disabilities by time.

treat one another as unique. The purpose of this chapter is to inform the reader of issues that may be relevant to the care of a person with learning disabilities who has been diagnosed as having a specific condition, within the more general condition known as learning disabilities.

INHERITANCE

Variation between individuals is a biological rule, resulting in the variety of the human species. Genetics could be described as the branch of science that is concerned with the study of heredity, i.e. the passing on of characteristics from parents to offspring.

Every human being originates as the result of the union of two gametes, the ovum and the sperm. The resultant individual is one of a kind, with a unique genotype. The individual's genetic make-up, or genome, represents the two sets of genetic instructions received, one from each parent.

Chromosomes

Each human cell contains 23 pairs of chromosomes, each pair consisting of one chromosome from each parent. During mitosis the cell replicates, ensuring that the same chromosomal pattern is achieved in each new daughter cell. The exception to this is in the gametes, where only one set of 23 chromosomes, one from each original pair, is represented. These will join to make up 23 pairs of chromosomes in the newly formed embryo.

Every chromosome is divided into loci, which contain the particular gene substance that determines the individual's inherited characteristics. Dutton (1975) has likened the relationship between chromosomes and genes to that of a string of beads, with the string being the chromosome and the individual beads representing genes.

Of the 23 pairs of chromosomes, pairs 1–22 can be matched and are described as autosomes. Pair 23 is known as the sex chromosomes. In the female these are matched and referred to as XX. In the male they are not matched and are referred to as XY. The chromosomes are numbered from 1 to 23 according to the Denver system, with the largest pair being number 1 and the smallest being number 22; pair 23 are the sex chromosomes (Fig. 2.2). Another method of organising chromosomes is to place them in one of seven groups labelled A–G according to size and shape. This enables the description of normal and abnormal karyotypes.

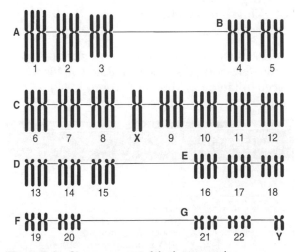

Figure 2.2 Chromosomes of the human male.

Genes

Genes are the units of heredity; they reside upon the chromosome and are responsible for many different traits, such as hair and eye colour. Like chromosomes they are matched (for the most part), and matched genes that are on the same locus of a homologous chromosome are called alleles. Therefore, when an individual inherits from each parent the same allelic form of a particular gene they are described as homozygous for that gene locus. However, if different alleles are present they are described as heterozygous. When a particular allele, when present in the heterozygote, gives rise to an obvious physical characteristic it is described as dominant. However, if the particular characteristic only appears in individuals when they are homozygous for the gene, it is described as recessive.

The individual's hereditary characteristics may then be described as chromosomal if they can be linked to one or more of the 23 pairs of identified chromosomes, and genetic if they are determined by one or more of the genes that reside upon those chromosomes. For example, an individual's sex is determined by a chromosomal hereditary characteristic (chromosome 23), whereas eye colour is identified as being caused by one or more genes and is referred to as genetic.

THE HUMAN GENOME PROJECT

In order to further our understanding of genetics a research project, which represents a collaboration of twenty research groups from around the world, is 'mapping' the human genome. This was achieved in June 2000, when the first draft of the human genome sequence was announced. The benefits of mapping the human genome are numerous: researchers will be able to look at how the human genome has evolved and suggest ways in which health can be promoted, and ill-health or genetic diversity can be better understood and tackled. However, genetic inheritance is only one part of the jigsaw that must be considered when trying to understand what makes an individual. The environment, and social and cultural factors all have a part to play. Therefore, although having a greater understanding of the human genome may increase our understanding of some of the causes and manifestations of learning disabilities, it is not the only factor that professionals should consider. There is much more work to be done with regard to the human genome project and as work progresses and knowledge increases so will the accompanying legal, ethical and moral dilemmas, therefore practitioners would be well advised to attempt to keep abreast of the advances that may have far-reaching implications for people who have learning disabilities.

CHROMOSOME ABNORMALITIES

Chromosomal abnormalities are estimated to be the cause of approximately one-third of the 50% of learning disabilities that are attributable to genetic factors (Mueller & Young 1998). However, this figure is constantly undergoing change as more is learned about genetics. An example of this can be seen in research conducted by Knight et al (1999) who identified that subtle chromosomal rearrangements were present in children with previously unexplained moderate to severe learning disabilities.

Autosomal

The incidence of autosomal abnormalities has been calculated and is reproduced in Table 2.1 (Mueller & Young 1998).

Autosomal abnormalities may be subdivided into three main categories:

1. Abnormality of number. Here there may be a loss (or more commonly a gain) of one or more chromosomes, for example Down syndrome, or trisomy 21, where there is an extra chromosome in pair 21, or Edwards syndrome, which has an extra chromosome present in pair 16, 17 or 18.

2. Abnormality of structure. Here there may be a loss of part of a chromosome (deletion) or a rearrangement (translocation) of the chromosomal material. For example, Cri-du-chat syndrome has a deletion of the short arm of chromosome 5. In Down syndrome an extra segment of chromosome may have been rearranged and attached to one of the following pairs: 13, 15, 21 or 22.

3. Mosaicism. Here individuals have cells with different numbers of chromosomes. This may occur as non-disjunction, or the accidental loss of a particular chromosome, usually during the first few cell divisions following fertilisation. Mosaicisms for autosomes do occur, but are encountered more frequently on sex chromosomes. Examples of mosaicism are Down syndrome and Klinefelter syndrome.

Sex chromosome abnormalities

As with autosomes, additions and deletions to the sex chromosomes may occur. Primary non-disjunction, if it occurs during the formation of the ova or the spermatozoa, gives rise to a gamete with an extra X or Y chromosome. Sex chromosome abnormalities can be divided into four main subgroups:

XO Turner syndrome
XXX Triple X syndrome
XXY Klinefelter syndrome
XYY syndrome.

The incidence of sex chromosome abnormalities in the new-born has been calculated and is reproduced in Table 2.2 (Mueller & Young 1998).

Table 2.1 Incidence autosomal abnormalities in the newborn

Abnormality		Incidence per 10000 births
Trisomy	13	2
	18	3
	21	15

Table 2.2 Incidence of sex chromosome abnormalities in the newborn

Abnormality		Incidence per 10000 births
Female births	45,XO (Turner syndrome)	1
	47,XXX (Triple X syndrome)	10
Male births	47,XXY (Klinefelter syndrome)	10
	47,XYY (XYY syndrome)	10

MANIFESTATIONS OF AUTOSOMAL DISORDERS

Down syndrome

Often referred to as the best known chromosomal abnormality, Down syndrome was first described in 1866 by Dr Langdon Down, from whom it derives its name. However, the chromosomal basis of Down syndrome was not established until 1959, when Lejeune and his colleagues discovered that people who had Down syndrome had 47 chromosomes, the extra chromosome residing with autosome 21 (trisomy 21).

The overall incidence of Down syndrome is approximately 1 in 650 to 1 in 700 (Mueller & Young 1998). The relationship between maternal age and the incidence of Down syndrome is well documented: in women aged 25 years and younger the incidence is under 1 in 1000, and the risk does not rise above that of the normal population until around 30 years. At the maternal age of about 40 the risk rises to 1 in 100, and thereafter continues to rise steeply. Antenatal diagnosis of Down syndrome can be made at around 10–12 weeks of pregnancy by chorionic villus sampling (Box 2.1) and at the 16th week of pregnancy by amniocentesis (Box 2.2).

Translocation Down syndrome

This group make up less than 5% of all cases of Down syndrome (Spitzer 1996). Where parents who are chromosomally normal have a child with

---

Box 2.1 Chorion biopsy

Chorion biopsy is a prenatal diagnosis that is carried out in the first trimester (10–11 weeks' gestation) to detect chromosomal defects and inborn errors of metabolism. Fetal tissue is obtained from the chorionic villi (fingerlike projections of the outermost membrane surrounding the fetus). With the aid of ultrasound, a small tube is inserted through the vagina and cervical canal and guided towards the placenta, where a sample of tissue can be removed. The sample contains large numbers of rapidly dividing cells that allow studies to be carried out within a few hours of sample collection.

Box 2.2 Amniocentesis

Amniocentesis is a prenatal procedure by which the diagnosis of a number of congenital abnormalities, such as chromosomal disorders and open neural tube defects, can be detected. The procedure is usually carried out by a skilled practitioner at an outpatients clinic, at around 15–16 weeks' gestation. The procedure commences with an ultrasound scan to locate the placenta and confirm the gestation (15–16 weeks is the earliest time that a satisfactory sample can be obtained). Then, under a local anaesthetic, a long thin needle is inserted into the amnion (the fluid-filled sac surrounding the fetus) via the mother's abdomen and a sample of the amniotic fluid withdrawn. The sample is then cultured, to provide enough cells for analysis. This process takes about 3–4 weeks, which means that the results are not available until 17–20 weeks' gestation.

---

translocation Down syndrome, the risk of having another affected child is low. However, chorion biopsy may be offered to diagnose translocation in high-risk cases (Box 2.1).

Characteristics

There are a large number of characteristics associated with Down syndrome and it should be remembered that not all people with this condition exhibit them all. However, the commonly known features usually allow identification of the condition in the neonatal period, with obvious floppiness (hypotonia) being a striking feature. In some cases chromosomal analysis may be the only method of confirming or excluding the condition.

The head is usually brachycephalic (small) and round, with a reduced cranial capacity. The brain appears 'simple' in structure and underweight. The higher brain functions are affected by the structural variations and accompanying malfunctions. However, the level of intellectual impairment varies between individuals. The achievement of developmental milestones may be slower and the child may appear to lag behind its peers, but with early intervention and support individuals may be allowed to work towards the achievement of their maximum potential.

Hair has a tendency to be dry, sparse and fine, with a possibility of recurrent focal alopecia in adulthood.

The face is flat (as is the occiput), and the ears are small with underdeveloped lobes. The eyes are usually upward- and outward-slanting, often with an epicanthic fold on the inner aspect of the upper eyelid. Strabismus, nystagmus and cataracts are common. Brushfield spots can be found flecked throughout the iris, which is often poorly developed. Owing to the lack of the enzyme lysozyme in tears, which acts as an antiseptic, conjunctivitis and blepharitis are common. The bridge of the nose is often poorly developed, and mouth breathing is common. The mouth is often small with a high narrow palate, whereas the tongue has a tendency to be large with horizontal fissures. As a result of this particular anatomy the mouth tends to be held open, with the tongue protruding. There is delayed development of the teeth, with an abnormality in their size, shape and alignment. Mouth breathing increases the risk of respiratory tract infection, which before the advent of antibiotics resulted in an increased mortality rate for this group of people. Atlantoaxial instability (a form of cervical spine instability) may also be present.

As an adult the individual may be small and broad in stature (usually not exceeding 1.5 m in height). Umbilical hernias are common. There is a tendency to hypotonia (reduced muscle tension), with the joints having an abnormal range of movement.

Hands and feet are distinctive, with the hands having a square palm with palmar crease, and a wide gap between the thumb and second finger. Fingers are short and stubby. Toes are shorter than normal and there may be a wide gap between the great toe and the second toe.

Genitalia in the male may be underdeveloped and there may be reduced fertility; however, males should not be assumed to be sterile. It is estimated that about one-third of women with Down syndrome ovulate, one-third have no evidence of ovulation, and that in the remaining third evidence of ovulation is indeterminate (Newton 1992).

Congenital heart disease affects around 40% of Down syndrome babies and thyroid disease occurs in about 20% of children (Gilbert 2000). As adults some individuals may experience some or all of the features of Alzheimer's disease.

Case illustration 2.1 shows how this information can be used to support the individual.

Case illustration 2.1   How can this information support the individual?

David has Down syndrome and congenital heart disease. Both David and his carers are aware that when he requires dental treatment, including routine descaling, oral antibiotics are prescribed before and after treatment to prevent endocarditis that may be caused by bacteria in the mouth entering the blood stream. Being aware of David's heart condition therefore allowed a course of preventive treatment that may otherwise have been overlooked.

Edwards syndrome

Edwards and associates first described Edwards syndrome in 1960. It is caused by the presence of an extra chromosome on pair 18 (trisomy 18). The incidence has been calculated as 1 in 5000 and increases with advanced maternal age (Mueller & Young 1998).

Characteristics

There is an elongation of the skull, with a receding chin. The face is characterised by hypertelorism (abnormal distance) of the eyes, with underdeveloped supraorbital ridges, eyebrows and eyelashes. The ears are low set and small, and abnormal in shape. The neck is short with redundant skin folds, or webbing. The fingers are flexed and have a tendency to overlap, with distally placed thumbs. The feet are described as 'rocker bottomed', with dorsiflexed great toes. Limited abduction of the hip may be evident and the individual may have some degree of spasticity. The frontal lobes of the cerebral hemispheres may not separate normally. The degree of learning disability is severe, with associated physical handicaps, including congenital abnormalities of the heart, nervous system, abdominal organs, kidneys and ears. The prognosis for affected individuals is poor, with 90% dying within the first 6 months (Russell 1996).

Cri-du-chat syndrome

Lejeune and his colleagues first described Cri-du-chat (or cry-of-the-cat syndrome) in 1963. It is caused by a deletion of the short arm of chromosome 5. The condition is rare, with an estimated incidence of approximately 1 in 50 000 (Mueller & Young 1998). The condition is characterised by a distinctive high-pitched wailing cry, believed to be caused by a laryngeal defect. It is not until the child begins to develop that the characteristics become more striking.

Characteristics

Affected individuals tend to be small in stature, with microcephaly being common. The face is characterised by hypertelorism and downward slant of the eyes. The chin is small and the ears are low set. The nose is broad at its base and has been described as beaklike. Birthweight is low, and in the early months there is a failure to thrive and a poor sucking reflex.

Prognosis is variable, with some individuals surviving into adulthood. The degree of learning disability is normally severe and the development of speech is limited.

MANIFESTATIONS OF SEX CHROMOSOME ABNORMALITIES

Turner (OX) syndrome

This condition was first described in 1938. It is characterised by diminished secondary sexual characteristics: the affected individual presents as female, but lacks ovarian tissue and sex hormones, is sterile and shows primary amenorrhoea. Short stature (average adult height of 145 cm), which becomes apparent by mid-childhood, webbing of the neck, a low hairline at the back of the neck and widely spaced nipples are also features. The incidence of Turner syndrome is low, with estimates ranging from 1 in 5000 to 1 in 10 000 (Mueller & Young 1998). Affected individuals who have learning disabilities are usually described as having a very low intellect. Oestrogen therapy may be initiated at adolescence to promote the development of secondary sexual characteristics and to prevent osteoporosis during later life.

Triple X (XXX) syndrome

Birth surveys have shown that approximately 0.1% of all females have a XXX karyotype (Mueller & Young 1998). These women usually have no physical abnormalities, but can show varying degrees of reduction in intellectual functioning. Women with more than three X chromosomes show a high incidence of decreased intellectual functioning. Skeletal and neurological problems have been identified in XXX women and psychotic disorders are thought to be more frequent than in the normal population.

Klinefelter (XXY) syndrome

This condition was first described in 1942, but it was not until 1959 that the presence of the additional X chromosome was identified. This is a relatively common condition with an incidence equal to 1 in 1000 male live births (Mueller & Young 1998).

Development until puberty appears normal; the syndrome then becomes apparent when the secondary sexual characteristics fail to develop: testes are small or undescended, body hair is sparse and approximately 30% of males show moderately severe gynaecomastia (enlargement of the breasts). Adults with Klinefelter syndrome tend to have long lower limbs and are slightly taller than average. There is an increased risk of leg ulcers, osteoporosis and carcinoma of the breast in adult life. Psychotic and personality problems have also been described. The development of secondary sexual characteristics and the prevention of osteoporosis can be encouraged with the use of testosterone from puberty onwards. Many people with Klinefelter syndrome are of normal intelligence; those with learning disabilities are mainly described as mildly affected.

XYY syndrome

XYY syndrome has a reported incidence of 1 in 1000 new-born males (Mueller & Young 1998). It must be noted, however, that most XYY males do not suffer from intellectual impairment or psychopathic and criminal behaviours, as was once thought. Physical appearance is normal, with an above-average stature. Learning disabilities, if present, are usually described as mild.

GENE ABNORMALITIES

It may be helpful to group abnormalities of the genes as autosomal dominant (Fig. 2.3), autosomal recessive (Fig. 2.4), sex-linked (Fig 2.5) and polygenetic.

Autosomal dominant inheritance

There are at least 1000 human traits that are known to have their genetic basis in dominant genes located on autosomes. Dimples and freckles are two examples of traits known to be dictated by dominant alleles.

Genetic disorders caused by dominant genes are fairly uncommon as lethal dominant genes are almost always expressed, resulting in the death of the developing embryo, fetus or child. There are, however, some conditions that are less severe, allowing the affected individual enough time to reproduce and pass on the affected gene. Achondroplasia, a rare form of dwarfism result-

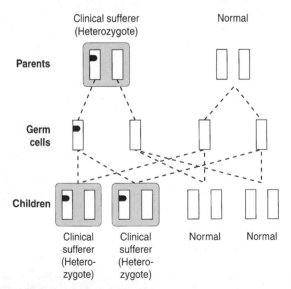

Figure 2.3 Dominant inheritance.

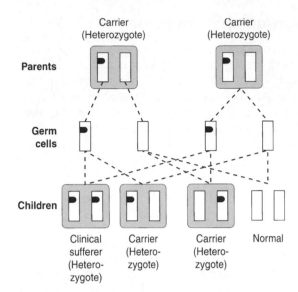

Figure 2.4 Recessive inheritance.

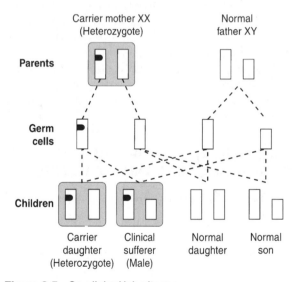

Figure 2.5 Sex-linked inheritance.

ing from the inability of the fetus to form cartilage bone, is one example.

Autosomal recessive inheritance

There are at least 600 human traits that are known to have an autosomal recessive pattern of inheritance. Many genetic disorders are inherited as simple recessive traits, for example phenylketonuria and Tay–Sachs disease. To be affected, individuals must receive the gene for a particular condition from both parents. Carriers of disorders do not express the disease themselves, but can pass it on to their offspring. Offspring from consanguineous marriages (marriages between close relatives, such as siblings and first cousins) have a greater chance of inheriting two identical recessive genes and thus expressing the disease. Advice from a genetic counselling service may be of use for relatives of affected persons, enabling them to discuss the chances of their being a carrier, or of having an affected child.

Sex-linked inheritance

The Y chromosome, which contains the genes for determining maleness, is only one-third the size of the X chromosome and lacks many of the genes present on the X that code for non-sexual characteristics. For example, the gene involved in the production of certain blood clotting factors is only found on the X chromosome. Genes found only on the X chromosome are described as being X-linked. Haemophilia is a classic example of a sex-linked disorder. If a male inherits an X-linked recessive allele (from his mother) its expression is not masked because there is no corresponding allele on his Y chromosome (inherited from his father), which results in the recessive gene being expressed. In contrast, a female must have two X-linked recessive alleles to express the disease.

An example of X-linked recessive inheritance is Hunter syndrome, a form of gargoylism.

Polygenetic inheritance

Polygenetic inheritance occurs when a number of genes act together, causing complex traits. The

Reader activity 2.1

There are a number of regional genetic counselling services. Find out where your nearest service is and identify what services are offered and how referrals are made.

estimated risk of inheritance is much less than in single gene inheritance, but the risk does increase with the number of first-degree relatives who suffer from the condition. Examples of congenital conditions that are multifactorially determined are spina bifida and cleft lip.

MANIFESTATIONS OF ABNORMAL GENES
Autosomal dominant genes
Tuberous sclerosis

Tuberous sclerosis, or epiloia as it is also known, was first clearly described by Bournville in 1880. It is a rare condition caused by a gene of poor penetrance, in that it varies in manifestation both physically and intellectually. The estimated incidence is one in every 30 000 to 40 000 live births (Gilbert 2000). The condition has a wide range of severity, with approximately 60% of affected individuals having some degree of learning disability.

Characteristics The distinctive features of the condition are skin lesions (adenoma sebaceum, achromic naevi and fibrotic plaques), learning disabilities of varying severity, and epilepsy.

In adults and older children there is a characteristic facial rash with a superficial resemblance to acne, caused by an overgrowth of the sebaceous glands. It appears over the bridge of the nose and the cheeks and is described as a butterfly rash. In childhood the rash first appears like grains of rice under the skin, but in later life red papules appear that slowly multiply and enlarge. Treatment with an argon laser can reduce the impact for the affected individual.

'Shagreen patches' – raised areas of skin – are sometimes present in the lumbosacral region. Tumours are often found in the muscle wall of the heart and in the kidneys, lungs and brain, and can become calcified.

Children who have tuberous sclerosis may be slow in reaching developmental milestones. Mental and physical deterioration may occur, resulting in loss or worsening of skills and abilities. Life expectancy for those severely affected is considerably reduced.

Neurofibromatosis

There are several forms of neurofibromatosis, the most common being type 1 with an incidence at birth of approximately 1 in 3000 (Mueller & Young 1998). The presence of six or more pigmented spots over 1.5 cm in diameter, and the characteristic *café-au-lait* appearance, is usually an indicator that the gene is present. Lisch nodules (harmless hamartomatous lesions) in the iris are a confirmatory clinical sign of the disease. About one-third of sufferers have one or more serious problems, including optic glioma, cerebral and spinal tumours, and mild or moderate learning disabilities, in comparison with two-thirds who are only mildly affected.

Prader–Willi syndrome

Although the specific mode of inheritance of Prader–Willi syndrome is uncertain, approximately 50% of affected individuals have been shown to have a small deletion on the long arm of chromosome 15. The syndrome also appears to be derived from the father (Gilbert 2000). Prader and colleagues first described the syndrome in 1956. It is associated with a variety of temperamental and behavioural characteristics, including feeding difficulties, insatiable appetite with temper tantrums triggered by inability to satisfy appetite, self-injury through skin picking and mood swings. The degree of learning disability is described as mild, but more severe impairments do occur.

Autosomal recessive genes

There are a number of autosomal recessive disorders, many of which are associated with learning disabilities, for example phenylketonuria, maple syrup disease, galactosaemia, Tay–Sachs disease, Hurler syndrome, hepatolenticular disease, Laurence–Moon–Biedl syndrome, true microcephaly, and Niemann–Pick disease.

Phenylketonuria

Asbjorn Folling, a Norwegian paediatrician, first described phenylketonuria in 1934. It is probably one of the best-known genetic conditions, and, if untreated, can result in learning disabilities and a number of associated conditions.

Phenylketonuria is a disorder of protein metabolism that can be detected by a blood test. The autosomal recessive gene causes a deficiency of the enzyme normally present in the liver which converts phenylalanine to tyrosine. This results in raised blood levels of phenylalanine, which are toxic to the developing brain. A blood test, or Guthrie test as it is known, is routinely carried out on all babies around the 5th or 6th day of life, provided that milk has been ingested. A child diagnosed as being phenylketonuric must be placed immediately on a phenylalanine-reduced diet. The effectiveness of the diet is monitored by regular urine tests for phenylketones and blood tests to ensure appropriate levels of phenylalanine.

Characteristics Affected children may have an increased incidence of vomiting, appear irritable, and are slow to reach developmental milestones. Hyperactivity and brain damage become evident in the second half of the first year of life. Autistic features, self-mutilation and a resistance to cuddling may be evident. Epilepsy is also characteristic in a number of children. Lack of pigmentation of the eyes, hair and skin is a result of the inability to convert phenylalanine to tyrosine, a precursor for melanin.

The degree of learning disability is dependent upon treatment, with untreated individuals being severely affected (Mueller & Young 1998).

Galactosaemia

Galactosaemia is an autosomal recessive condition in which there is an abnormality of galactose metabolism. The condition is caused by a deficiency of the enzyme galactose-1-phosphate uridyl transferase, which is essential for the metabolism of galactose (galactose is one of the sugars of milk and is contained in nearly all naturally occurring milks). When the enzyme is deficient galactose and galactose-1-phosphate accumulate in the blood and other tissues. This is thought to be responsible for the symptoms of the disease, which are usually evident during the first few weeks of life. Affected children present with jaundice, vomiting and failure to thrive. If the condition remains untreated liver failure occurs, and if the child survives learning disability is evident. Treatment uses a galactose-free diet and must be started as early as possible (Bonthron et al 1998).

Tay–Sachs disease

Tay–Sachs disease is an autosomal recessive disorder of the lipid metabolism that was first described by Tay in 1881 and by Sachs in 1887. The disease develops early in life, usually in the first year, and there is no treatment available that will prevent progressive mental deterioration.

With early onset of the condition death occurs in the 3rd or 4th year of life. With delayed onset, occurring in the 6th or 7th year of life, death is likely to occur in the mid-teens. The late-onset type is called Batten's disease.

Characteristics With early onset, spastic paralysis, blindness and convulsions accompany deterioration. A characteristic 'cherry red' spot can be found on the macula of the retina.

Hurler syndrome

Hurler syndrome is an autosomal recessive condition in which there is abnormal storage of mucopolysaccharides in the connective tissue. It is often referred to as gargoylism because of the physical appearance of those affected. The condition is not apparent at birth but becomes evident during the first year, with its distinctive features.

Characteristics The individual is short in stature, with limited extension of the shortened limbs. The head is large with frontal bossing, the supraorbital ridges are prominent and the bridge of the nose is depressed. The eyebrows are coarse and hairy, and the eyes are low set with corneal clouding in the majority of cases. Teeth are irregular and late in appearing. The neck is short and thick. Kyphosis develops owing to abnormal vertebral deposits. Death usually occurs in adolescence, as a result of physical and mental deterioration.

X-linked recessive genes

There are a number of genetically determined conditions associated with learning disabilities that are inherited in an X-linked manner. Females may be carriers of the conditions, with males being affected.

X-linked hydrocephalus

This is a rare form of hydrocephalus (Bonthron et al 1998) in which the aqueduct of Sylvius fails to develop fully. Without surgical intervention the cerebrospinal fluid accumulates in the ventricles and brain damage may occur.

Hunter syndrome

Hunter syndrome is a form of mucopolysaccharidosis (gargoylism). It is similar to Hurler syndrome except that it affects only males, no corneal clouding is evident and there is a much slower rate of physical and mental deterioration. Affected individuals usually survive into adulthood.

Fragile X syndrome

Fragile X syndrome was first described by Herbert Lubs in 1969. The term derives from the unusual appearance of the distal portion of the long arm of the X chromosome, which shows a fragile site. The condition causes a non-specific form of learning disability without major dysmorphic features or severe neurological abnormalities.

Fragile X syndrome has the unique and dubious distinction of being the most commonly inherited cause of learning disabilities, with an incidence of approximately 1 in 2000 males, and it accounts for 4–8% of all males with learning disabilities (Mueller & Young 1998).

Characteristics The clinical characteristics of this syndrome include a large forehead, ears and jaw, and following the onset of puberty macroorchidism (enlarged testicles) develops. Individuals may exhibit hyperactivity, autism and self-mutilating behaviour. The degree of learning disability is said to be moderate, with a few individuals described as profoundly disabled.

Polygenic inheritance

There are a large number of conditions, some of which are rare, that are considered to be of polygenetic origin.

Sturge–Weber syndrome

Sturge–Weber syndrome, or naevoid amentia as it is also known, is a rare condition of unknown cause characterised by a facial naevus, often referred to as a 'port wine stain'. Part or all of the trigeminal nerve is affected on one side of the face. On the same side as the naevus can be found a meningeal angioma. In some cases there may be calcification in the meningeal angioma and the cerebral cortex. Epilepsy and spasticity are common features. Hemiplegia occurs on the opposite side of the body to the facial naevus. The degree of learning disability encountered can be severe (Gilbert 2000).

Cornelia de Lange syndrome

The Dutch paediatrician Cornelia de Lange first described Cornelia de Lange syndrome in 1933. It has also become known as Amsterdam dwarfism. The incidence is approximately 1 in 10 000 with both boys and girls being equally affected (Gilbert 2000).

Characteristics The affected individual is dwarfed, with limb abnormalities, small hands and feet and underdeveloped genitalia. Microcephaly, facial hair, confluent eyebrows, downward-slanting eyes, small palate and irregular teeth are all characteristics.

All affected individuals have some degree of learning disability, which is often severe.

Hydrocephalus

Hydrocephalus is associated with an excessive amount of fluid in the brain. The rate of formation of cerebrospinal fluid (CSF) is often elevated, but more frequently the condition is caused by an obstruction to its flow. Hydrocephalus is often not recognised until the child is a few months old, and a considerable increase in head size can occur without evidence of significant brain damage. Severe damage to the brain substance occurs when the condition is untreated and the ventricles reach a critical point in their dilation. Surgical intervention may be required in a number of cases. The insertion of a ventriculoatrial shunt should allow the excess fluid to be drained off. Early intervention should ensure a positive outcome, but untreated cases could result in grossly distended skulls and severe learning disabilities. Strabismus, nystagmus, paralysis and epilepsy may also be evident. The reported prevalence of hydrocephalus averages 2 per 1000, but there is a higher incidence with increased parental age (Burns 1994).

Hypothyroidism

Hypothyroidism or cretinism is the name given to a group of conditions caused by a deficiency of thyroxine, which is secreted by the thyroid gland. A number of different metabolic errors result in a similar clinical picture. Although the precise cause is unknown the condition is treatable with thyroxine, usually given orally. Treatment should commence as early as possible, within the first few months of life.

The untreated individual frequently presents as apathetic, poor at feeding and sucking, a noisy breather owing to an enlarged tongue which protrudes, and also with delayed growth.

Characteristics The individual is small in stature, with severe learning disabilities, and speech acquisition is delayed until 7 or 8 years of age. The skin appears yellow in colour and is loose and wrinkled. There is thickening of the eyelids, nostrils, lips, hands and feet. Hair is usually scanty. Puberty is delayed and the external genitalia fail to develop.

ENVIRONMENT

The environment inextricably influences characteristics such as intelligence, health and body size. The individual who is deprived of food and vitamins is less likely to thrive than one who has an adequate supply. Similarly, the individual who is deprived of stimulation and education would appear to be at a disadvantage when developing intellectually, whatever their gene status. But what do we mean by environment? Like the term learning disabilities, the environment could be considered an umbrella term. Figure 2.1 shows the range of environmental factors that are considered important when studying the causes of learning disability.

ENVIRONMENTAL AND GENETIC CAUSES OF LEARNING DISABILITY BY TIME

The genetic causes of learning disability, although already identified, have been included here to demonstrate their relationship with the environmental causes of learning disabilities as identified in Figure 2.1.

Preconceptual

Preconceptual care and planning is for the most part a fairly new phenomenon. Good health prior to conception may not be an absolute guarantee of a healthy child, but there is statistical evidence (HC 1980, 1984; Sweet 1988) to show that unplanned pregnancies and perinatal mortality occur more frequently in the lower socio-economic groups, in young unsupported women and in women with pre-existing medical disorders and previous obstetric complications. It would therefore seem reasonable to consider the genetic and environmental factors that may be operating during the preconceptual stage. The organisation Foresight produces information including *Guidelines for Future Parents* (Dickerson 1980) and *Planning for a Healthy Baby* (Barnes & Bradley 1990). More information can be found at their internet website, details of which can be found at the end of this chapter.

Heredity

Genetic counselling, which will include obtaining a detailed family history or pedigree, may be necessary for some couples where there is a known or potential risk of abnormality (Box 2.3).

Environment

Nutrition is important at any stage in the lifecycle, and any nutritional deficiencies may take many months to correct. Prospective parents should be encouraged to maintain a healthy balanced diet,

---

Box 2.3   Genetic counselling

Genetic counselling is a service offered to patients or relatives who may be at risk from a disorder that may be hereditary in nature. During the process patients or relatives are advised of the consequences of the disorder, the probability of developing or transmitting it, and ways in which it may be prevented, avoided or ameliorated. However, the extent to which the information generated from genetic counselling either is unbiased or actually informs decision making has been drawn into question and remains an issue of some considerable debate (see Barr 1999 in Further reading). The Hospital for Sick Children in Great Ormond Street, London, was the first in the UK to develop a genetic counselling service in 1946. There are now a number of regionally based centres offering this service.

Reader activity 2.2

1. Find out the address and contact information for your local genetic counselling service.
2. Informing parents of the outcome of genetic testing is a skilled activity that requires a level of knowledge relating to chromosome anomalies and skill in communicating the results. However, recent research (Abramsky et al 2001) has suggested that there is great variation in professional knowledge and skill in conveying this information. You might like to consider and make notes of the kinds of knowledge, skills and attitudes a professional should have when giving parents the results of their tests. You should also consider the possible reaction parents might have to the results.

---

not only during pregnancy but also in preparation for conception. Children conceived during periods of poor nutrition, such as in Holland in the 'Hunger Winter' (October 1944 to May 1945), were found to have a high perinatal mortality rate. In those infants who survived there was found to be an increased incidence of congenital malformation. In addition to a healthy diet, vitamin supplements such as folic acid are advised prior to conception and up until the 12th week of pregnancy, to aid in the prevention of neural tube defects (Health Education Authority 1999).

Pre-existing medical disorders may have an adverse effect upon the mother and fetus (Alexander et al 1996): for example, a woman who was treated for phenylketonuria as a child but has now ceased taking her special diet would have high levels of phenylalanine during pregnancy. These high levels of phenylalanine are associated with abortion, intrauterine growth retardation, congenital heart defects, microcephaly and learning disabilities.

Prenatal

Heredity

As previously mentioned, there are a number of known conditions caused by genetic factors operating during the developmental cycle. Mothers falling into high-risk categories by virtue of age or known family incidence, who have not considered or received preconceptual care and advice, should be offered support, counselling and access to appropriate diagnostic tests, such as amniocentesis and chorionic villus sampling, should they require it.

Environment

There are numerous environmental influences that may affect the mother and the unborn child. Appropriate health education and antenatal care may go a long way in ensuring a greater understanding of the potential risk factors, and their effects upon the mother and child. Several factors operate during this developmental period that may have an effect upon the fetus.

Infections Maternal infections that may result in learning disabilities can be grouped under three main headings: viral, bacterial and protozoal.

Viral

1. *Rubella* (or German measles) is probably the best-known maternal viral infection which can cause learning disability. The degree of intellectual impairment, which can range from mild to profound, can be linked to the time of contraction of the virus; the earlier the exposure to the virus during the pregnancy, especially during the first trimester, the more affected the child will be, both physically and intellectually. After 16 weeks the risk of abnormality is very infrequent (Shaw et al 1998). Because congenital rubella may occur in the absence of overt maternal infection it may go undetected. The principal malformations seen

in congenital rubella include cataracts, deafness, congenital heart defects and microcephaly (Box 2.4) with learning disability (Frazier et al 1996).

2. *Cytomegalovirus* means 'large cell virus'. It belongs to the herpes family, along with the viruses that cause chickenpox (varicella zoster), cold sores and glandular fever. It is a common infection that usually has brief flu-like, or no symptoms. Without realising it, by the time they are middle-aged most people will have been infected. The most frequent times for contracting the virus are in early childhood and between 20 and 35 years. It is estimated that 4 out of every 1000 women who are pregnant become infected, and approximately half pass on the virus to the fetus, resulting in 10% of the infected babies having malformations (Shaw et al 1998). The principal malformations seen in cytomegalovirus are deafness, blindness, cerebral palsy and learning disabilities.

3. *Varicella zoster*, or chickenpox, poses a risk to the fetus if acquired during the first 5 months of pregnancy. The principal malformations include cataracts, microcephaly and learning disabilities (Harper 1998).

Bacterial congenital syphilis This is fortunately less common today than it was in the past. Improvements in general health education, antenatal care and the use of antibiotics have reduced the number of cases.

In the affected individual there is a general failure to thrive and growth is stunted. Physical manifestations include saddleback nose, pegshaped teeth, and opacities of the cornea, strabismus and nystagmus. The central nervous system is affected to various degrees and epilepsy may be present.

Protozoal When acute infection with *Toxoplasma gondii* occurs during pregnancy the parasite can

---

Box 2.4   Microcephaly

Microcephaly (abnormal smallness of the head) may result from a variety of intrauterine causes, including congenital infection, teratogens and maternal phenylketonuria. It may also be evident as part of a genetic syndrome, such as Cri-du-chat syndrome. True microcephaly is the result of autosomal recessive inheritance.

cross the placenta and infect the fetus. As with the previously described infections, the earlier this occurs in the pregnancy the more severe are the effects. Maternal infection is often asymptomatic and can result from contact with animal excrement (in particular cats), undercooked meat and unwashed vegetables. Only a small proportion of affected children would have severe manifestations, but learning disabilities and hearing defects do occur.

Maternal health

Maternal nutrition and health are known to be linked to fetal development. The supply of essential nutrients and oxygen to the fetus is totally dependent upon the mother, and any interruption of this process will affect the fetus. Good health for the pregnant mother should be thought of in the widest possible context, both on a physical and a psychological level, to maximise the development of a healthy pregnancy.

Toxic agents

There are a number of known toxic agents that can injure the developing fetus in some way. Smoking, alcohol, drugs and environmental pollutants have all been identified as associated factors in the causation of learning disabilities.

Smoking in itself may not be a direct cause of learning disabilities, but it does pose a preventable hazard to both the mother and the fetus. There is a wealth of evidence linking smoking during pregnancy with low birth weight, spontaneous abortion and perinatal death, as well as prenatal complications leading to handicapping conditions and deformity in the neonate (HEA 1999, Spitzer 1996).

Detailed accounts of the effects of alcohol consumption during pregnancy have only recently been described. However, alcohol consumption during pregnancy has been linked with spontaneous abortion, low birth weight and fetal alcohol syndrome (Gilbert 2000). Fetal alcohol syndrome is characterised by low birth weight, failure to thrive, reduced motor development and microcephaly. It is unclear how much alcohol needs to be consumed to have a detrimental effect upon the fetus, but there is a view that alcohol should not be consumed in large quantities (no more than one or two units once or twice a week) and that women should not get 'drunk' during pregnancy (Plant 1987, HEA 1999).

Drugs taken during pregnancy may have a teratogenic effect upon the developing fetus. The abnormality may, however, be the result of drug interaction with a nutrient, and not as a direct result of the drug action alone. The effects of the drug thalidomide have been well documented and reported. It has been suggested (Dickerson 1980) that the drug may have interacted with riboflavin (one of the heat-stable factors of the vitamin B complex), as similar effects have been recorded in riboflavin-deficient animals. Women taking anticonvulsant medication for the control of epilepsy have also been found to be at risk of producing children with malformations.

Environmental pollutants such as lead and mercury, and chemical agents such as solvents, pesticides, anaesthetic gases and ionising radiation, have all been identified as hazardous to the developing fetus. Lead pollution in the atmosphere is known to cause stillbirth and congenital damage to the brain and central nervous system, resulting in learning disabilities (FORESIGHT 2001).

Physical factors

Radiation in the form of excessive use of X-rays has been found to cause damage to the developing fetus, especially if exposure occurs during the first 3 months of pregnancy. Some pregnant women in Japan who survived the atomic bomb blasts were found to give birth to microcephalic children. Further studies of this group also identified chromosomal abnormalities and gene mutations. Ultrasound screening (a non-invasive technique that uses sound waves to visualise the position and size of the fetus and placenta) is a suitably safe alternative for examinations during pregnancy.

Maternal–fetal incompatibility (kernicterus)

Rhesus factor incompatibility occurs when a rhesus-negative mother is carrying a fetus that is rhesus positive (inherited from the father). The first child is usually unaffected, but in subsequent pregnancies the number of maternal antibodies increases. The antibodies then pass through the placental barrier and destroy the rhesus-positive blood of the fetus. An exchange transfusion can be given in utero if the blood is being destroyed, or immediately following the birth. At birth an affected child will be jaundiced, and if no action is taken brain damage will occur. Anti-D gamma globulin, if administered by injection to the rhesus-negative woman within 48 hours of the delivery of the first child, will prevent the formation of the dangerous antibodies.

Direct violence

Any trauma to the fetus may result in stillbirth, abortion or brain damage. The severity of the condition will depend upon the stage of gestation and the severity and nature of the violent act.

Anoxia

Should the brain be robbed of oxygen (anoxia) for a prolonged period of time then this will trigger irreversible changes in the brain. This is especially true for the developing fetus, which can only withstand very brief periods without oxygen before permanent damage occurs. Oxygen deprivation may be caused by a number of factors:

- Maternal illness, resulting in poorly oxygenated blood
- Reduction in respiration owing to maternal sedation
- Abnormal or premature detachment of the placenta.

Perinatal

The first 28 days of life are usually considered as the perinatal period (Hay et al 1999). Perinatal causes of learning disability that occur during this time include conditions such as prematurity, birth injury and/or abnormal labour.

Premature infants

These infants are born prior to 37 weeks' gestation. Although prematurity is not in itself a cause of learning disabilities, premature and low birth weight babies experience a significantly greater number of problems during labour and the birth process, including breathing difficulties and intraventricular haemorrhage, than do full-term infants, which places them at risk for subsequent developmental problems (Kitchen & Murton 1985).

Asphyxia

This is the primary cause of central nervous system damage before and after birth. Asphyxiation results in hypoxia, or decreased levels of oxygen and diminished cerebral blood flow. When the cerebral blood flow is diminished the self-regulation of the brain's blood supply is impaired, leading in turn to brain swelling and haemorrhage (Wyly 1995). Death or severe handicap occur in approximately 25% of all severely asphyxiated full-term infants (Rudolf & Levene 1999).

Birth trauma

Birth is a traumatic event under any circumstances, for both mother and baby, and full-term babies are also at risk from a number of factors operating during labour that can cause birth trauma or injury, including:

- Asphyxia: due to a prolonged second stage of labour, or the coiling of the umbilical cord round the child's neck
- Trauma: caused by instrumented delivery, i.e. forceps delivery. Excessive moulding of the head and breech presentation are also possible causes.

Damage or trauma to the brain may result in cerebral palsy, epilepsy or learning disabilities, depending upon the severity of the damage and the location within the brain.

Fetal monitoring, i.e. determining fetal size and presentation prior to and during labour with ultrasound and other monitoring equipment, can alert the attending professional to the signs of fetal distress and reduce the potential danger.

During the period immediately following birth, untreated hypocalcaemia, hypernatraemia and hypoglycaemia in the child can result in brain damage (Soothill et al 1987).

Postnatal

There are a number of factors that operate during the postnatal period that may result in learning disabilities, for example untreated genetic conditions, childhood infection, trauma, accidents, toxic agents, poor nutrition, and sensory and social isolation.

With appropriate health education and health promotion messages, increased awareness of these causative factors may help to reduce the incidence or promote early intervention to limit the severity of the learning disability.

Heredity

Many of the inherited conditions only become apparent in the postnatal period, for example phenylketonuria. As stated earlier, if this condition is not treated the child will become affected when the phenylalanine concentration rises above the critical level (Mueller & Young 1998).

Environmental

Infection A number of childhood infections carry the risk of brain damage as a complication, which may result in the affected individual having learning disabilities and/or an associated physical handicap. Encephalitis, meningitis and gastroenteritis are three examples of infections which, if untreated, can lead to intellectual impairment (Box 2.5).

Trauma Trauma to the head can be the result of accidental or non-accidental injury.

Accidental injuries may be sustained as a result of road traffic or general household accidents, or as a result of oxygen deprivation; or they may be the result of capillary haemorrhage caused by prolonged and severe coughing during whooping cough infection.

Box 2.5 Encephalitis

Encephalitis, or inflammation of the brain, can result from a viral infection, such as rubella, mumps or chickenpox. Encephalitis following vaccination (for example for whooping cough) is rare but does occur. The overall incidence of encephalitis is very low, but the effects and the degree of learning disability can be severe.

Meningitis, or inflammation of the membranes of the brain or spinal cord, can lead to brain damage and result in learning disability. Improvements in health care and early detection have reduced the number of recorded infections and associated complications.

Gastroenteritis, or inflammation of the mucous membrane of both stomach and intestine, can be especially dangerous in the very young. Dehydration, which may occur very rapidly, leads to brain haemorrhage, which can cause brain damage.

The main carer usually causes non-accidental injury, or battered baby syndrome. Injuries include depressed fractures of the skull, haematomas and blood vessel damage. The severity of the injury will determine the degree of intellectual impairment sustained. Children who are suspected of being at risk are placed on an at-risk register and will be closely monitored (Working Together Under the Children Act 1989).

Toxic agents As in the prenatal period toxic agents can damage the developing brain. Lead intoxication was once commonly known as a causative factor, but increased awareness of the potential problem has reduced the use of this damaging substance. Environmental pollutants are another cause for concern, and continued investigation to identify potential harmful substances is required. Mercury, copper, manganese and strontium are all seen as detrimental in the developmental period.

Nutrition Appropriate nutrition is a central element of health and wellbeing. The developing child who is malnourished may experience both physical and mental developmental delay.

Sensory and social deprivation Children learn and develop by interacting with their surroundings and environmental stimuli. Deprivation caused by impairment to any of the special senses (sight, hearing, touch, taste and smell) or social exclusion may have an effect upon the child's physical and intellectual development. Therefore, in order to prevent a secondary handicap professionals should have an understanding of the holistic needs of the developing individual and be able to educate and advise those who are not so well informed or who require assistance.

CONCLUSION

There is no easy or wholly satisfactory method for identifying and categorising the numerous causes of learning disabilities. Overlaps and anomalies exist that confirm or confound the known aetiologies. However, an understanding of the known causes and manifestations of learning disabilities may offer parents an opportunity to explore and conceptualise the ongoing needs of their child and may enhance the quality of professionals' practice in a number of ways:

- In the provision of appropriate person centered care
- As a means of improving the quality of life for the individual, rather than inhibiting or artificially limiting it
- By advising parents or carers as to the nature and potential effects of the individual's condition
- By answering questions or giving information to potential parents
- By recognising threats to the health of people with learning disabilities caused by a known disorder.

GLOSSARY OF TERMS

Allele Alternative form of a gene that may occupy the same site on homologous chromosomes

Autosome Chromosome other than the sex chromosome

Centromere A specialised region of a chromosome seen as a constriction under the microscope. This region is important in the activities of the chromosomes during cellular division

Chromosome Chromophilic body within the cell nucleus, visible as homologous pairs in dividing cells

Dominant trait One which is determined by the presence of a gene in heterozygous form

Gene The unit of inheritance, occupying a specific locus on a chromosome

Genotype An individual's genetic makeup

Heterozygous Having different alleles at a gene locus on each of a pair of homologous chromosomes

Homozygous Having the same allele at a gene locus on each of a pair of homologous chromosomes

Karyotype The chromosome characteristics of an individual arranged in pairs in descending order of size and according to the position of the centromere

Mosaicism The presence of more than one cell type in a single individual

Mutation A spontaneous or induced change in a gene or chromosome

Phenotype The way in which the genotype is expressed in the body

Recessive trait One which is determined by the presence of a gene in homozygous form

Sex chromosomes The pair of chromosomes responsible for sex determination

Sex-linked trait One determined by the presence of a gene on the sex chromosomes (usually X linked)

Translocation The transfer of a segment of a chromosome to a site on a different chromosome

Trisomy The presence of one chromosome additional to the normal homologous pair

REFERENCES

Abramsky L, Hall S, Levitan J, Marteau T M 2001 What parents are told after prenatal diagnosis of a sex chromosome abnormality: interview and questionnaire study. British Medical Journal 2001 322: 463–466

Alexander J, Levy V, Roach S (eds) 1996 Midwifery practice: core topics 1. Macmillan, London

Barnes B, Bradley S G 1990 Planning for a healthy baby. Foresight, Godalming

Bonthron D, FitzPatrick D, Porteous M, Trainer A 1998 Clinical genetics: a case based approach. W B Saunders, Bath

Burns J K 1994 Birth defects and their causes. Stress Books, Ireland

Clarke A M, Clarke A D B (eds) 1974 Mental deficiency, 3rd edn. Methuen, London

Department of Health 2001 Valuing people: a new strategy for learning disability for the 21st Century. Cm 5086, HMSO, London

Dickerson J W T 1980 Guidelines for future parents: environmental factors and foetal health. Foresight, Godalming

Dutton G 1975 Mental handicap. Butterworths, London

FORESIGHT 2001 The adverse effects of lead. Available from: http://www.foresight-preconception.org.uk/lead.html

Frazier M S, Drzymkowski J A, Doty S J 1996 Essentials of human diseases and conditions. W B Saunders, USA

Gilbert P 2000 A–Z of syndromes and inherited disorders, 3rd edn. Stanley Thornes, Great Britain

Harper P S 1998 Practical genetic counselling, 5th edn. Butterworth-Heinemann, Oxford

Hay W W, Hayward A R, Levin M J, Sondheimer J M (eds) 1999 Current pediatric diagnosis & treatment, 14th edn. Appleton & Lange, USA

Health Education Authority 1999 The pregnancy book. HEA, London

Health of the Nation 1995 A strategy for people with learning disabilities. HMSO, London

House of Commons Social Services Committee (HC) 1980 Report on perinatal and neonatal mortality (Short Report). HMSO, London

House of Commons Social Services Committee (HC) 1984 Follow-up report on perinatal and neonatal mortality. HMSO, London

Kitchen W, Murton L J 1985 Survival rates of infants with birth weight between 501 and 1000 g. American Journal of Diseases of Children 139: 470–471

Knight S J L, Regan R, Nicod A et al 1999 Subtle chromosomal rearrangements in children with unexplained mental retardation. Lancet 345 (9191): 1676–1681

Mueller R F, Young I D 1998 Emery's elements of medical genetics, 10th edn. Churchill Livingstone, Edinburgh

Newton R 1992 Down's syndrome. Optima, London

Plant M L 1987 Women, drinking and pregnancy. Tavistock Publications, London

Rudolf M C S, Levene M I 1999 Paediatrics and child health. Blackwell Science, Oxford

Russell P J 1996 Genetics, 4th edn. Harper Collins College Publishers, New York

Shaw I M, Morgan-Capner P, Pitt S J 1998 Viral infections of the foetus and neonate – a distance learning package. Jones-Sands, Coventry

Soothill P W, Nicolaides K H, Campbell S 1987 Prenatal asphyxia. British Medical Journal 294: 1051–1053

Spitzer A R (ed) 1996 Intensive care of the fetus and neonate. Mosby, USA

Sweet B R 1988 Mayes midwifery, 11th edn. Bailliere Tindall, London, pp 571–572

Working Together Under the Children Act 1989 1991 A guide for inter-agency co-operation for the protection of children from abuse. HMSO, London

Wyly M V 1995 Premature infants and their families developmental interventions. Singular Publishing Group, London

FURTHER READING

Barr O 1999 Genetic counselling: a consideration of the potential and key obstacles to assisting parents adapt to a child with learning disabilities. British Journal of Learning Disabilities 27: 30–36

Bellman M, Kennedy N (eds) 2000 Paediatrics and child health. Churchill Livingstone, Edinburgh

Harper P S 1999 Practical genetic counselling (5th edn) Butterworth-Heineman, Oxford

Health Departments of the United Kingdom 1998 Advisory committee on genetic testing: report on genetic testing for late onset disorders. Department of Health, London

USEFUL ADDRESSES

ASSERT (Angelman Syndrome Support Education and Research Trust)
PO Box 505
Sittingbourne
Kent ME10 NE
Tel. 01980 625616

The National Autistic Society
393 City Road
London EC1V 1NE
Tel. 020 7833 2299

Cornelia de Lange Foundation
'Tall Trees' 106 Lodge Lane
Grays
Essex RM16 2UL
Tel. 01375 376439

Cri-du-chat Syndrome Support Group
Penny Lane
Barwell
Leicestershire LE9 8HJ
Tel. 01455 841680

Down's Syndrome Association
155 Micham Road
London SW17 9PG
Tel. 020 8682 4001

SOFT UK (Edward's Syndrome)
48 Froggarts Ride
Walmley
Sutton Coldfield
West Midlands
B76 8TQ
Tel. 0121 351 3122

Foetal Alcohol Syndrome Trust
15 Wasdale Road
Aintree
Liverpool L9 8AS
Tel. 0151 284 2900

FORESIGHT The association for the promotion of pre-conceptual care
28 The Paddock, Godalming

Surrey, GU7 1XD
www.foresight-preconception.org.uk

Fragile X Society
53 Winchelsea Lane
Hastings
East Sussex TN35 4LG
Tel. 01424 813147

Klinefelter's Syndrome Association
56 Little Yeldham Road
Little Yeldham
Nr Halstead
Essex CO9 4QT
Tel. 01787 237460

The Research Trust into Metabolic Diseases in Children
(RTMDC)
Golden Gates Lodge
Weston Road
Crewe
Cheshire CW1 1XN
Tel. 01270 250221

Society for Mucopolysaccharide Diseases
46 Woodside Road
Amersham
Bucks HP6 6AJ
Tel. 01494 434156

Neurofibromatosis Association
82 London Road
Kingston-on-Thames
Surrey KT2 6PV
Tel. 020 8547 1636

National Society for Phenylketonuria (UK) Ltd
7 Lingley Lane
Wardley
Gateshead NE10 8BR
Tel. 01845 603 9136 (helpline)

Prader-Willi Syndrome Association (UK)
2 Wheatsheaf Close
Horsell
Woking
Surrey GU21 4BP
Tel. 01483 724784

Tay-Sachs and Allied Diseases Association
Golden Gates Lodge
Weston Road
Crewe
Cheshire CW1 1XN
Tel. 01270 250221

Tuberous Sclerosis Association of Great Britain
Little Barnsley Farm
Catshill
Bromsgrove
Worcestershire B61 0NQ
Tel. 01527 871898

The Turner Syndrome Society
c/o The Child Growth Foundation
2 Mayfield Avenue
London W4 1PW
Tel. 020 8994 7625 / 020 8995 0257

A history of learning disabilities

Helen Atherton

KEY ISSUES

- Throughout recorded history learning disabilities have been understood and accounted for in many different ways.
- A range of methods and materials may be accessed to understand the history of learning disabilities; these include photographs, central and local government reports, annual reports from past institutions, prose, art, poetry and autobiographical accounts.
- More recent history would seem to have perceived people with learning disabilities as a threat and this led to a segregationist policy in the UK and the construction of large institutions.
- During the closing decades of the 20th century a reversal of this policy was pursued. This was known as community care, and this policy is still actively being pursued through a new agenda of social inclusion.

INTRODUCTION

The study of history has been described as:

the best medicine for a sick mind; for in history you have a record of the infinite variety of human experience plainly set out for all to see; and in that record you can find yourself and your country both examples and warnings; fine things to take as models, base things rotten through and through, to avoid (Livy).

This chapter provides a concise history of the lives of people with learning disabilities from the time of Ancient Greece through to the present day. It will examine the range of attitudes and beliefs that have been held by different societies toward this group of people over this time, and how these, in combination with varying social and economic factors, have influenced the type and quality of care provided to them. The chapter will also explore key pieces of social policy and government legislation that have punctuated developments in this area.

Evidently, the content of this chapter can neither be definitive, nor indeed conclusive. The history of learning disabilities remains an emerging field of study and the range of evidence that we have at our disposal is steadily growing, and becoming more varied. What this chapter will aim to do, however, is to build on existing historical accounts of learning disabilities by marrying together a new range of evidence that has, up until now, been relatively disparate. This includes conventional sources of evidence taken from a number of different academic disciplines such as psychology, sociology, medicine and law as well as evidence taken from less conventional sources. This will include photographs, poems and representations of people with learning disabilities in literature. It is important to note that in some areas of the chapter, direct quotes from people with learning disabilities have been used to support statements made in the text. The purpose of this is to centralise the experience of people with learning disabilities, in order to respect their right to own a personal history; a right that in the past has more often than not been denied to them.

DIFFERENT SOURCES OF EVIDENCE

Providing an accurate and detailed account of the history of learning disabilities could be described as being synonymous with doing a jigsaw. You start off with an empty board and then start to put the pieces in place, first to form an outline and then to gradually fill it in. Sometimes the necessary pieces aren't easy to find, and for a time your picture may remain incomplete. Indeed on nearing the end of the jigsaw, you may find that you have a piece missing and that you are resigned to the fact that you may never have the luxury of see-

ing the complete image. For a great number of years, the history of people with learning disabilities was that empty jigsaw board. This group had an invisible presence within society, indistinct from other social groups. In addition to this, general stigmatisation of this group led to insufficient value being afforded to their lives to warrant any real interest in this area. However, in recent years there has been a surge of academic attention in this area. Atkinson et al (1997) have attributed this change to a range of factors that include:

- contemporary debates surrounding the merits of community care versus institutionalised care
- emergence of important archive material including personal records following the closure of long stay institutions
- growing influence of the self-advocacy movement in the UK
- increasing interest in the social history of devalued groups in general
- emergence of learning disabilities as a distinct medical speciality
- re-emergence of the genetics/eugenic debate.

A number of different sources of historical evidence are available in pursuit of an accurate portrayal of the history of people with learning disabilities. It is the case that a number of these sources, such as Acts of Parliament and local and national policy documents, have already been employed in the construction of previous historical accounts (Kirman 1975, Race 1995). Although these accounts in themselves provide a reservoir of accessible information, their approach has tended to be predominantly academic and analytical in style. Little attention has been afforded to the task of complementing these accounts with representations of the ways in which people with learning disabilities themselves have perceived the changing effects of service provision on their own lives. Indeed Ryan & Thomas (1980) have concluded that people with learning disabilities are: 'still hidden from history as they are from the rest of life. What history they do have is not so much theirs as the history of others acting either on their behalf, or against them.' (p. 85)

In recent years, however, attempts have been made to correct this imbalance. This includes the deliberate adaptation of research methods to be inclusive of the needs of people with learning disabilities, thereby enabling them to tell their own history (Atkinson 1997, Hussain 1997). In addition to this has been the active promotion of self-advocacy amongst this group. As a consequence, access has been facilitated to a rich source of evidence that has previously been untapped, i.e. the personal recollections of people with learning disabilities (Atkinson et al 1997, Barron 1996, Lewis 1997, Potts and Fido 1991). Indeed it could be argued such recollections represent the most legitimate form of evidence available to researchers in this field.

Atkinson et al (1997) have summarised the different archive material available to people wishing to undertake research in this area. This includes photographs, central and local government reports, annual reports from institutions and personal records. The recent publication *Harperbury Hospital, from Colony to Closure* (Brown 2001) is a good example of the effective use of a combination of archive material to compile a history of an institution. However, there exists a range of non-conventional material that can equally contribute to our understanding of this history. Atkinson & Williams (1990) have shown how the individual lives of people with learning disabilities can be documented through the use of prose, art and poetry. Another example of a non-conventional form of evidence is the representations of people with learning disabilities in fictional stories that have been written in different centuries (Bragg 1997, Davidson et al 1994). These include characters such as 'Lennie' in John Steinbeck's *Of Mice and Men* (Steinbeck 1937) who is described as being 'a huge man with a shapeless face, large pale eyes, wide, sloping shoulders; he walked heavily, dragging his feet a little . . . his arms did not swing at his sides but hung loosely'. Reid (1967) has concluded that Charles Dickens often used characters in his books that were considered to be children of god, mental inadequates, and simple minded or good in heart. One example of such a character is Smike from Charles Dickens' *Nicholas Nickleby* (Dickens 2000) who is described as being among other things 'a wretched creature with humble ability'. Other examples include Maggy from *Little Dorrit*, Tom Ping from *Martin*

Chuzzlewit and Toots from *Dombey and Son*. Much can be learnt about the social standing of these individuals by examining their interactions with other characters in the books. Knowledge can also be gained about the ways in which their disability was perceived and consequently treated by others. It is the case, however, that such sources of evidence have their limitations. One of these limitations has been recognised by McDonagh (2000) who has suggested that whilst novels are an important source of evidence, they may be deficient in terms of the amount of information they present about the actual day-to-day living of a person with learning disabilities.

To summarise, a wide range of evidence exists that has documented the lives of people with learning disabilities in different periods of time. To create as full a picture as possible about their history, it is important to marry together this range of evidence, whilst recognising both its strengths and weaknesses.

Reader activity 3.1

a) From your own personal experience, consider why the recognition of a past history is important for an individual with learning disabilities.
b) Suggest ways in which you might help someone with learning disabilities rediscover and record their own personal history.

A PROFILE OF LEARNING DISABILITIES FROM ANCIENT GREECE TO EARLY MODERN BRITAIN

It would not be unreasonable to assume that people with learning disabilities have, by their very nature, existed since the beginning of humanity. However, the extent to which they have been socially visible has differed over time, as has the way in which their existence has been understood by respective societies. Wolfensberger (1972) has summarised some of the terminology that reflects the range of attitudes and beliefs that have been held towards this group of people. These include subhuman organism, menace, unspeakable object of dread, object of pity, holy innocent, diseased organism, object of ridicule and eternal child. This chapter incorporates the range of 'statutory' terminology that has been used to define people with learning disabilities within different policy and legislative documents in history. Although these terms may appear derogatory by contemporary standards their inclusion is important in order to reflect changing attitudes toward this group of people.

To establish an accurate portrayal of the lives of people with learning disabilities in ancient times is problematic on two accounts. First is the obvious absence of written records from these periods, and second is the lack of any clear distinction between people with learning disabilities and those with other forms of disability. What is known, however, is that the existence of people with disabilities can be traced back to the time of the primitive savage who killed the weak and deformed as they were considered a burden on the tribe (Roper 1913). Indeed their existence can also be traced back to the time of Ancient Greece as reports of disabled people and their subsequent treatment feature in the writings of the Greek philosophers Socrates, Plato and Aristotle. It could be concluded from the following statement from Plato (427–347 BC) that people with a physical or psychological disability were not welcome entities in the development of civilised societies:

... then this is the kind of medical and judicial provision for which you legislate in your state. It will provide treatment for those citizens whose physical and psychological constitution is good; as for others, it will leave the unhealthy to die, and those whose psychological constitution is incurably corrupt it will put to death.

(Lee 1987, p. 114)

It was not until medieval times, however, that a distinction between people with learning disabilities and those with other forms of disability was established, thereby enabling a more precise understanding of their treatment by respective societies.

During medieval times, the absence of medical knowledge about the aetiology of disease led many to believe that the birth of a child with learning disabilities was the result of supernatural forces. This led people to both fear and worship those with learning disabilities, sometimes simultaneously, and as is suggested by the following statement this resulted in them being both persecuted and fostered:

mental illness and mental retardation (which were lumped together) were attributed to supernatural causes and considered in the province of priests and philosophers. Although a few retarded persons did have a career as 'court fools', others were exploited, persecuted and exorcised. The foundations of modern care of retarded people were laid in the nineteenth century (Szymanski & Crocker, cited in Wright & Digby 1996, p. 22).

Stratford (1996) has provided one example of where people with learning disabilities have been worshipped by a specific society. In reviewing the historical origin of Down syndrome, he draws attention to the reliefs, sculptures and other artefacts of the Olmecs, a tribe of people who lived around the Gulf of Mexico from 1500 BC to AD 300. These images were found to depict individuals with varying handicaps ranging from hunchback through to clubfoot. The most significant of these, however, were those that suggested that people with Down syndrome held religious meaning for the tribe. This was portrayed through images of senior female members of the tribe mating with a jaguar, the sacred totem of the Olmecs. The result of this was a child with the obvious characteristics of Down syndrome, portrayed in the reliefs as a god-human hybrid. This led Stratford to conclude that such children were probably given preferential treatment by the tribe, first because they were more than likely the offspring of its most senior members, and secondly because their survival at that time was probably something of a rarity. The religious significance of people with learning disabilities has also been prevalent in other cultures. From the late 17th century up until recent times, a shrine in Gurjrat, Pakistan was the location for a community of people with microcephaly, or 'chuas' (rats) as they became known. It was generally believed that their existence held some sort of special significance, and as a result the shrine attracted many visitors (Miles 1996). A further example is the community of 'cretins' (people suffering from hypothyroidism) who were found living below the walls of monasteries in Switzerland. Local belief suggested that they brought luck to the community by drawing God's wrath upon themselves thereby serving as scapegoats (Eberly 1988).

One of the most infamous examples of where people with learning disabilities have either been worshipped or persecuted, depending on the beliefs of individual communities, is in the legend of the 'changeling'. The changeling was considered to be an infant whose: 'head was too big for its body, its face was ugly and wrinkled, it looked old . . . it could not stand or walk but crept round like an animal. It drank greedily and insatiably and sucked four or five wet nurses dry. It did not laugh or talk but screamed and shouted interminably' (Haffter 1968).

Haffter draws attention to the similarities between the physical appearance and behaviour of some people with learning disabilities and the descriptions of changelings found within both folklore and other narrative works. These include William Shakespeare's *A Midsummer-Night's Dream* in which Titania, Queen of the Fairies, refuses to give up a little changeling boy. It was commonly believed that the changeling was an infant who had been left behind after the fairies or 'good people' stole a parent's true infant in a fit of jealousy over the beauty of mankind. Much can be learnt from such accounts about the treatment of these infants. According to Haffter, a number of methods were employed to persuade the creatures to remove the changeling and replace the original child. These tended to vary from place to place and included trying to outwit the changeling by making it laugh or talk in order to break the spell. This is demonstrated in an extract from the Fairy Tale *The Elves* by the brothers Grimm in Box 3.1 (see also Fig. 3.1).

Other methods employed, however, were more brutal and potentially harmful to the changeling. These included placing the child on a red-hot shovel, pressing it into red hot ashes, lying it on a red-hot grid, firing shots over it, feeding it leather and red hot iron or making it drink poison. Further to this notion of mysticism, Eberly (1988) has discussed the varying descriptions of fairies and hybrids (offspring resulting from sexual relations with non-humans such as supernatural forces or beasts) found within folklore and concluded that they were more likely than not based on the characteristics of individuals with congenital disabilities.

It is the case that despite the varying treatment of people with learning disabilities during this period, they were, generally speaking, integrated

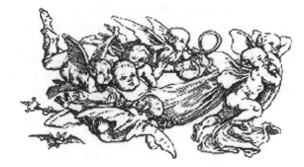

Figure 3.1 'The changeling' from the Brothers Grimm fairy story 'The Elves'.

Box 3.1 *The Elves*, The Brothers Grimm (1812) cited by Haffter (1967)

Fairies stole a mother's child from its cradle and in its place laid a changeling with a big head and staring eyes who wanted to do nothing but eat and drink. In her distress the mother went to a neighbour for advice. The neighbour told her to take the changeling into the kitchen, set it on the stove, make a fire and boil water in two egg-shells: this would make the changeling laugh, and if he laughed that would be the end of him. The woman did everything the neighbour had said. When she set the egg-shells of water on the fire, the changeling said:

I am as old
As the Wester Forest
Yet never have seen water boiled in an egg-shell,

And began to laugh. When it laughed, a troop of fairies came in, bringing with them the right child, which they set upon the stove, and taking the changeling away with them again.

within their communities without necessitating state support. In early modern Britain, however, their differences became more accentuated. De Prerogativia Regis 1325 (Kirman 1975) was the first piece of legislation that sought to exhibit some degree of state 'paternalism' toward both people with learning disabilities, who were at that time defined as 'idiots' or 'natural fools', and those suffering from some form of mental illness (lunatics). The principle aim of this legislation was to protect the lands of such individuals when it became apparent that they had neither the practical nor the intellectual ability to either sustain them, or to sensibly invest any profit gained from them. Determination of their abilities was based on a number of tests, the nature of which was to change over the proceeding two centuries. One example was the Fitzherbert's test (1534) that aimed to assess an individual's ability on the basis of being able to tell one's age, name one's parents and count out 20 pence. A later example was the Swinburne's test (1591) that aimed to assess an individual's ability on the basis of being able to name the days of the week and measure a yard of cloth (Kirman 1975). It is the case that the practical consequences of De Prerogativia Regis differed between people with learning disabilities and those with mental illness. For people with learning disabilities, the permanency of their condition meant that state control of their land was to continue until their death when it could then be transferred to their rightful heirs. In contrast, state control of the lands of people with mental illness could only be maintained until their recovery. Control of land of someone with learning disabilities could also, if deemed necessary, be transferred to the family whilst the person was still alive, as is shown by the following fictional story. Following the death of his wife and daughter, Walter Walkinshaw gave his estate to the daughter, not the son of his disinherited older brother. This action, along with others, convinced a court that he was suffering from intellectual incapacity, and as a consequence his estate was passed to his younger brother who had initiated the initial enquiry into Walter's behaviour (McDonagh 2000).

According to Neugebauer (1996), the permanency of state control over the lands of idiots, in comparison to its relative impermanency in respect to the lands of lunatics, was not the only differentiation between the two groups. For idiots, the law gave the crown the right to retain any revenue that was not required to provide the 'bare necessities' to them and their families. For lunatics, however, the law ensured that the crown returned any revenue that had not been used to maintain them and their family in a standard of life that did not reflect just bare necessities but equated to their social rank. These discrepancies were to remain unchanged until the 16th century when the law was modified to ensure that the rights of people with learning disabilities equated to those of people with a mental illness.

Although the care of idiots and lunatics was essentially the responsibility of the crown, their direct care was undertaken by private individuals who bought the right to this role. This, on the one hand, ensured that people could remain within their own community but on the other hand, the position inevitably lead to exploitation of the role for financial gain (Neugebauer 1996). This early example of community care was to continue until the 17th century when the responsibility for vulnerable groups was transferred from the crown to local parishes. Also, at this time social mobility became a significant feature of societies as people began to move around in search of employment. This led to one of the first pieces of segregative legislation, the Elizabethan Poor Law Act (1601). This act sought to restrict the movement of 'unattached groups' such as beggars, invalids and people with learning disabilities, who potentially threatened the stability of the establishment, by incarcerating them in workhouses (Kirman 1975). At this point the segregation of people considered to be a social and economic burden became a real option; however, it did not gather momentum until the beginning of the 20th century, when the threat of such groups amounted to a national crisis.

EUGENICS AND THE PROBLEM OF THE FEEBLE-MINDED

During the 18th century, the Western World was in the grip of the Industrial Revolution (from about 1760 onwards). The introduction of complex machinery ensured a demand for new technical skills amongst workforces. Race (1995) has suggested that this revolution brought about 'the measurement of people by their ability to cope with the new technological and commercial processes'. People with learning disabilities were singled out as one of a number of groups who were perceived as having neither the social nor the practical competencies to sustain themselves or any dependants in a developing society. As a consequence they were regarded, predominantly by the middle classes, as a financial burden. The Poor Law Amendment Act (1834) reacted to this situation by seeking to restrict state relief to only the able-bodied, and to continue to contain those who were either unwilling or unable to work within workhouses. This latter group included the urban poor, and people considered 'feeble-minded'. However, by the late 19th and early 20th centuries, the perceived threat posed to society by these groups of social deviants was not so much their financial burden, but the way in which they seemingly propagated their own kind, and hence spread many of society's social ills. It was believed that this would precipitate the degeneration of society through the erosion of its physical, intellectual and moral qualities, resulting in its eventual collapse. This view is reflected in the following statement: 'the danger lies in the fact that these degenerates mate with healthy members of the community and thereby constantly drag fresh blood into the vortex of disease and lower the general vigour of the nation' (Tredgold 1909). A number of political 'situations' served to strengthen this belief, the most significant of which centred on the process of imperialism. Imperialism became a key objective for many Western countries during the 19th century as they competed to become the most powerful and influential nations in the world. It was generally believed that the race for land largely depended on the 'survival of the fittest state' (Alaszewski 1988), the term 'fittest' implying both mental and physical vigour. This belief was theorised as 'Social Darwinism' (Bowler 1990). During the late 19th and early 20th centuries, however, the occurrence of a number of political crises served to cast doubt on the extent to which these desirable characteristics actually existed within defined populations. During the Boer War (1899–1902), for example, the British incurred an embarrassing defeat at the hands of a small group of Dutch farmers, whilst a significant number of conscripts to the army had been rejected on the grounds that they were medically unfit (Alaszewski 1988).

At the root of this problem was *differential fertility*, a concept that had been first introduced by T R Malthus in his *Essay on the Principle of Population* (1798). Malthus had concluded that the uncontrolled procreation of the working classes would cause an imbalance between population growth and the availability of food supplies, the result of which would be mass famine. Running concurrently with this was the debate surrounding the concept of degeneracy itself. A number of hypotheses were put forth at this time as to the exact cause of degeneracy within societies. Gelb (1995) cites the work of Morel (1857) who proposed the hypothesis that degeneracy was the result of poor or sinful living and included the ingestion of drugs and alcohol. He concluded that degeneracy in populations could be identified through the presence of a number of physical and behavioural 'stigmata' such as those presented in Box 3.2.

A second hypothesis was proposed by John Langdon Down (Borthwick 1996). Langdon Down had identified a group of people with learning disabilities within the asylum in which he worked. He believed this group to be representative of earlier forms of the human race, forms that had since developed through the process of evolution. He attempted to confirm his hypothesis by drawing comparisons between the characteristics of this group and those of existing 'underdeveloped' races such as the Mongolian tribes. He referred to the group as being 'throwbacks' although they were later identified as individuals with Down syndrome.

The 'feeble-minded' was a term applied to those individuals who were considered to be 'mildly handicapped and lacking physical stigmata' (Radford 1991). Using contemporary terminology, this group would probably have been labelled as having a 'mild learning disability'. It was believed that the feeble-minded were the

Box 3.2   Stigmata of degeneracy cited by Gelb (1995)

Physical Characteristics	Behavioural Characteristics
• Asymmetry of the head or face • Large and protruding jaws • Long arms • Open protruding mouths • High cheek bones • Hay fever • Suppressed noses • Narrow or arrest of the nasal cavity • Cleft palate • Club foot or hands • Shortened fingers • Hernias • Gout • Arthritis • Coarse skin • Jug-handled ears • Unusually large ears or very small ears	• Masturbation • Absence of shame • Impulsiveness • Egotism • Tendency to have a strong emotional response to music • Fearfulness • Reverie • Mysticism • Treachery • Vanity • Cruelty • Laziness • Vindictiveness • Indecisiveness • Enjoyment of the colours red and violet • The urge to collect things • Insensitivity to pain • Gambling • Fondness of animals • Enjoyment of slang • Tattooing

primary cause of many of the vices present within society, including prostitution, criminality, alcoholism and other conditions that resulted in diminished mental and physical vigour (Tredgold 1909). This fear was compounded by the perceived resistance of feeble-mindedness to any endeavours that sought its 'improvement' using contemporary methods of education and training. Because of these differing factors, control of the propagation of the feeble-minded was deemed imperative if national degeneracy was to be prevented. These beliefs were to coincide with the theory of eugenics that emerged to provide both the means and the justification for this control.

The term eugenics was first coined by Francis Galton in 1883 and was defined as being the 'science of improving inborn human qualities through selective breeding' (Galton 1883). Galton believed that feeble-mindedness was a single unit of inheritance that could be transmitted through generations of the same family, the nature of which was unaffected by environmental factors such as education. Information about inheritance at this time was often displayed as a 'pedigree chart'. This chart served to map how the gene for feeble-mindedness transmitted and manifested itself across each generation of the same family. This is demonstrated in Figure 3.2, which represents the infamous Kallikak Family (Goddard 1931), a family in which feeble-mindedness and the associated characteristics of alcoholism, prostitution and criminality were supposedly rife (see Chapter 23 for a fuller account). The specific afflictions of some members of the descendants of Martin Kallikak Jnr are displayed in Table 3.1.

Galton believed that nature was unreliable in selecting the most appropriate characteristics for the survival of the human race. These characteristics were summarised by Blacker (1945) as being:

Table 3.1   Type of afflictions affecting the Kallikak family (Goddard 1931)

Type of affliction	Number of people affected
Feeble-mindedness	143
Normality	46
Illegitimacy	36
Sexual Immorality	33
Alcoholism	24
Epilepsy	3
Criminality	3
Kept houses of ill fame	8
Died in infancy	82

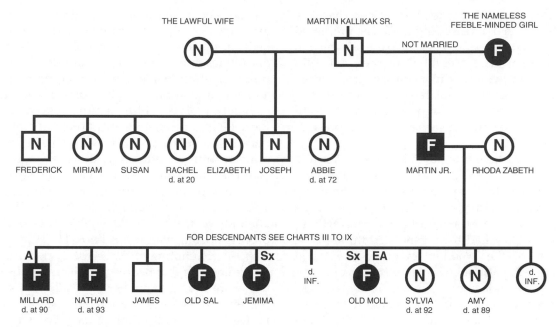

Figure 3.2   Pedigree of the Kallikak Family (Goddard 1931).

- Sound physical health and good physique
- Intelligence
- Social usefulness
- Free from genetic taints
- Membership of a large, united, well-adjusted family
- Fondness of children.

Galton therefore reasoned that the only way to prevent the degeneration of society was through artificial methods. He advocated two forms of eugenics: one was to promote procreation in the intellectual classes, a process termed *positive eugenics*, whilst the other was inhibition of procreation amongst classes that were considered to be socially deviant, a process termed *negative eugenics*. His theory was, however, not to be scientifically proven until the discovery of Mendel's laws of heredity in the early part of the 20th century. This resulted in the emergence of statistical tests that were to provide an objective measurement of the extent of the 'problem' of the feeble-minded (Mazumdar 1992).

In 1904 a Royal Commission was set up to investigate the 'problem' of the feeble-minded. It concluded that those individuals suffering from feeble-mindedness and the associated conditions of insanity, epilepsy, alcoholism, criminality and pauperism were a threat to the stability of society (Tredgold 1909). The commission advocated state intervention based on negative eugenic policy and this was to take the form of 'institutionalisation'. This choice of intervention can be contrasted with the negative eugenic policies of other European countries at this time. Germany, for example, favoured the mass genocide of those individuals who did not have typical Aryan characteristics (Burleigh 1994) whilst the Nordic countries favoured the method of compulsory sterilisation (Tannsjo 1998). This latter option had been debated in the UK at the beginning of the 20th century, but was subsequently rejected as a method of control following its appearance in the Mental Deficiency Bill of 1912.

It is the case that at the time of the recommendations of the Royal Commission, there was an absence of definitive criteria on which to base the identification of those individuals who presented a threat to society and of a legal basis on which to detain them. The Mental Deficiency Act 1913 sought to address these inadequacies. It identified four categories of mental defect and these were to provide the necessary diagnostic criteria for certification. These four categories have been presented in Box 3.3.

However, the implementation of this Act was largely delayed by the occurrence of the First World War, with the operation of its recommendations mainly taking place following the war's conclusion. At this time, further support for institutional policy had been generated through the findings of the Wood Committee. The Wood Report (1929), although initially set up to re-examine the education of children with mental defects, had extended its area of responsibility to the problem of all mental defects. Its investigations culminated in the recommendation for the immediate institutionalisation of 100 000 individuals suffering from this condition. This report was followed by an acceleration in the rate of institutionalisation of people with learning disabilities. In 1926 there had been an estimated 37 000 defectives under the care and control of the Mental Deficiency Act and this had risen to 90 000 by 1939 (Tredgold 1952).

LIFE IN AN INSTITUTION

The first institutions or asylums had accommodated people with both learning disabilities and mental illness, and they were introduced in the early part of the 19th century. The overriding belief at this time was that people with learning disabilities could, with appropriate education and training, return to live in their own communities and have a contributory role to play. The teaching techniques of the 19th century psychologists Itard, Pinel and Sequin were particularly influential at this time. They were based on the belief that if given sufficient attention, idiots and imbeciles could be taught simple tasks that would be useful to them in particular parts of society (Race 1995). The most famous example of this was Itard's attempts to teach a 'wild boy' simple skills, a process documented in his book *The Wild Boy of Averyon* (Humphrey 1932). However, with the increasing fear that people with learning disabilities were among a number of social groups contributing to the degeneration of society, asylums in the first part of the 20th century became more custodial and less reforming in nature. The main emphasis became one of containment as can be seen from the following statement:

You weren't allowed out of the hospital. You had to write up and ask could you leave the grounds. You had to ask the medical or write to the doctor and ask them. You couldn't just go across the road and look at the shops, it wasn't allowed unless you wrote up and asked. I didn't go out because I got so used to not going out. You'd get lost if you're not used to it (Mabel Cooper in Atkinson et al 1997, p. 27).

The Wood Committee (Wood Report 1929) had advocated the formation of self-sufficient 'colonies' that would cater for all groups of mental defect, regardless of age or level of disability. The term 'colony' was eventually to be replaced with the term 'subnormality hospital' with the implementation of the NHS Act 1946, under which control of colonies was transferred from local councils to Regional Hospital Boards. To ensure complete containment, the colonies were designed so that people lived, worked and undertook leisure activities on the same site, thereby minimising the amount of contact they had with the local community. Males and females were also separated to reduce the risk of sexual relations. More often than not, a colony would have its own farm, school, workshops, clothing store, laundry, shop,

---

Box 3.3   The Mental Deficiency Act 1913

- **Idiots** – persons so deeply affected in mind from birth or from an early age as to be unable to guard themselves against common dangers.
- **Imbeciles** – persons who whilst not being as defective as 'idiots' were still incapable of managing their own affairs.
- **Feeble-minded persons** – persons who whilst not being as defective as imbeciles still required care, supervision and control for their own protection or for the protection of others.
- **Moral defectives** – persons who from an early age display some permanent mental defect coupled with vicious or criminal propensities on which punishment has had little or no effect.

hairdressers and entertainment hall, as can be seen from the picture and map of Harperbury Hospital displayed in Figures 3.3 and 3.4.

It would appear from the following statement that the provision of leisure activities was central to maintaining the status quo of a colony:

Lastly, but certainly not of the least importance, is the organisation of pleasures and amusements for the mentally defective, which should be regarded as one of the ordinary duties of every member of the staff. No institution will be successful in making patients happy and contented to remain unless great attention is paid to this side of colony life (Board of Control Annual Report in Potts & Fido 1991, p. 81).

The self-sufficiency base of these colonies was dependent on the use of inmates as the main workforce. The Wood Committee (Wood Report 1929) had envisaged that a mixture of abilities would be necessary for the maintenance of the colonies. High-grade inmates (people with mild and borderline learning disabilities) would be required for jobs demanding skilled labour, medium grade inmates for simple routine work and low grades for those jobs that involved fetching and carrying. One significant feature of work

related to the colony was that it was unpaid, inmates only receiving literally 'token' recognition:

In them days you didn't have money. If they give you any money it's green, it's like little green coins. You can't use it outside, you can't buy anything outside, you can only use it in their canteen. You could just go down and spend it in the canteen. It was only for sweets (Mabel Cooper in Atkinson et al 1997, p. 25).

Admission to a colony could be at the request of the family, or of a number of people in the form of a petition, and was sanctioned on the basis of the signatories of two doctors, one of whom was officially approved for the purpose. Diagnosis and subsequent certification was undertaken using a number of 'tests' that aimed to disprove or in the main prove the inability of an individual to live in society. These tests included being able to differentiate between a fly and a butterfly or a stone and an egg, state the similarities between an apple and an orange, suggest how many feathers there were on a chicken or how many miles it was to America (National Council for Civil Liberties 1951, Potts & Fido 1991). It would appear that little attempt was made to assess a person's capabilities by taking

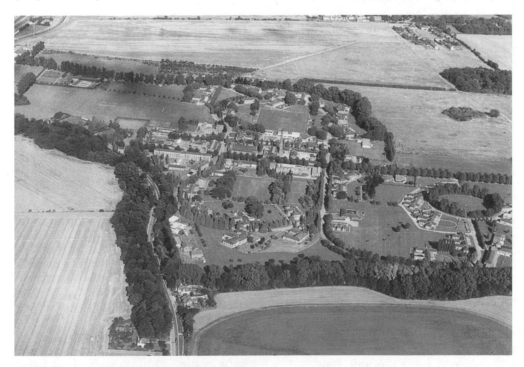

Figure 3.3   Aerial view of Harperbury Hospital (Brown 2001).

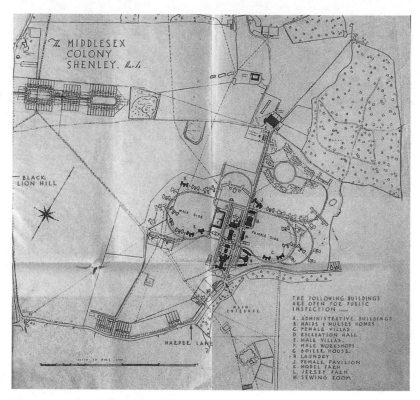

Figure 3.4 Map of Harperbury Hospital (Brown 2001).

account of their physical impairments, their social or educational history, level of disability, or even the distress that might have been incurred because of the tests themselves. It could be concluded from this that for many, institutionalisation was an inescapable outcome.

Following assessment, a person would be certified according to one of the four categories of the Mental Deficiency Act 1913. The certification order was to be renewed at 12 months, and then every 5 years, with any appeals being heard by the Board of Control for the institution. It is the case, however, that a person could not be admitted to a mental deficiency institution purely on the basis of being mentally deficient, although this inevitably ended up being the case, especially in instances where a family could no longer care for their dependent. One of the criteria was that they also had to be found to have additional degenerative characteristics such as inebriety, criminality, ineducability, or perceived promiscuity as can be seen from the following statement:

Mary did not understand the reason for this separation and what made it all the more distressing was that she was sent away, separated from her sister and family, while her sister remained part of the family. Mary realised that her family had not been pleased with her meeting a young man by the fire station some evenings, but could not see why her family had sent her away and not her sister, who had also been meeting a young man (Gray & Ridden 1999, p. 30).

For a number of people, reasons for their institutionalisation were unknown, whether because they were too young to understand or because they were never actually told:

I were at home with me mother and sister and brother. I must have been fifteen or summ'at like that when [I came in]. I left social services when I were fourteen years old . . . to work in t'mill. I did spinning and weaving. I only got ten shillings a week but to me it were worth it. I've no idea at [why I came to The Park]. I can never find out. Anyway, I am not bothered. I could be, as they say, I were the black sheep 'o' family. They've all died now that's why I get to know nothing (Grace in Potts & Fido 1991, p. 18).

For some, institutionalised life enabled the formation of lasting friendships both between inmates and between inmates and the members of staff who cared for them (Deacon 1974). However, for many the experience was tainted by negative memories. Institutionalised care carried with it a number of distinct characteristics. These have been effectively summarised through the work of Goffman (1961) as block treatment, rigidity of the system, depersonalisation and social distance between staff and residents:

They took mine away from me, the clothes I used to have. Put 'em away somewhere. I didn't see 'em again. I had to wear theirs. Old clothes! We had what they gave you. What they got from the sewing room. What wi' colony on; all marked, 'The Park Colony', inside 'collar. They were patched. On 'trousers at front and at 'back. Girls used to do that in'sewing room. Underclothes – they were marked 'n all (Frank in Potts & Fido 1991, p. 38).

Punishment was a common feature that ensured conformity to the system. Barron (1996) remembers that these punishments included:

- not being able to speak to the other patients on the ward
- removal of whatever possessions you had
- smoking, sweets, periodicals and other things that were normally allowed to patients were denied
- cutting meals by half
- scrubbing concrete with a brick and half a bucket of cold water.

It is undoubtedly the case that institutionalisation had profound effects on the lives of some people with learning disabilities, and their families. Some of these effects remain with them today and influence their ability to live in the community and form ordinary friendships and relationships, as can be seen from this final statement:

I've still got my memories and the pain. I sometimes find it hard being alone after so many years of being with others, never having to think for yourself, doing what you were told. I've got to watch that I don't slip back into institutional ways. They are hard habits to get out of and I still cling to some routines. We were compelled by institutional laws to turn our beds down. Every bed was turned down completely and the superintendent, or attendant in charge of the ward, went down with a line and everything had to be straight. To this day, in my little flat, I still turn my bed down, ready for inspection! (Barron 1996, p. 122).

Reader Activity 3.2

Try to imagine the main features of life for someone with learning disabilities living in an institution. Write down your ideas and then compare them with the main features of the lives of people with learning disabilities currently living in the community. Consider how, if at all, things have changed.

The closing sections of this chapter examine the pathway from institutional to community care.

THE INTRODUCTION OF THE CONCEPT OF COMMUNITY CARE AND THE PRINCIPLES OF NORMALISATION

Whitehead (1992) has suggested that the emergence of the concept of community care in Western countries can not be attributed to one single factor but is the result of a distillation of significant ideas, attitudes and social movements in the post-war years. First, there was an increased recognition of the inequalities faced by disabled people. Their profile within society had become more pronounced due to the effects of war and the polio epidemics of the 1950s. This in turn led to the formation of a number of human and civil rights movements and this subsequently led to the introduction of a number of policies including the European Convention on Human Rights (1950), although at this time there was no legislative backing. Secondly, changes also occurred within the content of sociological theories relating to the existence of devalued groups, and this included the effects of labelling (Goffman 1961). Goffman introduced the concept of the 'deviancy cycle', which suggested that devalued people often behaved in accordance with the 'deviant' label assigned to them by society. This behaviour, in turn, served to strengthen society's existing stereotypical beliefs about the group, the consequence being that behaviour exhibited towards such people reinforced their individual notions of being deviant. Also at this time there was a shift away from the 'problem' being one of a person's disability, to being the result of the person's physical environment. Race (1995) has drawn attention to a number of sociological studies undertaken during the 1950s that demonstrated that large numbers of individuals living in institutions at that time had the intellectual and social capabilities to sustain themselves in the community, and that institutional life did little to support personal development. These studies included the work of Tizard & O'Connor (1952) who discovered that some groups of people with learning disabilities, originally labelled as unemployable, did in fact have some of the necessary skills to sustain a job. In addition to this, the work of Clarke & Clarke (1959) confirmed the relationship between stimulating environments and a person's performance ability. This latter finding was consolidated by a number of reports issued in the 1960s that examined the conditions of a number of the long stay institutions in the UK. The most infamous of these was the *Report of the Committee of Enquiry into Ely Hospital* (Howe Report 1969). This identified impoverished and squalid living conditions, lack of privacy for patients, an emphasis on predominantly physical care, and custodial attitudes among staff. These reports were fuelled by a number of social activist groups that deplored the standards of the institutions and their blatant disregard of the human rights of both residents and their families (National Council for Civil Liberties 1951).

The changing social influences described above were to be consequently reflected in a modified political agenda. In 1957 the recommendations of the Royal Commission on the Law relating to Mental Illness and Mental Deficiency (Royal Commission 1957) were to pave the way for a new Mental Health Act in 1959. First, this act was to end compulsory certification, and hence provide the means by which those individuals with learning disabilities who were detained in hospitals for no legitimate reason could be discharged back into the community. Secondly, it replaced the term 'mental deficiency' with the term 'mental subnormality'. In 1971 the White Paper *Better Services for the Mentally Handicapped* was introduced (DHSS 1971). This advocated a 50% reduction in hospital places by 1991 and an increase in the provision of local authority-based residential and day care. It

also called for an end to custodial methods of care in hospitals and recommended the re-training of hospital staff. This paper represented one of the first pieces of social policy since the Mental Deficiency Act of 1913 that dealt specifically with the care of people with learning disabilities. It has been suggested, however, that its potential influence was thwarted by the absence of firm guidelines that would direct the future transfer of patients from hospitals to community settings and the absence of any legislative backing (Race 1995). In 1975 the Jay Committee was set up to further investigate service provision for people with learning disabilities. In its report (Jay Committee 1979) it re-emphasised the need for local authority-led care, and as importantly, a service philosophy based on the principles of normalisation.

The concept of normalisation, first introduced in Denmark in 1959 as part of the Mental Retardation Act, was initially used to define the creation of 'an existence for the mentally retarded as close to normal living conditions as possible' (Bank-Mikkelson 1980). This initial definition, however, tended to focus on securing normal housing, education and work and leisure conditions for people with learning disabilities. It was later adapted in Sweden to encapsulate patterns and conditions of living that equated to those of ordinary citizens and was redefined as 'making available to all mentally retarded people patterns of life and conditions of everyday living which are as close as possible to the regular circumstances and ways of society' (Nirje 1980). These included the rhythm of the day, the week, the month or year, the development of heterosexual relationships, economic and environmental standards and self-determination. It is the case that these initial definitions of normalisation have been criticised on the grounds that, although promoting equal rights for people with learning disabilities, they did not support the notion of integration (Emerson 1992). Their aims and objectives could be achieved without people with learning disabilities having to participate in any meaningful way within mainstream society. These limitations were recognised by Wolfensberger (1972), and normalisation was hence redefined as the 'utilisation of means which are as culturally normative as possible, in order to establish and/or maintain personal behaviours and characteristics which are as culturally normative as possible' (Wolfensberger 1972). However, the definition was to undergo a further modification in an attempt to emphasise the need for people with learning disabilities to fulfil socially valued roles, which Wolfensberger deemed to be the highest goal that could be achieved through normalisation. The term 'normalisation' was hence replaced by the term 'social role valorisation' and that referred to the creation, support and defence of valued social roles for people at risk of devaluation (Wolfensberger 1998).

The concept of normalisation or social role valorisation was underpinned by seven main service principles that are presented in Box 3.4.

In the UK, the principles of normalisation were adapted by O'Brien & Tyne (1981). In a bid to operationalise the concept, they identified five service accomplishments. These accomplishments provided services with a definitive framework on which to base care for people with learning disabilities and are presented in Box 3.5. These became the developmental goals which organisations then and organisations now strive towards.

Since the introduction of O'Brien and Tyne's five service accomplishments into the UK, there has been a steady stream of policy and legislative documents that have influenced service provision for people with learning disabilities. In 1989 the White Paper *Caring for people* (DOH 1989) confirmed the government's commitment to the development of locally based health and care services. Following on from this, the government introduced *The NHS and Community Care Act 1990*. The main aim of this act was to provide the necessary support structures to enable people to remain in their own homes where possible, thereby reducing the demand for long term care. These structures included an increase in the range of domicilliary, respite and day services including the promotion of independent care options and a greater emphasis on supporting informal carers. Central to these developments was the provision of a service that would be tailored to the needs of individuals and the introduction of community care assessments that would be undertaken by social services with the assistance of health care professionals.

Since the NHS and Community Care Act 1990 a continual improvement of services for people

---

Box 3.4   The seven underlying service principles of normalisation (Wolfensberger & Thomas 1983)

The role of the (un)consciousness in human services

- Role expectancy and role circularity to deviancy making and deviancy unmaking
- The conservatism corollary
- The developmental model and the importance of personal competency enhancement
- The power of imitation
- The dynamics of social imagery
- The importance of social integration and valued participation especially for those at risk of social devaluation.

Box 3.5   O'Brien & Tyne's five service accomplishments (1981) cited by Emerson (1992)

- **Community presence** – ensuring that service users are present in the community by supporting their actual presence in the same neighbourhoods, schools, workplaces, shops, recreation facilities and churches as ordinary citizens.
- **Choice** – ensuring that service users are supported in making choices about their lives by encouraging people to understand their situation, the options they face and helping them to act in their own interest both in small everyday matters and in such important issues as who to live with and what type of work to do.
- **Competence** – developing the competence of service users by developing skills and attributes that are functional and meaningful in natural community environments and relationships, i.e. skills and attributes which

significantly decrease a person's dependency or develop personal characteristics that other people value.
- **Respect** – enhancing the respect afforded to service users by developing and maintaining a positive reputation for people who use the service by ensuring that the choice of activities, locations, forms of dress and use of language promote perception of people with disabilities as developing citizens.
- **Community participation** – ensuring that service users participate in the life of the community by supporting people's natural relationships with their families, neighbours and co-workers and, when necessary, widening each individual's network of personal relationships to include an increasing number of people.

with learning disabilities has been sought through further policy and legislation, that has emphasised their social inclusion and attempted protection of their rights. *Moving into the Mainstream* (DOH 1998b) examined the range and quality of services provided to people with learning disabilities whilst *Signposts for success* (DOH 1998a) and *Once a day* (DOH 1999) set standards for the delivery of and access to health care for this group of people. Other policies and legislation have been more generic in nature, yet are still very applicable to people with learning disabilities. These include the Disability Discrimination Act 1995, the aim of which was to protect the rights of all individuals with disabilities with regard to their attainment of goods and services, buying and renting of land or property and employment. Another example is the Human Rights Act 1998, which aims to protect disabled and non-disabled groups alike by ensuring their rights to, among other things, freedom of expression, liberty and security, respect for private life, marriage, education, prohibition of discrimination and torture, and life itself.

 Reader activity 3.3

1. Draw a timeline that depicts the key milestones in the history of learning disabilities.
2. Consider ways in which the information on this timeline could be made accessible to someone with learning disabilities.

LEARNING DISABILITIES IN THE UK TODAY

It is undoubtedly the case that services for people with learning disabilities are significantly different from the model of institutionalised care that was a feature of most of the last century. The recent government White Paper *Valuing People* (DOH 2001) reports that most of the long stay hospitals have now closed, and that the residents of those that remain open will be transferred into community settings by 2004, yet the extent to which the individual needs of people with learning disabili-

ties are being met in a climate of true acceptance and inclusion is debatable. Although it could be argued that there has been a significant change in the actual physical make-up of services for this group, the rate of progress towards helping people with learning disabilities attain socially valued roles and valued lifestyles has been significantly slower. This is a view reiterated by Brown (1993) who suggests that the involvement of people with learning disabilities in community networks and the support required for them to make friends and maintain relationships, has proven to be more difficult to attain than the provision of ordinary housing, homely furniture and appliances. Haring (1991) refers to the former attainment as exemplifying social integration whilst the latter exemplifies functional integration. Evidence that suggests that current services for people with learning disabilities are based predominantly on the model of functional integration rather than social integration can also be found in the new White Paper *Valuing People* (DOH 2001). This concludes that people with learning disabilities still have little choice and control over their lives. Services tend to remain as large and predominantly segregated institutions offering little variety and, as such, generally do not meet the individual needs of clients. Access to inclusive services, including ordinary community activities, remains problematic with less than 10% of people with learning disabilities in some form of employment. Barriers to social inclusion are, at present, significantly more difficult to overcome for people with profound and complex needs and those from ethnic minority groups. The paper also reports that social relations formed by this group tend to be predominantly with paid carers, close family members or other people with learning disabilities as opposed to ordinary members of the local community. It would appear, therefore, that services are still predominantly based on a model of functional integration rather than one of social integration and this could be related to a number of different factors.

One issue of significant debate is the extent to which societal attitudes towards people with learning disabilities have improved alongside the change in service provision. First, evidence would suggest that people with learning disabilities are still amongst the least accepted 'disabled' groups in society, along with people with cerebral palsy, psychiatric illness and AIDS (Westbrook et al 1993). In addition to this, it has been found that societal attitudes towards community care for people with learning disabilities remains ambivalent (Myers et al 1998). More surprising, however, is research that indicates the prevalence of negative attitudes towards people with learning disabilities within the health care professions (Fitzsimmons & Barr 1997, French 1994).

Secondly, recent research draws into question whether or not society has relinquished eugenic attitudes of the past in favour of more accepting attitudes (Antonak et al 1995). Indeed, it has been suggested that eugenic attitudes continue to exist in contemporary society but in socially acceptable guises (Kobsell 1993). Furthermore, a number of parallels have been drawn between contemporary investigative techniques and eugenics. Indeed prenatal testing (Hubbard 1986), gene therapy (Harris 1993), IVF (Steinberg 1997) and prenatal selection techniques such as PID (preimplantation diagnosis) (Testart 1995) have all had their true objectives brought into question.

Reader activity 3.4

Identify the range of barriers to social inclusion that currently exist for people with learning disabilities, and consider the ways in which these barriers are currently being broken down at a local and national level.

THE FUTURE OF SERVICES FOR PEOPLE WITH LEARNING DISABILITIES

In order to attain a view of the future configuration of services for people with learning disabilities, it seems timely to refer to the directives of the recent White Paper *Valuing People* (DOH 2001). In this Paper, the government envisages a service based on four main underlying principles: rights, independence, choice and inclusion. Central to

this is the introduction of 'person-centred planning', an approach designed to ensure that the individual wishes and preferences of people with learning disabilities and their families are central to the decision-making process. Other areas of future work include the development of day-time opportunities, increasing the range of housing and employment opportunities, improving access to mainstream health care services, the development of advocacy services and improving the systems of support currently available to carers of people with learning disabilities. These will be achieved through:

- provision of a Learning Disability Development Fund of £50 million per annum from 2002
- joint working at the planning and implementation stages of service delivery with public, private and voluntary sector organisations
- meaningful involvement of people with learning disabilities in the design of services, including the development of a national forum for this group
- development of a national learning information centre and helpline for carers
- appointment of health facilitators to support people with learning disabilities in accessing mainstream health care provision.

It would be unrealistic at the time of writing this chapter to comment with any degree of certainty on the precise impact of this White Paper on the future of learning disability services. What can be said, however, is that its introduction appears to have been met with both enthusiasm and optimism amongst those who really count, that is people with learning disabilities themselves:

At last the Government is putting individual choice at the heart of learning disability services. We want to make our own decisions. We want the opportunities and all the basic services so that we can live the life that non-disabled people take for granted. Now is the time for the talking to stop and the changes to begin (Cramp 2001).

It is hoped that future revisions of this chapter will be able to comment on the fulfilment of these aspirations as a reality.

CONCLUSION

This chapter has provided an overview of the history of people with learning disabilities from Ancient Greek times through to the present day. Central to this overview has been an exploration of the changing attitudes and beliefs held by respective societies toward this group. These attitudes and beliefs have inevitably provided the foundations for varying social policy and law that has subsequently influenced the type and quality of services provided to people with learning dis-

abilities. It is suggested that the pace of change for people with learning disabilities has been most significant over the past 100 years, with an institutional model of care, which dominated most of the 20th century, being superseded by community care towards the end of the century. Although it is undeniably the case that services for people with learning disabilities continue to diversify, there is evidence to suggest that societies still have a long way to go if people with learning disabilities are to be accepted as fully included members.

REFERENCES

Alaszweski A 1988 From villains to victims. In: Leighton A (ed) Mental handicap in the community. Woodhead-Faulkner, Cambridge

Antonak R F, Mulick J A, Kobe F H, Fiedler C R 1995 Influence of mental retardation severity and respondent characteristics on self-reported attitudes toward mental retardation and eugenics. Journal of Intellectual Disability Research 39(4): 316–325

Atkinson D, Williams F (eds) 1990 Know me as I am. Hodder and Stoughton, London

Atkinson D, Jackson M, Walmsley J 1997 Forgotten Lives. BILD, Kidderminster

Atkinson D 1997 Auto/Biographical approach to learning disability research. Ashgate, UK

Bank-Mikkelson N 1980 Denmark. In: Flynn R J, Nitsch K E (eds) Normalization, social integration and community services. University Park Press, Baltimore

Barron D 1996 A price to be born. Mencap Northern Division, Harrogate

Blacker C P 1945 Eugenics in retrospect and prospect. The Galton Lecture. Eugenics Society, London

Borthwick C 1996 Racism, IQ and Down's syndrome. Disability and Society 11(3): 403–410

Bowler P J 1990 The role of the history of science in the understanding of social Darwinism and eugenics. Impact of science on society 40(3): 273–278

Bragg L 1997 From the Mute God to the Lesser God: disability in Medieval Celtic and Old Norse literature. Disability and Society 12(2): 165–177

Brown H 1993 What price theory if you cannot afford the bus fare: normalisation and leisure services for people with learning disabilities. Health and Social Care 2: 153–159

Brown K 2001 Harperbury Hospital, from Colony to closure, 1928–2001. Harper House Publications, London

Burleigh M 1994 Death and deliverance: euthanasia in Germany 1900–1945. Cambridge, Cambridge

Clarke A D B, Clarke M 1959 Recovery from the effects of deprivation. Acta Psychologica 16: 137–144

Cramp S 2001 Valuing people. The Link 11 (April) Mencap, London

Davidson I, Woodill G, Bredberg E 1994 Images of disability in 19th century British children's literature. Disability and Society 9(1): 33–46

Deacon J 1974 Tongue tied. National Society for Mentally Handicapped Children, UK

DHSS 1971 Better services for the mentally handicapped. Cmn 4683, HMSO, London

Dickens C 2000 Nicholas Nickleby. Introduction and notes by Cook T Wordsworth, Hertfordshire

DOH 1989 Caring for people: community care in the next decade and beyond. Cm 849, HMSO, London

DOH 1998a Signposts for success in commissioning and providing health services for people with learning disabilities. NHS Executive, London

DOH 1998b Moving into the mainstream: the report of a national inspection of services for adults with learning disabilities. Social Services Inspectorate, London

DOH 1999 Once a day. NHS Executive, London

DOH 2001 Valuing people: a new strategy for learning disability for the 21st century. Cm 5086, HMSO, London

Disability Discrimination Act 1995 HMSO, London

Eberly S S 1988 Fairies and the folklore of disability: changelings, hybrids and the solitary fairy. Folklore 99(1): 58–77

Elizabethan Poor Law Act 1601 HMSO, London

Emerson E 1992 What is normalisation? In: Brown H, Smith H (eds) Normalisation – a reader for the nineties. Routledge, London

Fitzsimmons J, Barr O 1997 A review of the reported attitudes of health and social care professionals towards people with learning disabilities: implications for education and further research. Journal of Learning Disabilities For Nursing, Health and Social Care 1(2): 57–64

French S 1994 Attitudes of health professionals towards disabled people: a discussion and review of the literature. Physiotherapy 80(10): 687–693

Galton F 1883 Inquiries into human faculty and its development. Macmillan, London

Gelb 1995 The beast in man: degeneration and mental retardation, 1900–1920. Mental Retardation 33(1): 1–9

Goddard H H 1931 The Kallikak family. Macmillan, New York

Godwin-Jones B 1999 The Changeling. In: The Elves. Available at http://www.vcu.edu/hasweb/for/grimm/wichtel_e_crane.html Retrieved 30/5/01

Goffman E 1961 Asylums: essays on the social situation of mental patients and other inmates. Penguin, Harmondsworth

Gray B, Ridden G 1999 Lifemaps of people with learning disabilities. Jessica Kingsley, London

Haffter C 1968 The changeling: history and psychodynamics of attitudes to handicapped children in European folklore. Journal of the History of the Behavioral Sciences 4: 55–61

Haring T G 1991 Social relationships. In: Meyer L H, Peck C A, Brown L (eds) Critical issues in the life of people with severe disabilities. Brookes, Baltimore

Harris J 1993 Is gene therapy a form of eugenics? Bioethics 7 (2–3): 178–187

Howe Report 1969 Report of the Committee of Enquiry into Allegations of Ill Treatment of Patients and other Irregularities at the Ely Hospital, Cardiff. Cmnd 3975, HMSO, London

Hubbard R 1986 Eugenics and prenatal testing. International Journal of Health Services, 16(2): 227–242a

Hussain F 1997 Life story work for people with learning disabilities. British Journal of Learning Disabilities 25: 73–76

Human Rights Act 1998 HMSO; London

Humphrey G M 1932 (transl) Itard. The Wild Boy of Averyon. New York Press, New York

Jay Committee 1979 Report of the Committee of Enquiry into Mental Handicap Nursing and Care. Cmnd 7468, HMSO, London

Kirman B 1975 Historical and legal aspects. In: Kirman B, Bicknell J (eds) Mental Handicap. Churchill Livingstone, UK

Kobsell S 1993 Testing, testing: the new eugenics. Disability, Pregnancy and Parenthood International 4: 11–13

Lee D (ed) 1987 Plato: The Republic, 2nd edn. Penguin, London

Lewis R 1997 Living in hospital and in the community. Pavilion, Brighton

McDonagh P 2000 Diminished men and dangerous women: representations of gender and learning disability in early- and mid-nineteenth-century Britain. British Journal of Learning Disabilities 28: 49–53

Malthus T R 1798 An essay on the principle of population. (Edited by Flew A 1970) Penguin, Harmondsworth

Mazumdar P 1992 Eugenics, human genetics and human failings: the Eugenics Society, its sources and its critics in Britain. Routledge, London

Miles M 1996 Pakistan's microcephalic "chuas" of Shah Daulah: cursed, clamped or cherished? History of Psychiatry 7(4): 571–590

Mental Deficiency Act 1912 HMSO, London

Mental Deficiency Act 1913 HMSO, London

Mental Health Act 1959 HMSO, London

Myers F, Ager A, Kerr P, Myles S 1998 Outside looking in? Studies of the community integration of people with learning disabilities. Disability and Society 13(3): 389–413

National Council for Civil Liberties 1951 50 000 outside the law: an examination of the treatment of those certified as mentally defective. National Council for Civil Liberties, London

National Health Service and Community Care Act 1990 HMSO, London

Neugebauer R 1996 Mental handicap in medieval and early modern England. In: Wright D, Digby A (eds) from idiocy to mental deficiency. Routledge, London

Nirje B 1980 The normalisation principle. In: Flynn R J, Nitsch K E (eds) Normalisation, social integration and community services. University Park Press, Baltimore

O'Brien J, Tyne A 1981 The principle of normalisation: a foundation for effective services. CMH, London

Poor Law Amendment Act 1834 HMSO, London

Potts M, Fido R 1991 A fit person to be removed. Northcote House, UK

Race D 1995 Historical development of service provision. In: Malin N (ed) Services for people with learning disabilities. Routledge, London

Radford J P 1991 Sterilization versus segregation: control of the feebleminded, 1900–1938. Social Science and Medicine 33(4): 449–458

Reid J C 1967 Dickens – Little Dorrit. Edward Arnold, London

Roper A G 1913 Ancient eugenics. Online. BH Blackwell, London Available from http://www.melvig.org/files/eugenics.html 27/10/97

Royal Commission 1957 Report of the Royal Commission on the Law Relating to Mental Illness and Mental Deficiency, 1954–57. Cmnd 169, HMSO, London

Ryan J, Thomas F 1987 The politics of mental handicap (revised ed). Free Association Books, London

Steinbeck J 1937 Of mice and men. Heinemann, London

Steinberg D L 1997 A most selective practice: the eugenics logics of IVF. Women's studies international forum 20(1): 33–48

Stratford B 1996 In the beginning. In: Stratford B, Gunn P (eds) Approaches to Down syndrome. Cassell, London

Tannsjo T 1998 Compulsory sterilisation in Sweden. Bioethics 12(3): 236–249

Testart J 1995 The new eugenics and medicalized reproduction. Cambridge Quarterly of Healthcare Ethics 4: 304–312

Tizard J, O'connor N 1952 The occupational adaption of high-grade detectives. Lancet 2: 620–623

Tredgold A F 1909 The feebleminded – a social danger. Eugenics Review 1: 97–104

Tredgold A F 1952 A textbook on mental deficiency. Baillière, Tindall and Cox, London

Westbrook M T, Legge V, Pennay M 1993 Attitudes towards disabilities in a multicultural society. Social Science and Medicine 36(5) 615–623

Whitehead S 1992 The social origins of normalisation. In: Brown H, Smith H (eds) Normalisation: a reader for the nineties. Routledge, London

Wolfensberger W 1972 The principle of normalisation in human management services. National Institute of Mental Retardation, Toronto

Wolfensberger W 1998 A brief introduction to social role valorisation: a high order concept for addressing the plight of societally devalued people, and for structuring human services, (3rd edn). Training Institute for Human Service Planning, Leadership & Change Agentry (Syracuse University), Syracuse, New York

Wolfensberger W, Thomas S 1983 PASSING: Program Analysis of Service Systems. Field Manual. National Institute on Mental Retardation, Toronto

Wood Report 1929 Report of the Mental Deficiency Committee, HMSO, London

Wright D, Digby A 1996 From idiocy to mental deficiency. Routledge, London

FURTHER READING

Bogdan R, Taylor S J 1994 The social meaning of mental retardation. Teachers College Press, New York

Brigham L, Atkinson D, Jackson M, Rolph S, Walmsley J 2000 Crossing boundaries. BILD, Kidderminster

Slater D, De Wit M 1999 Rediscovering our selves. Pavilion Publishing, Brighton *This is a useful teaching aid*.

Stuart M 1997 Looking back, looking forward – reminiscence with people with learning difficulties. Pavilion Publishing, Brighton *This is a useful teaching aid*.

Thompson M 1998 The problem of mental deficiency: eugenics, democracy and social policy in Britain c. 1870–1959. Clarendon Press, Oxford

Ward L 2001 Considered choices: the new genetics, prenatal testing and people with learning disabilities. BILD, Kidderminster

USEFUL ADDRESSES

Acts of the UK Parliament
http://www.hmso.gov.uk/acts.htm

An American history of mental retardation
http://members.aol.com/MRandDD/introhx-htm

Department of Health
http://www.doh.gov.uk

History of disabilities and social problems
http://barrier-free.arch.gatech.edu/

Image archive on the American Eugenics Movement
http://vector.cshl.org/eugenics/

Resources on the history of idiocy
http://www.personal.dundee.ac.uk/~mksimpso/

Perfect People? 2001 *This is a video made by people with learning disabilities that documents the past and future lives of people with learning disabilities.*
Available from Mencap National Centre (Gateway Division) 123 Golden Lane, London EC1Y 0R
Tel: 020 7696 5589

2

Services and support for people with learning disabilities

Chapter 4, by Jill Manthorpe, explores the nature of accessing services. Chapter 5, by Bob Gates, considers a range of residential alternatives. In Chapter 6, David Marsland presents a helpful overview of a range of issues around evaluating and monitoring services for people with learning disabilities. Next David and Linda Dickinson explain recent developments in the field of compulsory schooling. A chapter follows from Angie Walker exploring the role of further education in the lives of people with learning disabilities. Finally in this section, Tom Bush writes about the world of work and leisure as it relates to people with learning disabilities.

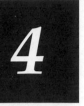

4

Accessing services and support

Jill Manthorpe

KEY ISSUES

- There are many barriers to services and support for people with learning disabilities and for disabled people generally.
- Some of these barriers are connected to the nature of services and attitudes of professionals and service providers whereas others relate to wider social and economic structures.
- There is also a range of other issues that impact on accessing services and these include: ethnicity, cost, geographical location and growing older.
- Accessing services should bring about inclusion and this may be understood within the context of the Government's modernising agenda.

INTRODUCTION

The chapter is divided into four main sections. The first outlines access problems in respect of their complexity and examines ways in which individuals can surmount such obstacles and how policy developments are seeking to revise service provision into more coherent and rational structures.

The second part of this chapter explores three themes arising from access issues:

- rationing and resources
- control and coercion
- facing up to discrimination.

A section that looks at particular experiences or difficulties in securing services or support follows this. This section commences with discussion on ethnicity, and moves to explore problems with paying for support. Also explored is the influence of geography, and finally consideration of life-course perspectives by examining relevant debates around growing up with learning disability and also getting old.

The final part of this chapter comprises an analysis of social inclusion in the context of the Government's modernising agenda. Foremost in such discussions are issues of employment but people with disabilities have also argued that these should be joined by debates about roles and relationships, social support and access to power.

Many of these debates relate to other chapters in this book but the main aim of this chapter is to portray access as a dynamic process that involves making use of services but also going beyond service arenas to build up other networks of support.

ACCESS PROBLEMS: THE SERVICE MAZE

One unifying element across the decades has been criticism by people with learning disabilities and their families that services are complex and difficult to access. A study of the Carers Act 1995, for example, reported that: ' . . . the dominant impression that parents and carers had was that access to services was a matter of chance . . . one parent commented: "I am very pleased, it's like winning the lottery, if you know what I mean." ' (Williams & Robinson 2000, p. 52.)

This complexity can arise from variation in local organisational patterns and their areas of responsibility. It can also be attributed to different structures that mean that services vary from one area to another in terms of where professionals are located and even what they are termed. In one area, for example, there may exist community learning disability teams while in others not, and their composition may also vary. In other areas, social services may use the term social workers or care managers. In almost every area, regular service reorganisation can change the landscape of care and organisations. Frequent staff turnover may result in continual requests for information and voluntary

sector groups may vary in their local priorities and activities. Parents, in particular, place high value on relevant and accessible information with Mitchell & Sloper (2000) proposing a three-dimension approach:

- in depth and informative guides
- shorter information material covering broad areas
- local key workers or facilitators.

Such information requires effort from professionals and organisations – particularly in keeping it up to date and monitoring its relevance.

This complex organisational world leads to frustration and disappointment among those who require support. Families, especially, have voiced numerous criticisms of services that are unable to respond to their individual needs. Their demands have generally been for a coordinator to help them negotiate the systems of care and access appropriate support. The practicalities of such a role have been explored by Mukherjee et al (1999) who questioned why this seemingly uncontested plea failed for so long to become incorporated into mainstream services.

In response to this concerted series of calls for such assistance, the White Paper *Valuing People* (DOH 2001a) made a commitment to providing families with a named individual to act as the first point of contact by July 2002. As it noted: 'Children and their families want services that are not only efficient and effective, but also joined up and responsive' (para 3.1, p. 30). Such key workers are intended to help coordinate services. Further developments place the onus on parents to seek out relevant information themselves with the establishment of the Contact a Family National Information Centre (p. 34, para 3.12) and the National Learning Disability Information Centre (para 5.9) under the auspices of Mencap. To this will be joined Care Direct as announced in the *NHS Plan* (Secretary of State for Health 2000) which will site a help desk in each local authority area to assist people to negotiate access to services. Telephone help-lines on a national basis have the advantage of expertise and authority: they are, however, by necessity 'distant' and do depend on families being able to articulate their needs and to work on the advice given. While some families may find this approach reasonable and dignifying, others may be better served by a more personalised approach in which relationships of trust can be built up over time. Other areas of study refer to the former approach as a form of 'do it yourself' consumerism, in which patients and parents are placed under expectations that they will do the 'work' entailed to solve their own problems and manage their own affairs.

As well as the possibility of coordinators or key workers to assist families, new policy developments permit parents to act as their own care managers in some respects, with direct payments and a voucher scheme becoming available to parents under the Carers and Disabled Children Act 2000 (implemented in 2001). Under these schemes parents' and their children's needs will be assessed and a cash (or voucher) sum will be allocated to be used flexibly and as parents choose. A family might, for example, use the money to pay for short-term care of their choice and to suit their own timing (subject to safeguards about children's protection). Such flexibility exists to a small degree in respect of the Motability scheme where disabled individuals or parents may choose to 'trade' their cash mobility allowance for a vehicle.

Parents, of course, will argue that they have always been the coordinators of care services for disabled children. They have negotiated around services that apparently do not communicate with each other and have managed household budgets to cover costs and fund support. Mothers, in particular, have identified that the extent of this coordinating role has been such that any employment outside the home has been difficult to juggle with their caring roles and that services have relied on them to act as conduits of information, repositories of knowledge and skill and as fall-back providers of care outside the very restricted hours of services – many of which have a limited concept of the working week and a generous definition of holidays.

It is not only families who are conceived of as being coordinators of care, for new moves in direct payments also mean that people with learning disabilities may increasingly find the

Reader activity 4.1   Carers' assessment

Is there a local Carers' Centre in your area? If so, what support does it supply and can you visit (if you have not already done so)? How do carers get to hear of the Carers' Centre? Are they involved in its management and plans? You will no doubt find information about Carers' Assessments at such a centre. If there is not one in your area then you may find similar support available to carers and can identify whether information is written in plain English and is available in a variety of formats and languages.

Community Care (Direct Payments) Act 1996 provides them with the choices and control they desire. Direct payments had their initial encouragement from the disability movement and have generally been thought of as allowing disabled people choice and flexibility over personal care services. People with learning disabilities who satisfy conditions of being willing and able may also find that employing personal assistants, for example, enables them to lead more fulfilling lives with more choice over the delivery of care or over activity and occupation (Ryan & Holman 1998). While some individuals may not wish to take on the 'paperwork' side of such employment relationships, arrangements are possible for voluntary sector organisations to take over some of this administration, in a 'broker' arrangement. As yet, we have little evidence from such schemes operating for people with learning disabilities. Relevant lessons are emerging, however, from evaluative studies of early schemes (see Leece 2000), including the important point that while direct payments were firmly rooted in payments for social care support, disabled people themselves have found that they can effectively be used to pay for nursing or therapeutic services, such as physiotherapy (Glendinning et al 2000). Empowerment, or facilitating people's choices, sometimes means that they will make different uses of resources than professionals anticipate. *Valuing People* (DOH 2001a) included specific commitments to developing the support structures to enable people to access direct payments (paras 4.12 – 4.15, p. 48) and noted that 'Schemes must be accessible to people with learning disabilities, so that they too have the right support to manage a direct payment and remain in control' (para 4.14).

Access to health resources

Few people would argue that life in long-stay mental handicap hospitals provided patients with sufficient and effective access to health care. Nominally under the control of superintendent physicians, the hospital could provide 'treatment' in the form of containment and activity, and medication was used with varying purposes. Some of the inquiries into abuses of care in long-stay hospitals provide an instructive picture of 'health care' (see, for example, the report of the Committee of Inquiry into Normansfield Hospital 1978, where many concerns were raised about medication and medical practice).

Health services continue to discriminate against people with learning disabilities. *Valuing People* (DOH 2001a) draws on such evidence to instruct community learning disability teams to identify a named health facilitator for people with learning disabilities to develop health plans (para 6.12, p. 63). It provided four examples of particular areas of concern:

- limited take-up of health screening
- inadequate diagnosis and treatment
- over-dependence on medication
- lack of recognition of health complications

and noted 'the wider NHS has failed to consider the needs of people with learning disabilities' (para 6.3, p. 60). Health facilitators are to be encouraged to assist people with learning disabilities to 'navigate their way around the health service' but also to 'advocate and ensure' that they 'gain full access to health care' (para 6.13, p. 64). They will also be responsible for completion of personal Health Action Plans (HAPs) (para 6.15, p. 64) which are to form an element of the person-centred plan. HAPs are to be offered and reviewed at key stages or transitions, times which often represent a movement from one set of services to another (for example, moving from education or to retirement). Health facilitators are to be in place by 2003 and HAPs by 2005.

This model of improving access leaves the structures of services largely unchanged and unchallenged. It has the advantages, still to be tested, of giving clear, central direction and a range of 'deliverables' that can be monitored. It will ensure the survival of specialist professional roles among nurses in particular, which have generally been welcomed by parents of people with learning disabilities as providing a source of support and expertise (see Alaszewski et al 2001). However, such a model is conservative and may run the risk of turning health surveillance into a bureaucratic or paperwork exercise. Much will depend on how broadly health facilitators conceive their role and how willing they are to challenge decisions and argue that access to health care is a matter of rights rather than special pleading. Recent research (Keywood, Fovargue & Flynn 1999) also pointed to a number of instances when professionals looked to relatives to be informants about health and to make decisions. This too can have the effect of denying people with learning disabilities access to health care.

The two-pronged approach of *Valuing People* (DOH 2001a) may be greeted with some optimism. As described above, individual personalised help is promised, a range of semi-independent advice appears to be developing at national level and, at the level of services, well-worn difficulties around organisational, legal and financial barriers seem to be dissolving. Interestingly, the issue of the professional standing of those working with people with learning disabilities appears relatively untouched, with learning disability nurses taking on new roles in respect of access to health care but little discussion as yet of their possible roles as care coordinators, advocates or service providers.

Access to technology

The personal element of key working and health facilitation to improve access to information and support can also be extended by technology developments. Assistive technology has frequently been seen as having potential to improve the quality of life of people with physical disabilities but its significance for people with learning disabilities is no less. The distinction between the two groups, of course, is often erroneous since increasing numbers of people have multiple disabilities, some at profound levels.

Technology has potential to improve aspects of the physical environment to enable people to remain in 'ordinary' housing. It can enhance access and security. It can take over tasks which may be difficult or unpleasant. It can facilitate communication between services and enable people who have communication problems to develop skills. Access to certain forms of technology, such as computers or mobile telephones, can be seen as part of 'care' but can also be part of ordinary life – used to maintain contact, access information or entertainment. Taylor (1998) added to a list of educational and assessment functions the potential for technology to:

- create personalised resources
- demonstrate hidden potential
- enhance interaction
- facilitate self-directed activities
- provide valued social experiences.

But there are questions to be asked about the purposes of technology, particularly its potential to increase control and surveillance. As with many developments there may be good reasons to look at the ethics of providing the means to curtail independence, risk and autonomy. Closed circuit television, for example, may provide a sense of reassurance when installed near people's homes but it can infringe people's rights to privacy and dignity. Many of these balancing acts have been explored in other areas of care, such as services for people with dementia (see Marshall 2000) and it may be helpful to discuss these across traditional 'client group' divides. The matter of consent when mental incapacity is involved is similar and there are common balances between duty of care principles and the right to take risks and be autonomous.

Policy developments

Assistive technology, like many other services and support systems, frequently requires people with learning disabilities and their families to do the 'spadework', either on their own or with

Reader activity 4.2   Accessing technology

You will find various sources of advice on technology – including professionals such as occupational therapists (in health or social services), organisations (often joint health/social services) promoting aids or assistance to independent living, and advice available from Healthy Living Networks. How easy would it be for people with learning disabilities to find out information and to try out the products on offer? What might make this equipment more accessible?

advice and suggestions from others in similar positions. This sense of struggle around welfare services and other help is evident from a number of studies, for example, Lambe 1998 describes the work required of families as 'daunting' (p. 167) and considers that to refer to their massive responsibilities as 'informal' care is insulting (p. 168). Over the years, a number of policy developments have sought to improve this matter. The NHS and Community Care Act 1990, for example, building on the proposals developed in the White Paper *Caring for People* (Secretaries of State 1989), saw great merit in providing a care manager to coordinate disparate services. At the end of the century, the Health Act 1999 considered structural matters needed reform, particularly the legal and financial barriers that caused difficulties in joint services and pooled budgets. This Act permits more integrated provision, establishes a lead in commissioning services and allows local authority and NHS budgets to be combined. The ethos of competition, exacerbated by purchaser and provider splits in functions, is being replaced by judgements about Best Value looking at quality and effectiveness, not simply cost. Development of Primary Care Trusts and proposals for integrated Care Trusts (involving social services functions) are further mechanisms designed to reduce the artificial barriers around service provision across the health and social care divide.

For adults with learning disabilities, *Valuing People* (DOH 2001a) outlined the role of Learning Disability Partnership Boards operating under the auspices of Local Strategic Partnerships, to bring together the providers of services, public and independent, in a quest for effective coordination at local level. As the White Paper observed, this type of coordination is envisaged to go beyond traditional social or personal care and will extend to transport, education, employment and housing (para 9.14, p. 109).

At the time of writing these changes are at a planning stage and it will be important to evaluate their effectiveness, mindful of the earlier reforms which thought that they had solved these problems. New policy developments will need to be integrated into commitments to quality, as outlined, for example, in *Better Care: Higher Standards* (Department of Health/Department of the Environment, Transport and the Regions 2000). This charter has encouraged local services to develop joint standards about information, referral and time-scales, together with details of how to complain. It remains a useful measuring tool to assess the extent to which services, in whatever constellation they develop, satisfy people's demands for structures that are understandable, personnel who are helpful and organisations that behave responsibly.

EMERGENT THEMES
Rationing and resources

The 1990s witnessed two major developments in respect of rationing and resources (payment and charges will be discussed later in this chapter). These consisted of the run-down and closure of much NHS long-stay provision for people with learning disabilities. This 'closing of the gates' represented a denial of access to the health service for families who perceived its institutions would provide a secure home for life for their relatives with learning disabilities, although many were cognisant of the problems of such institutions (see Barton's account of family perspectives on such moves, Barton 1998). The second development was the move to target community care services to those with greatest need, as determined by an assessment of their needs under Section 47 of the NHS and Community Care Act 1990. Targeting was explicitly designed to focus support on those with high levels of need and while one result of

this was greater levels of home care enabling people to stay at home or live with their families, another consequence was the withdrawal of services from those assessed to have moderate needs. These experiences, which can be described in policy language as a process of downward substitution, replacing institutional care with home care and this by support from other services and the community in general, resulted in changes to levels of support available from adult day centres, for example, which had offered activity or occupation but not always choice or skill development (McIntosh & Whittaker 1998).

Some people with learning disabilities, therefore, found themselves denied access to old forms of provision, in what was said to be their own interests, and in the policy desire to provide more resources to those in greatest need. In return for this, access to more 'ordinary' forms of activity and occupation has been encouraged, although some evidence suggests that such community provision has been woefully inadequate. Drawing on a research project developing individualised day opportunities, for example, Cole, McIntosh & Whittaker (2000) argued that such a move does not simply just happen but needs to be highly responsive, needs to be planned and supportive and requires skills in partnership work.

Concern about the impact of this on people with minimal or moderate learning disabilities has been expressed by a group of voluntary sector organisations (forming the MLD Alliance in 1998) who have argued that exclusion from contact with services can lead to crises and difficulties in ordinary living (Simons 2000). A preventive, low level response, they propose, might serve to support people who are vulnerable to exploitation and who yet may not be readily identified as having a form of disability.

However, there is also evidence that many people with learning disabilities have experienced a better quality of life with their greater integration into community networks. The example of tenants of Keyring, a supported housing network evaluated by Simons (1998), demonstrated people's greater participation in activities of ordinary life, despite their accommodation generally being sited in relatively deprived urban areas.

Such networks help people make connections with each other and their neighbours and community groups. In doing so, people are supported to make the break from a reliance on specialist services – a process that seems more effective than sudden moves to 'independence'.

Housing is not simply a matter of supporting tenants in their own accommodation, although the shift to integrating housing support planned by the White Paper, *Supporting People* (DSS 1998), may help lift restrictions on financial support to those living outside the arena of housing association and sheltered housing schemes and give greater flexibility. It is a key to helping people look after themselves or to support members of their family. Many children with learning disabilities also have physical disabilities and poor, unsuitable housing can increase the difficulties faced by their parents as well as restricting the extent to which disabled children can play, learn and socialise in the family home. Questions of such access have been explored by Oldman & Beresford (1998) who identified not only factors that made a home unsuitable but also what families did in response to such difficulties. They argued that 'the housing needs of families with disabled children are much broader than traditional issues of access in and around the home experienced by those with physical disabilities' (Oldman & Beresford 1998, p. 70). Adequate space inside the home was particularly important to those with complex disabilities and/or behaviour problems. Harsh local environments, disrepair and poor heating also contributed to unsuitable homes. Children's responses noted the limitations on their independence in unsuitable housing, with access to the kitchen identified as especially important in achieving some independence and in learning skills.

This research identified different dimensions to 'access', for it argued that while additional resources would be cost-effective and are urgently needed by families, changes in professional attitudes are also required. Professionals should be more conscious of and responsive to housing issues. Policies and service delivery should focus on the child's needs and wishes as well as those of carers. Housing officers need more training and closer links with children's disability services. Increasingly, research also identifies ways in which families and people with disabilities manage and cope with disabling barriers. This housing research, for example, noted that parents paid for many adaptations themselves, where they could, rather than suffer immense delay.

Control and coercion

Access to services is not universally seen as positive for some supports are controlling and coercive. People with learning disabilities have been a group over whom the interest of the state historically has been less directed to their welfare and more to an attempt to manage perceived problems of 'crime, illegitimacy and other social evils' (Walmsley & Rolph 2001, p. 64). Currently, placement of a small number of people with learning disabilities in forensic services such as Special Hospitals, for example, has been heavily criticised as incarcerating those who need conditions of highest security but who challenge existing services. Some commentators have warned against the closure of such facilities, arguing that these often contain concentrations of resources and experienced, skilled and motivated staff (Dickens 1998, p. 135). There are thus two arguments that raise issues of access to service planners and policy makers. Are people with learning disabilities best treated or contained in specialist facilities because this is more likely to provide them with appropriate support? Or, should they be treated or contained in more local facilities, perhaps with less expertise but nearer their communities and in less stigmatising environments? These questions often underlie many service models and also the specialisms of staff. People with learning disabilities who are detained because of their severe risk of danger to themselves or others are often not included in discussions about learning disability or in mental health debates. Thompson (2000) has shown, however, that it is wrong to conceive of people with learning disabilities as only vulnerable and never dangerous. Using as an example men with learning disabilities who sexually abuse, he noted that in the past services concentrated on the risks of pregnancy, with concerns accumulating about sexually transmitted diseases, sexual abuse and sexual abusers as the years passed. In a more 'enlightened era', sexual contact and activity has been encouraged at some levels but frequently is controlled. Staff are now asked to interpret relationships as unacceptable or empowering. This is a difficult judgement at times, involving invasions of privacy and a tension between rights of protection and self-expression.

Thompson found that in practice, responses to men with learning disabilities who sexually abused swung between control and indecisiveness. Legal proceedings were rarely used, particularly as victims were often other people with learning disabilities who made no official complaint. However, if the law was (eventually) resorted to, men with learning disabilities could receive disproportionately more severe treatment than other offenders – such as removal to a forensic unit. Men who abused received mixed messages about their behaviour: nothing might occur, or at times their social opportunities would be curtailed, or they might be excluded from services, face retaliation or be given severe sexually suppressant medication. Their victims, often people with learning disabilities, took on board the implications that their abuse was 'normal and acceptable, and that services will provide little protection and that their complaints will not be heard' (Thompson 2000, p. 38). Their access to justice and protection was ill defined and, while the men might be treated leniently initially, they too had limited access to support to help resolve their problems with sexuality and relationships.

Many of these problems relate to mental health and the artificial boundaries between the two services of mental health and learning disabilities, often compounded by different professional groupings, service settings and service principles. It is often forgotten that:

People with learning disabilities are more likely to experience risk factors associated with the occurrence of mental health problems (e.g. adverse life events), while having reduced access to protective factors (e.g. social support). As a result, they may be at greater risk of developing mental health problems (Foundation for People with Learning Disabilities 2001, p. 38).

It is estimated that among people with learning disabilities, 25–40% will have mental health needs (ibid. p. 39). The problem of dual diagnosis for services is a matter of boundaries: for service users it can entail being switched from service to service or a denial of learning disability as a factor that should be recognised in service responses. People with learning disabilities who have problems with their alcohol consumption, for example, may find that alcohol agencies feel inadequate to respond to their needs and that problems are left to reach crisis point.

Issues of control feature heavily around the stories of people with learning disabilities who wish to have children. The work of Booth & Booth (1994) has provided extensive evidence that such parents and their children would benefit from access to a range of advice and preventative services and that 'Support tends to be most effective when it is consistent, non-intrusive and non-threatening' (Booth & Booth 1994, p. 147). They found that the problems faced by parents tended to be made worse by services, not just by those professionals with 'moralistic, governessy, meddlesome instincts' (Booth & Booth 1994, p. 149) but by others who might define themselves as more supportive: '. . . even professionals whose sympathies are with the parents can find themselves trapped by the system into taking actions that oppress them' (Booth & Booth 1994, p. 149).

Illustrating these difficulties, Booth & Booth presented a detailed case study that provided indications of possible reasons why an individual (Molly Austin) might not make use of services:

Molly has received little parenting support from the health and welfare services. Services delivery tends to be crisis-orientated: Molly has been left to cope as best she can until things go wrong. Her past experience has taught her to be wary of social workers who, in any case, tend to move on so frequently as to prevent the formation of trusting relationships. The community nurses have provided valuable practical and emotional support but often too little and too late (Booth & Booth 1994, p. 80).

Such accounts provide a view of access issues that needs to be listened to by practitioners and policy makers. Rather than blaming people for their failure to engage with services, it should be possible to identify the risks they perceive in seeking help and in admitting they have problems. When the likelihood of negative judgements is high, as in the case of parents who fear losing their children, it is easy to understand reluctance to seek support.

Facing up to discrimination

Access to justice has been a central part of debates about citizenship and human rights. This has been particularly driven by evidence of abuse of people with learning disabilities and has resulted in a series of recommendations and reforms around procedural justice. It has also stemmed from accounts of discrimination in many other areas of life. One of the first cases brought under the Disability Discrimination Act 1996, involved people with learning disabilities who had been asked to leave a pub restaurant. Engagement with discrimination issues has brought a new emphasis on rights in the context of work with people with learning disabilities who have often been portrayed as in need of help and protection. A rights-based perspective has also forged links with the disability movement, which, until recently, has generally been led by people with physical disabilities. Simone Apsis (Campbell & Oliver 1996, p. 97) has commented that the coming together of the British Council of Disabled People with People First has not been easy because of disabled people's fears of being seen as incapable.

Walmsley (1997) has argued a need to be cautious in seeing this as a solution to problems of exclusion. She proposed that there are still differences in the way people with learning disabilities perceive themselves and think about their situation and the way disabled people take up issues of identity and inclusion. It is not enough to point to involvement and self-advocacy because people with learning disabilities rely more on human intermediaries to participate in political life than many other disabled people. The self-advocacy and advocacy movements have had to work in a different context and at a time when decision-making is receiving new attention in respect of those who are said not to have mental capacity.

This umbrella term is increasingly encountered in respect of adults (typically people with dementia, severe learning disabilities and brain injury), and there is pressure to develop formal, court-based systems of substitute decision-making in respect of people in such groups.

It is generally professionals and family members who have been behind such pressures. As the campaigning group Values into Action has observed (Bewley 1997) substitute decision-making often becomes seen as a means of limiting people's choices and can be disempowering. An artificial distinction can be made between those with mental capacity and those without, rather than seeing this as a continuum. Substitute decision-making can take over, rather than support. Whatever new systems evolve in respect of mental capacity and decision-making, it will be important that they respond to the needs of people with problems with capacity rather than to the problems of those who provide support.

Only a minority of people with learning disabilities may be affected by reforms in this area (proposals for which are summarised by the Lord Chancellor's Department's documents *Who Decides?* (1997) and *Making Decisions* (1999)). Many more, however, are affected by access to systems of advocacy containing elements of:

- a personal relationship
- communication of the person's expressed wishes, not what is thought to be in their best interests
- speaking up on the person's behalf.

For many people with learning disabilities, however, it has not been possible to choose the support of an advocate, still less to choose between different forms of advocacy. *Valuing People* (DOH 2001a) stated a commitment to developing this service and access to advocacy will be a means of measuring the extent to which such commitment has been translated to actual groundwork. Likewise learning disability service users and their carers have much to teach other service users about models and advocacy and what it feels like to be in partnership with such a volunteer or member of staff.

FURTHER ISSUES AFFECTING ACCESS

Ethnicity and access

Valuing People (DOH 2001a) placed great emphasis on the needs of people from minority ethnic communities, with a specially commissioned report *Learning Difficulties and Ethnicity* drawing together a range of evidence and opinion. Its key findings relate to the needs of both people with learning disabilities and their families and included:

- delayed diagnosis and inadequate information for parents
- language barriers and negative stereotypes and attitudes
- high levels of stress among carers
- inadequate understanding by services of cultural and religious practices (para 1.18, p. 20).

This was set in the context of greater need; the prevalence of learning disability in some South Asian communities is greater by a factor of three than in the general population (para 1.18). While many families suffer social exclusion, ethnic minority families appear to experience these disproportionately (para 3.2). Thus proposed measures to alleviate poverty among families with disabled children, such as increases in benefits, should positively impact on minority families in particular (para 3.29).

Hatton et al (1998) have presented specific ideas, drawn from the experiences of South Asian carers, about practical measures to improve access to services and their quality. These included:

- help with interpretation and information in translation
- more staff from South Asian backgrounds
- greater cultural sensitivity
- stronger support networks (p. 832).

These recommendations encompass the area of communication and a proactive approach to this. Their evidence was that this group of carers was often under severe stress, and that their lack of familiarity with services placed them at a disadvantage. Second, the message that services should be culturally sensitive may help to improve service use and acceptability to both family carers and people with learning disabilities themselves. Third, this research argued that flexibility was necessary in order to enable communities to help themselves and to find support that was appropriate.

Experiences of racism and cultural insensitivity also impact on people from minority ethnic groups in contact with health and welfare services generally. The Parekh Report (Parekh 2000), for example, argued that 'access to health care is crucial to inclusion' (p. 183) but observed that ethnic monitoring of services was inconsistent and the data poorly analysed and acted on. It also noted the under-development of interpreting services generally, a point that is relevant for services trying to develop practical initiatives and training.

Ethnic minority issues are not only concerned with access problems arising from communication in spoken or written English. This would not explain the difficulties experienced by families where English is widely spoken. As Craig & Rai (1996) observed in relation to social security, there are structural problems as well as communication issues (p. 138). Specific problems around attitudes to claiming and stereotypical responses may be 'submerged' in studies focusing on language and cultural problems, ' . . . which sometimes inadvertently contribute to common perceptions of 'ignorant' ethnic minority communities' (p. 141).

Policies which seek to limit social security expenditure and to review disabled people's entitlements may seem at odds with those seeking to maximise take-up, particularly at local level. People with minimal disabilities, in particular, may find their classification as job seekers instead of disability claimants, welcome in some respects but not all. For those from minority ethnic communities, there may be continual need for explanation as systems and policies evolve, and for their views and circumstances to be taken into account when policies are evaluated.

 Reader activity 4.3

What information for parents in your area is available in different languages? Where would you go for an interpreter?

Paying for support

There is now much more evidence about the cost of disability, in financial terms, and who pays for care and support. Baldwin (1985) identified the heavy costs of caring incurred by families and this analysis has been furthered by studies of specific costs, at particular periods of the life-course, and differences between families, as well as similarities. So, while there is general agreement that large numbers of families fail to claim benefits to which they are entitled, such as Disability Living Allowance (Roberts & Lawton 1999), there is evidence that single parent families and families from ethnic minorities experience particular hardship. Single mothers, for example, may have no wage coming into the household and expenditure on transport and equipment may be especially difficult for them (Cigno & Burke 1997). Many may find it difficult to find employment that permits them to take time off for appointments and, if they are earning low wages, it may not be in their financial interests to move from benefits to earnings and to commitments to work-related expenditure on child care, travel and meals. This can also be complicated by loss of 'passport' benefits such as free school meals, help with travel costs and health charges, which can make employment a risky option.

Families where children have left full-time education may find that charges for services impact on the family budget. For some families, this will be a reversal of the situation where adult training centres used to offer a token 'wage' for attendance and industrial type work. This deprivation has been particularly resented by people with learning disabilities, who, almost overnight, could see a 'wage' replaced by a bill: 'Why all these years have I not had to pay . . . and then all of a sudden everybody having to pay something?' (Chetwynd & Ritchie 1996, p. 16). Families too, could be asked to pay for respite when provided or arranged by the local authority under community care arrangements, when previously hospital respite stays incurred no charge. Means testing, or financial assessment, is often resented as intrusive and a charge on disability (Bradley & Manthorpe 1997). There are arguments, of course, in the main from service providers, that paying for services gives the consumer dignity and some greater sense of control over the agency and the service. Such arguments would be easier to validate if people did not live on very small incomes in the main.

Payment for services, however, brings into play a range of other related issues, such as access to money and resources. People living in residential care, for example, are often reliant on the very small income of their personal allowance to fund expenses and to participate in ordinary life activities. For them, and for others living on income support, the benefits trap can mean that work is financially not worth it. Many people, however, may wish to participate in forms of employment, not least because living on income support or disability benefits means very restricted choices about activities, food, clothing and entertainment. While it is appreciated that carers may have extra costs because of their caring work, it is often forgotten that people with learning disabilities may pay more for items because they are unable to buy in bulk or travel to supermarkets, they lack secure or adequate storage facilities, or they have not had the opportunity to develop skills in managing budgets or making savings. Major purchases can be difficult to fund and easy credit, official or unofficial, can seem a tempting solution.

Unlike other poor people, some people with learning disabilities do not have direct control over their money. As Bewley (1997) observed, the benefits claimed by a person with learning disabilities can be seen by some families as part of the family income and this can prevent people taking up opportunities or moving out of the family home because of the impact on family finances. Illustrating this, Bewley reported on the experience of one woman: 'Dorothy's mother collects her benefits from the local post office, without any involvement from Dorothy. The family has a car, paid for by Dorothy's mobility money, but do not use it for her benefit' (p. 10). In such circumstances, it is likely that Dorothy's mother has been made Dorothy's appointee, a system applying only to benefits and pensions. Many people with learning disabilities have their income claimed in this way and there is some concern that they have little say over such benefits and thus do not learn how to manage money. There is also evidence that people with learning disabilities may be financially abused by acts of deliberate exploitation and suffer betrayals of trust. New government guidance on the protection of vulnerable adults is clear that financial abuse is, like other forms of abuse, a violation of a person's civil and human rights (DOH 2000a). Hilary Brown (Brown 1999, p. 26), however, noted that financial or material abuse is not often reported as abuse by practitioners, who seem more accepting of irregularities than their colleagues working with older people and condone a variety of arrangements in respect of people with learning disabilities.

Reader activity 4.4   Accessing income

What benefits might be available to the following case examples:

- a person with learning disabilities considering part-time seasonal work
- a single mother with a child aged 5 who has profound disabilities
- a person with learning disabilities (18 years) studying full-time in further education and living with his parents
- an older person with Down syndrome moving into a residential care home?

You may find it helpful to check out your replies (having consulted a useful publication such as the *Disability Rights Handbook* (Disability Alliance 2001) with the local Citizens Advice Bureau, Mencap, a local authority welfare rights advisor (if there is one) or a Disability Advice agency (these will vary in availability locally) or the Benefits Agency. In your area, where would you recommend people to go for expert advice?

Geographical influences

Services for people with learning disabilities have long recognised that place (or geography) is an important factor in systems of support. Urban areas have been identified as centres for services and expertise but have drawbacks in terms of possible poor housing and urban deprivation. Rural communities have been identified as supportive but also potentially restrictive. As locations of mental handicap hospitals, they were also seen as places of containment.

Recent attention to rural community care developed a series of five standards for local social care services. These included:

- responsiveness – to rural communities and their needs
- accessibility – services being available without undue travel time or expense, or alternatives available
- information and communication – broadly spread through local networks
- equal opportunities – including respect for rural lifestyles
- management arrangements – such as consultation, local commissioning and range of choice (Brown 1999, pp 57–60).

However, rural provision is often underdeveloped and reliant, unjustifiably, on positive images of rural life. Pugh (2000) observed that travel costs could affect take-up of support and that service users could often be required either to travel long distances or to move to services and become dislocated from community networks. Rural isolation was a significant problem for carers, particularly for mothers and for people from ethnic minorities.

Problems have been identified with rural services around access and the difficulty of moving from centres and centralised support to more community based provision. In this respect they are similar to the difficulties of many urban areas. However, rural areas appear to have less resources to fund such a shift, partly because of national policy decisions about the distribution of resources and partly because of frequent longstanding local allocations of resources to institutional provision. Rural social care has generally relied heavily on informal or community networks (Craig & Manthorpe 2000), many of which have depended on the local economy. Disruptions to this way of life may impact on people with disabilities disproportionately since their mobility and resources may be restricted.

Rural and urban areas, different parts of the country and the different countries of the UK all experience variations in services. Debates over territorial justice draw attention to this tension between locally responsible and locally determined resource allocations versus centralised planning and models of service delivery. The All Wales Strategy, for example, was a national development, which inspired other shifts to community services and family support. Criticism of service variation (the postcode lottery), however, is central to *Valuing People*, which promises attention to this inequality in access to care and support (DOH 2001a, pp 18 and 20).

Growing up and growing old

In this section we consider access to services on the basis of age, an analysis that has achieved greater popularity in recent years. A range of criticism has been levelled at children's services that they marginalise disabled children. Similarly, older people's services may fail to recognise the needs of older carers and the needs of people with learning disabilities as they age.

In relation to children's services, Middleton (1999) has argued that there is a discriminatory and harmful 'conceptual distinction' between children and disabled children. She found that child protection workers could feel de-skilled when working with disabled children and that practitioners working with disabled children conceived their work to be less risky, more family-focused and more supporting. This division can mean that disabled children are further vulnerable to abuse. Child protection workers may find it difficult to communicate with disabled children and may misinterpret behaviour. They may over-empathise with the parents or care staff and miss signs of abuse. They may be unable to identify alternative care settings if a disabled child has to leave the family. Middleton also warned that child protection workers might share disablist values and not give sufficient priority to disabled children's needs. This suggests that those working with disabled children need to advocate for them at times, within services and with their colleagues. Childcare skills need to be applied to all children. This means listening to and observing children. As Middleton recalled: ' "Challenging behaviour", which was once translated for me as "eloquence" may be an attempt to communicate unhappiness' (Middleton 1999). She has drawn attention to the need for all practitioners to be alert to the possibility of abuse but this is set within the context of including all children within protective frameworks. This is a part of an equality agenda.

Access to education, however, is more commonly addressed in respect of disabled children. The Education Act 1987 abolished the category 'ineducable children' (Bridge 1999), to be followed by a series of educational reforms and procedures (outlined elsewhere in this book) which have focused on access to integrated schooling, obtaining a statement of need and the resources to meet this, and on education as part of a more general plan for a child's welfare. Bridge (1999) however, has thrown light on the different abilities of parents to manage access to educational support for their children. In her study of children with cerebral palsy, she found many parents exhibited great determination and tenacity, but 'The most articulate and the wealthiest families are likely to take legal action against LEAs (Local Education Authorities)' (Bridge 1999, p. 165). She found disabled children and their families made use of both specialist and mainstream provision before school age. Access to pre-school provision, therefore, can involve a complex set of arrangements with play groups, nurseries, Portage, toy libraries and opportunity groups. As Bridge observed, of the families she studied: 'Their experiences mirror those of able children but are exacerbated by patchy, under-funded provision and what appears to be limited commitment to promoting these facilities for disabled children with communication and mobility problems' (Bridge 1999, p. 181).

Such research points to the variety of learning and educational experiences of children and the need to see education more broadly than simply full-time schooling. Access to education may involve commercially provided opportunities, such as private pre-schooling, voluntary sector groups' provision, ranging from self-help to commissioned services, and statutory or public services. Parents' own resources, notably those arising from their class or educational advantages, appear to be able to assist them in drawing down resources and enabling them to make informed choices between alternatives. Those parents with limited resources are further disadvantaged.

At the other end of the life-course, access to support is important for the growing numbers of people with learning disabilities who survive into old age. The situation of older people with learning disabilities has been described as one of 'double jeopardy' (Walker et al 1996). Many will be 'too young' for older people's services and may not have much in common with people whose life experiences have been so different. Thompson's research (2001) has found that the average age of people with learning disabilities who live in old people's homes is 65 – a full 20 years younger than other residents, whose average age is 85 years. *The National Service Framework for Older People* (DOH 2001b) suggested that it was poor practice to 'misplace' people with learning disabilities in old people's homes if they are aged 75 or under. They may, however, have been excluded or 'retired' from learning disability services on the grounds that they were too 'young'. Grant (2001) has presented the result as meaning that older people with learning disabilities often live on the 'fringe of society', with limited resources and restricted social networks. He has further identified that they may be disadvantaged in their access to psychiatric services in old age, despite the evidence that they may benefit from help with a variety of problems, not simply the increased risk of dementia associated with Down syndrome. These problems include possible depression, hearing loss, visual difficulties and hypothyroidism.

Older people with learning disabilities do not simply have needs in respect of their own health, for they may be acting as carers for members of their own families, particularly their parents. Much attention was given in *Valuing People* (DOH 2001a) to older parents of people with learning disabilities, but there is increasing evidence that people with learning disabilities provide care and support to their ageing parents at times. This may be particularly so for those who are women and those with moderate learning disabilities. In some instances relationships become those of interdependency and mutual care. Opportunities to access carer support services may be limited and carers' assessments will need to be sensitive to family circumstances and possible planning over what support and resources will be available to the person with learning disabilities when or if the person they are looking after moves to residential care or dies.

Walmsley (2000) has provided accounts of the lives of women with learning disabilities who have taken on aspects of the caring role. Beryl, for example, looked after her elderly mother who was ill and housebound. Such life histories demonstrate the interrelationships between caring and being cared for. As people with learning disabilities grow older so do their circles of families and friends. Walmsley found that some women with learning disabilities could find a place in the world through caring. This place, of course, may be welcome or restrictive, or a mixture of the two. Services and support can link together ageing and care so that the interaction between the two is considered rather than ignored.

 Reader activity 4.5

If an older person with learning disabilities wanted to join older people's groups which, in your area, might be welcoming?

INCLUSION NOT ACCESS

Social inclusion is a concept that brings together many of the issues discussed in this chapter. It is a helpful concept since it places responsibility for social exclusion on the shoulders of those who control power not on those who are excluded from participation in society on the basis of discrimination for whatever reason. People at the margins of society, in particular, may benefit from joined up thinking around social problems and joined up government. Equally, as Becker (2000) has suggested, there may be some point in thinking about the position of carers as one of social exclusion since they are often denied equal opportunities by services and in respect of employment. He argued that it is possible to identify certain vulnerability factors to social exclusion among carers, in respect of their own personal circumstances, their caring work and wider family indicators, which may suggest a need for higher levels of support. Such support would need to be a joining up of cash and care.

Social inclusion is thus more than an attempt to involve everyone in the world of work, although much of its emphasis is in respect of making people employable in a global economy and to reduce perceived reliance on state welfare. This fits with the expressed views of people with learning disabilities who, when asked, say that they would like to work (Mental Health Foundation 1996, p. 34). Work has long been identified as a place of status, of social support and a demonstration of independence. Supported employment has been one way of promoting work and building up people's confidence and skills. Such schemes can also challenge the discrimination against people with disabilities. However, as Beyer (2000) has observed, most of the 7 000 or so people with learning disabilities who participate in supported employment schemes have mild or moderate learning disabilities. People with high support needs can be included in such schemes providing suitable adaptations are made. These can be practical, in terms of matching the person, the task and the work environment. Support may have to be more fine-tuned, with perhaps some form of assistance, technical or personal. People with high support needs may have a range of personal care requirements that also need to be planned around. Beyer has identified attitudinal barriers as the greatest obstacle to developing support in this area and yet sees the alternative of intensive day care as having few advantages over a well thought out employment scheme.

It is employment's social functions that are often identified as important for people with learning disabilities, because of their limited access to other informal networks. Access to peers can be limited to special or segregated provision from early years and families can be wary of allowing people with learning disabilities to experience the risks of hurt and rejection. Again, people with high support needs may find it more difficult to access informal friendship networks and services may have to work with people to find a way of reducing isolation. Circles of support have been one way in which barriers to friendships have been broken down, with one project, the Friendship Train, offering a range of suggestions about this very challenging area of work (Foundation for People with Learning Disabilities 2000).

Other research has illustrated how people's access to their locality may be restricted in an attempt to minimise perceived harm. People can be warned against going to various places or taking certain journeys, they can also be limited to only going out in day time or safe times. Heyman, Huckle & Handyside (1998), for example, demonstrated that parents could encourage 'spatial autonomy' or freedom within the locality for their adult children with learning disabilities: alternatively, they could monitor their activities closely and constrain them to defined, often accompanied, journeys. Brenda, for example, had been warned against going out in the dark: 'Because people in cars might take me away . . . You don't know what they are like. They might hurt you. They might kidnap me' (Heyman, Huckle Handyside 1998, p. 205). Such discussions raise the perceived and real problems of the victimisation of people with learning disabilities who may be subject to bullying, gang abuse and intimidation when out of their homes. Their access to their neighbourhoods can be curtailed through fear.

Social inclusion can also mean other forms of participation, notably involvement in political life. Access to self-advocacy groups and pressure groups has undoubtedly increased and many users' councils are developing around services. Participation in the democratic process is still limited for people with learning disabilities. Although one million have the vote, it was estimated that only 5% used it in the 2001 General Election (Pring 2001, p. 26). Elections themselves may exclude people with disabilities since most parties produce inaccessible literature and make little or no attempt to reach out to people with learning disabilities. Exercising the responsibilities of citizenship may be a way of moving the debate on from narrow associations between people with learning disabilities and services.

This chapter has drawn on a variety of evidence to argue that access is not a simple matter of finding the right key to unlock services. Access may be better conceived as a process of social inclusion. This puts the onus on those in powerful positions to respond to the rights of people with learning disabilities to participate in and contribute to society.

REFERENCES

Alaszewski A, Gates B, Ayer S, Manthorpe J 2001 Educational preparation for learning disability nursing: outcomes evaluation of the contribution of learning disability nurses within the multi-professional, multi-agency team. Research highlights. English National Board for Nursing, Midwifery and Health Visiting, London

Baldwin S 1985 The costs of caring: families with disabled children. Routledge and Kegan Paul, London

Barton R 1998 Family involvement in the pre-discharge assessment of long-stay patients with learning disabilities: a qualitative study. Journal of Learning Disabilities for Nursing, Health and Social Care 2(2): 79–88

Becker S 2000 Carers and indicators of vulnerability to social exclusion. Benefits 28: 1–4, (April/May)

Bewley C 1997 Money matters: helping people with learning disabilities have more control over their money. Values into Action, London

Beyer S 2000 Choosing work. Introduction. In: Everyday lives, everyday choices for people with learning disabilities and high support needs, The Foundation for People with Learning Disabilities, London, pp 44–48

Booth T, Booth W 1994 Parenting under pressure: mothers and fathers with learning difficulties. Open University Press, Buckingham

Bradley G, Manthorpe J 1997 Dilemmas of financial assessment: a practitioner's guide. Venture Press, Birmingham

Bridge G 1999 Parents as care managers: the experiences of those caring for young children with cerebral palsy. Ashgate, Aldershot

Brown D 1999 Care in the country – inspection of community care services in rural areas. Department of Health, London

Brown H 1999 Abuse of people with learning disabilities: layers of concern and analysis. In: Stanley N, Manthorpe J, Penhale B (eds) Institutional abuse: perspectives across the life course. Routledge, London, pp 89–109

Campbell J, Oliver J 1996 Disability politics. Routledge, London

Chetwynd M, Ritchie J 1996 The cost of care: the impact of charging policy on the lives of disabled people. Joseph Rowntree Foundation, York

Cigno K, Burke P 1997 Single mothers of children with learning disabilities: an undervalued group. Journal of Interprofessional Care 11(2): 177–186

Cole A, McIntosh B, Whittaker A 2000 We want our voices heard developing new lifestyles with disabled people. Policy Press, Bristol

Committee of Inquiry into Normansfield Hospital 1978 Report of the committee of inquiry into Normansfield Hospital. Cmd 7357, HMSO, London

Craig G, Manthorpe J 2000 Fresh fields: developing an agenda for rural social care. York Publishing Services, York

Craig G, Rai D K 1996 Social security, community care – and 'race'. In: Ahmad W, Atkin K (eds) 'Race' and community care. Open University Press, Buckingham pp 124–143

Department of Health 2001a Valuing people: a new strategy for learning disability for the 21st century. Cm 5086, The Stationery Office, London

Department of Health 2001b National service framework for older people. The Stationery Office, London

Department of Health/Department of the Environment, Transport and the Regions 2000 Better care: higher standards, Department of Health, London

Department of Social Security 1998 Supporting people: a new policy and funding framework for support services. Produced for the inter-departmental review for supported accommodation. DSS, London

Dickens D 1998 Learning disability in the special hospitals. In: Kaye C, Franey A (eds) Managing high security psychiatric care. Jessica Kingsley, London, pp 123–135

Disability Alliance 2001 Disability rights handbook. Disability Alliance, London

Foundation for People with Learning Disabilities 2001 Learning disabilities: the fundamental facts. Mental Health Foundation, London

Glendinning C, Halliwell S, Jacobs S, Rummery K, Tyrer J 2000 Buying independence: using direct payments to integrate health and social services. Policy Press, Bristol

Grant G 2001 Older people with learning disabilities: health, community inclusion and family care giving. In: Working with older people and their families: key issues in policy and practice. Open University Press, Buckingham

Hatton C, Azmi S, Caine A, Emerson E 1998 Informal carers of adolescents and adults with learning difficulties from the South Asian continent, service support and carer stress. British Journal of Social Work 28(6): 821–838

Heyman B, Huckle S, Handyside E 1998 Freedom of the locality for people with learning difficulties. In: Heyman B (ed) Risk: health and health care, Arnold, London

Jones C, Wright K 1996 Public expenditure on services for people with intellectual disabilities. Journal of Applied Research in Intellectual Disabilities 9(4): 289–306

Keywood K, Fovargue S, Flynn M 1999 Best practice? Health care decision-making by, with and for adults with learning disabilities. National Development Team, Manchester

Lambe L 1998 Supporting families. In: Lacey P, Ouvry C (eds) People with profound and multiple learning disabilities. Jessica Kingsley, London, pp 167–175

Leece J 2000 Making direct payments work in Staffordshire. Practice 12(4): 37–48

Lord Chancellor's Department 1997 Who decides? Making decision on behalf of mentally incapacitated adults. Cm 3803, The Stationery Office, London

Lord Chancellor's Department 1999 Making decisions: the Government's proposals for making decisions on behalf of mentally incapacitated adults. Cm 4465, The Stationery Office, London

McIntosh B, Whittaker A 1998 Days of change: a practical guide to developing better day opportunities with people with learning difficulties. King's Fund, London

Marshall M 2000 Astrid: a social and technological response to meeting the needs of individuals with dementia and their carers. Hawker Publications, London

Mental Health Foundation 1996 Building expectations: opportunities and services for people with a learning disability. Mental Health Foundation, London

Middleton L 1999 Disabled children: challenging social exclusion. Blackwell Science, Oxford

Mitchell W, Sloper P 2000 User-friendly information for families with disabled children: a guide to good practice. York Publishing Services, York

Mukherjee S, Beresford B, Lightfoot J, Norris P, Sloper P 1999 Implementing key worker services: a case study of promoting evidence-based practice. Joseph Rowntree Foundation, York

Oldman C, Beresford B 1998 Homes unfit for children. Policy Press, Bristol

Parekh B 2000 The future of multi-ethnic Britain (The Parekh Report). Profile Books, London

Pring J 2001 Crossed off. Community Care, 26 July, 1383: 26–27

Pugh R 2000 Rural social work. Russell House Publishing, Lyme Regis

Roberts K, Lawton D 1999 Reaching its target? Disability allowance for children. Social Policy Research Unit, University of York, York

Ryan T, Holman A 1998 Able and willing: supporting people with learning difficulties to use direct payments. Values into Action, London

Secretaries of State 1989 Caring for people: community care for the next decade and beyond. Cm 849, HMSO, London

Secretary of State for Health 2000 The NHS plan. Cm 4818–1, The Stationery Office, London

Simons K 1998 Living support networks: an evaluation of the services provided by Keyring. Pavilion/Joseph Rowntree Foundation, Brighton

Simons K 2000 Life on the edge: the experiences of people with a learning disability who do not use specialist services. Pavilion, Brighton

Taylor J 1998 Technology for living and learning. In: Lacey P, Ouvery C (eds) People with profound and multiple learning disabilities. David Fulton, London, pp 156–166

Thompson D 2000 Vulnerability, dangerousness and risk: the case of men with learning disabilities who sexually abuse. Health, Risk and Society 2(1): 33–46

Thompson D 2001 People with learning disabilities in residential services for older people, Foundation for People with Learning Disabilities, London

Walker A, Walker C, Ryan T 1996 Older people with learning difficulties leaving institutional care – a case of double jeopardy. Ageing and Society 16: 125–150

Walmsley J 1997 Including people with learning difficulties: theory and practice. In: Barton L, Oliver M (eds) Disability studies: past, present and future. The Disability Press, Leeds, pp 62–77

Walmsley J 2000 Caring – a place in the world? In: Traustadottir R, Johnson K (eds) Women with intellectual disabilities: finding a place in the world. Jessica Kingsley, London, pp 191–212

Walmsley J, Rolph S 2001 The development of community care with learning difficulties 1913 to 1946: Critical Social Policy 21(1): 59–80

Williams V, Robinson C 2000 In their own right: the Carers Act and carers of people with learning disabilities. Policy Press, Bristol

FURTHER READING

Brigham L, Atkinson D, Jackson M, Rolph S, Walmsley J (eds) 2000 Crossing boundaries: change and continuity in the history of learning disability. British Institute of Learning Disabilities, Kidderminster

Foundation for People with Learning Disabilities 2001 Learning disabilities, the fundamental facts. Mental Health Foundation, London

Malin N, Manthorpe J, Race D, Wilmot S 1999 Community care for nurses and the caring professions. Open University Press, Buckingham

Ramcharan P, Roberts G, Grant G, Borland J (eds) 1997 Empowerment in everyday life. Jessica Kingsley, London

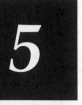

5

Residential alternatives for people with learning disabilities

Bob Gates

KEY ISSUES

- Historically, in the UK, residential care has been much influenced by political, ideological and economical factors. Given that people with learning disabilities have been and still are often misunderstood, this has sometimes resulted in inappropriate residential care alternatives being offered to them and their families.
- The recent White Paper says that local authorities should consider a range of housing care and support options for people with learning disabilities, and that no option should be routinely disregarded (DOH 2001).
- There is a range of residential alternatives for people with learning disabilities and these currently include: group homes, residential units, hospitals, village communities and/or intentional communities, tenancy agreements, supported living, home ownership and family placements.
- Recent research by Emerson et al (1999) would seem to suggest that there are to be found some differences in benefits, measured in terms of quality of care and costs, between different types of residential care provision.
- It is likely that new forms of residential care provision will be pursued, even without an evidence base, and that the emerging form of preferred residential provision will be that of supported living.
- The Care Standards Act has established councils that will set and monitor standards in residential care for England and Wales.

- **The introduction of direct payments may make it easier for people with learning disabilities to explore a range of housing opportunities based on individual choice, and the introduction of person-centred planning will act as the vehicle through which choice can be facilitated.**

INTRODUCTION

There are numerous and well-rehearsed debates that can be found in nearly all text books on learning disability concerning the most appropriate forms of residential care provision for people with learning disabilities. In 1980 it was estimated that there were as many as 55 000 people with learning disabilities who lived in 'long-term residential care' and that by 1999 this number had fallen to approximately 12 000. A similar scale of movement of people with learning disabilities from large residential provision to other more community oriented alternatives can be found across Europe (Mansell & Ericsson 1996). Currently, Emerson et al (2001) have suggested that 63% of adults with learning disabilities live in private households whereas 37% live in communal or residential care. Interestingly this ratio seems to reverse once people reach the age of 55 and over. Whereas professional and caring agencies have little or no control as to how private households are configured, this is not the case when it comes to communal residential care provision. This single area has the potential to cause heated and protracted arguments between the proponents of different forms of residential provision, each thinking that their position is the more defendable and realistic and that positions adopted by others are untenable, oppressive and so on. It is possible to find arguments about the optimum size of the 'home', how many people should live there, whether it should be staffed, and if so by whom. Should it be 'ordinary' in the sense that it should look the same as other homes in the street? Should it be isolated, in the country, or fully integrated in an urban setting?

In 1997, this author published an editorial which explored a number of issues, including the assertion that village communities might be a realistic residential alternative for people with learning disabilities (Gates 1997). I concluded thus:

> As ordinary people appear to have a multiplicity of preferences for where they live, why should it be the case that people with learning disabilities should be any different? It does seem somewhat strange that the ideologies of normalisation that we have inherited from another era should still be dictating where and how people with learning disabilities should live. Perhaps it is time to adopt a new, more balanced posture to this issue. Perhaps it is time for people with learning disabilities and their carers or advocates to decide where and how they wish to live (Gates 1997, p. 3).

The response to this editorial was a salvo of written rebuttals, two of which were published (Collins 1997, and Brandon 1997). It was the case that a seemingly inoffensive editorial that merely sought to raise as problematic the issue of where people might wish to live caused a furore disproportionate to the issue being discussed. This brief chapter will attempt to outline a number of different residential options that people with learning disabilities and/or their carers might wish to consider. It will also explore issues around quality and cost and will identify the importance of direct payments, and the possible impact this could make on the choice of residential alternatives within the context of person-centred planning. Importantly, it will attempt to present a balanced portrayal of residential alternatives for people with learning disabilities.

BACKGROUND

In Chapter 3 an excellent and comprehensive account was provided of the historical development of one type of residential provision that has dominated much of the European and North American care provision for some 100 years: institutional care. In the UK this model of service provision was rooted in the development of workhouses prior to the 19th century. Similar structures (institutions, asylums and colonies) were used from the late 19th century to the middle of the 20th century to contain people who were certified as 'mentally deficient'. These places of segregation were developed and structured specifically for containment and segregation. It was not until the introduction of the NHS Act 1946 that many of these places were designated as hospitals. Their continued existence and use was, by and large, determined by the prevalent social attitudes of the time, rather than by an objective view as to whether that type of residential accommodation was appropriate. However, academic interest began to emerge regarding the appropriateness of this form of residential provision. In 1958 Jack Tizard undertook a pioneering piece of work that was to compare the development of children at Brooklands, an experimental small residential unit, with children at Fountain Hospital, a nearby large institutional facility for people with learning disabilities (Tizard 1964). This research had three overriding objectives:

- to serve as a pilot scheme in which a particular technique of care and education could be studied
- to compare the development, over a 2 year period, of children in the small unit with that of a matched control group of children living in the parent hospital
- to explore the administrative and social implications of a system of residential care for mentally subnormal children deprived of normal home life, based as far as possible on the type of care offered to normal children who require it.

Essentially this experiment placed 16 children in a small residential unit and then compared their development, with a matched control group of 16 children back at the parent hospital. The children were matched for gender, age, measured intelligence and, wherever possible, diagnosis. This chapter cannot describe the intricacies of this experiment in detail, rather it will present the main findings and hopefully serve to illustrate the origins of more systematic ways for determining the merits or otherwise of different types of residential support provided for some people with learning disabilities. Readers who wish to read further in this area should refer to Tizard (1964, pp 86–137). At the end of 2 years, perhaps not surprisingly, the children at the Brooklands unit demonstrated superior development over the children back at the hospital. Findings of the

study can be described both quantitatively and qualitatively. Tizard reported:

The quantitative findings are clear-cut. There was a marked and significant rise, averaging fourteen months, in the verbal mental age of the Brooklands children during their two years residence in the unit, as compared with only six months for the control group (Tizard 1964, p. 130).

These results are shown in Figure 5.1; however, it can be seen that there was not a significant difference between the two groups in non-verbal mental age. Concerning qualitative findings the Brooklands children changed enormously. Tizard reported that:

They kept in good physical health and, living much of the time out of doors engaged in gross motor activities, they looked healthy, sun-tanned and alert. They ate and slept well, and we had little sickness...emotionally they became much less maladjusted (Tizard 1964, p. 133).

Tizard reported on the significant global effects of this non-institutionalised form of care on the development of the children. He observed that the children at Brooklands developed strong attachments to care staff and other children. They played cooperatively, and they appeared

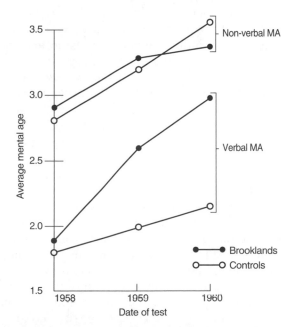

Figure 5.1 Intelligence tests for Brooklands and control groups. Reproduced with kind permission from Oxford University Press.

affectionate and happy. He also noted that the older children helped with household chores. He concluded:

It was these differences which constituted the success of the experiment, and we should have continued to call the study a success whether or not any quantitative changes had occurred in the level of the children's abilities as measured psychometrically (Tizard 1964, p. 134).

These findings, when understood within a temporal context that also included the emerging scandals and enquiries of the 1960s into the conditions of some of Britain's long stay institutions (Ely in 1969, Normansfield in 1969), added fuel to the need to move away from this type of residential alternative. This period of time also saw the beginnings of the normalisation movement, the growth of consumerism and the development of human rights activists. All of these separate but nonetheless interrelated factors conspired to challenge the appropriateness of institutions to provide residential services for people with learning disabilities.

By the early 1970s a new vision had begun to emerge of different types of residential alternatives, and this was finally articulated in a White Paper for people with learning disabilities (DOH 1971). This provided a central policy initiative for the reduction in the number of 'beds' in institutions in order to pursue more appropriate 'community oriented living arrangements' and support for families. By 1990 the move toward 'community care' was almost complete and resulted in the NHS and Community Care Act (1990), which advocated an internal market that sought to establish purchasers and providers, thereby removing the monopoly from health and social services in the provision of residential care. This has resulted in a mixed economy of care which now includes independent, private, charitable and housing association as well as statutory providers. This move to community care took place with considerable confusion and even difference of opinion as to what it meant. For example, did it mean care in the community or care by the community? Did it refer to the size and configuration of services? What parts of the community were people to move to?

Tracing the development of services for people with learning disabilities is fascinating and the reader is directed to three texts that illustrate the *Zeitgeist* in the development of residential services. In Craft & Miles (1967), the reader should note the terminology and the unquestionable dominance of a medical model. An inherently interesting book by Heron & Myers (1983) captures, in Chapter 3, the universality of the movement away from institutional care to 'community care'. Finally, Williams (1995) provides a very helpful summary of some of the arguments around residential care in an excellent chapter on residential and day services. The reader might also wish to refer back to Chapter 3, which provides a historical account of the development of services for people with learning disabilities.

DIFFERENT TYPES OF RESIDENTIAL ALTERNATIVES

This next section briefly describes a range of residential options that people with learning disabilities currently use. It is the case that each option has both strengths and weaknesses, but the relative merits, or otherwise, of different types of residential alternatives should ultimately be decided upon by those people with learning disabilities who will use them, and their families; where any of us live is, relatively, a matter of choice. With the advent and slowly emerging nature of person-centred planning it will be the needs, wishes and aspirations of people with learning disabilities as to where they wish to live that are paramount rather than the views of professionals and/or statutory agencies. This chapter does not present information concerning that group of people who may have offended or have special needs that are more appropriately met in other establishments. For this the reader is referred to Chapter 14.

Supported living

This might best be thought of not as a single model, rather as a range of residential alternatives for people with learning disabilities. Central to any of these alternatives would be living in one's own home, participating in one's own community and with all planning centred around the individual concerned. In an excellent publication by the Scottish Executive, *The view from Arthur's Seat* (Simmons & Watson 1999), supported living is described as 'a form of intensive domiciliary service (support provided to people in their own home).' Supported living represents a way of constructing services that takes services to people's own homes, and then develops around them the kinds of support that they will need to live as independently as possible. There is some evidence that supports this form of residential alternative as a viable and successful way of living (Simmons and Watson 1999). It is important to remember that supported living does not imply that all people with learning disabilities no longer require the support of qualified and highly skilled assistance, simply to place people in residential settings without appropriate support systems in place might be both dangerous and self-defeating. Within this type of residential alternative a range of options might include rented or leased accommodation, or ownership of one's own property. In a sense supported living might be a direct consequence of person-centred planning. This is because the type of residential alternative offered to people is constructed around their needs, wishes and aspirations. For those readers wishing to pursue this area further there is an excellent contribution offered by Sanderson et al (1997).

Village and intentional communities

The recent White Paper has defined village communities as '[a] service operated by [an] independent organisation comprising houses clustered on one site together that share facilities'. An intentional community is defined as 'services operated by [an] independent sector organisation comprising houses and some shared facilities on one or more sites based on philosophical or religious belief' (DOH 2001, pp 132–133). The origins of such communities lie in the Camphill Village movement, which was established by Dr Karl König who founded the movement in Scotland during the 1940s. This movement is based upon the educational theories of Rudolf Steiner (1861–1925), and it was from his philosophy that

the idea of therapeutic communities was developed (Jackson 1999). Therapies are supported by anthroposophical ideas and homeopathic medicines, which along with the community experience are designed to 'foster the harmonious development of the whole human being – body, soul and spirit – to create a healthy balance between thinking, feeling, and will activity and to engender morality, social co-operation and responsibility' (Fulgosi 1990, pp 40–41). In such communities each person, according to that person's abilities, contributes what he or she can toward the wellbeing of other members of the community. The idea is to foster mutual help and understanding in an environment that seeks to counter some of the supposed harmful ways of modern life. Non-disabled members of the community are not referred to as carers. Rather they are known as co-workers, in that they do not receive financial remuneration for their efforts and that the nature of the relationship between village members is based on equality. One problem with the description 'village communities' is that not all such communities can properly be described as villages, therefore a newer term has arisen, 'intentional communities', that perhaps more correctly describes them. Other types of residential community include L'Arche, a federation of communities in the UK, France, Denmark, Belgium, Norway, and the USA as well as in countries like India (see further resources at the end of the chapter), and Cottage and Rural Enterprise and the Home Farm Trust. For an interesting account of a range of different types of residential communities the reader is advised to refer to Segal (1990).

 Reader activity 5.1

Either individually, or in a small group, make arrangements to visit a village community. Spend time preparing before your visit; whilst there spend some time with the villagers to ascertain how happy they are living there and what kinds of things constitute quality of life for them.

NHS provision

Despite the closure of the long stay learning disability hospitals, some residential care provision has remained on site and this has become known as 'residential campuses', usually run by NHS Trusts. Generally speaking these campuses have retained nursing and medical staff and therapists, and provide a specialist focus of care. In addition, it should be remembered that some dedicated learning disabilities hospitals remain. For example, in England there are still some 1 500 people with learning disabilities who reside in hospitals (DOH 2001), and in Wales, Scotland and Northern Ireland there still remain the last vestiges of an era now past. The learning disability hospitals, as explained in Chapter 3, were originally large asylums and were simply transformed into hospitals by the introduction of the NHS Act of 1946. Across the UK their planned closure is predicted to be: Scotland by 2005, England by 2004, Wales by 2006. Although no specific date has been identified in Northern Ireland a planned programme of reduction in beds is being pursued. It is not the intention of this chapter either to attack or defend these establishments. Simply, the provision of hospitals as a residential alternative represents an era that poorly understood the needs and aspirations of people with learning disabilities and their families. This form of residential provision went perversely wrong representing in the end a form of social control and with the inevitable underfunding and other associated resource problems the eventual demise of these hospitals became assured. This type of residential provision, when compared with others such as village communities and dispersed housing schemes, has failed to demonstrate quality service and there appears to be no easy answer as to why (Emerson et al 1999).

Hostels

These emerged during the 1960s and 1970s. Typically they catered for approximately 12–30 people, were often referred to as 'half-way houses' and were usually run by social service departments. The 'half-way' referred to them being half way between a hospital and independent community living. Despite being much smaller than the institutions, many of these establishments were still very institutionalised, and sometimes continued to perpetuate systems that provided block treatment and depersonalised forms of care (Heron 1982). Although not a preferred option, some still exist today. A development of the provision of hostel accommodation was that of 'core and cluster' arrangements. In this form of residential provision a number of smaller 'ordinary' types of houses were clustered around a larger residential unit, which was able to offer an administrative base and back-up for people with learning disabilities if the nature of their dependency changed and they required greater support.

Family (adult) placements

Adult placements seem to have evolved from the fostering of children with special needs from the 1970s. There are many adult family placement schemes to be found across the country. Essentially, people with learning disabilities are placed in families, other than their own, as an alternative to residential care. The families are approved and trained by an official agency, which continues to provide support and assistance both to the adult who has been placed, and the carers.

Such schemes are in fact quite complex and because of the vulnerability of some people with learning disabilities they are highly regulated, with extensive procedures and policies. These typically include policies on: recruitment; selection, assessment and training of carers; registration and inspection; selection panels; referrals of clients; matching; placement agreements; carer's support; reviews; and various documentation required. This has resulted in the past in this type of residential provision being offered by people with a professional background in caring (Dagnan & Drewett 1988). Whereas this is not in itself problematic, it does seem to tie people with learning disabilities to a lifetime of dependency on those who wish to care for them, precluding the exploration of other more independent forms of residential care provision.

To conclude, there are numerous configurations for different types of residential care provision that can be made available for people with learning disabilities. Where people with learning disabilities live should ultimately be a matter of their choice; all too often it is not.

Reader activity 5.2

Spend some time researching different types of residential services in your area. See if it is possible to visit at least some of these, in addition to the already suggested village community. Try to imagine what it might feel like to live there. Try and identify how these services are monitored for quality.

WHICH IS THE BEST RESIDENTIAL ALTERNATIVE?

This section of the chapter does not seek to replicate the already excellent contribution exploring the monitoring and evaluation of services provided by David Marsland in Chapter 6. Rather, it will attempt to confine itself to recent research and other contemporary literature on the range and extent of evidence that we have at our disposal concerning different types of residential alternatives. For some considerable time attention has been paid to discovering the form of residential provision that offers the highest quality of care at the lowest price or, as it is now known, 'best value'. Given the estimated amount (some £2.5 billion) from the public purse that is spent on residential provision, this is clearly an area that ought to be subjected to empirical scrutiny (Emerson et al 2001, p. 53). It has been known for some time that there are considerable variations in both the quality of care and the costs associated with different forms of residential provision across the UK (Raynes 1994), and it would seem inappropriate to purchase residential services when the costs are known to be high and the quality questionable.

Over the years all manner of variables have been included in studies of what constitutes quality and what the benefits of one type of residential care are when compared with another. These variables have included studying the effects of the residential setting on changes in behaviour, participation in the community, contact with staff, participation in domestic chores and choice (Simmons & Watson 1999). Here in the UK a series of studies has been undertaken over a long period of time to establish the effects of moving people with learning disabilities from institutional care into smaller more community-oriented settings. Collins & Halman (1996) have reported on a study that concentrated on 16 people who moved from an institution to small 4-bedded units. They found that aggression towards other residents was reduced and that self-injurious behaviour showed a downward trend, but this trend was not statistically significant. Hatton et al (1996) studied 40 people with learning disabilities who had moved from an institution to small staffed community homes. Amongst other things, they found more positive staff–resident interactions, and a high level of scheduled activity. Felce & Perry (1997) undertook a study in Wales that compared family homes, specialist community homes and traditional residential services. This study involved 39 people with learning disabilities and it was found that the highest levels of engagement took place in community homes. They were also associated with a higher percentage of qualified staff. Community services seemed a preferable option when compared with the other options on a range of outcomes. In another study Dagnan et al (1998) found that 29 individuals who moved from an institution to 3–4 bedroom homes demonstrated increased levels of social interaction.

More recently, Emerson et al (1999) have undertaken an extensive and sophisticated piece of research that sought to compare the quality and costs of care in village communities, residential campuses and dispersed housing schemes. These included five village communities, five residential campuses and ten services that sought to provide community-based residential support in dispersed housing schemes. These were studied by investigating the 'characteristics and needs of supports provided to, and outcomes experienced by 500 people with learning disabilities' (Emerson et al 1999). Of the people in the study, those living in village communities were younger than those living in residential campuses or dispersed housing schemes. For the variable age and ethnicity, there was no significant difference between the three forms of residential provision under scrutiny. People living in village communities were more likely to have moved from family homes or other communities and they were more likely to have been living in their current home for longer and to have experienced fewer moves than those in dispersed housing or residential campuses. Those people who lived in residential campuses were more disabled than those who lived in dispersed housing, who in turn were more disabled than those living in village communities. There were no significant differences between the models of residential provision with regard to additional impairments and it was noted that people living in village communities were more likely to have Down syndrome. There were no differences in mental health between the people in the three different settings. Finally, those living in residential campuses had greater health needs and were reported to show more severely challenging behaviour than those living in both the other forms of residential provision. In this study achieving minimal variation between the profiles of the populations being studied was important, because any subsequent findings related to cost and quality of care could then be attributed to the type of residential environment in which individuals were living, rather than to some other variable. When a number of 'quality' variables were explored as the preferred model, then on almost every measure dispersed housing and village communities were significantly superior to residential campuses, though it must be remembered that this was not the case in all instances and there were a number of variables where no clear difference appeared between any of the residential alternatives. When the variables of age, ability and challenging behaviour were statistically controlled for, the total costs associated with village communities and residential campuses were significantly lower than those associated with dispersed housing schemes. Interested readers are advised to access the complete study (Emerson et al 1999).

One might surmise that there now exists sufficient and overwhelming evidence that smaller more community-oriented residential services have brought about significant improvements for people with learning disabilities, compared with institutional settings (Emerson 2001). To conclude, there is a range of alternative residential provision and some might be thought of as being superior in quality to others. However, the relationship between quality and cost is still a problematic area, and the evidence is not unequivocal. What is important is that people with learning disabilities should be offered choice.

FUTURE RESIDENTIAL TRAJECTORIES

Notwithstanding the need for a range of residential alternatives for people with learning disabilities, some are predicting that, as the remaining long-stay learning disability hospitals close, there will be an unprecedented move towards supported living. It is likely that this form of residential provision will also replace a number of existing and discredited (at least by some) forms of residential care provision, for example hostels and group homes. A recent letter from the Department for Transport, Local Government and the Regions sought to establish, through the use of private finance initiatives, local authorities who would be interested in providing additional social housing (DTLR 2001). It suggested long-term service contracts for potentially socially excluded groups and specifically identified people with learning disabilities as a group who might benefit from such a scheme. With a commitment to using direct payments more imaginatively, and enabling more people with learning disabilities to use such payments, it is hoped that this will result in an increasing number of people determining for themselves the kind of home they want. There is an excellent publication by the Department of Health which fully explains the benefits of such schemes (DOH 2000) and is very accessible to people with learning disabilities. It is likely that new and exciting forms of residential provision will begin to emerge that can provide people with learning disabilities, should they wish, with their own homes. Whatever the future brings in terms of the range of residential alternatives, it is to be hoped that people with learning disabilities and their families will have the right to choose the type of accommodation that they would like to live in.

CONCLUSION

This chapter has presented a range of residential alternatives and has alluded to some of the evidence we have at our disposal concerning the relative merits, or otherwise, associated with the different arrangements. Throughout, it has been argued that people with learning disabilities need to be afforded choice when it comes to where and how they wish to live. However, to facilitate this it is likely that in the future we will require a greater range of alternatives that people with learning disabilities can access without encountering ideological obstructions to their wishes.

REFERENCES

Brandon D 1997 Correspondence to the author. Journal of Learning Disability for Nursing, Health and Social Care 1(3): 157

Collins G, Halman F 1996 The move from hospital: a long-term follow-up of challenging behaviour levels. Journal of Applied Research in Intellectual Disabilities 9: 4

Collins J 1997 Correspondence to the author. Journal of Learning Disability for Nursing, Health and Social Care 1(4): 203

Craft M, Miles L 1967 Patterns of care for the subnormal. Pergamon Press, Oxford

Dagnan D, Drewett R 1988 Community based care for people with a mental handicap: a family placement scheme in County Durham. British Journal of Social Work 18: 543–575

Dagnan D, Ruddick L, Jones J 1998 A longitudinal study of the quality of life of older people with intellectual disability after leaving hospital. Journal of Intellectual Disability Research 42: 2

DOH 1971 Better services for the mentally handicapped. HMSO, London

DOH 2000 An easy guide to direct payments. DOH, London

DOH 2001 Valuing people: a new strategy for learning disability for the 21st century. CM 5086. The Stationery Office, London, pp 70–75

DTLR 2001 Local government private finance initiative: providing additional social housing and making local authorities more accessible to the public. DTLR, London

Emerson E, Robertson J, Gregory N et al 1999 A comparative analysis of quality and costs in group homes and supported living schemes. Hester Adrian Research Centre, University of Manchester, Manchester

Emerson E, Hatton C, Felce D, Murphy G 2001 Learning disabilities: The fundamental facts. The Foundation for People with Learning Disabilities, London

Felce D, Perry J 1997 A PASS 3 evaluation of community residences in Wales. Mental Retardation 35(3): 170–176

Fulgosi L 1990 Camphill communititres. In: Segal S (ed) The place of special villages and residential communities. AB Academic Publishers, Oxon, pp 39–48

Gates B 1997 Where to live and how to live: Zeitgeist and learning disabilities. Journal of Learning Disabilities for Nursing, Health and Social Care 1(1): 1–3

Hatton C, Emerson E, Robertson J et al 1996 Factors associated with staff support and resident lifestyle in services for people with multiple disabilities. Journal of Intellectual Disability Research 40(5): 466–477

Heron A 1982 Better services for the mentally handicapped? Lessons from the Sheffield evaluation studies. Kings Fund Centre, London

Heron A, Myers M 1983 Intellectual impairment: the battle against handicap. Academic Press, London

Jackson R 1999 The case for village communities for adults with learning disabilities: an exploration of the concept. Journal of Learning Disabilities for Nursing, Health and Social Care 3(2): 110–117

Mansell I, Ericsson E 1996 Deinstitutionalization and community living: intellectual disability services in Britain, Scandinavia and the USA. Chapman and Hall, London

Raynes N 1994 The cost and quality of community residential care. David Fulton, London

Sanderson H, Kennedy J, Ritchie P, Goodwin G 1997 People, plans and possibilities: exploring person centred planning. SHS Ltd, Edinburgh

Segal S 1990 The place of special villages and residential communities. AB Academic Publishers, Oxon

Simmons K, Watson D 1999 The view from Arthur's Seat: a literature review of housing and support options 'Beyond Scotland'. The Scottish Office Central Research Unit, The Stationery Office, Edinburgh

Tizard J 1964 Community services for the mentally handicapped. Oxford University Press, London

Williams P 1995 Residential and day services. In: Malin N (ed) Services for people with learning disabilities. Routledge, London, pp 79–110

FURTHER READING

Atkinson D, Jackson M, Walmsley J 1997 Forgotten lives: exploring the history of learning disability. British Institute of Learning Disability, Worcestershire

Duffy S 1996 Unlocking the imagination. Choice Press, London

Jack R 1998 Residential versus community care: the role of institutions in welfare provision. Macmillan Press, London

Pietzner C 1990 A candle on the hill: images of Camphill life. Floris Books, Edinburgh

Segal S 1990 The place of special villages and residential communities. AB Academic Publishers, Oxon

USEFUL ADDRESSES

Readers are advised to search the world wide web sites extensively. There is a wealth of fascinating alternatives that can be found internationally in the ways in which residential services are constructed for people with learning disabilities.

Australia The Australian Society for the Scientific Study of Intellectual Disabilities
http://www.rmit.edu.au/departments/ps/assid/

Belgium Inclusion International
http://users.skynet.be/incluit/

Canada Individualised Funding Information Resources
http://members.home.net/bsalisbury/

Finland National Research and Development Centre for Welfare and Health
http://www.stakes.fi/english/index.html

Germany Lebenshilfe
http://www.lebenshilfe.de/

Netherlands Bisschop Bekkers Instituut
http://www.bbi-utrect.nl/

Norway Full Rulles
http://www.fullrulle.no/index.en.htm

United Kingdom a range of providers randomly selected from the internet
www.intercareresidentaail.co.uk
www.theorchardengroup.co.uk
www.richmond.gov.uk
www.residentail-care-placements.co.uk
www.brookdale-healthcare.co.uk
www.orchard-trust.org.uk
www.larche.org.uk

USA American Association on Mental Retardation
http://aamr.org/

Contact the Department of Health for a free copy of 'An easy guide to Direct Payments', which also comes with audiotape and CD.
Department of Health Publications
PO Box 777
London
SE1 6XH

6

Evaluating the quality of support services for people with learning disabilities

Dave Marsland

KEY ISSUES

- Government policy is increasingly demanding that support services demonstrate their effectiveness in meeting the needs of people with learning disabilities. Practitioners face the problem of how best to explore and demonstrate this effectiveness.

- Different approaches to exploring service effectiveness and evaluating quality focus on different features of the support environment. For example, an evaluation might focus on examining the practice of direct care staff, or it might instead choose to highlight the quality of lifestyle being enjoyed by the people being supported. Choosing an evaluation approach therefore presents something of a dilemma to practitioners.

- This dilemma is further complicated by the context for this kind of quality evaluation. The key ingredient of a support service is a relationship, or set of relationships, between staff and people with learning disabilities. Therefore an evaluation should address the difficult and complex task of exploring and assessing the kinds of relationships that exist within a service.

- Many technologies and methods have been developed for evaluating the quality of support services for people with learning disabilities. Evaluation in itself does not, however, improve services and help people with learning disabilities to enjoy better, fuller lives. Evaluation should be seen as a tool to be used in the overall process of service development and the enabling of people with learning disabilities. An evaluation system can be positively employed as a means to an end and should not be allowed to become an end in itself.

INTRODUCTION

In August 2000 the Department of Health published a consultation paper entitled *A Quality Strategy For Social Care* (DOH 2000). The title and content of this document reflected ongoing concern at central and local government level with monitoring and measuring quality within social support and health services. This concern with quality has been a growing feature of policy and guidance since the early 1990s, but this focus has grown enormously over the last 3 years in particular (DOH 1998, 1999a, 1999b, 1999c, 2000a, 2000b). Other commentators have linked this policy development with a wider social and economic phenomenon described as the growth of consumerism with emphasis on the message of 'Listen to your customers' (McConkey 1996).

This policy development has led to pressure being put on those who commission, as well as those who provide, social and health support services for people with learning disabilities, to demonstrate that services delivered are effective and appropriate. This pressure to demonstrate effectiveness has also been increasingly apparent from the self-advocacy movement, and groups such as CHANGE and Mencap (CHANGE 1998, Mencap 1999). Researchers who seek to work alongside people with learning disabilities have been concerned to develop, and use evaluation to highlight the limitations in the services developed for people with learning disabilities as a consequence of 2 decades of hospital closure. Support services may be better, but they are still not good enough (Emerson 1999).

This growing interest in finding out how good services are, has in turn led to the development of a significant subsection of research and development devoted to improving and implementing evaluation and monitoring systems. For the purposes of this chapter it will be suggested that the definitions of Whittaker and McConkey should be combined. Whittaker's definition reflects a concern to demystify evaluation, and therefore help explain the process to a wide cross-section of people. Therefore, her description of evaluation is 'Looking at how services are working and giving your opinions about what is good and what is not so good' (Whittaker 1997, p. 5). McConkeys' definition highlights that evaluation should seek to explore beyond the surface appearance of things, and in doing so help us to gain a greater understanding of services. He has argued that the goal of evaluation is to 'cast new light on the familiar, and to deepen our insights of the world about us' (McConkey 1996, p. 3). When these definitions are combined therefore, evaluation involves studying the complex sets of circumstances and relationships that make up services and using the knowledge revealed to make a judgement on the effectiveness of those services.

This chapter explores the differences between some of the approaches to evaluation that have been developed, and comments on their potential usefulness to those people involved in providing and commissioning support services. This exploration will be undertaken by considering the issue from the viewpoint of two imaginary professionals (Margaret and Mark, see Box 6.1), who work within a service for adults with learning disabilities.

Our imaginary evaluators have met for an initial meeting to discuss aims and objectives of the

Box 6.1   Milburn Close

Margaret is a manager of small group home for four adults with learning disabilities, known as Milburn Close. She is a qualified Learning Disability Nurse, and has been managing the service since it opened three years ago.

Mark is Quality Assurance Officer for a local authority Social Services department. He has been given responsibility for monitoring and reviewing the services delivered to the people living at Milburn Close. Mark has little experience of residential services for people with learning disabilities but has worked extensively within performance monitoring in both the public and private sector.

The people living in this service had previously lived for most of their lives in a hospital for people with learning disabilities, and their ages range from 35 to 47 years old. Two people are described as having no verbal communication, the other two have difficulties with communication, but are able to use a limited number of words to good effect. One person has no living relatives, but the other three all have families, who take an active interest in the development of the service, some of them visiting weekly.

There are two shifts or teams of direct support staff working at Milburn Close, each with a different shift leader.

One team is made up entirely of staff from the long-stay hospital where the people with learning disabilities had previously resided. The staff in the other team come from a more varied background of community residential and day services for people with learning disabilities. Each team appears to enjoy a different kind of relationship with the people they support. Some of the people living at Milburn Close have clear preferences for individual staff members and prefer different teams.

The local authority has asked all providers of support to develop quality monitoring systems which demonstrate service effectiveness. The local authority is also keen to work in partnership with service providers to promote the development of appropriate monitoring systems. As a result, Margaret and Mark have been asked to work together on a pilot project, which addresses the question of whether evaluation systems can help to indicate how good the service is. At Milburn Close, it is their job to consider the relative merits of the different evaluation systems available and to recommend which system, if any, should be adopted.

---

project and resources available. At this meeting they identified six criteria (see Box 6.2), which they hope will guide them through this process, as well as helping them to make clear and reasoned recommendations to the local authority and regional service manager.

Each of these six criteria are now discussed and explained.

Box 6.2   Criteria governing this evaluation project

- The scope of the evaluation project should not be too large, and should focus on the daily lives and experiences of the people being supported
- The approach adopted should help to compare the quality of support delivered with services of a similar size and design elsewhere
- The evaluation system adopted should involve the direct observation of staff practice
- The evaluation approach adopted should provide some real detail about the lifestyles enjoyed by the people being supported
- The approach adopted should offer everyone concerned the opportunity to take part in the evaluation, especially service users
- The approach adopted should be based on sound research methods and be fair and independent of all interested parties

Reader activity 6.1

Imagine you are receiving long-term support services. What are the most important features of your lifestyle? Which relationships, activities and experiences would you need to maintain in order to ensure your emotional and physical wellbeing?

'THE SCOPE OF THE PROJECT SHOULD NOT BE TOO LARGE AND SHOULD FOCUS ON THE DAILY LIVES AND EXPERIENCES OF THE PEOPLE BEING SUPPORTED'

Margaret and Mark are concerned to ensure that the process of evaluation does not itself become one of the main tasks of the service. They are aiming to achieve a balance in making certain that the process adopted is relatively time-limited but still focuses on exploring the essential elements of the service being delivered. They are also conscious that the project should complement and not duplicate other monitoring and evaluating systems already in existence. For example, the local authority has been developing its Best Value systems in respect of community support services, and these focus on certain aspects of local service provision as a whole (Cambridge 2000).

A question which arises, therefore, is what should the evaluation seek to focus on and measure. What are the essential elements of the support service that affect and influence the daily lives and experiences of people living at Milburn Close? Or more precisely, what is a support service? What does it entail and therefore what should evaluators be seeking to measure?

On one level the answer to this question may be simple and uncontroversial. The service to be evaluated might be described as a staffed group home for four people with moderate to severe learning disabilities. The aims of this service are framed in terms of O'Brien's accomplishments (O'Brien 1987, see Chapter 3) and refer to supporting people to live a valued life in the community. The aims also refer to the service supporting people to participate fully in the running of their home and making full use of ordinary nonsegregated community facilities.

These statements begin to tell us something about what the support service aims to help people to achieve. However, they do not tell us what the mechanism or resource is that helps people with learning disabilities to accomplish their chosen lifestyles. So what is this resource or mechanism? What is it that supports these four people with learning disabilities living at this home to achieve their chosen lifestyles and therefore what is it that our evaluators should seek to measure?

The answer of course is people. The direct support delivered to the people in our example can be viewed as the end result of a number of different individuals' efforts and relationships which all affect and influence the daily lives and experiences of those concerned. Some of these relationships will be close and easily recognisable, whereas others may appear distant, and of little immediate significance. For example, there are paid carers who provide direct support to enable service users to work towards and achieve their chosen lifestyles. Then there are managers of services, such as Margaret, whose relationship with people with learning disabilities is slightly more

distant and less immediate. At the very broadest perspective there are perhaps those individuals with responsibility for commissioning and planning the delivery of learning disability services for the region as a whole. All of these relationships can in some way be shown to have an effect on the daily lives of the people living at Milburn Close.

People and relationships: the context for quality evaluation

Our evaluators are clearly not about to embark on a project that will seek to explore all these different sets of relationships. It is suggested that what is necessary is a framework for describing such sets of relationships which will help them to make an informed choice as to the limits of their project in terms of relationships and people. One way of conceptualising relationships is to imagine layers of increasing complexity surrounding each one of us. These layers are interconnected, and within each layer the people concerned and their mutual relationships are enmeshed together like nests (see Fig. 6.1).

Bronfenbrenner has developed a framework for exploring the position of individuals in the context of systems, or nests of relationships (Bronfenbrenner 1979). In this framework there are four interconnected systems, or nests of relationships, of which the individual citizen is a member. This can help provide a framework for

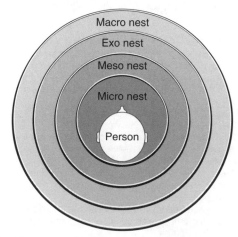

Figure 6.1

considering evaluation approaches, since different systems of evaluation seek to focus on different nests or levels of relationships (Fig. 6.1).

If we apply this model to our example then the Micro nest of relationships refers to an individual service user living at Milburn Close, and the people who have direct and regular contact with that service user. This will encompass each person with a learning disability, the other people who live in the house with them, and the staff who support them.

The Meso nest refers to the other people that these specific service users might encounter in other social settings alongside their primary, or most common social setting. This Meso layer or nest could include, for example, relationships with people who work at day centres, colleges and places of supported employment. A person may be seen to move between a small number of Micro nests or systems during an average week. The Meso system therefore refers to the group or cluster of Micro systems that each individual living at Milburn Close is directly engaged with or participates in.

The Exo system, or nest encompasses individuals or groups of people who work for the local authority social services or education departments, or people who are senior managers in the organisation, delivering staff support to the service users. These individuals may be directly linked to one or more of the Micro systems that service users are engaged in but may never in fact meet the people who live at Milburn Close. This direct link or interconnection with Micro systems ensures that their decisions, policies and actions have a significant impact on the lives of people with learning disabilities.

The final nest identified by Bronfenbrenner is referred to as the Macro nest or system. This Macro system encompasses the predominant culture and social climate in which the Meso systems of a particular region or class exist. This prevailing culture or climate is regarded as having an overarching effect on the relationships and environment within the Micro and Meso systems. For example, the value a society attaches to socially disadvantaged groups, such as people with learning disabilities, is seen to affect the kind of relationships

and lifestyle experienced within each Micro system. This concept of Macro system also explicitly recognises the relationship between the actions of policy makers and the lifestyles enjoyed by people with learning disabilities, since policy is seen to reflect the prevailing social climate.

 Reader activity 6.2

Think about the relationships in your own life and the complex layers, systems and subsystems that you are part of. Can you identify 'nests' for your own context, for your working life and your personal life? Is it easy to see where one system ends and another one begins?

How does this framework help our evaluators to identify an approach or focus?

Margaret and Mark have stated clearly that one of their priorities is to focus on the daily lives and experiences of people with learning disabilities. In light of Bronfenbrenner's model it might be suggested that they should concentrate on approaches to evaluation which focus on relationships within the Meso and Micro nests or levels. They do not have the resources, nor is it necessary, to undertake large regional or national evaluations, such as those undertaken by Social Services Inspectorate or the Department of Health (DOH 1998). Nor do they wish to duplicate the monitoring work being done at the Exo level in their locality in respect of the performance of overall systems and groups of organisations (DOH 1999a, 1999b, Cambridge 2000). Having given consideration to the scope of the project, they will use the remaining five criteria, therefore, to highlight evaluation approaches that address relationships with service users at the Micro and Meso levels.

'THE APPROACH ADOPTED SHOULD HELP TO COMPARE THE QUALITY OF SUPPORT DELIVERED, WITH SERVICES OF A SIMILAR SIZE AND DESIGN ELSEWHERE'

Our imaginary evaluators want the approach adopted to address two central issues in respect of this criterion. First, they hope to achieve some measure of the size and nature of the task being addressed by the team working at Milburn Close. They are interested to find out whether or not it is possible to quantify the demands placed on the staff team by this particular group of service users. Secondly, they hope the approach adopted will provide a picture of the level of resources available, and an indication of the way in which these resources are organised. In the theoretical development of evaluation research methods this interest in resources and their organisation has been usefully described as the study of structure (Donabedian 1980). Evaluation approaches that successfully address these two issues can help to compare the quality of support delivered across a range of different services in a region or locality by ensuring that like is compared with like (Oakes 2000).

Is it possible to measure the size of the task or the job of care support?

Research has identified a number of methods that can be used to explore the levels of need of service users, and by implication, quantify the amount of support necessary. These methods go beyond the more commonly found approaches of classifying services as being high, medium or low dependency, or classifying people as being severely, moderately or mildly disabled. For example the studies of Perry et al have identified four different methods of measuring and describing 'resident characteristics' (Perry et al 2000). These are listed below:

- The Adaptive Behaviour Scale (Nihira et al 1993) has been used to gather information about individuals' skills and abilities across 10 aspects of lifestyle or functioning. For example, a persons' domestic skills can be explored and then given a score or rating reflecting the answers given to a number of set questions.
- The Aberrant Behavior Checklist (Aman & Singh 1986) can be used to gather information about the frequency and/or severity of an individual's perceived behaviour under five headings: irritability, lethargy, hyperactivity, stereotypy, and inappropriate speech.

- The Psychiatric Assessment Schedule (PASAD) for Adults with a Developmental Disability Checklist (Prosser et al 1998) is a checklist used to help to identify people who may already have, or are at risk of developing, mental health problems.
- The Disability Assessment Schedule (Holmes et al 1982) was used by Perry et al to gather information on an individual's social impairments. This schedule of questions contains sections that focus on social interaction, engagement in symbolic activities, stereotypic behaviour and echolalia.

The level and organisation of resources

In keeping with the analysis above it is clear that the most significant resource to be measured and commented on is the staff team. This resource can be considered in many ways but commonly studies consider the total number of staff hours per week available, the numbers of staff on duty at different times of day, the length of their hours and their levels of qualification, training and experience (Cragg and Look 1994, Oakes 2000, Perry et al 2000). A limited number of studies have also tried to identify the length of time that staff have worked alongside service users, and turnover rates across the team. It seems sensible to suggest that the length of time that staff have known service users will affect the depth of the relationship that has been developed.

Perry's study also made use of a number of different ways of examining other aspects of resources available to meet the needs of service users (Perry et al 2000):

- The Characteristics of the Physical Environment Scale (Rotegard et al 1981) can be used to rate the homeliness of each room in the service concerned.
- Programme Analysis of Service Systems 3 (Wolfensberger & Glenn 1975) can be used to assess the physical integration of services into the local community. This measure might address issues such as the service having a sign outside that identifies the house and its occupants as service users. It might also focus atten-

tion on the location of services. For example, it might encourage those concerned to consider whether or not the service is in an area known for a cluster of services associated with socially devalued groups.

- The Working Methods Scale (Felce et al 1997) can be used to gather information about the extent to which the service adopts consistent frameworks and structures to underpin the delivery of its service. For example, individual planning mechanisms for service users are explored and staff supervision systems examined.
- The Group Home Management Schedule (Pratt et al 1979) can be used to measure the extent to which management practices support the delivery of either institutionalised, or individually oriented services. This schedule therefore explores issues such as the extent to which people are treated as a group, and the extent to which daily lifestyles are governed by rigid routines.

Summary

Apparent from the detail above is that there are evaluation measures available that can assist in making comparisons of quality of support across different services. Some of these measures can provide the kind of quantitative information that is required to help compare quality across different services.

However, since many of these measures are reliant on the perceptions of staff and managers it is important to consider the reported reliability of each approach (Perry et al 2000) and its potential usefulness. Some of the systems available may not actually be measuring what they say they are measuring but may be recording the perceptions of staff. For instance, as you may remember, the people living in our example service enjoyed very different relationships with each of the two teams supporting them. Perceptions and attitudes were not consistent across the whole staff team. It is likely, therefore, that different staff may interpret similar behaviours in different ways, according to their relationship and feelings about the person

Reader activity 6.3

Can measures that focus on perceived negative features of people's personalities be positive in outcome for that person? How can people who use measures such as the Aberrant Behavior Checklist ensure that service users have given consent to being measured in this way? Would you agree to being 'measured' in this way?

concerned. These differences in interpretation may affect the validity of some of these measures.

'THE EVALUATION SYSTEM ADOPTED SHOULD INVOLVE THE DIRECT OBSERVATION OF STAFF PRACTICE'

Evaluation should involve focusing on the actual point of contact between service provider and service user. If our imagined evaluators' first criterion reflected an interest in the structure of services, then this criterion focuses on the actual process of support, or point of delivery (Donabedian 1980, Oakes 2000). As has been highlighted already above, this point of delivery takes the form of a relationship, or set of relationships. In effect this criterion means that the evaluation system chosen should involve some attempt to observe and comment on the quality of relationship between staff and service users. Approaches that give emphasis to this difficult and complex task will be considered here, although it should be noted that few studies have addressed this issue (Golden and Reese 1996, McConkey et al 1999, Oakes 2000, Purcell et al 2000, Raynes et al 1979).

Observing staff interaction with service users

The study of care organisations for people with learning disabilities by Raynes, Pratt & Rose (1979) was one of the first studies to recognise the significance of direct observation of staff practice. They regarded staff interaction with service users as one of the key aspects or dimensions of care to be measured. Their approach suggested that staff communication can be coded according to its content, and therefore be commented on as to its effectiveness in supporting service users. They recorded their observations of interaction under the following headings:

1. *Information exchange* referred to occasions when staff gave service users information or explanation.
2. *Controlling speech* referred to occasions when staff gave positive or negative commands.
3. *Other speech* referred to occasions when staff engaged service users in casual conversation.
4. *No talk* was a measure of the amount of time when staff did not interact with service users at all.
5. *Did the service user reply?* Represented an attempt to gauge the possible comprehension of the person with learning disabilities.
6. Other details such as the room they were in and the number of other staff present were recorded.

Later approaches to research in this area have built on this early example and extended aspects of the observation method, which may be of relevance to the service being considered in this chapter. For instance, the evaluation system developed by Oakes (Oakes 2000) has sought to modify the approach of Raynes by coding examples of nonverbal interaction observed as well as recording the language-based communication. Alongside this adaptation to Raynes' formal coding system, the system developed by Oakes also asks the observer to comment on the social communication styles used by staff. For example, the extent to which communication observed is characterised by give and take, and equal participation between partners. This interest in social communication partnerships reflects an attempt to incorporate findings from developmental psychology and specifically the work of MacDonald (1990).

The work of David Felce and others at the Welsh Centre for Learning Disabilities has developed the observation of staff to observation of resident interaction, the better to explore the issue of service user engagement in leisure, domestic and household activities (Felce 1996). Their approach has highlighted the amount of interaction received by residents, and evaluated the content of that communication with respect to whether or not it supported service users to take part in activities (Felce 1999).

Summary

It is suggested that Margaret and Mark could indeed identify approaches to direct observation that would help them to gain an important insight into the practice and particularly the communication styles of staff. If, as it is argued here, these relationships are taken to be the fundamental component in a support service, then it is crucial to find some way of observing these relationships in action. The methods developed for this kind of enquiry are far from perfect and further refinement is necessary, particularly with regard to observing staff interaction with people who do not use verbal communication. The process of observing staff practice is dependent on an open and consenting partnership between the evaluator and the people being observed. Therefore, the process adopted will need to be carefully explained and be introduced to the direct care staff and service users concerned.

'THE EVALUATION APPROACH ADOPTED SHOULD PROVIDE SOME REAL DETAILS ABOUT THE LIFESTYLES ENJOYED BY THE PEOPLE WITH LEARNING DISABILITIES BEING SUPPORTED'

Margaret and Mark have identified two possible benefits that may be achieved as a result of the evaluation project producing information describing the lifestyles enjoyed by the people supported by this team. First, they wish to be able to compare the lifestyles of the people living here with those enjoyed by service users elsewhere. Secondly, it is hoped that this detail of daily life will help staff to reflect on the differences between the lifestyles that they themselves enjoy, and the contrasting experiences of people with learning disabilities. Their concerns reflect the sensible priority that much of the information produced should be meaningful and understandable to all people involved. As has been written elsewhere, they are keen to work in way which provides a 'down-to-earth look at services from the point of view of a person using the service – what is happening in people's lives now – how do they feel about their lives – what do they want in the future' (Whittaker et al 1991, p. vii).

There are potentially an infinite number of different ways in which lifestyle outcomes can be measured. For the purposes of this chapter, however, it is suggested that two main areas or types of enquiry be considered. Firstly, it is suggested that research-based approaches that explore the quality of life and/or life experiences should be considered. Secondly, it is suggested that approaches that have been developed involving extensive input from service users should be considered. These evaluation systems or projects have very often sought to highlight the observable lifestyle outcomes for people with learning disabilities (Ager 1990, Raynes et al 1994, Schalock et al 1989, Schalock 1996).

Quality of life measures

Attempts to develop ways of measuring the quality of life enjoyed by people with learning disabilities have proliferated over the last 2 decades. The appeal of these approaches seems to stem from their attempt to bring in some experiential or real life evidence to the study of quality. A study by Perry & Felce (1995), which explored different quality of life assessments, has suggested that the supporters regard measuring quality of life as something of a Holy Grail: 'The quality of life of service users has been increasingly proposed as the ultimate criterion for the assessment of the effectiveness of social care delivery in the field of learning disabilities' (Perry & Felce 1995).

This study by Perry & Felce (1995) identified six different groupings for the quality of life measures explored. These were quality of housing, social and community integration, social interactions, development, activity, and autonomy and choice (Perry & Felce 1995). Each measure might involve a researcher asking a set of questions of service users or staff, or making judgements in respect of physical or structural aspects of the environment. For instance, the Index of Community Involvement is a short checklist designed to measure the extent to which service users are involved in social and community based activities. Respondents are asked about which activities they have taken part in over the last 4 weeks from a predetermined checklist. This checklist, for example, refers to going shopping or to the cinema and asks whether service users have been on holiday in the last year (Perry & Felce 1995, Myles et al 2000).

It is suggested here that if our evaluators chose one aspect to prioritise such as 'community integration' then they could identify a quality of life measure that could give them evidence of lifestyle outcome that they desire. However, despite the advantage of producing information that can be understood and related to by all concerned, there are some critical issues that should be considered. Is it possible to reach agreement on what constitutes a good quality of life? Can people really sit down with their neighbours and say that their own quality of life is better or worse than theirs? There are those who have argued that the attempt to measure quality of life should be abandoned altogether due to such conceptual difficulties and other problems (Hatton 1998).

Hatton (1998) has made two fundamental criticisms of quality of life measures. First, he has suggested that there are unresolveable methodological problems associated with measuring or assessing subjective indicators of quality of life, which mean that results for one person or one service cannot meaningfully be compared with results elsewhere. Moreover, he has argued that the emphasis within quality of life measures on combining subjective with objective indicators tend to exclude those who cannot verbalise their preferences and feelings (Hatton 1998, pp 105–107). Secondly, he has pointed out that the apparent scientific basis to quality of life evaluation can be used to the detriment of people with learning disabilities. There is a danger that the concept of quality of life can be applied to compare the possible outcomes of decisions within the health and welfare services. Hatton cited the example of treatment being denied to children with Down syndrome since it might be perceived that their quality of life would be less than a child without learning disabilities (Hatton 1998).

Service user led outcome measures

...structures and systems are only a means to an end. The end, after all is what matters, and the end is outcomes for service users (Beresford et al 1996, p. 12).

As this quote demonstrates, some would clearly advise evaluators to focus their undivided attention on exploring the lifestyle outcomes for the people with learning disabilities concerned. It is, after all, good outcomes that interest service users and not necessarily the processes employed by an organisation in bringing about such outcomes. The paper by Beresford et al also proposes that service users should have a key role in defining what a good outcome might be (Beresford et al 1996). In other words, it is also crucial to identify and then measure the lifestyle outcomes that really matter to the people being supported. What is a desirable outcome for a service user may be very different from a desirable outcome from the perspective of the social worker involved.

A number of different projects have sought to address this issue and have generally devised questionnaire-based approaches which seek to explore the feelings and perceptions of those who receive services (Leeds Coalition 1996, The Quality Network 1998, Question Time Group 1997, Whittaker et al 1991). These service user focused approaches to evaluation usually comprise two key stages which reflect the concerns highlighted by Beresford above.

The first stage entails meeting with people with learning disabilities and helping them to identify what matters to them. Most often this has been done with an external group of people with learning disabilities, perhaps a self-advocacy group, rather than the recipients of the specific service in question. These issues of importance are then written up in the form of lifestyle standards or desirable outcomes. For example, the work done by the Question Time Group in Leeds identified thirteen such standards to check. These included:

- 'People go to work'

- 'People do their own shopping'
- 'There are parties or social nights with music' (Question Time Group 1997, p. 6).

Another project known as the Quality Network worked with people with learning disabilities and other stakeholders to identify ten outcomes to be explored. These included:

- 'I have friendships and relationships'
- 'I am part of my local community'
- 'I make everyday choices' (Quality Network 1998).

It is interesting to note that when this kind of exercise has been carried out the issues identified have been remarkably consistent (CHANGE 1998, HELP 2001, Leeds Coalition 1996, The Quality Network 1998, Question Time Group 1997, Whittaker 1997). This consistency supports the notion that any list of outcomes identified is likely to reflect overarching human concerns, rather than highlighting issues that may be of significance only to people with learning disabilities. This should be of no great surprise as some people with learning disabilities have long argued that their needs and priorities are no different from anyone else's.

The second stage in this type of process involves using these outcomes as a guide against which to measure people's lifestyles. In some situations this has meant independent groups of people with learning disabilities being supported to explore the lifestyle outcomes of their peers. (Question Time Group 1997, Whittaker et al 1991). In other situations the evaluation process is explicitly internal and based on the premise of self-review. For example, the Quality Network approach involves the service provider taking the lead in setting up a reviewing process that involves service users, staff, family members and other stakeholders. This reviewing process uses the outcomes developed in stage one to provide a framework with which to ask people questions about their lives (Quality Network 2000).

The service user focused approaches described above can be readily adapted to provide interested parties with information about lifestyles and the priorities of individuals or specific groups of people with learning disabilities. The process of identifying the priorities of people with learning disabilities might in itself help staff involved to reflect upon the similarities between their own aspirations and wishes and those of the people they support.

Most evaluation or service review systems attempt to incorporate some measure of lifestyle outcome for the service users concerned (CHANGE 1998, Cragg & Look 1994, Oakes 2000). The preceding examples already described are useful, in that they place great emphasis on measuring outcomes and providing details as well as recording perceptions of service users.

'THE APPROACH ADOPTED SHOULD OFFER EVERYONE CONCERNED THE OPPORTUNITY TO TAKE PART IN THE EVALUATION, ESPECIALLY SERVICE USERS'

Our evaluators are keen to involve everyone who is directly linked to the service in the quality monitoring project. For example, they will seek to involve all staff who work in the service, and invite parents and friends to take a role. However, their overwhelming concern is to ensure that the people being supported by the service are helped to take part in the process.

It has been demonstrated, in this chapter, that some evaluation systems do encourage and to some extent even rely on the active participation of service users. For instance, some of the quality of life measures outlined earlier are based on questionnaire type interviews with service users, which explore key aspects of a person's lifestyle. The same is true of many of the service user led lifestyle measures previously described. These kinds of evaluation system can be effective in involving people with learning disabilities who are able to comprehend and then answer questions or take part in interviews or discussions. However, two of the people in our example service do not use recognisable language to communicate their thoughts and feelings. Of the remaining two people, there may be significant differences in their level of understanding and ability to put their feelings into words. Many people with learn-

ing disabilities are not used to being asked for their comments on their service, and may not therefore have the confidence to express negative opinions. Therefore, an approach that relies heavily on service users being able to answer a questionnaire will be unlikely to satisfy our evaluators' criteria.

Their concern to focus on direct practice (criterion 3) may have already identified some evaluation methods that do involve the participation of service users, regardless of communication or intellectual abilities. Any system of evaluation that focuses on the interaction between staff and service users will inevitably involve the participation of the people being supported. This participation, however, can at best be described as passive, and may be indicated solely by the fact that service users have not chosen to withdraw from the place of observation or withdraw their consent.

Two other tentative, albeit imperfect, evaluation options are suggested here in response to the issue of involving people who need the highest levels of support. First, it is suggested that one way of ensuring a limited amount of participation from people who are non-verbal is to spend time being with them and gaining a picture of their lifestyles, their priorities and their wishes. There are a small number of systems that do ask evaluators to devote a high proportion of their time to being with service users and getting to know them.

For example, the approach to evaluation developed by Oakes places significant emphasis on the need to 'build a working relationship with the people who live and work in the house' (Oakes 1998, p. 7). To this end he has suggested that evaluators should visit the service and meet people on a number of separate occasions and take advantage of any opportunity to make informal contacts. This contact should include taking part in the daily routines of life, perhaps sharing an evening meal, or taking part in other activities (Oakes 1998, p. 7).

Secondly, some systems of quality evaluation have explicitly aimed to secure the participation of the people who receive services, regardless of skills and abilities (Millner 1991, Quality Network

2000). For example, the Quality Action Group approach developed in the late 1980s suggested that all those concerned with a service should come together to address consumer satisfaction in a meaningful and dynamic way. It was suggested that the Quality Action Group would:

provide one mechanism for considering service quality from the point of view of the service user. They provide a framework in which service users meet regularly with staff, relatives, professionals, advocates and members of the local community to look at quality of the service they are getting (Millner 1991, p. 13).

The purpose of a Quality Action Group is to bring all stakeholders together to think about what the service should be doing and then to monitor and review the service being delivered. This reviewing process then identifies areas of development for the team, which are then worked upon by all concerned and then re-evaluated. People who are non-verbal or who need help to communicate are helped to take part in Quality Action Groups by the involvement of independent advocates. Many of the principles of this participative, cyclical approach have been taken up by the current Quality Network system (Quality Network 1998, 2000).

Summary

Pressure from people with learning disabilities has begun to ensure that service users are increasingly involved in research and development (Barnes 1992, 1996). This imperative now includes research into methods of evaluating services. Recently developed approaches to evaluation have acknowledged and acted on this imperative and recognised the importance of working alongside people with learning disabilities (Oakes 2000, Quality Network 1998, 2000).

However, people who are described as non-verbal or who have difficulty communicating still find themselves excluded from such processes. It is unlikely that our evalautors will come across some magical technical innovation which will make this possible. At present the most positive approaches are based on ensuring the involvement of an independent advocate. However, large numbers of people with learning disabilities who

might benefit from receiving support from an advocate may never be able to secure such help. The challenge remains for evaluators of services and service providers to work with people with learning disabilities to develop better ways of involving people who need most support to communicate.

'THE APPROACH ADOPTED SHOULD BE BASED ON SOUND RESEARCH METHODS AND BE SEEN BY ALL CONCERNED TO BE FAIR AND INDEPENDENT OF ALL INTERESTED PARTIES'

It is essential for our evaluators that the project's findings should be seen as legitimate by all concerned and therefore enjoy the support of all interested parties. If these findings are seen to be biased, or to closely reflect the agenda of one of the professional groups involved, then it is unlikely that any conclusions will be acted upon successfully. Indeed, it is partly this desire for objectivity that has led Margaret and Mark to consider research-based approaches to evaluation as a response to the question of how good the service is. Within this central theme of legitimacy there are two aspects that should be addressed.

First, it is necessary to reassure all parties concerned that any research-based evaluation system recommended has been proven to be valid and reliable. Valid means that the evaluation system measures that which it is designed to measure. Reliable, in this context, means that the system has been proven to be consistent, and therefore will highlight the same findings regardless of who is undertaking the evaluation, or when it is taking place. For instance, if one wants to measure homeliness of services, then the criteria used must enjoy a broad level of support and agreement amongst all interested parties for it to be valid. For the measure to be reliable one must demonstrate that when used on separate occasions the results gained in respect of this homeliness were broadly similar.

It has been argued that the Programme Analysis of Service Systems, PASS3, (Wolfensberger & Glenn 1975) has been shown to be reliable and valid despite apparent difficulties in its use and application (Oakes 2000). Another approach developed in America, the Multiphasic Environmental Assessment Procedure (Timko & Moos 1991), has been shown to be reliable and valid, and for this reason has been used as a component in longitudinal studies of lifestyle change for people with learning disabilities (Conroy 1996). In Britain a system known as Quest (Oakes 1998, 2000) has been shown to be valid and reliable and has been applied to the evaluation of community-based services, as well as larger institutional provision.

Secondly, it may be necessary and beneficial to involve an independent external agency to help to reassure people of the validity and fairness of the approach and findings. There are a number of agencies and approaches that might be worthy of consideration in this context. Some learning disability organisations with a national focus offer support to people wishing to evaluate services. For example, the Quality Network system has been developed with support from the National Development Team and the British Institute of Learning Disabilities (Quality Network 1998). Other systems have been developed with support and scrutiny from Universities and Research Institutes (Felce et al 1991, Oakes 1998, 2000).

Our evaluators might also consider approaching local self-advocacy or citizen advocacy groups to ask them if they would be prepared to act as external independent verifiers of the project. Established groups such as People First have been successfully engaged in evaluation projects for some years, and many individual members have gained much expertise and knowledge (Whittaker et al 1991, Whittaker 1997).

An important issue to consider at this point might be the potential cost of securing support from an external agency. In this respect a locally based self-advocacy group may have some clear advantages when compared to other options.

Summary

This last criterion raises some significant problems for our evaluators. Few evaluation systems that might be appropriate have, in fact, been vigorously tested for reliability and/or research validity. This is particularly the case in respect of approaches developed by those within the self-advocacy movement where emphasis has understandably been placed on exploring the lifestyles and feelings of service users. However, as noted earlier, such approaches are often reliant on service users being able to comprehend and verbally respond to questions. On the other hand those approaches that have proven research robustness may involve greater cost to the service, or to social services. Therefore, if Margaret and Mark wish to pursue this criterion they may either have to abandon key aspects of it, or they may have to work hard to secure the resources necessary to buy in external support.

CONCLUSION

Most of the methods of evaluation described in this chapter could help those concerned to reflect on how good the service is at Milburn Close. Different approaches clearly choose to highlight different aspects of the service and the outcomes for service users. However, it is evident that no single system will meet all our desired criteria for evaluation. For example, the service user focused approaches that identify real lifestyle outcomes for people do not involve the direct observation of staff practice. There are similar limitations to most of the research-based quality of life measures. Other systems such as the Quest system (Oakes 2000) may not highlight enough detail of lifestyle outcomes to help staff reflect on the differences between their experiences and those of the people they support. Therefore, recommendations for any envisaged evaluation project will probably need to adopt a combination of systems or approaches.

Such a combination of methods might have the advantage of encouraging those concerned to reflect on the quality of the service from a number of different perspectives, rather than focusing on one dimension of quality. A possible disadvantage might be that such a combination approach could prove to be expensive and use a lot of staff time. It is inevitable that the application of evaluation systems to explore the quality of a support service will involve an input of staff hours, and some extra costs to the service. However, it does not seem sensible to make demands on staff teams to such an extent that they are impeded in their daily duties, thus actually helping to detract from the service offered. This would seem to undermine the purpose of evaluation.

Consideration of this implicit purpose of evaluation should be the true guide to people like Margaret and Mark. What must be remembered is that the aim of evaluation is to provide information to those concerned so that improvements can be made, and the support service made better. Evaluation should be seen as the means to an end, and not an end in itself. For example, if the information provided does not help stakeholders to identify the need for potential changes in the process of service delivery, or in the underlying structure of the service, then it is unlikely that outcomes for those being supported will be enhanced. Many outcomes-based approaches will indeed be able to identify what is and what is not happening in the lives of the people with learning disabilities. However, these approaches often do not attempt to consider the reasons why certain lifestyle outcomes are not being achieved. On the other hand, other studies have concluded there is little evidence to suggest that process- or practice-focused approaches to evaluation are any better at addressing this core purpose of achieving positive change (Oakes 2000).

It has been maintained throughout this chapter that a key determinant of service quality is the relationships that exist between staff and the people they support. This notion is supported by examples from service users groups which have found that what is most important is not so much what staff are doing, but the way that they are doing it, and also who is delivering the support (HELP 2001). Therefore, to achieve change in the quality of support service it follows that the nature of these relationships must change in some way. For instance, it may be that an evaluation identifies that direct support staff in a service do little to enable or empower those that they support. In essence they might be working in a controlling and protective manner and consequently offer people few choices or opportunities to take decisions. It is one thing to identify that relationships are characterised in this way, but it is a far more difficult and complex task to begin to change the nature of these relationships.

It is suggested that those considering the possible application of evaluation methods should hold these difficult and complex issues in mind from the outset. If an evaluation system can be found which can help all concerned to reflect on their relationships then that might be a positive place to begin. If this system can also highlight, recognise and perhaps reward staff for their effort to develop positive, empowering relationships then this added dimension might be of immense benefit. The problem is that although some evaluation systems have begun to address this issue, most have concentrated instead on aspects of quality that can more easily be measured and addressed. There are many evaluation systems that can assist service providers and commissioners to explore quality of support services, from numerous different perspectives. If a suitable approach cannot be found that focuses on exploring the relationships between the people concerned, then perhaps it would be wiser simply to ask those being supported whether or not they are happy with their service, and spend the money and time saved on other things.

REFERENCES

Ager A 1988 Life experiences and quality of life in the general population: a study of undergraduate students using the life experiences checklist. Mental Handicap Research Group Working Paper 3, University of Leicester

Ager A 1990 Life experiences checklist. NFER Nelson, Windsor

Aman M, Singh N 1986 The aberrant behavior checklist. Slosson Educational Publications, New York

Barnes C 1992 Qualitative research: valuable or irrelevant? Disability Handicap and Society 7: 115–124

Barnes C 1996 Disability and the myth of the independent researcher. Disability and Society 11: 107–110

Beresford P, Croft S, Evans C, Harding T 1996 The quality that matters – enabling service users to define successful outcomes. Care Plan September 1996

Bronfenbrenner U 1979 The ecology of human development: experiments by nature and design. Harvard University Press, London

Cambridge P 2000 Using 'best value' in purchasing and providing services for people with learning disabilities. British Journal of Learning Disabilities, 28: 31–37

CHANGE 1998 Our lives our standards: national quality standards. CHANGE, London

Conroy J 1996 Results of deinstitutionalization in Connecticut. In: Mansell J, Ericsson K (eds) Deinstitutionalisation and community living: intellectual disability services in Britain, Scandinavia and the USA. Chapman and Hall, London

Cragg R, Look R 1994 Compass : a multi-perspective evaluation of quality in home life. Wolverley NHS Trust, Kidderminster

Department of Health 1998 Modernising social services. Department of Health, London

Department of Health 1999a Personal social services performance assessment framework. Department of Health, London

Department of Health 1999b Better care, higher standards – a charter for long-term care. Department of Health, London

Department of Health 1999c Facing the facts: services for people with learning difficulties. Department of Health, London

Department of Health 2000 A quality strategy for social care. Department of Health, London

Department of Health 2000a Performance assessment 2000–01 – a guide. Department of Health. Available online at www.doh.gov.uk/scg/pssperform

Department of Health 2000b Guide to quality schemes and best value. DETR, IDeA and DOH, London

Donabedian A 1980 Explorations in quality assessment and monitoring. Vol 1 The definition of quality and approaches to its assessment. Health Administration Press, Ann Arbor, Michigan

Emerson E 1999 Good but not good enough. Community Living (October/November)

Felce D 1996 Quality of support for ordinary living. In: Mansell J, Ericsson K (eds) Deinstitutionalization and community living: intellectual disability services in Britain, Scandinavia and the USA. Chapman and Hall, London

Felce O 1999 The Gerry Simon Lecture, 1998: Enhancing the quality of life of people receiving residential support. British Journal of Learning Disabilities 27: 4–9

Felce D, Repp A, Thomas M, Ager A, Blunden R 1991 The relationship of staff : client ratios, interactions and residential placement. Research in Developmental Disabilities 12: 315–331

Felce D, Lowe K, Perry J, Emerson E 1997 The working methods scale (revised). Welsh Centre for Learning Disabilities, Cardiff

Golden J, Reese M, 1996 Focus on communication: improving interaction between staff and residents who have severe or profound mental retardation. Research in Developmental Disabilities 17(5): 363–382

Hatton C 1998 Whose quality of life is it anyway? Some problems with the emerging quality of life consensus. Mental Retardation 36(2): 104–115

HELP Helping Empower Lincolnshire People 2001 Our meetings: what are good services. HELP, Lincoln

Holmes N, Shah A, Wing L 1982 The Disability Assessment Schedule: a brief screening device for use with the mentally retarded. Psychological Medicine 2(4): 879–890

Leeds Coalition 1996 What would make services good? Quality standards in services for people with learning disabilities – a user perspective. Leeds Coalition, Leeds

McConkey R 1996 New perspectives on evaluation. In: McConkey R (ed) Innovations in evaluating services for people with intellectual disabilities. Lisieux Hall, Chorley

McConkey R, Morris I, Purcell M 1999 Communications between staff and adults with intellectual disabilities in naturally occurring settings. Journal of Intellectual Disability Research 43(3): 194–205

MacDonald J 1990 An ecological model for social and communicative partnerships. In: Schroeder S (ed) Ecobehavioural analysis and developmental disabilities: the twenty first century. Springer-Verlag, New York

MENCAP 1999 (video) What's good support? Helping people to speak out. Mental Health Media and MENCAP, London

Millner L 1991 Collective action. LLAIS 22: 13–14

Myles S, Ager A, Kerr P, Myers F, Walker J 2000 Moving home: costs associated with different models of accommodation for adults with learning disabilities. Health and Social Care in the Community 8(6): 406–416

Nihira K, Leland H, Lambert N 1993 AAMD Adaptive Behaviour Scale, 2nd edn. American Association on Mental Deficiency, Washington DC

Oakes P 1998 Quest: users' guide. University of Hull, Hull

Oakes P 2000 Quest: a system of evaluation for residential support services for people with learning disabilities. Journal of Learning Disabilities 4(1): 7–26

O'Brien J 1987 A guide to lifestyle planning. In: Wilcox B, Bellamy G T (eds) Comprehensive guide to the activities catalog. Paul H Brookes, Baltimore

Perry J, Felce D 1995 Objective assessments of quality of life: how much do they agree with each other? Journal of Community and Applied Social Psychology 5: 1–19

Perry J, Lowe K, Felce D, Jones S 2000 Characteristics of staffed housing for people with learning disabilities: a stratified random sample of statutory, voluntary and private agency provision. Health and Social Care in the Community 8(5): 307–315

Pratt M W, Luszcz M A, Brown M E 1979 Measuring the dimensions of the quality of care in small community residences. American Journal of Mental Deficiency 85: 188–194

Prosser H, Moss S, Costello H, Simpson N, Patel P 1998 The psychiatric assessment schedule for adults with a developmental disability (PAS-ADD) checklist. Hester Adrian Research Centre, University of Manchester

Purcell P, McConkey R, Morris I 2000 Staff communication with people with intellectual disabilities: the impact of a work-based training programme. International Journal of Language and Communication Disorders 35(1): 147–158

The Quality Network 1998 Our lives: a framework of outcomes for services used by people with learning disabilities. British Institute of Learning Disabilities and National Development Team, Oxford

The Quality Network 2000 Introduction to the quality network. Available online at www.qualitynetwork.org.uk

Question Time Group 1997 Report of service checks. Question Time Group/Leeds Coalition, Leeds

Raynes N, Pratt M, Roses S 1979 Organisational structure and the care of the mentally retarded. Croom Helm, London

Raynes N, Wright K, Shiell A, Pettipher C 1994 The cost and quality of community residential care. David Fulton, London

Rotegard L L, Bruininks R H, Hill B K 1981 Environmental characteristics of residential facilities for mentally retarded people. University of Minnesota, Minneapolis

Schalock R (ed) 1996 Quality of life: vol 1: Conceptualisation and measurement. AAMR, Washington

Schalock R, Keith K, Hoffman K, Karan O 1989 Quality of life: its measurement and its use. Mental Retardation 1: 25–31

Timko C, Moos R H 1991 Assessing the quality of residential programs: methods and applications. Adult Residential Care Journal 5: 113–129

Whittaker A (ed) 1997 Looking at our services: service evaluation by people with learning difficulties. Kings Fund Centre, London

Whittaker A, Gardner S, Kershaw J 1991 Service evaluation by people with learning difficulties. Kings Fund Centre, London

Wolfensberger W, Glen L 1975 Programme analysis of service systems: handbook and manual, 3rd edn. National Institute on Mental Retardation, Toronto

FURTHER READING

'Innovations in Evaluating Services for People with Intellectual Disabilities' edited by Roy McConkey (1996) is an excellent collection of studies highlighting approaches to and methods of evaluation. The collection includes perspectives on evaluation from a number of different countries as well as focusing on identifying the main stakeholders to involve.

'Looking At Our Services: Service evaluation by people with learning difficulties' edited by Andrea Whittaker gives very useful advice and guidance to those who might wish to support people with learning disabilities to take part in service evaluation. This book is useful in that it does discuss some of the problems and difficulties involved in service user evaluation whilst emphasising throughout that involvement of people with learning disabilities is possible and necessary.

'Our Lives Our Standards: National Quality Standards (1998)' produced by CHANGE is a useful publication since people with learning disabilities identified the standards contained in it themselves. These CHANGE standards have been used frequently by the author to help staff teams and other professionals to think about what matters most to people receiving support services.

USEFUL ADDRESSES

www.qualitynetwork.org.uk
www.jrf.org.uk
www.learningdisabilities.org.uk

www.rnld.co.uk
www.doh.gov.uk
www.bris.ac.uk/Depts/NorahFry/

7

Compulsory school education

David Dickinson, Linda Dickinson

KEY ISSUES

- The provision of effective education for young people with learning disabilities continues to be the subject of considerable debate and development.
- The right of access to an education that meets an individual learner's needs has placed far-reaching demands upon professional knowledge and practice since that right was originally enshrined in UK legislation in the mid 1940s. It has taken several decades to reach the levels of sophistication of approach to education for all learners that we recognise and expect in the 21st century, and there is still a significant pace of development, particularly in the provision of effective special education for children with learning disabilities.
- Effective education is a complex process. Teaching is far more than the imparting of knowledge and skill: it relies upon sophisticated approaches to assessment and intervention that recognise the particular learning needs of the individual.
- This chapter explores how educational legislation and the development of professional practice currently supports the process of meeting the individual and special educational needs of children with learning disabilities.

INTRODUCTION

Since the late 1970s there have been significant developments in special education. There have been major changes in thinking about how to provide education for children with learning disabilities, and these changes have had far-reaching effects upon professional practice.

The concept of special educational need: Warnock and the 1981 Education Act

The Warnock Report (1978) and the 1981 Education Act marked fundamental changes in approaches to the education of children with learning disabilities. Establishing a government committee of enquiry into special education, chaired by Mary Warnock was, in large part, a response to concerns that:

- Special education had focused for many years upon children's 'handicapping' conditions, rather than individual needs. This focus often detracted attention from the children's abilities and aptitudes and served to set children with learning disabilities apart from those considered to be learning normally.
- This approach had led to the formation of statutory categories of handicap into which children with disabilities were placed. The development of special schools designed to cater for the categories of handicap led to the further separation of children with disabilities from those considered to be learning normally. This segregation of children with disabilities potentially limited their access to a broad and balanced curriculum.
- There were many more children with learning disabilities in the education system than the relatively small number attending special schools.
- The support professionals (medical, psychological, educational and social) employed to identify and categorise children's handicaps might be better deployed in the long-term support of their education.
- There was limited formal involvement of parents in the educational decisions taken for their children.

The key recommendations of the Warnock report included the following:

- Abolition of the statutory categories of handicap and an end to the distinction between 'handicapped' and 'non-handicapped' children.
- The introduction of the concept of 'special educational need', focusing attention on the individual learning needs of children rather than their handicapping condition. Special educational needs should take into account the child's existing abilities and the need for special facilities and resources in order to maximise the child's learning.
- The recognition that approximately 20% of children will experience some form of special educational need at some time in their school career.
- Wherever possible, children's special educational needs should be met in ordinary schools. There was also a recognition that approximately 2% of children may experience significant learning difficulties that would require their special needs to be met in a special school.
- Special schools should continue to play an important role in meeting the special educational needs of those children for whom the facilities and resources did not exist in ordinary schools. This role should broaden to include active collaboration with ordinary schools.
- The introduction of a staged approach to the assessment of special need, initially involving the child, parent and the teacher and moving through the stages to involve outside agencies and local education authority resources.

The 1981 Education Act responded to the Warnock Committee recommendations in a number of ways. Legislation did indeed abolish the statutory categories of handicap, and these were replaced by a formal recognition of a concept of special educational need (this will be explored in more detail later in the chapter). Furthermore, the 1981 Act instituted a process of assessment, based upon the Warnock 'stages'. Local education authorities were charged with the duty to identify the needs of children (aged 2–19) through a process of multidisciplinary assessment involving parents, teachers, educational psychologists, medical professionals and the social services. If a child was identified as having a significant level of need, then the LEA was required to make appropriate arrangements for provision. The making of a statement, a legally binding document identifying the needs of the child and stating how the LEA intended to meet those needs, safeguarded these arrangements. Significantly, the 1981 Act also gave formal recognition to the Warnock recommendation that, wherever possible, the special educational needs of children should be met in ordinary schools.

In many senses, therefore, the Warnock Committee and the 1981 Education Act served to change the emphasis of special education away from where the child's needs should be met to how they should be met. The focus was now more upon the facilities and resources required to meet identified needs, and more attention was turned to the capacity of ordinary schools to provide for children with learning disabilities.

INTEGRATION/INCLUSION VERSUS SEGREGATION/EXCLUSION

The term 'integration' was coined in the Warnock Report to refer to the processes involved in meeting special needs in an ordinary school. There has been much debate (e.g. Portwood 1995) since the Warnock Report about the ways in which integration can be achieved, and the continuing purpose of segregation (i.e. the process of meeting needs in special schools etc.). Some have argued that all needs could be met in ordinary schools, given appropriate levels of resources (Dessent 1987, Sayer 1983a, 1983b), yet segregation continues to be a feature of the educational system. Although the statutory categories of handicap were abolished by the 1981 Education Act, special schools in many areas of the country continue to provide for categories of learning difficulty (e.g. severe and moderate learning difficulties, emotional and behavioural difficulties).

The capacity of ordinary schools to respond to wider ranges of special educational needs has undoubtedly increased since the 1981 Education Act. Parents are more aware of their rights to expect access to ordinary schools for their children (reinforced by the 1993 and 1998 Education Acts and the Special Educational Needs and Disability Act 2001 – see later in the chapter). Consequently there are more children in ordinary schools with a wider range of learning needs. This has placed considerable demands upon the processes of multidisciplinary professional support for children, their schools and parents.

In order to ensure that children receive appropriate support in an integrated setting, it is important that all professionals involved understand precisely what is meant by 'integration'. Warnock outlined three fundamental aspects of integration:

- Locational integration. This is where a special school or class is located on the same campus as an ordinary school.
- Social integration. This is where children with special learning needs may enjoy contact with children with ordinary learning needs, but there are no formal arrangements for them to learn together in the same classes.
- Functional integration. This form of integration is the most sophisticated. Children with a wide range of learning needs across the spectrum from ordinary to special learn together in the same classes. At its most sophisticated, functional integration demands the provision of differentiated approaches to the teaching of individual children. These differentiated approaches recognise the learning needs of individuals and provide the right level of access to a curriculum that all children in the class are following. This, of course, places considerable demands upon teachers' skills and approaches to learning needs.

The demands created by functional integration (mainly upon resources, teacher skills and organisation in ordinary schools) have meant that for some children the most appropriate place for their education has continued to be in a segregated special school. It is important to remember, however, that there is formal and legislative recognition that, wherever possible, children should have their needs met in ordinary schools. This continues to provide an impetus to the process of enhancing the capacity of ordinary schools to meet a wider range of needs.

The concept of 'inclusion' has more recently superseded that of 'integration'. Given formal recognition by central government in the late 1990s as a wide ranging human right, inclusion and more particularly social inclusion, has been a driving value for much of UK social legislation. The National Curriculum Inclusion Statement (see below for detail) outlines three key principles for inclusive education:

1. setting suitable learning challenges
2. responding to pupils' diverse learning needs
3. overcoming potential barriers to learning and assessment for individuals and groups of pupils.

Special Education has benefited from this drive, with the universal right to social inclusion underpinning the provisions of the Special Educational Needs (SEN) and Disability Act 2001. This legislation provided;

- strengthened rights for all children to be educated in a mainstream school
- new duties on Local Education Authorities to provide advice, information and processes for resolution of disputes regarding SEN, for parents and children
- a duty for schools to prohibit discrimination against disabled children in any of its policies and procedures for admissions, general education and exclusions
- a duty for schools to take reasonable steps to ensure that children with disabilities are not disadvantaged or treated less favourably than children who are not disabled
- a right for schools to request a statutory assessment of a child's special educational needs.

MULTIDISCIPLINARY ASSESSMENT AND STATEMENTS

The replacement of categories of handicap with a more sophisticated process of defining special educational need required the development of professional practices that could respond to new expectations. The 1981 Education Act outlined new responsibilities for LEAs to identify special educational needs, and to specify the provision necessary to meet those needs via a statutory process of 'multidisciplinary assessments' and 'statements'. The Warnock Report, however, recommended that the statutory identification of special need should be preceded by a less formal and staged approach to assessment, as outlined below.

- **Stage 1** Where a teacher identifies that a child may have a learning difficulty then the parents and the headteacher should be informed. Special arrangements are made for teaching such children in the mainstream classroom and for assessing their progress.
- **Stage 2** If the child continues to demonstrate special learning needs in the classroom, then the school should inform the parents and involve more specialist teaching from within existing school resources, perhaps by providing individual teaching for key skill areas.
- **Stage 3** Where the school feels that the child's needs are not adequately met by the stage 1 and 2 approaches, then the parents should be informed and advice or input should be sought from outside agencies (e.g. peripatetic specialist teachers, educational psychologists, speech therapists etc.).

The next two stages were those formally introduced by the 1981 Act.

- **Stage 4** If the child is considered to be demonstrating special learning needs that are beyond the resources deployed at stages 1–3, then a request can be made to the LEA to make a statutory multidisciplinary assessment of the child's needs. If the LEA decides that there is a case for such an assessment to be made, then, with parental consent, requests are made for reports from the school, an educational psychologist, the health authority and social services. Representations are also sought from the parents regarding the needs of their child. Once the reports are received then it is the duty of the LEA to consider the advice and to decide whether a statement is necessary. A statement is a legally binding document that lists the child's special educational needs and indicates how and where they are to be met. Parents are given 15 days to agree or disagree with its contents before it is finally issued. The LEA is then committed to the provision of the facilities and resources promised in the statement. The statement must be reviewed annually.

• **Stage 5** The statement is now put into operation. The process of annual review should involve the parents and the professionals in consideration of the effectiveness of the provision. If there is general agreement that the child's needs have changed, then the LEA can decide to change the provision or cease to maintain the statement. All children with statements must be reassessed formally between the ages of $13\frac{1}{2}$ and $14\frac{1}{2}$.

These latter two stages have come to be known commonly as 'statementing'. However, it is important to draw a distinction between stages 4 and 5 and to recognise that 'statementing' should refer only to stage 5. The stage 4 multidisciplinary assessment is, by law, a non-prejudicial process where no assumption should be made that a statement will be issued at the end.

Over the decade following the introduction of the 1981 Education Act there were many problems encountered in the operation of the staged approach to assessment. Special educational legislation over the next 2 decades attempted to address many of these. Before detailed consideration of this legislation, however, it is important to examine another development in educational legislation that had significant effects upon the education of children with learning disabilities – the 1988 Education Act and the National Curriculum.

THE 1988 EDUCATION ACT AND THE NATIONAL CURRICULUM

The introduction of the National Curriculum by the 1988 Education Act provided a structure for the education of all children throughout their school careers (ages 5–16) and a set of expectations for what a child should be able to achieve within core and foundation subject areas. These expectations were based upon a detailed breakdown of the skills and knowledge (statements of attainment) that the child should learn within four key stages of learning development (key stage 1 being up to age 7, key stage 2 up to age 11, key stage 3 up to age 14 and key stage 4 up to age 16).

The introduction of national testing of children (standard assessment tests) was intended to provide a picture of a child's attainments against the expectations of the National Curriculum. At each key stage there are expected levels of attainment, and these are intended to give an indication of how a child is performing at the end of that stage. To illustrate: at key stage 1 (up to age 7) if children are performing at level 2 then they are considered to be attaining at the expected level (average range) within the National Curriculum. Performance at level 1 (or lower) or level 3 (or higher) gives some idea of variation either side of the expectation.

The National Curriculum has important implications for the education of children with learning disabilities. Some of these implications can be seen as advantageous, others not so.

Advantages:

• A clear structure of expectations exists against which to gauge a child's learning development.
• An outline is provided for the teaching of skills and knowledge.
• The National Curriculum provides a basic assessment tool for parents, teachers and other professionals to help identify children's learning needs.

Disadvantages:

• The National Curriculum expectations may be too broad to cater for the specific needs of many children with learning disabilities.
• This may reinforce a picture of 'failure' against national expectations.
• The statements of attainment may be too broad or too steeply graded to cater for the more finely graded achievements of children with learning disabilities.

Many children with learning disabilities will, throughout their school careers, perform well below the National Curriculum expectations, and the lack of finely graded steps might call into question the relevance of the Curriculum for such children. In recognition of this, the 1988 Education Act provided for children with special educational needs to be exempted from following the National Curriculum. This exemption can be provided for all or part of the Curriculum, and must be confirmed by a statement of special educational need.

In many cases nationally, however, this path has not been followed. There appear to be three main reasons for this:

- In a context of inclusion the child has an entitlement to the same curricular access as all children.
- If a child is exempted from the National Curriculum, then the school and LEA must formally outline an alternative. If the child is not exempted then the concept of 'working towards' a level of attainment can replace the need for a formally rewritten curriculum. In this case it is up to the teacher to identify the more finely graded steps required for a child to be taught effectively.
- In an inclusive classroom the teacher can provide the same curriculum for all children, but differentiate the ways in which information is presented, in recognition of individual learning needs. Assessment of progress can similarly be differentiated and delivered.

The National Curriculum Inclusion Statement incorporated into the National Curriculum documentation revised in 2000 provides clear advice to schools about the principles that they must follow to ensure that all pupils have a chance to succeed, including advice on how the National Curriculum might be modified to meet individual need.

The introduction of the National Literacy Strategy and National Numeracy Strategy to primary school classrooms in 1998 and 1999 respectively, provided teachers with frameworks for teaching literacy and numeracy to children from age 5 to 11. (Similar frameworks were introduced at key stage 3 for children aged 11–14 from 2001). These strategies provided further sophisticated guidance and benchmarking against which to judge educational need, along with an emphasis and expectation that as wide a range of learning need as possible should be included and addressed in literacy and numeracy lessons.

Since the introduction of the National Curriculum and the Literacy and Numeracy Strategies, approaches to assessment have continued to develop, in recognition of the complex processes involved in defining the special needs of children with learning disability. The provisions of the 1993 Education Act and the introduction of the *Code of practice on the identification and assessment of special educational needs* (DFE 1994) marked a significant and relatively early step forward in this latter respect.

THE 1993 EDUCATION ACT AND THE CODE OF PRACTICE

In the years following the passing of the 1981 Education Act there were many criticisms of the ways in which LEAs and schools carried out the new statutory expectations. These criticisms centred on:

- a lack of national consistency in the ways in which the processes of identification, assessment and meeting of special educational needs developed. This was highlighted by a survey carried out by the Audit Commission and Her Majesty's Inspectorate of Schools (Audit Commission 1992), where 13 LEAs were investigated in terms of their implementation of the 1981 Act
- delays in the processing of multidisciplinary assessments and the issuing of statements
- a lack of guidance from the Department for Education regarding effective implementation of the 1981 Act
- a lack of rigour in the implementation of the five-stage Warnock model of assessment.

In late 1992 the Audit Commission and Her Majesty's Inspectorate of Schools published their recommendations, based upon the preceding survey, of how LEAs might improve their processes of assessment and identification of special educational needs (Audit Commission 1993). Many of these were embodied in the 1993 Education Act, which introduced the requirement for a national code of practice on the identification and assessment of special educational needs. LEAs and schools were expected to give 'due regard' to this code of practice. A new rigour was introduced to the whole process of identifying and meeting special educational needs, with clear timescales for statutory processes of assessment and statementing. The roles and responsibilities of schools in carrying out the staged model of assessment, originally instituted by the 1981 Act, were also introduced.

Following extensive consultation over the 4 years between 1997 and 2001, central government enacted the Special Educational Needs and Disability Act 2001, a key feature of which was the duty of schools and LEAs to have due regard to a redrafted code of practice. The increased emphasis on duties to include children in rather than exclude them from educational opportunity is embodied in this new code, along with a reformulation of the approaches to assessment and identification. The staged approach that had been a key feature of SEN processes for 2 decades was replaced by new concepts that were intended to avoid the dangers inherent in that staged approach, i.e. that a child placed at stage 1 would be assumed inevitably to progress to stage 5 and a highly specialist form of provision through a statement. This tendency was neither naturally inclusive nor did it place the emphasis upon the duty of the school to meet a child's needs in as inclusive a way as professionally possible.

Detailed consideration of the requirements of the code of practice is given later in this chapter. Before moving on to this, however, it is important to explore the concepts and methods that underpin effective professional practice in meeting the needs of children with learning disabilities.

Individual need and special need

Changing the emphasis of teaching, from an approach based upon a child's handicap to an approach based upon special educational need, has important implications for professional practice. All those concerned with the child should share a common perspective of how best to help with the child's individual and special educational needs.

At first it may seem difficult to separate these two concepts: surely individual needs are the same as special needs, particularly if the child has a learning difficulty? Difficult as it may seem to draw a distinction between the two, however, it is important to develop a clear picture of both.

A definition of individual need

All children, regardless of ability, have individual educational needs. All children have a need to:

- acquire the skills and knowledge that will give them effective access to the world
- gain access to a curriculum that will provide the experiences necessary to enable learning of these skills and knowledge.

For most children, access to ordinary schools and the National Curriculum will provide for their individual educational needs. With effective teaching and classroom management schools can respond effectively to most children's educational needs, and provide an environment and curriculum which enables children to make the most of what is on offer.

However, for some children this is not the case, particularly where there is a degree of learning disability or difficulty.

Defining special educational need – a model for practice

Special educational needs can be defined as those that arise from a child's difficulty in accessing the curriculum ordinarily offered in mainstream schools. These special needs will, of course, be highly individualised and require a very sensitive approach to assessment and teaching. Later in this chapter we describe how the Special Educational Needs and Disability Act 2001 and the *Code of Practice* provide a framework for effective assessment, intervention and teaching of children with special educational needs. First, however, it is important to consider the general processes involved in defining the special educational needs of the individual child.

It is tempting and easy to ascribe a child's difficulty in accessing the ordinary curriculum solely to factors 'within' the child. In other words, it is possible to 'blame' the child for not learning effectively on the grounds of, for example, limited cognitive ability, lack of motivation, physical difficulties or emotional and behavioural difficulties. This may lead to an exclusive impression that there is something 'wrong' with the child that is preventing access to the curriculum. This may then lead to the belief that a 'cure' for 'within-child' problems might overcome the learning difficulties. This is not to say that within-child factors are unimportant: of course they are, but cures are extremely rare. As yet there is very little understanding of the neurological processes involved in learning that might lead to an understanding of how to cure learning disabilities.

Special education is a far more complex and interactive process than merely diagnosing a within-child problem and prescribing a cure. It must involve not only the within-child factors, but also factors in the child's learning environment.

It is possible to describe the educational process as an interaction between the child, the teacher/adult, and the curriculum. This interaction can be portrayed as a triangle (Fig. 7.1), where the relationships or dimensions between each of the points are seen to be vital to the effectiveness of the educational process. Effective education relies upon the integrity of the relationships or dimensions between each of the three points.

Dimension (a) in Figure 7.1 describes the relationship between the teacher and the child. The teacher's understanding of the child will involve some knowledge of within-child factors (e.g. medical conditions or physical disabilities which may affect learning). The teacher will also need to have a clear picture of the child's current levels of attainment and past progress in learning. In some cases it may be important for the teacher to have some awareness of the child's past emotional and behavioural responses to certain learning situations. An understanding of all the above will enable prediction of the child's likely response to planned teaching. For the planned teaching to be effective, it is also vital that the child understands what the teacher requires in response.

Dimension (b) in Figure 7.1 describes the relationship between the teacher and the curriculum. It is obviously important that the teacher understands the framework and content of the curriculum to be delivered to the child. However, it is also vitally important that the teacher understands how best to tailor teaching approaches in order to enable the child to access the curriculum effectively. This is commonly known as the 'differentiation' of teaching approaches, and will rely upon the teacher's understanding of both the child and the curriculum.

Dimension (c) in Figure 7.1 describes the relationship between the child and the curriculum. The curriculum provided for the child must recognise both individual and special educational needs. The child must be able to access the curriculum effectively and demonstrate learning through appropriate response to the demands of the curriculum.

The child's assessed or measured response to the curriculum, in terms of learning progress and attainment, completes the relationships in the learning triangle. In other words, the quality and integrity of the relationships in the triangle are tested by the child's assessed progress in learning.

This interactive model, therefore, enables the analysis of all the factors involved in effective learning. A child's learning disability cannot be exclusively ascribed to inability or within-child limitations. The model demands that consideration is also given to the effectiveness and sensitivity of the assessment and teaching approaches provided for the child. Where a child's learning disability is causing concern, the model enables detailed analysis not only of what is 'wrong' or 'right' with the child, but also of what might be 'wrong' or 'right' with the learning environment. Parents, teachers and support professionals can then contribute to the analysis of the factors in the learning environment which are vital for learning progress.

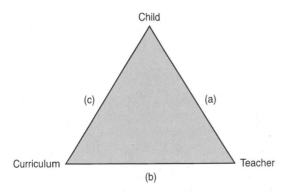

Figure 7.1   The interactive nature of the educational process.

ASSESSMENT AND INTERVENTION

An important aspect of good teaching is that the teacher is continuously assessing the child's response to the teaching. This enables the teacher to plan and adjust approaches to the child's learning on the basis of a developing picture of his or her special educational needs. In this way intervention and assessment become one and the same process.

This is an important issue when considering ways in which to help with the education of children with learning disabilities. The special educational needs of such children demand far more than a process of 'teaching first and assessing later' in order to see how the child has progressed. Any intervention designed to meet a child's learning need must be very sensitive to the child's response, otherwise the teaching may not achieve its aims.

The successful integration of assessment and intervention into one complete process relies upon the analyses made possible by the learning triangle described above. In other words, successful education of children with learning disabilities must take into consideration all the factors, both child-centred and in the learning environment, that might need attention and change.

For many children with learning disability this process of assessment and intervention needs to be a daily aspect of teaching. As the education progresses small changes may be required in the direction and emphasis of the teaching in order to respond adequately to the child's needs. If a child appears to be 'getting stuck' in the learning of a skill or knowledge, then consideration should be given to the ways in which the teaching might be changed to help the child to progress. It may also be that the assessment is not enabling the child to demonstrate the newly acquired skill effectively. This approach is a far cry from one which assumes that the child's failure to learn is solely a within-child problem.

If the teaching approach is based upon the concept of the learning triangle and an integrated process of assessment and intervention, then the input of outside professionals (support teachers, medical professionals, psychologists, learning disability nurses etc.) can be focused upon how to help with the teaching, rather than simply upon diagnosing what might be 'wrong' with the child.

Syndromes and conditions – educational implications

Many children with learning disabilities may also have been diagnosed as having some form of medical condition or syndrome (for example, Down syndrome, autism, attention deficit disorder, and cerebral palsy). There is not the scope in this chapter for a detailed consideration of the implications of such diagnoses (see Ch. 2); however, it is important to look at the general implications of the existence of syndromes and conditions.

These diagnoses often cause teachers great concern in terms of their planning of effective teaching. There may be a fear that the condition or syndrome may require a specialist approach, and that there is a danger that the 'wrong' approaches may be adopted. It is vitally important, therefore, that any such diagnosis should (where appropriate) be communicated to the educational professionals concerned in terms of the implications that conditions or syndromes may have for teaching and learning; this is especially the role of the learning disabilities nurse.

A word of warning, however: there is the danger that diagnoses of conditions may imply limitations in the child's ability to learn, which might reduce expectations in the teaching approach. This is commonly referred to as the 'self-fulfilling prophecy', and can result in a reduction in people's expectations of the child's capacity to learn. There are many examples where children with conditions or syndromes which might have severely restricted their capacity to learn have responded positively to effective teaching (e.g. Feuerstein 1980). Such approaches have been based upon the sensitive assessment of need within the learning triangle, not solely upon the within-child factors which a diagnosis of a condition or syndrome might imply.

The concepts and methods outlined above are significant features of the educational approaches described by the Code of Practice (DfES 2002), to which all schools and LEAs must have due regard.

We turn now to a detailed consideration of the requirements of the *Code of Practice*.

Applying the *Code of Practice*

The *Code of Practice* provides schools and local education authorities with clear information regarding their responsibilities for all children considered as having learning disabilities. The basic principles are founded upon the Warnock recommendations and the 1981 Education Act. The *Code of Practice* should be considered as a valuable working document designed to guide the practice of all those involved with the education of children with special learning needs.

 Reader activity 7.1   The learning triangle

Select a skill or area of knowledge which you have attempted to learn, but with which you have experienced difficulty. Now consider the three dimensions of the learning triangle. How might changes be made along the three dimensions in order to enhance the quality of your learning?

The Special Educational Needs and Disability Act 2001 and the *Code of Practice* require all schools to publish a policy document relating to the meeting of special educational needs. This should give clear information as to how resources are allocated to special needs, and how the school's systems respond to the demands of the *Code of Practice*. The schools' governing bodies have responsibility for all pupils with special needs, and should appoint a governor whose role it is to oversee the operation of the special needs policy. Schools are also required to have a designated member of staff with responsibility for special needs, known as the 'special needs coordinator' (SENCO) who should be a member of the senior management team of the school and thus be positioned to influence whole school policy and practice. The code also indicates that sufficient time should be made available for the SENCO to carry out the duties associated with the post. The definition of sufficiency will always be subject to scrutiny by external audit through OfSTED inspection (Office for Standards in Education).

A school having regard to the *Code of Practice* will be using an approach to meet the needs of pupils with learning difficulties that is based upon the principles of early identification and intervention, fundamentally emphasising the school's role in these processes. The involvement of parents in these processes is considered to be of vital importance.

An approach to assessment and intervention

'School Action': teacher, parent and child

The *Code of Practice* promotes early identification of need, and 'School Action' describes the processes required to meet a child's special educational needs, usually identified by the class teacher. However, parents may express a concern regarding their child's progress, and this must be considered as being equally important.

A child may be identified as having a special educational need by referring to the child's progress as defined by:

- results from baseline assessments and progress against these results
- progress against National Literacy and Numeracy objectives
- attainments within the statements of attainment in the National Curriculum
- performance in standardised or norm referenced tests of basic skills.

If a child is identified as having a special need, this need should be carefully documented and plans outlined that are intended to address this need. If the identification of a need has come from the class teacher, the parents should be informed immediately. Records of action and intervention should be kept, together with records of strategies adopted to meet the identified need.

'School Action': teacher, parent, child and SENCO

If the strategies of intervention used by the class teacher/subject teacher appear to be failing to meet the child's needs (i.e. satisfactory progress is not being made), then the teacher may decide to seek the involvement of the school's special needs coordinator (SENCO) in the planning and provision for the child's needs. The teacher and SENCO review the evidence from earlier intervention and from parents. The SENCO and the teacher may then draw up an individual education plan (IEP) for the child, and the parents are informed. (A detailed description of the structure and format of IEPs is given later in the chapter.)

The IEP will focus upon the skills and knowledge to be developed by the child, and the strategies to be employed by the school to help the child. The IEP will usually run for approximately one school term (although this could be longer) before being reviewed. Parents should be involved in these reviews.

It is important to note that 'School Action' requires the school to use its own resources to run the IEP. In reality this means that the class teacher continues to take responsibility for the education of the child, perhaps with additional teaching input from others, and with the continuing advice of the SENCO.

The child's response to the IEP should yield important information as to the appropriateness of the strategies being used by the school, and about the child's continuing quality of need. Queries may arise regarding, for example, the child's vision, hearing, language or physical development, which might need to be checked by outside professionals (e.g. by referral to medical professionals, speech therapists or physiotherapists). The results of such checks will then inform future IEP planning.

The review of the IEP may result in:

- continuation with 'School Action' with a revised IEP
- consideration of 'School Action Plus'.

'School Action Plus': involving outside support agencies

A decision to move to 'School Action Plus' is taken when the teacher, SENCO and parents feel that the child's needs require the input of specialist professionals in order to contribute to the implementation of the IEP. The responsibility to compile, implement and review the IEP remains with the teacher and SENCO, but the contribution of outside professionals should be formally noted.

A range of outside professionals may be called upon, according to the nature of the child's needs. Specialist teachers with skills in the areas of learning disability, sensory impairment, emotional and behavioural difficulty and so on are often involved in advice or direct specialist teaching. Educational psychologists may also play a key role in assessment and intervention with regard to special need. Such people are usually employed by the local education authority and provide a service to schools as part of their routine delivery. They may also give advice to schools about ways in which the teacher and SENCO might meet need during 'School Action' without becoming directly involved with the child. In addition to the services provided by LEAs, schools may also call upon the advice and guidance of medical and other professionals, according to the nature of the child's needs. School medical officers, learning disabilities nurses and therapists, along with social services personnel, may all have relevant inputs to make. The availability of such support will, of course, be affected by local policies of provision and funding, and it is vital that the SENCO is fully aware of the extent and quality of available help. The Health Act 1999 (section 31) provides for partnership arrangements between health providers and local authorities, linking more closely the health related functions of both forms of authority. The impact of the Act should be clearly seen in the increased clarity available to schools about the nature of support services available.

Reviews of IEPs should be carried out on at least a twice-yearly basis, involving the views of parents, school and involved outside agencies. The review of the IEP may result in:

- a return to 'School Action' only
- continuation with 'School Action Plus' with a revised IEP
- a decision to request a move to formal statutory multidisciplinary assessment.

Statutory multidisciplinary assessment

The decision to move to a statutory assessment must be taken in light of the evidence of the child's progress as a result of 'School Action Plus'. If there is concern and evidence that the child's needs place demands upon the school's resources which the school cannot fully meet, then a decision is taken to approach the local education authority to request a multidisciplinary assessment of those needs. The LEA will make this decision in the light of all the available evidence of assessments and interventions made thus far. IEPs should still continue to be devised and implemented while the statutory assessment is being made.

The *Code of Practice* and the 2001 Act impose time limits on the statutory assessment process, requiring that the whole procedure be completed within a 6-month period. Once the LEA agrees to proceed with a statutory assessment the parents are formally consulted, and written advice regarding the nature of the child's special educational needs is sought from those professionally involved.

There is a fundamental requirement for the LEA to formally seek the views of:

- the parents
- the school
- other educationalists involved with the child
- educational psychologists
- medical professionals: the child will be required to be medically examined, and reports should be submitted from those medical and therapeutic professionals involved in ongoing support
- social services personnel
- any other person whose views are considered to be important and, of course, the child.

Once these reports are received the LEA has a duty to consider all the advice and to determine whether a statement of special educational needs is required in order to meet the identified needs appropriately.

Statement of special educational need

A statement is a statutory document compiled by the LEA which:

- outlines the nature of the child's special learning needs

- identifies the special educational provision, which the LEA considers to be necessary to meet these needs. This provision is described in terms of the learning objectives for which the provision is intended, the quality of provision (e.g. details of school-based support, special school placement etc.) and arrangements for monitoring progress
- names the place where education is to be carried out
- lists non-educational needs agreed by social services, health professionals etc., and how provision for these is to be made.

Parents are consulted about the contents of the statement and the received professional advice before the statement is finally issued. If parents disagree with any aspect of the advice they can discuss their concerns with the professional in question. This is particularly important if the parents feel that an aspect of advice has led to decisions about resourcing in the statement with which they disagree. Likewise, if the parents disagree with the outlined provision then they have recourse to arbitration from the Special Needs Tribunal system provided by central government.

Notes in lieu of a statement

There may be occasions where the statutory assessment process has contributed evidence to the LEA that the child's needs can continue to be provided for within the existing resources of the school. If this is the case the LEA may issue a note in lieu, which indicates that strategies for provision need to be developed in light of the advice received, without the provision of enhanced or additional resources. Again, should the parents disagree with this perspective they have the right of appeal to the Special Educational Needs Tribunal.

Annual reviews and transition plans

Annual review Once the statement is issued it is the responsibility of the school to review the appropriateness of the provision at least once a year. This is known as the annual review process, where the school, with the advice of appropriate outside agencies and parents, reassesses the child's progress and the effectiveness of provision. Should there be significant changes in the level of need or appropriateness of provision during the year, then the LEA should be informed in order to request a revision of the statement.

Transition plans The annual review of a statement in the period following a young person's 14th birthday is a significant event in the process of statutory provision for special educational needs. In order to ensure that effective plans are made for the young person's future beyond school age, the headteacher must convene a meeting to review any special needs and provision, involving appropriate representatives from the Connexions Service who will manage the transition plan for the child during transition into adulthood. The aim of the meeting is to compile a transition plan, which will help to meet the needs of the young person in the final years of school and beyond. The meeting must be attended by the Connexions Service Personal Adviser who will work with the child, the parents, appropriate school staff, social services personnel and any other relevant support professional who might have significant input to the continued meeting of the child's special educational needs. Consideration should be given to statutory assessments which may be necessary under legislation other than the 2001 Special Educational Needs and Disability Act (i.e. the Chronically Sick and Disabled Persons Act 1970, the Disabled Persons Act 1986 and the NHS and Community Care Act 1990). The transition plan should incorporate the views of the young person, the school, appropriate outside agencies and the family as to the young person's needs and appropriate resources for the future.

Pre-school/early years assessment

Much has been written in this chapter so far relating to school-based assessment and intervention in the area of special educational needs. However, many children have special needs that are identified long before their eligibility for full-time education at the age of 5. This may have been the result of health or social service interventions and

involvements, or from parents' own observations and assessments. The *Code of Practice* outlines the roles and responsibilities of early years providers of childcare and education, LEAs, social services departments, health bodies and voluntary organisations in meeting the special needs of pre-school children. All LEAs have a duty to establish Early Years Development and Childcare Partnerships involving all the bodies described above, and whose task it is to review and plan child care and educational provision for children aged 3 to 5 years. This phase of education is described as the 'foundation stage' and is seen to be a vital platform upon which to base school-based education.

As central government increases the resources available to provide educational opportunity for all children aged 3–5, so the sophistication of provision for special educational needs develops. Area SENCOs are funded by LEAs to provide advice and support to groups of childminders, playgroups and nursery providers.

The *Code of Practice* outlines a set of processes for the identification of and provision for special educational needs of pre-school children that mirrors those described above for schools. 'Early Years Action' and 'Early Years Action Plus' mirror 'School Action' and 'School Action Plus'.

Rights to statutory assessment for all pre-school children, and provision for need through statements, are endorsed through the *Code of Practice* and the 2001 Act.

Reader activity 7.2   Informing parents

Imagine that you have to explain to parents how their child's special educational needs will be assessed and met. Which key points will you emphasise in your discussion in order to inform parents effectively about this complex process? Remember that these key points should be easily remembered after your discussion, and should help the parents to help the child.

Individual education plans

Target setting for children As the term 'individual education plan' suggests, all children considered as having special educational needs require a detailed individual plan of how their special educational needs are to be met. The plan should set out:

- nature of the child's learning needs that are special and beyond those ordinarily expected
- action – the special educational provision – staff involved, including frequency of support, specific programmes/activities/materials/equipment, involvement of outside professionals
- help from parents at home
- targets to be achieved in a given time
- any pastoral care or medical requirements
- monitoring and assessment arrangements
- review arrangements and date.

The statements relating to action, targets and monitoring require careful planning by the professionals involved. In setting out the targets to be achieved it is vital that appropriate action is taken in an attempt to meet the needs of the individual child.

A good individual education plan will set specific targets for the child to achieve. These targets can only be reviewed effectively if they are expressed in terms of learning behaviour, i.e. skills, which can be directly observed and assessed. Precision in thinking and planning are important aspects of the process of setting realistic targets, therefore a target to 'improve reading' could be considered to be far too broad; it may be better to focus upon particular component skills involved with reading, such as letter recognition, basic sight vocabulary or blend use etc. To enable precise targets to be set it is important to consider the abilities of the child and to know what they can already do in the selected targeted skill area. The class teacher or SENCO may have to carry out 'baseline' assessments to establish a starting point. It should be possible to identify specific skills to be targeted in all major areas of learning activity, both academic and social.

In choosing a precise target the professionals are setting out an expectation for the child to achieve within a certain time limit, usually by the next review date. The targets should be observable and assessable in order to establish whether the child has made progress. It is important to specify the activities that will be carried out during the plan, and the setting in which these will occur (i.e. the child may be in a small group situation for some activities, or even receive some individual tuition). If outside agencies are involved they should be part of the planning process and their involvement should be recorded as part of the individual education plan.

In the mainstream school a child will be educated for the majority of time in a larger class-based setting. It is important, therefore, to identify those subject areas where differentiation is required in order for the child to access the curriculum. Precision is also vital in the planning of how this is to be achieved. In a secondary school setting the subject teachers will be mainly responsible for this differentiation, but the plan should reflect how it would occur. A record should be made in the plan of the materials and approaches to be used in recognition of the individual child's skill level. In a primary school setting the class teacher will probably be responsible for differentiation in many curriculum areas, and will need to be aware of the levels of skills in order to do this appropriately for each individual child.

A review date should then be set. At the review reference should be made to what the child has achieved in the previously targeted areas. These achievements should be recorded in as precise terms as the original targets – if the targets were not reached, it is still important to note what the child is now able to do in that area. Discussions at the review will lead to decisions about where to go next. All the professionals involved in the delivery of the plan should be invited to attend, as well as the parents. If the original targets were achieved then decisions should be made about making a new individual education plan. If the targets were not reached, questions need to be asked about the nature of the targets, the consistency of the delivery and demands being placed upon the resources.

Pupils who have been issued with a statement will have that statement reviewed annually. However, they will still need an individual education plan, with short-term targets that can assess the progress being achieved.

Target setting for professionals The role of the professionals in setting precise and accurate targets for an individual child is a crucial aspect of assessing progress. The professionals involved must be fully aware of each individual child's abilities, and have knowledge of strategies that may help the child to reach the learning targets. It is important to consider not only the child's apparent progress but also the factors listed in the individual education plan that relate to its professional delivery. An analytical and critical approach is required to determine whether all aspects of the plan were delivered as originally anticipated. For example, certain materials or equipment may not have been as readily available as initially planned. The plan cannot then be considered to have been fully delivered, thus contributing to the child not having achieved the set targets. This reflects the notion of the triangular model described earlier, where the interaction between the child, the teacher and the curriculum is vital to the process of learning. An effective individual education plan is therefore dependent upon the relationship between the targets set for the learner, and the targets set for the deliverer.

Even where all aspects of the plan have been delivered, however, if the child has not reached the set targets there needs to be careful consideration of the quality and appropriateness of the strategies employed by the professionals in the operation of the plan.

As mentioned earlier in the chapter, it is all too easy to blame the child for failing to achieve the targets without carefully considering:

- whether the targets were appropriate in the first place
- whether smaller 'steps to targets' are required
- whether the strategies were appropriate for helping the child to reach the targets.

The professionals involved in the delivery of the IEP should therefore regularly consider whether the targets set for their own delivery were appropriate in the first place.

Careful management of the individual education planning process, which concentrates upon the effectiveness of the interaction between learning targets and delivery targets, should ensure

sensitive and effective special educational provision.

Figure 7.2 presents a proposed outline for an individual education plan, which follows the requirements of the *Code of Practice*.

CONCLUSION

Current approaches to the education of young people with learning disabilities focus upon the interactive nature of the educational process rather than solely upon what might be 'wrong' with the learner. There has been a change of emphasis in the latter half of the 20th century, from an approach based upon the 'categorisation of handicap' to an approach which attempts to define special educational need. This has enabled all those who work with children with learning disabilities to consider how best to respond to individual learning needs by analysing the ways in which the learner responds to new learning targets. This chapter has presented a working model (the learning triangle) that enables the analysis of all the major features of the learning environment; this should help with the process of identifying individual *and* special needs in ways that lead to an effective meeting of those needs.

Recent educational legislation has recognised the importance of the interactive nature of learning, and the *Code of Practice* on the identification and assessment of special educational needs endorses the interactive model by outlining the professional responsibilities required to ensure that such needs are properly met. The individual education plan, as required by the *Code of Practice*, should be a practical reflection of the interactive processes involved in identifying and meeting the needs of a child with a learning disability.

 Reader activity 7.3   Compiling individual education plans

Using the IEP format presented in Figure 7.2, compile an IEP for a child with a learning disability. Remember to select observable learning targets which can be reviewed after one term, and consider how you as a health professional might be incorporated into the delivery of the IEP.

INDIVIDUAL EDUCATION PLAN

Name: Period of plan:

School: Review date:

Date of birth: Year: 1 2 3 4 5 6 7 8 9 10 11

Compiled by:

Specific skills to be delivered by this plan _____

_____

_____

_____

_____

_____

What can the pupil do in skill area (s) at beginning of plan? _____

_____

_____

_____

_____

_____

_____

_____

Details of specific teaching/assessment activities to be delivered in individual or small group setting (including parental involvement) _____

_____

Who will carry these out? _____

_____

When will they be carried out? _____

_____

Hours per week devoted to these activities _____

_____

_____

Details of class-based differentiation

List areas of National Curriculum where differentiation is necessary and identify how this is to be achieved _____

Curriculum area/ Subject area	Differentiated approach (materials/teacher method)
_____	_____
_____	_____
_____	_____
_____	_____

IEP REVIEW

Date of review: People attending:

What can pupil do now in targeted skill area? _____

_____

_____

_____

Observations regarding the success of the plan:
Did the plan reach its targets? _____

Were all aspects of the plan delivered? _____

_____

Is a new IEP necessary?   *yes/no*

Relevant comments arising from review (Include comments regarding effective strategies to be continued, possible medical investigations necessary, etc.) _____

_____

_____

_____

Signed: _____ *Special Needs Coordinator*

Figure 7.2 Proposed format for an individual education plan.

REFERENCES

Audit Commission 1992 Getting in on the Act. HMSO, London

Audit Commission 1993 Getting the Act together. HMSO, London

Department for Education 1994 Code of practice on the identification and assessment of special educational needs. HMSO, London

Department for Education and Skills 2002 Code of practice on the identification and assessment of special educational needs. HMSO, London

Dessent T 1987 Making the ordinary schools special. Falmer Press, London

Feuerstein R 1980 Instrumental enrichment. University Park Press, Baltimore

Portwood P F 1995 An experience of integration. Children Nationwide Medical Research Fund, London

Sayer J 1983a A comprehensive school for all. In: Booth A, Potts P (eds) Integrating special education. Blackwell, Oxford

Sayer J 1983b Assessments for all, statements for none. Special Education 10: 4

Warnock M (Chair) 1978 Special educational needs. HMSO, London

FURTHER READING

Advisory Centre for Education 1994 Special education handbook; The law on children with special needs, 6th edn. ACE, London

Department for Education 1995 Innovatory practice in mainstream schools for special educational needs. HMSO, London

Department for Education and Employment 2000 Curriculum 2000. HMSO, London

Website; www.dfes.gov.uk

8

Post-compulsory education

Angie Walker, Chris Parkin

KEY ISSUES

- Learning makes a positive contribution to the wellbeing of the community it serves, as a mediator for socialising its members, and people with learning disabilities are increasingly accessing further education provision.
- The development of educational provision for people with learning disabilities has undergone a slow but gradual metamorphosis away from segregation toward inclusion. Key educational reports that have helped to shape this are the Dearing (1996), Elton (1989), Kennedy (1997), Moser (1999), Tomlinson (1996), and Warnock (1978) Reports.
- Inclusive education needs to be student-centred to meet individual needs.
- In the future there will be increased emphasis on inclusive learning in Further Education and this will continue to be supported by central national policy. This will occur within the context of a need for frequent skills updating.

INTRODUCTION

Learning and training are important and positive contributions that people can make to being part of the community in which they live. They are an ideal, which many people aspire to for the contribution they can make to peoples' own wealth creation capabilities as well as to enhancing the wealth and skills base of the community. Learning and training can also contribute to the enrichment of the community's cultural core. In sociological terms they are also a community's way of socialising its members through education to the norms established in that community. This is an important facet of a pluralistic society. Implicit in this is the recognition that adults post-16 have a right to learn and make choices about their learning. At the further education stage this is embodied by the onus being placed on individuals to choose their own paths for educational achievement and to seek professional guidance in order to make the correct choices. Many of the national policy developments that have emerged over the last 25 years, both in the compulsory and post compulsory education sectors, have gradually worked towards this ethos. Such developments have had an impact on young people with additional learning needs, such as those with learning disabilities. National policy has evolved from two consecutive viewpoints:

1. The earlier perspective entailed a concentration on identifying special educational needs within the individual learner, and in doing so made a distinction between the handicapped and the non-handicapped.

2. Evolving out of this more recently has been the view that we should make further education accessible to all learners and in doing so widen participation in education and move away from the earlier distinction. Attempts should be made to integrate the learner with special educational needs, with additional support as appropriate. In doing this, we put the learner at the centre of the education process. However, as will be seen, this scenario cannot be achieved overnight, there being numerous examples of institutional, cultural and attitudinal factors weighing against it.

 Reader activity 8.1

Many Careers and Guidance Services have Specialist Careers Officers. Their role is to track learners who have additional needs through the education system and beyond, to ensure that their needs are met. Contact them and find out how many colleges are in your area.

This chapter will explore how this development has occurred against the background of a complete reappraisal by society of what it expects from the further education system and the learners within it. Looking at some of the historical aspects of this development will therefore provide a context for understanding why these attitudinal changes are beginning to take place.

HISTORICAL CONTEXT

Prior to the Second World War people with learning disabilities had largely been segregated away from society and viewed as having a medical problem. Even the passing of the 1944 Education Act did not completely remove the input that local health authorities could make on the suitability of a child to be educated at school or, because of the degree of his mental handicap, in a junior training centre.

Although this Act stipulated that it was the duty of local education authorities to make provision for full- and part-time education for people over compulsory school age who were able and willing to profit by the facilities provided for that purpose, in effect it meant that mentally handicapped learners on reaching the age of sixteen were excluded from further education. Therefore, a proportion of mentally handicapped people were excluded from any form of statutory education.

The 1971 Education Act brought the then junior training centres under the control of local education authorities, but the assessment of mental handicap was still undertaken largely by professionals located within health authorities. There came a growing realisation, however, that educational assessment was as important as medical assessment. Moreover, there was an increasing belief that education for handicapped learners did not necessarily stop at the end of compulsory schooling.

Warnock (1978) recognised this, stating that where it was in the interest of pupils with special educational needs they should be able to stay at school beyond sixteen. The 1981 Education Act embodied this in law by stating that all young people had a right to full-time education up to their nineteenth birthday on request, either at school or college (the authority could decide which). This legal duty could now be enforced on colleges of further education (then under local education authority control), not just on special schools.

Consequently many further education colleges rose to this challenge and began establishing links with predominantly special schools within their neighbourhoods, which led to a multiplicity of national provision of further education for people with learning disabilities. Some colleges had already established some form of provision for learners with special educational needs even prior to the Warnock Report, notably Richmond-upon-Thames College of Further Education.

Despite the legal framework conferring responsibility for special educational needs post-16, the Act did not state what form this provision should take.

Moreover, funding levels varied greatly between local education authorities. Provision was predominantly discrete, often with accommodation for students with learning difficulties being separate and distant from that for other learners within the college, so the two groups rarely met.

After several of Mary Warnock's conclusions were incorporated into the Education Act the way was set for change. Prior to this people with learning difficulties had been labelled mostly in medical terms, since many of them were still under health authority jurisdiction. Terms such as educationally subnormal and maladjusted still existed. Hence as the new Act came into being 70 000 people were labelled as educationally subnormal and 21 000 were identified as maladjusted in the education system (Newell 1983).

The Warnock Committee indicated that special education should help children to be independent, the extent of which would depend on the individual's capabilities. The Committee abandoned the labelling of children but instead looked at the continuum of need. They indicated that maybe 2% of school-aged children might need a particular form of educational provision and that a further 20% would require special provision to be made within normal schools. Findings also indicated

that education should start as early as possible, i.e. playgroups and pre-school provision, and should end as late as possible, i.e. further education after the age of 16 years.

Warnock had stated that all children should be educated in mainstream schools unless their educational needs could be more 'efficiently' met in a special school. The report had therefore championed the concept of 'integration'. Examples of integration of children with special educational needs within mainstream school began to develop, but only on an ad hoc basis. However, the integration concept did not so readily spread to the further education sector. The 1981 Education Act, although a starting block for further education colleges to offer provision for learners with special educational needs, did not confer any pressure to integrate, possibly because of the colleges' more examination-biased curriculum.

The 1981 Education Act stipulated that assessment would focus on identifying educational need involving a five stage process in which a multidisciplinary approach would be adopted involving schools, social services, other professionals and parents. The inclusion of parents in this process is significant in that it was the first time that parents had been given the right to influence the decision-making process.

This move towards integration should be seen in the context of other changes at that time. For example care in the community (DHSS 1981) commenced and long-stay hospitals were beginning to move their resources out into the community. A major shift was also beginning that would affect social services and health as well as education.

This shift in policy was viewed as a human rights issue by many pressure groups at the time. For the relatively new Conservative administration it was arguably viewed as a means to reduce state participation and hopefully funding. Not surprisingly, the move towards greater integration was often undertaken in a rather cynical way, with the aim of reducing costs rather than more effectively meeting the needs of the learner. The Centre for Studies on Integration in Education in 1989 set up an Integration Charter following the Centre's statistical report on segregation in that period (CSIE 1989). The Centre for Studies on

Integration in Education was an independent educational charity that monitored local education authority practice and collated and disseminated information on good practice. They found that there had been little progress toward integration between 1982 and 1987, and that eleven local education authorities had actually increased segregated provision in that time. Thus it was evident that a more cohesive national approach was required.

The Elton Report of 1989, although predominantly directed towards secondary schools, was to have an effect on the further education sector. The report suggested that educators should look at their own practice and, through their initial and continuing training opportunities, further develop their class management skills. Elton further suggested that the modelling of behaviour and attitudes of individual staff members (and the whole school) were important. Elton stressed the relationship between the organisation, parents, outside agencies and the community as a whole. This underlined the need for a multi-agency approach to meeting special educational needs.

More directly related to the further education sector was the Dearing Report of 1996 which reviewed qualifications awarded to 14–19 year olds. The Dearing Report identified four groups – low attainers, under-achievers, those with learning difficulties and those with exceptional abilities – who may need help to maximise their potential. Dearing suggested that entry-level qualifications and courses, which accredit skills for independent adult life, could improve motivation for learners through providing a vocationally relevant curriculum. Elton and Dearing both influenced the further education sector, in so far as there was a need to introduce new courses to cater for the four client groups identified.

In 1993, a committee headed by Professor John Tomlinson was asked to review the range and type of further education available in England for people with learning difficulties or disabilities. Its remit was to recommend to the Further Education Funding Council how it could best fulfil its legal responsibilities to this group of students. This was the only group of learners identified in the 1992 Education Act, which initially set up the Further Education Funding Council. The committee was concerned with the extent and quality of what was then provided, together with the role of other agencies in that provision, and how that might be funded effectively. This was the first inquiry of its kind in Britain to examine special educational needs uniquely concerned with further education. Since the committee reported to the Further Education Funding Council and not the government, the committee was viewed as national, independent and able to bring a fresh view to the subject (Hewitson-Ratcliffe 1995).

In Helen Kennedy's Report, *Learning Works: Widening Participation in Further Education* (Kennedy 1997), Kennedy has argued that participation should be widened, rather than simply increased. It was felt that qualified people go on to get more education and earn more than those who fail first time around. People never really make up for this failure either educationally or economically, which has a knock-on effect on them and their families. This Report saw the further education sector as a place to address these issues. Kennedy also suggested that the Further Education Funding Council should reform their funding policy to better accommodate learners from more deprived areas and that new groups of learners would learn new skills, from a wider range of staff, who would need to be supported to adjust their teaching strategies to respond to individual requirements and learning strategies.

The Moser Report (Moser 1999) aimed at improving basic numeracy and literacy skills among the adult population, set against a background of technological innovation, which is demanding new skills and a higher level of basic skill. Statistics show that 20% of adults (7 million people) have severe problems with basic skills. These problems close doors on opportunities for them and their families. A lack of basic skills can limit opportunities in the employment market. For those already in the market it can limit opportunities for promotion and with it a higher earning and spending capacity. The ability to read and write is an economic issue that is beneficial for the individual and the country. Moser also suggested the implementation of a massive staff development programme of basic skills training, thus ensuring quality throughout the further education sector, rather than having a relatively small group of staff whose role (the teaching of basic Maths and English) was seen as separate to the vocational areas such as catering or construction. Moser also considered the particular educational needs that adults with learning disabilities and people with dyslexia have but recognised that this was an area that needed further consultation and that there should be a special study following his report.

Hence specific demands were being made on the further education sector to meet the needs of all learners, whatever their level of attainment.

Lifting the level of basic education in Britain has now become a national priority, starting with the Government's launch of the National Strategies for Literacy and Numeracy for schools. 'The Literacy and Numeracy Hour' as it has been termed, has been put into place to help to ensure that the adult population in 15 years time do not face the same disadvantages, through lack of basic skills, as they do now.

The Further Education Funding Council was established in 1992 to fund further education colleges. This meant that colleges became self-governing and were taken out of the control of local education authorities (this was known as incorporation). Through the Further Education Funding Council successive governments have been able to exert some degree of control and therefore have established a national policy for this sector of education. Hence, in the 3 years after incorporation the then Conservative Government expected a 25% increase in participation in the further education sector, or 500 000 extra students by the year 2002. Through a change in funding methodology, further education colleges were encouraged to increase their student numbers to include those learners identified by Dearing (1996) as low attainers, under-achievers, those with learning difficulties and those with exceptional abilities. Such an inclusive policy was encouraged by the recommendations of the Tomlinson Report (Tomlinson 1996). The main thrust of this report was embodied in the concept of inclusive learning. The report defined inclusive learning as the match between learning goals, learning style and the learning environment for each learner. The concept of inclusivity therefore focuses on learning and places the learner at the centre of that process. As with Elton, it demands the need to match how individuals learn best with the curriculum, which inevitably has an impact on teaching.

Inclusive learning brings this historical perspective on the development of further education for people with a learning disability up to date. How the inclusive learning concept has affected further education colleges since Tomlinson will now be reviewed. In doing this, more pragmatic problems and dilemmas arising out of the inclusive learning approach on both local and national levels will be explained. Specialist colleges will not be described or discussed as they do not per se fall into the inclusive model.

THE CONCEPT OF INCLUSIVE LEARNING

The core purpose of further education colleges in common with other education providers is the successful promotion of learning through a range of education and training programmes. This chapter has already shown how the various developments in recent years have emphasised the importance of learning at an individual level. This has necessitated an increasing need for learners to take responsibility for their own learning. There needs to be a certain level of self organisation and a sharply focused approach to self-evaluation of educational needs, enabling learners to prioritise, evaluate and plan their learning more effectively.

The concept of inclusive learning encapsulates this trend by promoting an equality of opportunity for all learners to do this, whatever their ability. The need to do this has been enshrined in law, the most recent piece of such legislation being the Learning and Skills Act 2000. This has set up a new body, the Learning and Skills Council, which took over from the Further Education Funding Council. The Learning and Skills Council is responsible for the planning and funding of all post-16 education and training, excluding higher education. The Act signals a strong emphasis on commitment to equality of opportunity and to achieve this the Learning and Skills Council will ensure that learners who need additional support will get the help that they need.

As was seen earlier, the Tomlinson Report argued that if inclusive learning was to be adopted fully, then learners who had learning difficulties should not be segregated by the way in which their learning was managed. Learners should only be recognised by their particular support needs, also by the level of their participation in learning.

The meeting of individual and particular needs necessitates a college or institution-wide approach which the Government has encouraged with the setting up of Lifelong Learning Strategic Partnerships which have a requirement to consider the needs of under-represented and disadvantaged groups in the communities that they serve.

Other government inspired policies and documents that encourage widening participation have also been published; these include *The Learning Age* (DEFF 1998), local Lifelong Learning Development Plans and The Teaching and Higher Education Act 1998.

Yet inclusion is not without controversy. Some observers believe that inclusion should be regarded as the right of all children with learning disabilities (Oliver 1996), whereas others (Kauffman & Hallahan 1995) believe that the widespread adoption of inclusive models could lead to deterioration in the education provided for many learners with learning disabilities. In the long-term these models may lead to the demise of special education. Lindsay (1997) has admitted that in the short term inclusive learning does raise concerns, for example about the ability of teachers to cope within the classroom with learners who have learning disabilities.

Hornby (1999) has concluded that the theory and practice of inclusion is being adopted wholesale, without adequate research evidence about its effectiveness. He goes on to say that in the seven major reviews of the literature that he analysed, apart from the lower cost of inclusive practices, there was very little evidence to suggest that the goals of inclusion were being met. Thus greater educational attainment, increased social skills, reduced stigma, increased self-esteem, greater social interaction, improved parental involvement and individualisation of the institution did not necessarily result from including learners with special educational needs in mainstream schools.

However, public policy both in the UK and in the USA supports the principle of including as many children with learning disabilities as possible in mainstream educational provision. This action has been underpinned by the United Nations Education Agency in the Salamanca World Statement on Special Needs Education (UNESCO 1994), which called on governments to adopt the principle of inclusive education, enabling all (learners) to access regular education unless there are some compelling reasons for doing otherwise (Hornby 1999).

Perhaps, therefore, it is not so surprising that in accordance with this trend Professor Tomlinson in his report whole-heartedly adopted the inclusive learning model. The report was also written against the background of prevailing British attitudes in which there was a very carefully calibrated hierarchy of worthwhile achievement, which has clearly established rules that reward academic success well above any other accomplishment (Sternberg 1997). The Tomlinson Report, therefore, together with the Kennedy Report, simply attempts to embed the inclusive learning philosophy into the field of further education against a possible academic backlash that states that there is evidence both for and against its overall success.

If the concept of inclusive learning is to be a viable educational strategy that tackles poverty and helps to promote equality of access, then there needs to be a whole new set of social attitudes to offset the ones that previous governments and the media have tried to embed.

Further education establishments, therefore, have to initiate more flexibility in their educational provision if they are to deal effectively with the behaviours that new learners may now bring to the classroom. This will entail different teaching styles and attitudinal changes to emotional and/or behavioural difficulties. Hence further education colleges are slowly coming to terms with the understanding that they are of major importance in this concept of an inclusive society. In achieving this there will need to be a college-wide approach in meeting the needs of learners. The outcome is that inclusive learning has shifted the focus to the learner, focusing on how people learn so that they can be better helped (as appropriate, and on an individual level) to learn. Experience has shown that people who have additional educational needs use the further education system at various times in their lives, but unfortunately many accredited courses have been neither accessible nor relevant to their needs.

Kennedy's view of the need to widen participation in the further education sector should help to address these issues, as the sector will be able to promote new courses to meet a variety of need, notably for people who have emotional and/or behavioural difficulties, profound and complex needs, as well as people recovering from mental health problems. People with these additional needs are currently under-represented in the further education sector. Providing access on to the educational ladder is the key to widening participation and this should have a knock-on effect for all learners.

In an attempt to ensure that new learners access the system successfully, a well constructed pastoral care system is seen as a major prerequisite to successful learning, as opposed to the often more ad hoc arrangement previously employed. This will include a tutorial system that facilitates both individuals and curricular groups, giving each time to work through action planning and other issues. College counsellors have become more widespread to counsel learners. These counsellors have the ability to refer learners to outside support agencies if necessary, and indeed work in collaboration. College policy should recognise the interaction between intellectual and emotional factors in learners.

It is generally agreed that the emotional and behavioural difficulties of learners should be combated constructively. Learners with additional needs have often experienced 'managed moves' that have displaced them from the National Curriculum, thus strengthening an already negative self-image and reinforcing their failure within the 'normal' system. Smith (1991) has argued against displacing the National Curriculum. The modification of certain aspects of the curriculum is not applicable within the further education sector. Validating bodies set the standards and criteria of achievement nationally. However, colleges can offer courses divided into short, achievable modules. This can help to raise an individual learner's self-esteem and promote more positive expectations of the education system. The inclusive learning approach also dictates that further education colleges should provide non-accredited courses primarily as a stepping stone provision for students who do not currently have either the academic qualifications or the requisite social skills to access their chosen programme straight away.

It should be noted that society as a whole has a role to play in promoting inclusivity, if it is to become anything other than an expectation of the education system. Thus all organisations, both statutory and voluntary, should ensure that they provide an equality of access to their services regardless of age, disability or ability if we are to achieve a truly inclusive society.

THE WAY FORWARD

There has in the past been an inconsistent approach to implementing inclusive learning within colleges; some of the reasons behind this are that each college reflects the community that it serves. Hence in some areas where large long-stay hospitals closed down, colleges in the locality may well have already developed an inclusive culture, working as a partner over the years alongside social services and the health authority. Other colleges may not have developed such a culture, since provision is often demand-led. Case illustrations 8.1 and 8.2 give examples of how one college has developed its provision. It must be realised that this college is very large, compared to many colleges of further education, though there are strategies now in place to help to ensure that there is a more uniform provision of inclusion across the further education sector.

The Further Education Funding Council (1998) has provided colleges with an *Inclusive Learning – Quality Initiative Prospectus* and has allocated funds to develop resource materials to assist staff and organisational development. The Prospectus has guided colleges through the planning stages to work towards an inclusive learning environment, using the quality initiative materials and working with a facilitator, whose role it is to go into colleges to advise and guide staff. This qual-

Case illustration 8.1   Hull College: discrete provision

Hull College runs a part-time course for older learners who have specific learning difficulties. Learners attend for three sessions per week, a session being 3 hours; there are eight students per class with one lecturer and one support worker. The Learning and Skills Council at present supports this small staff/student ratio. The programme runs through an academic year of three terms and each student's course can run for up to 3 years. As we emphasise the need to work with other agencies and parents we have a referral system that incorporates information from the learner's Individual Programme Plan (IPP). The learners choose programmes to suit their needs. After an initial assessment learners also choose personal targets such as to recall their telephone number or work on telling the time. This target is then attempted at each session, the lesson being the vehicle through which learning takes place both via the aims and objectives of the lesson and the personal learning aims of the learner. Thus progression can be monitored in two ways. This concept is used as a tool for carers, staff and learners to understand why they are coming to college and that it is a process in their own personal development (learning for life) rather than college as an open-ended, free 'minding' service, which it is admitted it has been misused as in the past. Our provision is needs-led rather than accreditation-led, thus we have the freedom to write the curriculum to accommodate the learning group, and where appropriate the class is accredited by the normative awarding body, for example The City and Guilds -333/1 Cookery Preliminary level award. This provision was commented upon at the last Further Education Funding Council Inspection in late October/November 2000, when it was awarded a grade two, which indicates provision that has many strengths and a few weaknesses:

A focused programme for part-time students with Learning Difficulties. It clearly links with other agencies in the use of learners' IPPs to influence the college learning programme. A standard minimal attendance of three sessions ensures that there was time for learning targets to be achieved.

The provision also has a time limit of three years, which means students are focused towards progression and this prevents recycling of students. Some accreditation was available for this group of learners. (FEFC Inspection report 2000)

Case illustration 8.2   Hull College: inclusive provision

All learners who ask via the college enrolment form or who are referred for support are assessed and consulted as to their preferred way to be supported. The class tutor is made aware of the provision that the learner has access to and works with the support worker if and when necessary. The support is reviewed at regular intervals.

Good practice example 1

Three learners who had learning difficulties and were in discrete provision transferred on to a National Vocational Qualification (NVQ) course in Motor Vehicle. A support worker supported the learners by making sure that the curriculum had been understood by them. This entailed going over the work set in class or redrafting worksheets. These learners got help with portfolio building and were encouraged to work as independently as was individually possible. They took the course over 2 years instead of 1 year.

Good practice example 2

This learner had suffered a traffic accident which had affected mobility and short-term memory. This learner preferred to have the support of a 'note taker' in the class. The class tutor also photocopied the lesson notes. This learner had access to specialist equipment when required.

Good practice example 3

This learner had a mental health problem. The class was A Level English and the learner was supported by a mentor who was available for a set period of time each week to support the learner and talk through any difficulties that may have arisen. This learner also had extra time allocated in an exam situation and had support for University place interviews.

ity initiative originated from the findings of the Tomlinson Report. Since inclusive learning originated in work about learners who have additional learning needs, this approach is relevant to all learners. The good practice that has been nurtured in isolated corners of the further education sector must now be disseminated to maximise the benefits for all learners; thus what was good practice for learners with learning difficulties should be good practice for all learners. Inclusive learning is one of a number of strategies that can help colleges to improve their provision. Colleges may use the *Inclusive Learning – Quality Initiative*

Prospectus in ways that suit their particular situation; thus this initiative is not a blanket proposal for the whole sector.

It should be remembered that the Further Education Funding Council which had control over funding, and the new Learning and Skills Council (which has taken over from the Further Education Funding Council) has a commitment to equality of opportunity. It should be said that colleges have a vested interest in following these guidelines and implementing the inclusive philosophy as far as is practicable.

The further education sector is clearly relevant to the market place, as it allows the learner easy access to learning and updating skills, so as to increase employability. This can include people returning to work after a period of child rearing, or retraining after having been made redundant. The increased importance of Information Technology has caused many people to realise that the acquisition of skills in order to use this technology and so re-enter employment is essential. Governments over the last 15 years have promoted the concept of lifelong learning as a means of developing a multi-skilled flexible work force, for whom a job for life is a thing of the past. Instead workers may be expected to change careers two or three times during their lives. This demands flexibility on the part of the learners as well as the educational institutions.

Lifelong learning is a term that in some quarters has been interpreted as a 'right' to education if and when the individual requires it, even though that right to a place on an educational course may have been taken up for merely social reasons, rather than for educational purposes. Perhaps a more practicable interpretation of lifelong learning is to think about it as learning for life.

Learning for life can be viewed in parallel to inclusive learning. The latter places an onus on the institution to provide the right supportive environment in which all people may learn. Learning for life places an onus on learners to gain a better insight into their individual skills and abilities so as to be able to transfer skills and respond flexibly to whatever situation arises.

The process of responding flexibly to one's environment, or to a challenging situation, and indeed shaping the situation, is a skill that gives a person the ability to change and succeed over time. This flexibility constitutes the key to lifelong learning. It is now understood that individuals learn in different ways and that people who did not score highly on the traditional tests, which require a certain kind of narrow ability, were systematically excluded from higher educational opportunities and, in time, professional areas. This system that our society has upheld with great reverence may cause learners who score badly at school but then achieve later in life, to view themselves as having achieved in spite of the system rather than because of it (Sternberg 1997).

The understanding that people learn in different ways, and therefore teaching must be differentiated accordingly, hopefully leads to an increase in learning. This is better than merely looking at the Intelligence Quotient (IQ) of an individual, which only considers the ability of the learner on one level (Howie, in press) and may result in low expectations by the facilitator and indeed by the learners themselves. When individuals know and work with their own preferred learning styles they will not automatically become Einsteins but will be enabled to work towards their full potential. Thus society needs to encourage an attitudinal change, so that our perception of what constitutes intelligence develops to embrace a more inclusive approach.

New perspectives on learning, led by Professors such as Lev Vygotsky, Reuven Feuerstein, Howard Gardener and Robert Sternberg, have begun to be recognised within the British education system. Their work has shown that for the educator there is a need to understand that there are a variety of learning styles (Squires 1999), and that educators need to teach in ways that recognise all talents. This is important to help to fulfil educational potential and career needs. We therefore have to measure success on an individual basis (Gipps & Tunstall 1998) to help enhance a person's sense of self-esteem, rather than compare learners with classmates or adults with workmates who have different sets of natural or nurtured attributes.

As the teaching of thinking skills is on the educational agenda at all levels, and the effects of teaching these skills should last a lifetime (Carvel 2000), staff will need to draw on certain strategies and ideologies to ensure success, and they need to work consistently together in enforcing these strategies. Fogell & Long (1997) state that staff teams need to have clear goals, be open and honest, set high standards, plan well together, be flexible enough to support colleagues in difficulties, have effective leadership, be resourced appropriately, communicate with people inside and outside of the team, have clear induction strategies, recognise and celebrate achievement and include support staff as an integral part of the team if they are to support and flourish. This applies to teaching and learning in all educational settings.

The further education sector is able to accommodate learners who have different learning styles because the curriculum is more vocationally biased and hence more practically and creatively based. This may be a reason why young people who have become disaffected with the statutory education system, or people who did not fulfil their potential the first time around, achieve more within the further education sector. Motivation is enhanced, as people can usually choose which specialist area they would like to access, be it catering or engineering. Hence people start at a point where they may have experienced success or at least have an interest. Confidence should grow as learners achieve in small steps; there is time to work out success and to analyse failure within a supportive network, as other learners are also experiencing the same process.

There are, however, some threats to the concept of inclusion. As stated earlier there was to be a 25% increase in student numbers under the last government. Added to that is this government's commitment to lifelong learning and its social inclusion initiatives (such as New Deal, which aims to get thousands of 16–19 year olds who are neither working nor studying into full-time education). This should leave no doubt as to how the further education sector will look in the future. This has inevitably resulted in a learner base that has shifted from having a motivated, work-ethical background to being a demotivated, vocationally unsure student body, many of whose basic and/or social skills hinder their employability.

Reader activity 8.2

Colleges usually have a named person who oversees inclusive learning provision. This person coordinates and enables access and support. Invite the named person to your next group meeting to explain what is available for your prospective learners; or telephone and talk to the person on an individual basis.

With a client base that is changing to include people of all ages with varying degrees of social problems as well as the more vulnerable people within our society, there have been concerns about the safety of the more vulnerable, especially during non-teaching times. Many colleges have tackled these issues through such measures as employing their own security staff or installing closed circuit television cameras. Some colleges have systems of security that are more suited to a prison than to an educational institution. Each college has dealt with this issue in its own way; however, it should be remembered that people who are vulnerable are at risk in any social situation. This issue needs to be looked at on the basis of individual colleges and their prospective learners, then strategies can be put in place within the college to ensure, as far as is possible, the safety of all learners.

Reader activity 8.3

Make arrangements to visit your local further education college. When you visit try to empathise with your prospective learners. How far is it for them to travel? Would learners cope with the hustle and bustle of college life? Could learners physically access the facilities? Remember the information that you need to gain is two-fold, you need to know that the learners will succeed, and the learners need to know that they will cope.

There are many voices from the education sector as a whole calling for caution, as Crace (2000) points out. Some people are beginning to suggest that the reason that we are losing students in the further education sector is due to the practice of social inclusion. There was a 3% decrease in numbers in further education between November 1998 and November 1999 – a decrease for the second year running. The argument put forward is that providing for lower level groups results in the middle level groups staying away or choosing sixth form colleges instead.

Indeed the 'market place' ethos is paramount to all colleges since incorporation. When it comes to choosing a college place it should be noted that parents still have an important input in deciding where their teenagers should study (Corbett & Norwich 1997). The post-sixteen sector is vulnerable in this market place, no matter how individual colleges market themselves.

Other threats are prevalent. Labelling is on the increase, since the 'market place' puts a price on to a difficulty. Dyslexia is one example that is often highlighted, though the bright side to this is that colleges have been quick to test, support and claim through their cross-college basic skills assessment, which picks up on this and indeed on any basic skill difficulties quickly, as well as allowing extra funding to be claimed. College enrolment forms may now ask all learners many questions about particular needs, and it could be argued that this takes away articulate parents getting extra support to improve the quality of their children's education (Corbett & Norwich 1997). Perhaps it is more equitable to have a system where additional support can be obtained based on personal assessment of an individual, rather than relying on more articulate others.

The long-term aim of inclusion is for all staff to manage student needs with the support of a cross-college team to advise and guide. This can cause difficulties, as inclusion will bring changes of responsibility and often additional responsibilities to staff. Not all staff are equally open to change. Moreover, further education may be working alongside external agencies to support learners' needs, but these organisations are not always working fully with each other. Even with inclusive practice it is envisaged that there will be a need for provision for discrete groups for learners who require that type of provision. This may be seen by some as internal exclusion but what is perhaps needed is a system that ensures that Warnock's 20% do not receive less support than

Reader activity 8.4

Colleges of further education and specialist colleges provide varied courses. Contact your local colleges and find out what provision they have for your prospective learners. They should send you information leaflets.

their peers (Feiler & Gibson 1999) and yet still gives importance to the match of learning needs and teaching styles that is inclusive learning.

A further problem is that the very terminology used, be it inclusive education or inclusion, has been interpreted differently within local education authorities and within schools themselves (Sebba & Ainscow 1996), so learners may reach the further education sector with very different sets of ideas as to how their needs are likely to be met. In 1987 the Centre for Studies of Integration in Education found that local education authorities had increased segregated provision. Ten years later a study of the role of local education authorities in developing inclusive polices suggested that inclusive practice should be given priority and be well integrated into all local government policy if the term inclusive education was not to come to mean traditional but parallel systems of special and mainstream education (Ainscow et al 1999). Observers hope, therefore, that Professor Tomlinson's recommendations will be adequately funded rather than simply becoming an echo of Warnock's attempts to change attitudes, since the further education sector has the capacity to take on a new lead in inclusive provision (Corbett &

Reader activity 8.5

Having visited your local further education college you might like to undertake the following activities. List the social/coping skills that your prospective learners will need to be able to access the further education sector successfully. How can you help learners to find strategies for coping if they do not already have them? What other agencies are supporting the learners? Is a local multi-agency approach operational?

Braham 1997). It may be argued that Tomlinson's conclusions are in many ways a modern version of Warnock and that if change could not be implemented over the years for those with 'deserving difficulties' (those with obvious special needs), then how probable is it that change will occur for those with 'undeserving difficulties' (those without obvious special needs).

CONCLUSION

Educational provision for people with learning disabilities has changed considerably over the last 100 years. This has been especially so in the further education sector where, prior to Warnock, provision for 16-plus learners was virtually non-existent. Warnock was viewed as a major threshold not merely in recognising that the learner will have individual educational needs, but also in stating that these should not necessarily be met through a policy of segregation. In the days of Warnock there was no national policy dictating the type of provision for people with a learning disability post-16, yet the period saw a huge expansion in this type of provision within the further education sector.

The 1980s and 1990s witnessed a greater centralisation of policy with regard to the education of those with learning disabilities; witness the establishment of the National Curriculum in schools and the Future Education Funding Council. Numerous reports have also adopted a more utilitarian stance towards education, highlighting the basic skills shortages in the UK as a whole and indicating that this would need to be rectified if the UK was to have the flexible, multi-skilled workforce that is necessary in today's global economy.

A logical conclusion from Warnock's interpretation of integration has been the concept of inclusive learning, in which a more holistic view of the learner is embodied. Identifying the needs of the learner and trying to meet them within a mainstream setting is coupled with a desire to modify the educational provision so as to achieve a match between learner and learning material.

Arguably society is still unsure of the true meaning of inclusion, as far as providing services for people with additional needs goes. There have been many interpretations placed upon the concept but no definition seems to have been given that will adequately cover them all. The trouble with change is that not all people are open to it at the same time.

Inclusive learning should provide wider access to learning for young people with a learning disability, indeed for all learners, with expert tuition at a level that they require. There should also be an increase in provision throughout adult life, to enable us to manage our changing world and to aid inclusion into society, though this should not be at the expense of other groups, whether this be the more vulnerable or the middle level groups mentioned earlier. However, labelling should be seen at present as an advantage, in that it attracts funding on behalf of the individual learner, which the further education sector uses to educate staff to facilitate the learner rather than to exclude individuals or groups. It is generally felt that there will always be a need for a wide provision and that this will include discrete groups of learners if this best meets their individual needs. Until there is an overall understanding of inclusion that is adopted throughout society for all age groups, then the further education sector will continue to lead a process that should remove boundaries.

REFERENCES

Ainscow M, Farrell P, Tweddle G, Malki G 1999 The role of LEAs in developing inclusive policies and practices. British Journal of Special Education 26(3): 136–140
Carvel J 2000 Pupils to learn how to think. The Guardian 6th January 2000
Corbett J, Norwich B 1997 Special needs and client rights: the changing social and political context of special educational

research. British Educational Research Journal 23(3): 379–389
Crace J 2000 But is it the right policy? The Guardian Education 25th April 2000
CSIE 1989 The integration charter. The Centre for Studies on Integration in Education (now the Centre for Studies of Inclusive Education), Bristol

Dearing R 1996 Review of qualifications for 14–19 year olds. SCAA, HMSO, London

DEFF 1998 The learning age. The Stationery Office, London

DHSS 1981 Care in the community – a consultative document on resources for care in England. HMSO, London

Elton (Lord) 1989 Discipline in schools; report of the committee of enquiry. Department of Education and Science. HMSO, London

Feiler A, Gibson H 1999 Threats to the inclusive movement. In: British Journal of Special Education 26(3): 147–152

Fogell J, Long R 1997 Emotional and behavioural difficulties. NASEN, Tamworth, Staffs

Further Education Funding Council 1998 Inclusive learning – quality initiative prospectus. FEFC, Coventry

Gipps C, Tunstall P 1998 Effort, ability and the teacher, young children's explanation for success and failure. Oxford Review of Education 24(2): 149–161

Hewitson-Ratcliffe C (ed) 1995 Current developments in further education. The third John Baillie Memorial Conference: report of a national conference. National Bureau for Students with Disabilities, SKILL, London

Hornby G 1999 Inclusion or delusion: can one size fit all? Support for Learning: British Journal of Learning Support 14(4): 152–157

Howie D (In Press) Thinking about the teaching of thinking. Council for Educational Research, Wellington, New Zealand

Kauffman J, Hallahan D 1995 The illusion of full inclusion: a comprehensive critique of a current special education bandwagon. PRO-ED, Austin, Texas

Kennedy H 1997 Learning works; widening participation in further education. Further Education Funding Council, Coventry

Lindsay G 1997 Values, rights and dilemmas. British Journal of Special Education 24: 55–59

Moser C 1999 Improving literacy and numeracy: a fresh start. Department for Education and Employment publications, Sudbury, Suffolk

Newell P 1983 ACE special education handbook. The new law on children with special needs. Advisory Centre for Education, London

Oliver M 1996 Understanding disability: from theory to practice. Macmillan, Basingstoke

Sebba J, Ainscow M 1996 International development in inclusive schooling: mapping the issues. Cambridge Journal of Education 26(1): 5–18

Smith C J 1991 Behaviour management: a whole-school policy. In: Hinson M (ed) Teachers and Special Educational Needs, 2nd edn. Longman, Harlow pp 165–166

Squires G 1999 Teaching as a professional discipline. Falmer Press, London, p. 119

Sternberg R 1997 The concept of intelligence and its role in lifelong learning and success. American Psychologist (October 1997) 52(10): 1030–1037

Tomlinson J 1996 The learning difficulties and disabilities committee: inclusive learning. Further Education Funding Council. HMSO, London

UNESCO 1994 Salamanca statement. Report of the World Conference on Special Educational Needs. UNESCO

Warnock M 1978 Special educational needs. Report of the committee of enquiry into the education of handicapped children and young people. HMSO, London

USEFUL ADDRESSES

Advisory Centre for Education, (ACE)
18 Victoria Park Square,
London
E2 9PB

Centre for Studies on Inclusive Education, (CSIE)
1 Redland Close,
Elm Lane,
Redland,
Bristol
BS6 6UE
Website: http://inclusion.uwe.ac.uk

National Institute for Adult and Continuing Education (NIACE)
21 De Montfort Street,
Leicester
LE12 7GE

SKILL (National Bureau for Students with Disabilities)
336 Brixton Road,
London
SW9 7AA

The Learning and Skills Council
Cheylesmore House,
Quinton Road,
Coventry
CV1 2WT

Professional publications of FEFC include:
Tomlinson J 1996 The learning difficulties and disabilities committee; inclusive learning
Kennedy H 1997 Learning works: widening participation in further education

The National Association for Special Educational Needs (NASEN)
NASEN House,
4/5 Amber Business Village,
Amber Close,
Amington,
Tamworth
B77 4RP
E-Mail: welcome@nasen.org.uk
Website: http://www.nasen.org.uk

Professional publications of NASEN include:
British Journal of Special Education
British Journal of Learning Support

9

Employment, leisure and learning disabilities

Tom Bush

CHAPTER CONTENTS

KEY ISSUES

- This chapter explores employment and leisure in relation to the general population and then more specifically in relation to people with learning disabilities.
- In particular there will be an exploration of what individuals gain from employment and leisure, and how a lack of both employment and leisure can affect the perceptions of others about an individual's circumstances and abilities.
- National and European law and convention are explored, which are increasingly impacting on access to employment for people with disabilities.
- As we enter the 21st century there is real opportunity for more people with learning disabilities to experience aspects of life that many take for granted.

DEFINING EMPLOYMENT

It is important to make a distinction between employment and work. In everyday usage the terms 'employment' and 'work' are used interchangeably. People speak of getting 'work' when what they actually mean is getting 'employment'. A client who packs screws sitting at a bench in a sheltered work setting might arguably be working but is not employed. Why is this?

To be employed, in the true sense of the word, one has to:

- receive a wage in relation to work done
- have terms and conditions of employment and

Reader activity 9.1

Spend a few minutes thinking about what is meant by the terms 'employment' and 'work'. Following this it is suggested that you spend some time looking up definitions in a good sociology textbook, and make some notes.

Reader activity 9.2

Spend some time with a colleague discussing what the terms 'leisure' and 'recreation' mean. You might also find it useful to look up some definitions of these terms in a dictionary.

- be able to be dismissed from the place of employment (Grint 1992, p. 10).

Thus a client attending a social education centre is not earning a wage, but is in receipt of benefits; the client, who has no terms and conditions for working in the centre, and is not able to be dismissed, is working but not employed. For the purposes of this chapter, work is defined as, 'Being engaged in activities for which one receives remuneration and that could not be considered as leisure or recreation' (Grint 1992, p. 11).

Another term used specifically in relation to people with learning disabilities is 'meaningful employment'. This term comes from the Canadian Service Brokerage system (Marlett 1988) and attempts to define an intermediate stage between employment and work. The main characteristics of 'meaningful employment' are that it:

- provides a wage on which one could live
- has worth to the community in which it takes place
- has worth to the individual undertaking the task
- provides social interaction with non-handicapped people in society.

DEFINING LEISURE

Just as work and employment are terms used interchangeably so too are the words 'leisure' and 'recreation'. At its simplest, leisure might be defined as 'time not spent in employment'. However, there are things that we do away from employment that we would not consider leisure, for example decorating or gardening. These might be perceived by some to represent work. They are things that have to be done for their own

sake, and hold little or no enjoyment for some individuals.

Brooman (1976), in his seminal paper on the subject, has defined leisure as: 'Time not required for employment or work of any kind' (Brooman 1976, p. 21). This definition might be thought of as problematic. Can we really say that all the time not used in work or employment is leisure? Roberts (1991) has defined leisure as a type of experience where doing things for their own sake gives the individual intrinsic satisfaction. Thus the enjoyment gained from gardening, cooking or playing games is the total reward. We allot time to undertake these activities to give us enjoyment and satisfaction. What can be seen from this are the three key elements that define leisure, namely time allocation, type of activity and the quality of experience. Added to this, leisure may also be seen as something undertaken singularly or in small groups. So, for the purposes of this chapter, leisure is defined as: 'An activity outside work or employment for which time is allocated that provides the individual with a quality experience'.

So how does this differ from the term 'recreation'? In the main, recreation is used to describe those activities that fall into the above definition but rather than being activities that take place individually, they are undertaken in small or large groups. Thus gardening would be a leisure activity and playing or watching football at a match would be recreation. However, if one watches football at home on the television this would constitute leisure. This simple distinction does, however, raise some anomalies. For example, hiking by oneself might be seen by many as a recreational pursuit, but according to the definitions advanced in this chapter it would be seen as leisure. As stated previously, the key difference between leisure and recreation is the number of people involved. Others have also added that recreation may have an enhancing effect on one's health or on the culture of a given community (Beresford et al 1984, Brooman 1976, Potterfield 1985). This would mean that to physical activities, such as playing football, could also be added cultural activities, such as the performance of plays and concerts. Thus it would be possible to define recreation as: 'An activity outside work or employment for which time is allocated that provides a group of individuals with a quality experience that enhances life and the wellbeing of an individual or a community'.

You might like to reflect on your discussions and the definitions you have previously identified in relation to the above.

WHY ARE EMPLOYMENT AND LEISURE IMPORTANT?

In a 1997 interview Sir John Hannam MP, then chair of the all party committee on disability, said the following: 'If we look at our lives they are built on three key building blocks, our employment, our pursuit of leisure and recreation and family life. If any one of these are missing or impaired then a major imbalance in the social functioning of the individual will occur' (Bush 1997).

Some might believe that if there were less time devoted to employment then there would be more time for leisure and recreation, work and the family. Studies have shown that in the early stages of unemployment this is true (Archer & Rhodes 1987, Brooman 1976). Jobs that have been waiting to be done around the house for some time get done. People also spend more time undertaking activities that they enjoyed doing outside the hours of employment, for example fishing, walking or working on the car. There is also delight in being home with the family.

However, studies have also shown that as time progresses and no employment is found, there is no more work around the house and the fun and enjoyment of leisure and recreation become boring, often because the activities become solo activities (Burgess 1999, Murray 1996). In interviews with long-term unemployed people it becomes clear that the family are perceived as an irritating fact of life, mainly because of the pressure they place on the individual to find employment. Some studies have shown that long-term unemployed people exhibit major social dysfunction, not wanting to go out or mix with other people (Burgess 1999, Murray 1996). They appear to lose the work habit, and see a major change in their waking time from day to night. In interviews the author has undertaken with long-term unemployed people from the general population, and with people with learning disabilities, it is striking to note the similarity in social dysfunction in both groups. For example, both report difficulty in making choices; also making social contact with others is very difficult; they experienced difficulty in articulating feelings, as well as losing the will to work or participate in any social activity. This may explain why some studies have shown that long-term unemployed married males have a higher than average divorce rate (Brooman 1976, Grint 1992, Wedderburn 1965).

THE ROLE OF EMPLOYMENT IN SOCIETY

A measure of status

Beresford et al (1984) have pointed out that we live in a wage-based society where people are largely defined and valued according to whether they have employment and what kind of employment they have. Brooman (1976) has stated that it is instilled into us from a very early age that individuals should practise the virtues of industry and thrift. Thus, not to work as a general rule is seen in the UK as being wrong, deviant and antisocial, unless there are overriding reasons why this should be so, for example due to a disability. Thus, by implication, income and status are accorded to people by their employment. The value placed on employment does not seem to have been undermined by the rising rates of unemployment that have existed in past decades. Long-term unemployment is still seen by many in society as being the fault of the individual, rather than due to the economic climate prevailing at the time (Burgess 1999). It could be argued that the reason why both British and other European governments have invested in training schemes for unemployed young people has been to preserve the work ethic. For people with learning disabilities, high unemployment has had two major effects.

First, it has meant that job opportunities were radically reduced. In interviews with the author for his PhD study in the mid-1990s, various employment agencies such as the Shaw Trust and Mencap's Pathway Employment Scheme spoke of the difficulty in getting jobs for people with disabilities. In the main this was because employers perceived the needs of the so-called 'normal population' as being greater than those of people with a disability. As a consequence, at a time of moderate unemployment levels they were more inclined to give jobs to the non-disabled many, on the grounds that they had more family and financial commitments.

Secondly, as youth and long-term unemployment rose, places on government training schemes became more difficult to obtain. To alleviate this shortage there was a tendency to exclude people with learning disabilities from them. In April 1995 the Department of Employment allowed 27% of all places on government sponsored training schemes to be 'protected', i.e. they would be specifically reserved for people with a disability; of these 1% were to be for people with learning disabilities. In April 1996 the Department for Education and Employment reduced the 'protected' starts to 26% and no allocation for special groups within that total was allowed. Added to this there was a general reduction in funding for training places and a reduction in the time training programmes could last. In 1990 training programmes lasted between 12 and 24 months; by 1998 the average length of a course was 16 weeks. This had the effect, nationally, of allowing only people who had an 80% chance of gaining employment to start the courses. This virtually ruled out anyone with a learning disability for they were perceived to have a much lower chance of gaining employment by the schemes' organisers (Bush 1997).

It has been stated that employment has a profound effect upon our lives (Roberts 1991, Rusch & Schutz 1981). For most people employment is the main source of income, status, occupation and purpose in life. For many it is the main time consumer of our day; it provides us with life chances; it provides a means to live. For many minority groups, and in particular people with learning disabilities, finding employment is much more difficult than for the average member of the general population (Potterfield 1985). When jobs are found they tend to be at the lower end of the employment spectrum: poorly paid, poorly valued, less secure and less pleasant (Bush 1991). Unlike the majority of these groups, people with learning disabilities have no national body safeguarding their employment prospects. Wolfensberger & Tullman (1989) have explained that the lack of paid employment is one factor that has added to the devalued way that industrialised societies perceive people with learning disabilities. They also stated that without employment that was valued by society, people with learning disabilities would have difficulty adjusting to the demands of society, as well as this having a detrimental effect on their self-image. By making people with a disability dependent on benefits to finance their lifestyle, we ensure that they will always be dependent on others to make their life choices.

Reader activity 9.3

Imagine that you are at a party by yourself and you know none of the other people there. Usually in such situations, when meeting someone for the first time, it is not long before the question is asked, 'What do you do for a living?' Often the reason for asking this question is to place the person in context and to measure their status against yours. Imagine then, being at such a party and using your current employment status, how you would feel if the other person introduced themselves as:

- the chief executive of a major company
- a person with the same job as you
- a student
- a long-term unemployed person?

Discuss with a colleague and compare how knowing what their occupation was affected your perception of them.

A means of earning money

Besides being an index by which one is judged by society, money also provides opportunities to participate in a range of activities, both leisure and social. It also provides access to a wide range of opportunities and experiences that potentially integrate one into society. A fundamental feature of income for people with learning disabilities is their reliance on social security benefits. When attending social education centres people with learning disabilities might be offered a system of reward payments for work undertaken at the centre. These rewards bear little or no relation to the actual rate that should be paid for the job. In fact the amount is well below what one would expect to earn if doing a similar job in a normal work situation, or even the minimum wage. The usual justification for the low level of pay is that to pay people at a higher rate would cause their benefits to be cut. However, by maintaining this state of affairs, the net effect on individuals is to keep them socially dependent and devalued. In contrast, in Denmark people with a learning disability are paid a non-contributory disability pension equal to £800 per week. The Danes believe, as stated in their constitution, that 'Any person unable to support themselves or their dependants shall . . . be entitled to receive public assistance' (Bush 1991, p. 44).

The Danish Central Council for the Handicapped has interpreted this to mean that benefits paid should be at a level that will enable an individual to live as normal a life as possible, i.e. their benefits should not be a means by which discrimination could be exercised. Benefits should also not be a means whereby the state could intervene in the autonomy of an individual. This means that people with learning disabilities living in Denmark have a much higher standard of living and financial independence than their British counterparts. Where earnings from employment are gained, the reduction of benefits is on a graded scale. This means that an individual will not lose money when moving from benefits to earnings. In the UK we have no such system. Instead there are cut off points that mean if you earn a wage just above the benefit level, you will lose the total benefit, which has the effect of the individual receiving less money. This is often referred to as 'the benefits trap'. To overcome this the Conservative government in the mid-1990s introduced Disabled Working Allowance. This allowance was paid at the rate of £50 per week, indexed to the rate of inflation, to those who had been on Disability Living Allowance and were attempting to move off benefits and go into full-time employment. Even with this benefit the situation has changed little. The Disability Working Allowance was replaced in October 1999 by the Disabled Persons Tax Credit, which appears more flexible in its approach to bridging the poverty trap, being linked to earnings as opposed to being a fixed rate, which was the case with the former allowance.

Under the new national strategy the government has made two major commitments (DOH 2001). The first is that Job Brokers established under the New Deal for Disabled People, set up jointly between the Department of Social Security and the Department of Education and Employment in 2000, who offer work-focused help to the disabled, will have to work with people with learning disabilities. Secondly, so as to assist with the overcoming of the 'benefit trap', people with learning disabilities should not automatically lose their right to DLA. The new national strategy makes it clear that decision-makers in relation to benefit payments do not have to stop DLA once a person with a disability starts work.

A means of structuring our lives

As human beings, order and structure play an important part in our lives. Many studies have shown that without employment to structure our day life becomes meaningless. (Archer and Rhodes 1987, Sinfield 1985, Wedderburn; 1965). Without employment the need for a structure to our day disappears. We also accept, as part of the work ethic, that if we are in employment and do not adhere to a structure then penalties may be incurred, such as losing pay for being late. It is a general myth that people with learning disabilities have no need for structure or order in their lives. Indeed, some members of the general public would suggest that they have little drive or ambition, this is not the case. A publication by Mencap based on interviews conducted in England called *Empty Days, Empty Lives* (Mencap 1991) clearly demonstrated that people with learning disabilities want order and structure in their lives and for that to happen by being given meaningful employment. What they actually receive is a very poorly coordinated approach to life, often changed at the whim of an individual for no apparent reason. Social education centres often have late starts and early finishes, where no attempt is made to match the day to a normal working schedule. In most other northern European countries the approach to this problem was to set up training centres on industrial estates. The programmes for the day were to match the usual work patterns of factory life. Staff employed in such units would be an equal mix of skilled craftsmen and social pedagogues (teachers of social skills). In doing this it was hoped that this would ease the integration of people with learning disabilities into open employment (LEV 1992).

Control

By having money and status people are in some ways able to influence the courses that their lives are likely to take. A key part of that control is the range and extent of choices that are open to them. A lack of money often reduces the range of choices available. Arguably, this might mean that choice is exercised by those who control one's flow of cash. People with learning disabilities often have a marked lack of income. What income they gain from benefits is often in the control of others, mainly due to the benefits being paid to a nominated person on their behalf. The lack of income and the lack of control over their benefits often places individuals with learning disabilities into a dependent relationship: they never have a chance to prove that they can make choices or handle money. In most other northern European countries all benefits are paid to the individual concerned. Only if it can be demonstrated that the individual is unable to handle money, will the benefit be paid to a nominated person. With benefits paid to the individual and at the same level as

other citizens, the income for a person with learning disabilities is broadly comparable with the average wage. The effect of having at least the equivalent of the average wage is to give similar choices to individuals with learning disabilities about how they live their lives (Mead 1997).

Image and self-image

Several studies have highlighted the psychological effects of unemployment on the individual (Sinfield 1985, Wedderburn 1965). In Wedderburn's study, informants recalled how it felt to be unemployed: 'I feel ashamed. I go around the back streets, and I don't meet people'; 'I have the feeling of being totally unwanted, rejected and abandoned by society'; 'I miss the company of my work mates; when I see them now I have little in common to talk with them about'. In 1991 Mencap undertook a similar study amongst people with learning disabilities who wanted to work, but were unable to gain employment. Similar responses were found: 'There is no life after 19 . . . all that education was great. But what for . . . I have no job'; 'All I do all day is jigsaws and watch telly'; 'At home you feel bored . . . having your own family is not enough . . . we need more . . . we need cheering up.' Both these sets of quotations are from long-term unemployed people. Both demonstrate low levels of self-esteem because of lack of work. Having a disability of any form does not stop one losing self-esteem, indeed it could aggravate it. The general image projected about people with learning disabilities is one of a dependent non-worker who is incapable of all but the simplest employment (DOH 2001). The type of employment offered and the environment in which it takes place often compound this view (Bass & Verlangi 1995, Bush 1991).

A similar view of people with learning disabilities existed in the 1970s in the Danish system. In an interview John Moller, Director of Landforenningen Evnesvages Vel (LEV) (the Danish equivalent of Mencap), commented on the general lack of a positive image of people with learning disabilities in Denmark. In 1980 all the charities who cared for people with any kind of disability decided to form the Central Council for the Handicapped, to evaluate the conditions of the handicapped and to act as a unified pressure group to improve the conditions and image of the disabled. This attempt to display a positive image for the disabled had a major impact upon services provided to people with learning disabilities and upon the attitude of the providers of these services.

Relationships

John Moller, Director of LEV, made the following comment:

Examine your own life and look at your relationships and you will see that they are founded on three key aspects of your life, i.e. your work; your leisure; your family. All these take place in a community context. If you have no employment, no leisure, no life set in your local community how can you ever expect to have normal relationships (LEV 1992).

Beresford (1984) has pointed out that it is through employment that we have the opportunity to meet a variety of people in different walks of life and social settings. It is through these encounters that we measure, absorb and reflect our own performance and image against others and, in so doing, become accepted within the social culture of our community. By removing this opportunity to work with so called 'normal people', society curtails the opportunities for people with learning disabilities to build relationships with ordinary people. Studies have shown that when we evaluate what people with learning disabilities get from work, high on the list are social relations and interactions with the general populous (Mank et al 1998, Rusch et al 1997). If their opportunities to mix socially through leisure are reduced, either because of lack of money or segregated opportunities, then they are further isolated, creating what Wolfensberger (1980) referred to as 'devalued people'.

A sense of achievement

It is often the case that through our chosen careers we obtain a sense of achievement in our lives, sometimes by stepping up rungs on a promotion ladder. For the majority in our society the need to achieve is part of an inculcation process through our education systems and through our parents at home.

However, in the case of people with learning disabilities, this normal pattern of expectation is not fostered (Beyer et al 1996). In general the expectations of parents and teachers tend to be very low, with the resultant effect that low expectation produces low achievement in the child. It also leads, in later life, to the parents and professionals not expecting much in the way of employment for the person with learning disabilities.

In Britain, the usual criterion for employability is that the applicant has demonstrated some achievement in either the academic or the vocational field, in the form of formal qualifications or through vocational qualifications achieved whilst working. For most people with learning disabilities these qualifications are never obtained, mainly due to lack of opportunities to prove themselves and low expectations of carers.

The northern European experience has been a little different. To overcome the problem of demonstrating employability, training centres adopted a different approach to providing meaningful employment. This approach was to identify niches in the market for quality products. Once the product was identified it was to be manufactured for sale on the open market. Work done by clients would be remunerated as a wage paid out of the income from product sales. When people with learning disabilities demonstrated that they could produce a high quality product on a consistent basis, and handle normal factory plant in a factory-type setting, employers could see the quality of work that clients could do. How this actually works in practice will be outlined later. This is in marked contrast to British social education centres where production processes have been largely removed. This has happened for a variety of reasons, the most important of which has been doubt about the clients' abilities to operate machinery, and fears about the safety of clients.

To summarise, it is work and the money generated from it that give us many of life's chances and experiences and make us the individuals that we are. If society takes away the opportunity to work and earn a wage, as has been described, not only do people lose their means of income but they also lose a whole raft of psychological states and support mechanisms that allow them to operate effectively in society. Often self-image and confidence are dented and people are unable to hold their heads up in social settings. It is often noted how difficult long-term unemployed people find it to make choices and be motivated (Brooman 1976). Similar findings have also been demonstrated with people with learning disabilities working in social education centres (Mencap 1991).

EMPLOYMENT AND PEOPLE WITH LEARNING DISABILITIES

Types of employment

At the beginning of this chapter the term employment was defined. It will be remembered that this definition comprised of the following elements:

- to receive a wage in relation to work done
- to have terms and conditions of employment
- to be able to be dismissed from the place of employment (Grint 1992, p. 10).

Another term also used at the beginning of the chapter was 'meaningful employment'. This was defined as:

- provides a wage on which one could live
- has worth to the society in which it takes place
- has worth to the individual undertaking the task
- provides a social interaction with non-handicapped people in society.

The reason for reviewing these two terms is that it is possible for people with disabilities to have all of the elements in the first definition and still not have a worthwhile job, and therefore still be disadvantaged in society by their employment. Using the first definition it is possible for a disabled person to be working entirely with other disabled people, earning a wage and creating a product that only really sells through sympathy for a particular disability, e.g. craft goods made by the blind. If the other criteria from the definition of meaningful employment are added, i.e. a wage to live on, mixing with other non-disabled people and doing a job that is valued by society, then the whole quality of the employment experience is improved. With this in mind, a list of employment options in the UK are identified.

Employment opportunities for people with learning disabilities

It is possible to group employment opportunities for people with learning disabilities under several headings.

Open employment

Open employment refers to the individual who has gained employment on a full or part-time basis, and is working independently without support from services, once established in post. According to Whelan (1985), it is likely that the majority of people with mild learning disabilities who work have this kind of employment. However, people with learning disabilities are not a homogeneous group, so people with moderate, severe or profound learning disabilities might also be included in this approach.

Job sharing

The usual concept of job sharing is where a full-time post is divided amongst a number of people each of whom is unable to contract for the full number of hours, but who can do so when their time availability is put together.

In relation to people with learning disabilities, job sharing has the advantage of letting more clients sample work in an open employment situation, particularly when such jobs are scarce. Beresford et al (1984) have pointed out that job sharing can be used to divide skills amongst people, e.g. domestic help posts can involve shopping, cleaning and food preparation. These tasks could be divided between several clients at the same or at different times of the day.

Options for job sharing could be as individual as the people prepared to accept the posts. It has been found by many employers who use such job sharing arrangements, that they actually gain more from the shared post than if they had only employed one person (Bush 1997). However, in the case of people with learning disabilities, it is important to ensure that this does not result in exploitation.

Sheltered work employment

This can be present in several different forms, the most common being when disabled people work in units specifically established for them. However, in more recent years the idea of segregated workshops has given way to 'enclave' schemes. These are where groups of disabled workers are employed within a normal work setting, as a small group, within the organisation of a larger factory or place of work.

Such groups allow people with learning disabilities to experience a work situation without being exposed to the full conditions of a normal contract of employment. It is usual to find such schemes being developed as a bridge to full employment, or as a means to providing employment for people with more severe learning disabilities (Beresford et al 1984).

Work experience

These tend to be short-term placements that allow people with learning disabilities to sample the working environment without necessarily being offered a full-time post. They are usually part of a training programme to equip an individual with the necessary skills so as to undertake full-time employment.

However, such places might also be used to give the employer the opportunity of experiencing what a person with learning disabilities could undertake. In this way individuals are given a useful 'foot in the door' opportunity to demonstrate what they are capable of doing to a reluctant employer (Whelan & Speake 1981).

Finally, work experience can also be used to overcome the benefit trap by allowing employment to take place on a short-term basis without adversely affecting the benefit payments for individuals. Various organisations such as the Shaw Trust and Mencap's Pathway to Employment Scheme have used this approach with varying degrees of success.

Job shadowing

This allows an individual with learning disabilities the opportunity of working alongside a fully skilled worker. As such the individual has the opportunity to work as a 'mate' and assist in whatever is appropriate.

This type of work experience often allows the less able client the opportunity to experience work. It is also of great value in allowing the individual to network through a whole circle of new relationships with non-handicapped people (Beresford et al 1984).

Training schemes

In the 1980s and early 90s, when unemployment was high amongst young people in the UK, the Manpower Services Commission provided a whole variety of training schemes for the unemployed, and still does today. Such schemes are often designed to train people for work and, as such, provide an ideal training medium for people with learning disabilities.

However, because the number of places on such schemes often outstrips demand, there is a reluctance on the part of managers of such schemes to offer places to people with learning disabilities. To overcome this, some training agencies have, as part of their funding strategy, placed in their plans for course development specific training schemes for people with a 'social, mental or physical disability'. Unfortunately such schemes tend to be time-limited and only provide a short-term option for employment.

Cooperatives

Much of the development of cooperatives arose out of the late 1970s employment policy of the last Labour Government. Such cooperatives are usually on a small scale and allow the ownership of a particular facility and any resultant profits to be shared amongst the entire work force. This work has been further developed under the auspices of the European Community, through its Social Development Fund.

In the majority of cases such cooperatives appear to develop a niche market for a service or a product. These have included 'whole food' products, fabric design, printing and craft products. The aim of the majority of such cooperatives is to lift the employment of people with a learning disability away from the mundane. By giving them jobs that have status it is hoped to raise their status in the eyes of the community. Good examples of these are the Hope Nursery, based in Hertfordshire, and the Wharf Bakery in the East End of London. Schemes also exist in other parts of the country such as the Saw Doctors in Newcastle and Quinn Foods in South Devon.

Adult training/social education centres/resource centres

For a majority of people with learning disabilities this is still the major provider of day services (Bush 1991). Often such centres provide work experience through line assembly tasks. So as to gain contracts for such work, centres quote prices that do not allow the client to be paid a living wage for the work undertaken.

The usual type of assembly work ranges from packing screws in boxes to packing and labelling cosmetics for major companies. In the main such centres cater for people with more severe and profound learning disabilities and, as a consequence, achieving strict delivery times and quality control might be difficult.

The Department of Health's recently published strategy for learning disabilities (DOH 2001) challenges this and provides a 5 year plan to support local councils in modernising their day services. The aim will be to provide services and activities that will allow people with learning disabilities to lead full and purposeful lives in their chosen communities. The strategy sees a much closer link developing between social education centres and supported employment schemes, so as to ensure seamless progress between the two services. To aid this modernisation, under the new strategy the government have agreed to give additional funding through the Learning Disability Development Fund, in order to provide bridging finance to support the change. Development work on the new day service provision has to be completed by 2006.

EMPLOYMENT, DISABILITY AND THE LAW

The Disability Discrimination Act 1995

The Disability Discrimination Act 1995 has slowly been making an impact on how employers see disability, and how they are looking at ways in which disabled people, including people with learning disabilities, can be incorporated into the general workforce. Under Section 4 of the Act it is illegal for an employer to discriminate against a disabled person:

- in arrangements for what determines who should be employed
- in terms of employment
- by refusing to offer employment to disabled people on the grounds of their disability.

If the disabled person is already employed it is unlawful for the employer to discriminate:

- in terms of employment undertaken
- in opportunities for promotion
- by refusing training
- by dismissing the person on the grounds of disability.

Also under the Act employees with a disability are entitled to the same full pay and conditions offered to other employees.

This Act, coupled with a shrinking pool of labour, has meant that employers have been looking for new sources of labour. At the last time of near-full employment in the 1950s and 60s, the new sources of labour were women and workers from the new commonwealth. As we approach near-full employment again, the new source of labour may be those with a disability.

Employers appear to view favourably the work of such people as Gold (1981) from the USA. Gold found that, following training, people with learning disabilities on average took 50% longer to pick up a skill when compared with other employees. However, once the skill was learnt, their efficiency rating (ability to do the task correctly) was on average 90%. This compared favourably with those without disability, whose efficiency rating was reported to be around 75%. Thus, the smaller number of rejects in production, compared with the normal worker, offset the cost of longer training. In a longitudinal study conducted in the USA it was found that people with learning disabilities stayed with their employers longer, had no greater sickness record than the average worker and were generally viewed by employers to be 'good employees' (Kraus 1982). Work undertaken more recently in the UK seems to support these findings (Beyer et al 1996, Bush 1991).

There is also a growing body of anecdotal evidence that the introduction of the Disability Discrimination Act 1995 is beginning to influence how people with disabilities are being placed into employment. Two trends already evident are:

- Employment agencies for people with learning disabilities are moving from job coaching to acting as consultants in how such people can best be used by companies such as Sainsbury's, Forte and McDonald's.
- Major companies are looking at how to provide 'in house' support for people with learning disabilities, to meet their obligations under the Act.

In so doing, many companies are finding that employing a person with learning disabilities is not an act of charity but a sound business decision.

European Convention on Human Rights (Human Rights Act 1998)

Far less clear is what effect the incorporation of the European Convention on Human Rights will have in relation to employment and disability, now that it is part of UK law. The convention sets forth a number of fundamental rights and freedoms. These are:

- the right to life
- prohibition of torture
- prohibition of slavery and forced labour
- right to liberty and security
- right to a fair trial
- no punishment without law
- right to respect for private and family life
- freedom of assembly and association
- right to marry
- the right to an effective remedy
- prohibition of discrimination.

As can be seen, there is no direct mention of the right to employment. However, running parallel with the convention is the European Social Chapter (1961). Within part 1 of the Chapter it is clearly stated what rights citizens of the European Community can expect. This Convention states that all people should have the opportunity to earn their own living in an occupation freely entered upon. Also, that workers should receive fair remuneration, sufficient for a decent standard of living for themselves and their families. Workers also have the right to appropriate vocational training. The Chapter states specifically that disabled persons have the right to vocational training, rehabilitation and resettlement whatever the origin and nature of their disability. As yet there has been no major testing of the Convention and Chapter in a British Court, but this may only be a matter of time.

LEISURE AND RECREATION IN THE LIVES OF PEOPLE WITH LEARNING DISABILITIES

At the beginning of this chapter leisure was defined as being: 'An activity outside work or employment for which time is allocated that provides an individual with a quality experience', and recreation as: 'An activity outside work or employment for which time is allocated that provides a group of individuals with a quality experience that enhances life and the wellbeing of the individuals or community.' Various studies, such as that undertaken by Mencap, *Empty Days, Empty Lives* (Mencap 1991), have been carried out over the years that have looked at how people with learning disabilities spend their leisure time. In the main such studies have consistently demonstrated that most spend their time in solitary activities that require little energy. When activities are carried out in groups, often these are with their own families, or with similar people from the residential homes where they live. Where people with learning disabilities live in residential homes, most leisure time is spent undertaking group activities such as minibus trips; clients rarely undertake leisure or recreational activities on an individual basis.

The main problem in providing leisure and recreational activities for people with learning disabilities is the danger of such activities becoming 'therapy sessions'. This is not to say that therapy might not be a secondary issue, but the overriding aim should be to provide satisfaction and enjoyment. This can often be achieved by making sure that staff who carry out therapy sessions do not take the lead in sessions that are for leisure or recreation. The reason for this is that having the same staff leading therapy as well as leisure and recreation sessions can lead to confusion in the minds of people with learning disabilities, taking away the enjoyment of a leisure or recreational activity. Equally, undertaking such activities when the rest of the community might undertake them, i.e. in the evenings and at weekends, helps to make the distinction between therapy and recreation and leisure more clear.

Leisure as a means of integration

Providing leisure and recreation for specialist groups away from mainstream groups has had the effect of segregating people with learning disabilities from society. In years past it was rare to see groups of disabled people joining in with so called 'normal' people in leisure and recreational activities. However, with the adoption of the view that people with learning disabilities should be socially valued, the role of leisure and recreational pursuits as a means of socially integrating people with learning disabilities has become increasingly recognised. Added to this has been the growth in leisure and recreational centres offering a wide range of activities for the general population.

With the vast majority of people with learning disabilities now living in the community, rather than in large residential institutions, it is to the local community that clients and carers should look initially to have their leisure and recreational needs met. There are now many organisations that welcome people with learning disabilities, from the very young to the old, into their midst. Organisations such as the Scout movement and Guides have active policies of encouraging disabled children into their groups, and have special programmes that allow them to get the full benefit of belonging to such organisations. Many sports clubs now enrol people with disabilities and develop their strengths, often encouraging them to prepare for events such as the UK Mini Olympics, held for people with learning disabilities, or even international events such as the recent Paraplegic Olympics in Sydney 2000.

Often there is a lack of information as to where clubs and organisations that welcome disabled people meet. A useful source for such information is the local public library; however this often relies on the organisations posting their information to the library services, and as such it is a passive way for people to gain information. In some parts of the country groups that work with people with disabilities have tried a more active approach by developing information booklets on what is available in given local communities. In the main these have been very successful but the task of keeping the information up-to-date has, at times, been problematic.

Choosing activities

It goes without saying that choosing activities very much depends on what a person with learning disabilities wants to do. Research has shown that people with a learning disability have clear ideas as to what they enjoy doing and how they would like to spend their leisure time (Mencap 1991). Evidence from such research shows that most want to undertake activities that are age appropriate. In some cases this might be difficult, as the intellectual ability of a person with learning disabilities may preclude them from fully understanding what has to be done, or what is going on. However, this should not bar them from being involved with that activity. Where this is a problem, many groups and organisations provide 'buddies' or 'friends' to help individuals understand and cope with what is going on.

The key to achieving meaningful occupation and leisure is allowing individuals to choose their own leisure and recreational activities. This assumes that people with learning disabilities have a clear idea as to what they want to do. This is not always the case and it is at this point that carers, relatives and advocates have a valuable role to play. They can make suggestions and, as they often have their own leisure and recreational activities, can introduce the person with a learning disability to what they enjoy doing. A good example of this would be taking a friend to a football match, or accompanying a friend on a fishing trip; the list could be endless. So often ordinary opportunities are overlooked, and yet they represent a valuable resource for people with learning disabilities.

Types of activities and pursuits

Writing about activities and pursuits is very difficult, mainly because the number and type of activities are many and varied. However, it is possible to group activities undertaken by people with learning disabilities under four main headings:

- Domestic leisure
- The arts
- Technology
- Physical activity

Domestic leisure

As far back as 1991, research was showing that the majority of people with learning disabilities spend much of their leisure time at home (Mencap 1991). Ten years on the new national strategy still sees this as the case (DOH 2001). As stated earlier, domestic leisure activity is mainly watching television or undertaking solo activities such as reading, doing puzzles or playing on a computer. If these are the only leisure activities the person with learning disabilities undertakes, opportunities to network with other people outside the family are severely restricted. According to the new national strategy document *Valuing People*, (DOH 2001), this is why so many people with learning disabilities become socially isolated. This also places greater pressure on carers, who do not get a break if the person with learning disabilities is never out of the house (Emap 2000).

The arts

There exist throughout the UK a number of performing arts companies that either cater exclu-sively for people with a disability or have mixed abled and disabled groups. All have found that by including people with a learning disability into their performances they have been able to enrich their activities. There have been several international events that have had a major impact in this area. Of particular note was the opera Madam Butterfly performed at Sydney Opera House in the 1970s by people with learning disabilities miming to record. The performance was recorded by Australian television and seen throughout the world to great acclaim. The new national strategy (DOH 2001) mentions a good example of one such company. Heart n' Soul is a national touring company with 10 people with learning disabilities and four professional musicians. Based in London, they run a night club and have toured the UK with 10 full-scale musical productions as well as producing their own television programme, Breaking the Rules, on BBC2. A fuller list of drama groups can be found at the end of the chapter.

Technology

The development of modern technology, mainly through computer and micro technology, has opened new doors for people with learning disabilities. Just as for other members of the community, computers hold great fascination for people with learning disabilities. Several companies, such as Widgit and Inclusive Technologies Ltd., have specialised in developing computer programmes especially for people with learning disabilities. The author's main objection to these has been that, as stated earlier, the line between therapy and leisure is difficult to define. In the main, many of the computer programmes and much of the web technology can be accessible with help.

Physical activities

It is in this area of activity that major strides have been made in perceptions of what people with learning disabilities can do. There are several examples of activities that would have been unthinkable several years ago. In 1998 a group of people with learning disabilities from England went with an Everest trekking group to Everest

Base Camp. They out-walked the other members of the group and were often found keeping up with the sherpas (Massey & Rose 1992). A second example comes from the Paraplegic Olympics where a person with Down syndrome from the West of England was found to be lifting weights just under the world record for his class. This demonstrates that learning disabilities need not be a barrier to the physical activities that people can undertake.

CONCLUSION

In this chapter employment and leisure, in relation to the general population and also to people with learning disabilities, have been explored. It has been suggested that people with learning disabilities have the same needs as other members of the communities in which they live. In years past they have been discriminated against on the grounds of their disabilities and this has led to marginalisation. However, research demonstrates that some people with learning disabilities are able to undertake a day's work at the same standard as or at an even better standard than the average person, providing the training and conditions are right.

This chapter has also explored what is meant by employment and leisure, and how these concepts apply to the lives of people with learning disabilities, as well as to our own lives. From this it has been demonstrated that the effects of unemployment and lack of money and choices are similar in the long-term unemployed and in people with a learning disability who have never been fully employed.

In particular this chapter has explored what people gain from employment and leisure and how a lack of both employment and leisure can affect the perceptions of others about an individual's circumstances and abilities. This leads to the question of what it is that disables a person with disabilities. Seemingly it may be the lack of meaningful employment and of contact with other people in normal community settings that causes social isolation and further disables a person with learning disabilities.

National and European law together with European Conventions are increasingly having an impact on access to employment for people with disabilities. Employers are much more serious about fulfilling their obligations under the Disability Discrimination Act 1995 and the European Social Chapter. Seemingly employers are looking anew at people with learning disabilities and seeing that there is a new and valuable source of labour that is ready for developing.

The leisure industry is growing, and with the right to refuse disabled people access to such resources now outlawed, new and exciting opportunities are opening up. Most holiday companies welcome all client groups, although some still ask to be notified if the customer has a physical disability. Companies are realising that the market for providing leisure pursuits and recreation for people with learning disabilities is an area ready for development. It has been exciting to see the range of leisure pursuits that have been undertaken, ranging from sedate horse riding to hiking to Everest Base Camp in Nepal.

As we enter the 21st century there is real opportunity for more people with learning disabilities to experience aspects of life that many other people take for granted. However, in so doing, they will still only be catching up with many of their European counterparts who have had these opportunities for many years.

The new National Strategy, as part of its objectives, has identified the importance of employment and leisure in the lives of people with learning disabilities. It aims to increase the number of people with learning disabilities participating in employment by a variety of strategies and initiatives. It also intends to broaden the range of leisure and recreational activities by ensuring that planning for leisure and recreation is built into individual and community care plans. To enable all this to happen the government has allocated new money, as well as reviewing the work of government agencies involved in the provision and support of employment, leisure and recreation.

REFERENCES

Archer J, Rhodes V 1987 Bereavement and reactions to job loss. A comparative review. British Journal of Social Psychology 26(3): 211–224

Bass M, Velangi R 1995 The employers – what they think of supported employment. European Journal of Supported Employment 1(1): 14–18 (Oct 1995)

Beresford P 1984 An ordinary working life: vocational services for people with mental handicap, Project Paper 50. King Edward's Hospital Fund for London, London

Beyer S, Goodere L, Kilsby M 1996 The cost and benefits of supported employment agencies. Welsh Centre for Learning Disabilities (Applied Research), Cardiff

Brooman F S 1976 Employment and unemployment. In: Sarre P (ed) The limits of everyday thinking. The Open University Press, Milton Keynes

Burgess C 1999 The class of '81. Centre for Policy Studies, London

Bush T 1991 It's off to work we go: a research monogram. University of Portsmouth Library, Portsmouth

Bush T 1997 Recorded interview transcript with Sir John Hannam. House of Commons. Available from author

DOH 2001 Valuing people. A new strategy for learning disabilities for the 21st century. Cmd 5086, HMSO, London

Emap 2000 Learning disabilities and the care of the older person. Emap Health Care, London

Gold M 1981 Try another way manual. Champaign 177. Research Press, Wisconsin

Grint K 1992 The sociology of work. An introduction. Polity Press, Cambridge

Hannam J 1996 Unpublished recorded interview with author, 24th July 1996

Kraus M 1982 Competitive employment training for mentally retarded adults: the support work model. American Journal of Mental Deficiency 76: 653–656

LEV 1992 Scandinavia – normalisation and integration. LEV, Copenhagen

Mank D, Cioffi A, Yovanoff P 1998 Employment outcomes for people with severe disabilities: opportunities for improvement. Mental Retardation 36(3): 205–216 (June 1998)

Marlett N 1988 Independent service brokerage, Dinsdale Centre, Alberta, Canada

Massey P, Rose S, 1992 Adventurous outdoor activities: a review and description of a new service delivery package for clients with learning difficulties who have behaviour which challenge services or society. Journal of Advanced Nursing 17(12): 1415–1421 (December 1992)

Mead M 1997 From welfare to work. IEA, London

Mencap 1986 Day services – today and tomorrow – Mencap's vision. Mencap Publications, London

Mencap 1991 Empty days, empty lives. Mencap Publications, London

Murray C 1996 Charles Murray's underclass. The Institute of Economic Affairs, London

Potterfield J 1985 The employment of people with a mental handicap: progress towards an ordinary working life. Project Paper 55, King Edward's Hospital Fund for London, London

Roberts K 1991 Youth employment. In: Thomas K 1991 Work, employment and unemployment. Open University Press, Milton Keynes

Rusch F R, Schutz R P 1981 Vocational and social work behaviour.

Sinfield A 1985 Being out of work. In: Littler C (ed) The experience of work. Gower, Aldershot

Wedderburn D 1965 Redundancy and the railway men. University of Cambridge Department of Applied Economics, Occasional Paper 4, Cambridge University Press, Cambridge

Whelan E, Speake B 1981 Getting to work. Human Horizon Series, Souvenir Press, London

Whelan P 1985 Competitive employment for persons with mental retardation. Mental Retardation 23(6): 274–281

Wolfensberger W 1980 The definition of normalisation: update, problems, disagreements and misunderstandings. In: Flynn R J, Nitsch K E (eds) Normalisation, social integration and community services. Baltimore University Press, Baltimore

Wolfensberger W, Tullman S, 1989 A brief outline of the principle of normalisation. In: Brechin A, Walmesley J Making connections. The Open University Press, Milton Keynes

FURTHER READING

Employment

McIntosh B, Whittaker A 1998 Days of change: a practical guide to developing better day opportunities with people with learning disabilities. The Kings Fund, London

Wertheimer A 1991 Employment opportunities for people with severe learning disabilities: report of two conferences held at the Kings Fund Centre. Kings Fund, London

McConkey R, McGinley P 1992 Innovations in employment training and work for people with learning disabilities. Lisieux Hall, Dublin

Council of Europe 1995 Employment strategies for people with disabilities: the role of employers. Council of Europe Publishing

Leisure and Recreation

Cordes K 1999 Applications in recreation and leisure for today and the future. McGraw-Hill, London

Cotton M 1983 Outdoor adventure for handicapped people. Human Horizon Series, Sovereign Press, London

Social Services Inspectorate 1995 Opportunities or knocks: national inspection of recreation and leisure in day services for people with learning disabilities. Social Services Inspectorate, Central Inspection Group, London

USEFUL ADDRESSES

Employment

The Pathway Employment Scheme
The Royal Society for Mentally Handicapped Children and
    Adults
123 Golden Lane
London
EC1Y 0RT
Tel 020 7454 0454

Project Scheme
The National Autistic Society
393 City Road
London
EC1V 1NE
Tel 020 7833 2299

The Shaw Trust
Shaw House
Epsom Square
White Horse Business Park
Trowbridge
Wilts.
BA14 0XJ
Tel 01225 716350

Arts and Drama Groups

Prism Arts
Carlisle Enterprise Centre
James Street
Carlisle
CA2 5BB
Tel 01228 625700 ext 228

CandoCo Dance Company
Dawn Prentice
2L Leroy House
436 Essex Road
London
N1 2QP

Graeae Theatre Company
Interchange Studios
Dalby Street
London
NW5 3NQ

Heart 'n Soul
Website www.heartnsoul.co.uk

Computer software for people with special needs

Computer Kids Library
Woodene

Nottingham Road
Herts
WD3 5DN
Tel 01923 282720

Inclusive Technology Ltd
Gatehead Business Park
Delph New Road
Delph
Oldham
OL3 5BX
Tel 01457 819790

Widgit
23 Queen Street
Cubbington
Leamington Spa
CV32 7NA

Physical activities

The British Mountaineering Council
Crowford House
Booth Street
Manchester
M13 9RZ

The British Ski Club for the Disabled
Corton House
Corton
Warminster
Wilts.
BA12 0SZ

The British Sports Association for the Disabled
Sir Ludwig Gutterman Sports Centre
Harvey Road
Aylesbury
Bucks.
HP21 8PP

The Jubilee Sailing Trust
Beauvior Lodge
Effingham Lane
Copthorne
Sussex

Riding for the Disabled Association
Avenue R
National Agricultural Centre
Stoneleigh
Kenilworth
Warks.
CV8 2LY

3

Distressed states of learning disability

In this section, a range of factors that are experienced by some people with learning disabilities are explored. This section includes a chapter by Mick Wolverson on challenging behaviour; here he provides a useful overview of the subject along with some very practical ways of working with such people. Next Maggie Anderson provides a comprehensive chapter on Autistic Spectrum Disorder. In Chapter 12, Ibrahim Turkistani provides an overview of mental ill health as it affects people with learning disabilities. A chapter follows by Bob Gates, that specifically explores self-injurious behaviour, a distressed state that is found in some people with learning disabilities. Finally, Dermot Rowe and Odete Lopes present a comprehensive overview of people with learning disabilities who have offended in law.

Challenging behaviour

Mick Wolverson

KEY ISSUES

- This chapter offers a comprehensive overview of definitions, causation and interventions associated with challenging behaviour.
- A wide range of historical, sociological, psychological and contemporary sources are used to support the major theme of the chapter: that much challenging behaviour is created and maintained, rather than being an integral part of a person's personality.
- Discussion of therapeutic interventions and the use of case studies offer examples of how challenging behaviour can be 'deconstructed' and therefore ameliorated.

INTRODUCTION

The overall aim of this chapter is to explore the phenomenon that has come to be described as challenging behaviour. During the course of this chapter the major concurrent theme will be an explanation of how challenging behaviour is created and maintained by powerful macro and micro factors which shape the lives of those labelled as 'challenging'. This discussion will include an exploration of a facile assumption that challenging behaviour is, in most instances, an innate part of a person's character, and the assertion that this view pathologises individuals so labelled. This dangerous assumption has led to the symptoms, rather than the underlying causes of challenging behaviour becoming the main focus of service interventions. This chapter will therefore offer explanations of how challenging behaviour has been socially constructed; this basic premise will allow discussion of how challenging behaviour can be 'deconstructed' and will ultimately lead to enlightened and constructive ways of working with people who have been ascribed such labels.

DEFINITIONS

It is necessary to discuss various definitions of challenging behaviour in order that certain parameters can frame the theoretical content of this chapter. This will assist direct carers, who help people with challenging behaviour to identify those who are so labelled. Whereas it is necessary to discuss definitions, it is vitally important that a caveat relating to labelling is applied. The label 'challenging behaviour' has the potential to have a hugely negative impact on those so 'defined'. This caveat is, therefore, that any explanation of the definitions of challenging behaviour must be conducted with an understanding of the profound power of labelling (this will be discussed in more depth later in the chapter).

Slee (1996) has discussed how words bring assumptions, represent history and define practice. Slee's comments are important when considering the term 'challenging behaviour' as few definitions can be associated with so many negative assumptions; similarly people defined as challenging often carry an associated personal history, that largely dwells on their behavioural difficulties, and their symptoms rather than their causation. Finally, Slee's observation is crucial because what Slee refers to as practice, should be interpreted as how a person labelled as having challenging behaviour will be treated and where they will be treated. Increasingly people labelled as challenging will be offered treatment in specialist treatment and assessment units which, paradoxically, have the potential to maintain rather than relieve the symptoms associated with challenging behaviour. Thus the term 'challenging behaviour' should be used carefully. Blunden & Allen (1987) have acknowledged the potential for negative labelling by stating that:

We have decided to adopt the term challenging behaviour rather than problem behaviour or severe problem behaviour since it emphasises that such behaviours represent challenges to services rather than problems which individuals with learning difficulties in some way carry round with them. If services could rise to the 'challenge' of dealing with these behaviours they would cease to be 'problems'. The term challenging behaviour places the focus of discussion on services rather than on the individuals showing the behaviours. (Blunden & Allen 1987, p. 14)

This definition suggests that the word 'challenging' is used to place an obligation on care givers to offer constructive ways of working with people with problematic behaviour. Blunden & Allen also sought to emphasise that challenging behaviour is not necessarily an innate part of an individual's personality. Whereas these issues are fundamental to any definition and understanding of challenging behaviour, it is also necessary to identify the range of behaviours included under this increasingly 'umbrella' term. Emerson et al (1988a) have offered a succinct definition that has become widely regarded as both useful and accurate and is that:

Severe challenging behaviour refers to behaviour of such an intensity, frequency or duration that the physical safety of the person or others is likely to be placed in serious jeopardy, or behaviour that is likely to seriously limit or deny access to the use of ordinary community facilities. (Emerson et al, 1988a, p. 16)

This often used definition focuses on how the negative effects of challenging behaviour impact on the individual and others without mentioning specific challenging behaviours. The term challenging behaviour encompasses a wide spectrum of behaviours that are shown in Box 10.1.

Box 10.1 The spectrum of challenging behaviour adapted from Nihira et al (1993)

- Violence
- Destructiveness
- Rebelliousness
- Untrustworthiness
- Stereotyped behaviour
- Peculiar mannerisms
- Inappropriate interpersonal manners
- Unacceptable or eccentric habits
- Hyperactivity
- Sexually aberrant behaviour
- Self injury
- Psychological disturbances

All of the above behaviours might be perceived to be overtly difficult and damaging, and most people asked to define challenging behaviour would include some of them in their definition. It must be noted that of an equally challenging nature and with the potential to limit an individual's lifestyle are the phenomena associated with 'withdrawal'. Within the population of people with learning disabilities are many people who display symptoms of withdrawal; some such individuals are electively mute, refuse to engage with their environment, refuse to leave familiar surroundings, seek comfort in seemingly meaningless repetitive behaviours, such as twirling string, or display a profound regression in previous social and personal skills. These individuals also present major challenges to care givers, and their needs can often be overlooked as priority is instead given to those with overtly challenging behaviour.

General definitions have been further developed in recent years to include individuals who may enter the criminal justice system, and those diagnosed with learning disabilities and personality disorder; the following definition from the Department of Health (1992) acknowledged this fact and attempted to explain the wide range of people and their behaviours by commenting that:

People with learning disabilities who have challenging behaviour form an extremely diverse group; including individuals with all levels of learning disability, many sensory or physical impairments and presenting quite different kinds of challenges. The group includes, for example, people with mild or borderline learning disability who have been diagnosed as mentally ill and who enter the criminal justice system for crimes such as arson or sexual offences: as well as people with profound learning disability, often with sensory handicaps and other physical problems, who injure themselves, for example by repeated head banging or eye poking. (DOH 1992, p. 3)

Thus the term challenging behaviour has come to define a disparate group of people and behaviours that seem to be ever increasing. It is worthy of note that some behaviours that originally would not have been included under the umbrella term challenging behaviour now are so included, for example Attention Defect Disorder. In many

respects it would appear that the term challenging behaviour has become a convenient label attached to those people who deviate, even if only slightly, from accepted norms. The preceding discussion has focused on the original intention behind the term challenging behaviour; however, many people are unaware of the implications of terminology and therefore the label challenging behaviour is frequently misused (Gates 1996, pp 7–8). It may well be that the term is used as a euphemism for or an attempt to sanitise what some regard as unacceptable behaviour, implying that the ownership of such behaviour therefore must reside with the individual displaying it. It is hoped that this overview has drawn some parameters around the behaviours associated with the term challenging behaviour. Importantly, this overview should serve to highlight the original meaning of the term and the necessity of using it cautiously, accurately and with an understanding of the negative connotations the words challenging behaviour can convey. Attempts have been made by some organisations to exclude offending or forensic behaviours from definitions of challenging behaviour. This trend is potentially constructive; however while these behaviours can, and in most instances still do, fall under the term challenging behaviour, reference is made to them in this chapter.

CAUSATION OF CHALLENGING BEHAVIOUR

The previous section offered definitions of challenging behaviour and alluded to how it is often the symptomology, and not the causes of behavioural difficulties that interventions are focused on. This 'inverted' approach offers no long term fundamental change to a person's behaviour. Conversely, if the causes of behavioural difficulties can be ascertained, then constructive interventions can be appropriately employed to alleviate the causes and the symptoms of challenging behaviour and hopefully bring about a long lasting amelioration of such behaviour. This section of the chapter offers brief outlines of the causative factors that contribute to the development of challenging behaviour. Causation of challenging behaviour is often an amalgamation of several, or all, of the following factors: physical/biological, behavioural, environmental and psychological. It is often the powerful interactions of a combination of these that coalesce to form a picture of someone being labelled as having behavioural difficulties.

Phenotypes and biological dysfunction associated with challenging behaviour

A vast spectrum of manifestations is covered by the term learning disabilities. Within this spectrum are specific conditions that will result in an individual displaying behavioural difficulties. Murphy (1994) has stated that: 'There are only two known conditions which can be biologically defined and which always lead to a specific behavioural difficulty, Lesch–Nyhan syndrome and Prader–Willi syndrome'. (Murphy 1994, p. 39)

Both of the conditions identified by Murphy are extremely rare. Christie et al (1982) have explained that Lesch–Nyhan syndrome will always result in those affected displaying self-injurious behaviour that will involve biting both the lips and hands. Prader–Willi syndrome involves the inability to suppress appetite, resulting in obsessive gorging of food and consequently morbid obesity. Murphy (1999) has commented further on these phenotypes stating that they are also associated with self-injurious behaviour, which of course presents challenges to care givers. Self-injurious behaviour is dealt with more fully in Chapter 13.

Murphy (1994) was accurate in her observation that these two conditions always result in challenging behaviour, however there are other conditions associated with learning disabilities that can also result in the person affected displaying challenging behaviour. One such condition is phenylketonuria (PKU) which is an inborn error of metabolism. If left untreated in infancy, PKU results in learning disabilities and an increased likelihood of those affected displaying frequent challenging behaviours such as hitting, slapping, scratching and hair pulling. PKU is easily identified now by the Guthrie test at birth and subsequently controlled by diet.

Another chromosomal aberration, Fragile X syndrome, is also usually associated with challenging behaviour. Fragile X syndrome is a genetic abnormality which disproportionately affects males. Those affected will have some degree of learning disabilities and generally some persistent challenging behaviour involving destructiveness and, on occasions, self-injurious behaviour such as head slapping. It is thought that these behaviours subside by early adulthood. One other condition cited as causing challenging behaviour is the so-called 'super-male syndrome', or XYY syndrome. Some males have a chromosomal abnormality whereby they have an extra Y chromosome, hence the term XYY syndrome. The usual male chromosomal configuration is XY, therefore those with an extra male chromosome have been categorised as being potentially more aggressive than the average male. Craft (1984) has demonstrated by analysing pertinent research that the correlation between XYY syndrome and aggressive behaviour is possible but unproven.

Another condition commonly associated with learning disabilities is epilepsy. Epilepsy affects 0.5% of the general population, however, epilepsy may affect 75% of those with severe learning disabilities. Challenging behaviour can be associated with pre- and post-epileptic activity, and with temporal lobe epilepsy; during these transient periods mental functioning and consciousness are impaired and altered, and individuals may display dangerous and/or bizarre behaviour over which they have no control or subsequent recollection.

Autistic Spectrum Disorder (ASD), like epilepsy, is not always associated with learning disabilities or challenging behaviour; however ASD is more prevalent in this client group than the general population, and it can result in those affected displaying some degree of challenging behaviour. It is the case that challenging behaviours are associated with ASD. Such behaviours may include an obsessive adherence to routine(s) that can appear meaningless and bizarre. While slavish adherence to routine may in itself not constitute a major behavioural problem, interfering with these routines may cause seemingly irrational emotional distress resulting in the behaviour being perceived to be challenging. A further phenomenon associated with ASD is the belief that those affected can 'objectify' care givers, and view them as inanimate objects without human emotion and feeling. If this belief is accurate, it accounts for the occasions when some people with ASD may harm care givers and then fail to respond to the hurt they may have caused. Autistic Spectrum Disorder is dealt with more fully in Chapter 11.

Reeves (1997) has stated that some people with learning disabilities may have identifiable neurological dysfunctions which are often misinterpreted as challenging behaviour and are therefore left untreated. Reeves has suggested that such dysfunctions include visual agnosia (an inability to recognise objects and their shape), apraxia (inability to carry out purposeful voluntary movement without losing muscle power) and proprioception (difficulty in judging the position of one's body and limbs in space). Verri et al (2000) have described how rhombencephalosynapsys (a cerebellar malformation), although extremely rare, can result in behaviour that is likely to be interpreted as challenging.

Some conditions, as highlighted above, are either specific to learning disabilities or more prevalent within this client group. It should be noted that other conditions that affect the general population can also cause challenging behaviour in those with learning disabilities, and these are as follows:

- Hypo/hyper glycaemia. Diabetes can result in those affected experiencing periods when their blood sugar levels are either low (hypoglycaemia) or high (hyper-glycaemia). During these periods consciousness is impaired and people may display behaviours that are perceived as being challenging.
- Urinary tract infections (UTIs). UTIs can result in acute confusional states due to the infection entering and infecting the blood stream.
- Uncontrolled pain. People with learning disabilities can have difficulties in communication. When such people are experiencing pain they may display behaviours that are seen to be challenging in an attempt to convey that they are in pain.

- Dementia and other degenerative conditions. These conditions are a result of organic changes in the brain and the resulting behaviour is dependent on which area of the brain has undergone change. An example of this is changes to the frontal lobe which can result in poor judgement and lack of insight which may lead to disinhibited behaviour.

Alyward et al (1997) have commented that the decline in functioning associated with dementia may be different from the general population. These differences may include reduced ability in self-help skills and the onset of dementia at a younger age, associated with Down syndrome.

This list is not exhaustive; its purpose is to demonstrate that some conditions can result in those affected displaying behavioural difficulties of either a transient (e.g. hyper-glycaemia) or more permanent nature (e.g. dementia). These conditions are invariably treated if the person experiencing them does not have learning disabilities. However, in people with learning disabilities symptoms of some illnesses can be often missed or attributed to their learning disabilities or an associated condition such as epilepsy; this is known as 'diagnostic overshadowing'. A common example of this in people with learning disabilities is undiagnosed pain. People with learning disabilities may lack the appropriate communication skills to indicate they are experiencing pain and instead display challenging behaviour which is then interpreted as being due to their 'learning disabilities'.

This exploration of the physical causations of challenging behaviour indicates that some phenotypes and biological dysfunctions may result in behavioural difficulties. The important message from this is that these physical causations only account for a limited number of behavioural difficulties. Any person or service wishing to help those with learning disabilities and challenging behaviour should first assess if individuals have a physical cause for their behaviour. If a physical cause can be ascertained, then appropriate interventions should be conducted to alleviate its symptoms. If a physical cause is not apparent then the behaviour must be attributable to some other causative factor(s) that will now be discussed.

Behavioural explanations for the development of challenging behaviour

A crucial point to consider when seeking to understand seemingly inexplicable behaviours is that all behaviour has meaning. The behaviourist approach to understanding challenging behaviour offers plausible explanation as to why some people may use inappropriate behaviours to express themselves. Care givers need to skilfully interpret the meaning of such behaviours, and these behavioural interpretations may serve to help understand both the development and meaning of inappropriate behaviours.

The behaviourist interpretation of challenging behaviour rests on the central premise that all behaviour, either appropriate or inappropriate, has been learned. That behaviour can be learned has been experimentally proven by early, and well-known psychological theorists such as Pavlov (1927) and Skinner (1953). Behaviourism rests on the assumption that behaviour will be repeated if reinforced in some way. This assumption is easily vindicated when obviously appropriate behaviours are reinforced and their frequency increases. The assumption can seem far less plausible when considering the development of challenging behaviour. To explain how behaviour is learned, theorists have proposed the antecedent–behaviour–consequence sequential triad. An example of this is shown in Box 10.2.

A child would therefore learn to repeat this behaviour as it is rewarded by being fed. It is proposed that undesirable behaviours are learnt in the same way and an example of this is shown in Box 10.3.

Box 10.3 provides an example that demonstrates how the basic need for attention results in disturbing behaviour, this is reinforced and therefore repeated by often well-intentioned attempts to prevent the behaviour.

Box 10.2   The ABC sequential triad

Antecedent – A child is hungry
Behaviour – The child cries
Consequence – The child is fed

Box 10.3   The development of undesirable behaviours

Antecedent – A person with learning disabilities is feeling the need for attention from care givers which is not forthcoming while the person is passive
Behaviour – The person bangs their head on the wall until it bleeds
Consequence – Care givers intervene in an attempt to stop this undesirable behaviour

---

It is often suggested that inappropriate behaviour can be vicariously learned Bandura (1977). Historically, and in many instances, contemporary attempts to alleviate or contain challenging behaviour have resulted in those displaying it residing together. In such environments it is entirely feasible that some people have learned to use inappropriate behaviour to gain what they need, by observing the behaviour of their peers.

That inappropriate behaviour can be learned suggests that appropriate behaviour can also be learned through positive reinforcement and this will be discussed in a later section.

Environmental explanations

We are all to some extent products of our environment. For the majority of the general population, choices about such things as where to live, how to spend leisure time, what job to pursue and who to live with allow a degree of control over the environment. For some people with learning disabilities the opportunity to control such fundamental issues is denied them for a variety of reasons. Historically, and to some extent within contemporary services, the world of people with learning disabilities and particularly those with challenging behaviours was, and continues to be, a narrow one with little opportunity for control. The lives of this group of people are often prescribed within limited boundaries in terms of both resource allocation and philosophies of care.

Any exploration of the environmental causation of challenging behaviour needs to acknowledge the massive impact of 20th century institutionalisation on this client group, fully outlined in Chapter

3. The characteristics of institutionalisation are well documented (Barton 1960, Goffman 1961) and these are shown in Box 10.4.

Past environments, by their very design, have created and maintained challenging behaviours. The behavioural explanation offered for 'head banging' in Box 10.3 could be a learned behaviour used to gain attention. Many inappropriate behaviours have developed in institutional settings, as they were often the only mechanism available to obtain attention, even if this attention was negative, for example restraint and seclusion. Should attempts be made to ignore inappropriate behaviours then often disturbing behaviour was 'ratcheted' up, until staff intervention was inevitable in order to prevent physical harm to self, or others.

Many challenging behaviours developed as a result of institutionalisation are of an overtly aggressive nature (Borthwick-Duffy (1994a), Qureshi (1994)), however the withdrawn states discussed previously were also created and maintained by such environments. Many people who experienced institutionalised care became electively mute, selectively withdrew from interaction with their (unrewarding) environment, or sought stimulation in bizarre stereotypic behaviours such as twirling threads and repetitive behaviours such as projectile vomiting. The realisation that the gaunt Victorian institutions dehumanised those they were designed to care for has almost led to their closure; however they still exert a powerful legacy as the people who were housed in them still exhibit the challenging behaviours created and maintained by them. They may also be cared for by the same people who worked in these asylums, whose values and visions may not have developed from their custodial past. Many challenging behaviours developed in institutional settings were caused by the physical environment; however some behaviour was attributable to poor staff training, controlling staff attitudes and organisational priorities. These factors may still exert a powerful influence over contemporary services, leading to the development of 'mini-institutions' in smaller group home settings.

A further point to consider in relation to institutional environments is that behaviours once tolerated within them due to their often typical geographical isolation and their 'closed' nature, are now not acceptable in new community-based units. A common example of this, and a recurring problem, is stripping and masturbating in public places. Another example is persistently shouting, screaming or making strange noises. These behaviours often cause concern for those living close to people relocated into community settings. It should be noted that challenging behaviours such as these may not constitute a problem for the person displaying them, rather they are perceived to be inappropriate and unacceptable by others.

Sociological factors

When attempting to explain causation of challenging behaviours, it is helpful to examine some sociological factors. These factors may not be directly responsible for the development of behavioural difficulties, however they contribute to the development of a milieu conducive to creating and maintaining inappropriate behaviour. In the majority of instances a powerful combination of poor expectations, stigma/labelling, abuse and poor parenting skills coalesce to create conditions in which behavioural difficulties develop; each of these are briefly discussed.

Poor expectations

Bicknell & Conboy-Hill (1992) have explained the profound effect of poor expectations of people with learning disabilities by proposing a model known as the deviancy career. This model

---

Box 10.4   Characteristics of institutionalisation

- Dehumanising
- Impersonal
- Controlling
- Devaluing
- Disempowering
- They encourage inappropriate behaviour
- They seek homogeneity
- They validate the medical model
- They cause learnt dependency
- They encourage inappropriate attention seeking

demonstrates how the limited ability associated with learning disabilities leads to society at large, and care givers, having relatively low expectations for the individual and client group. This, in turn, leads to limited provision of opportunity, which further compounds the initial developmental delay resulting in poor achievement. This cycle culminates in people with learning disabilities assuming such prescribed roles in self-fulfilling prophecies. This deviancy career is applicable to learning disabilities in general, however it is magnified if the person also has challenging behaviour. In such instances challenging behaviour is often expected as an inevitable part of a person's personality, leading to care in specialist units which maintain, rather than alleviate the causes of behavioural difficulties. Seemingly the person in this cycle has become 'crystalised' in a static position of being challenging. Once in this position the person's continued challenging behaviour and receipt of specialist services is perceived as justifying the original decisions taken by service providers that placed the person in this position. Responsibility must rest with services, professionals and other care givers to break the links in this deviancy cycle, by aiming at positive rather than negative outcomes.

Stigma and labelling

Goffman (1963), in his seminal work on stigma, has described the phenomena associated with the hugely negative effects of stigmatisation. This has also contributed to those with challenging behaviour experiencing a 'narrow existence' based on discrimination born out of stigmatisation.

Stigma attached to those with learning disabilities and challenging behaviour has a similar effect to the deviancy career, as it reinforces an expectation that an individual will be challenging. It also limits or precludes attempts to understand and alleviate the causes of behavioural difficulties as stigma encourages a perception that challenging behaviour is an inevitable component of that person's make-up.

Goffman has asserted that a stigma is a personal characteristic that 'discredits' the individual in the estimation of mainstream society. Goffman stated

that society views people with a stigma as being: 'Of a less desirable kind in the extreme, a person who is quite thoroughly bad, or dangerous . . . ' (Goffman 1963, p. 12). Goffman did not make explicit reference to challenging behaviour, he discussed the negative consequences of stigmatisation in universal terms. It is, however, appropriate to suggest that challenging behaviour is a stigma that can lead to those so labelled being seen as being less than human and Goffman states that: 'By definition, of course, we believe the person with stigma is not quite human. On this assumption we exercise varieties of discrimination, through which we effectively, if often unthinkingly, reduce his life chances' (Goffman 1963, p. 15). This concept is important, as such an assumption first allows some people with challenging behaviours to be treated, on occasions, in ways that would not be acceptable for the general population; and secondly, it may be used to justify conditions that compound and maintain behavioural difficulties.

Stigma directly leads to negative labelling. Without specifically mentioning challenging behaviour, Pilgrim & Rogers (1999) have discussed labelling theories in some depth; however, their fundamental contention is that, as with stigma and the deviancy cycle, labelling can reinforce a view that people with a label (such as challenging behaviour) will inevitably continue to exhibit it. Pilgrim & Rogers (1999) have discussed how labelling theorists maintain that powerful sociological forces are responsible for ascribing labels to groups of people who in some way deviate from expectations of normality, and that deviancy can therefore be socially constructed. This is an important issue as it contributes to the notion that much challenging behaviour is socially constructed and can therefore be 'deconstructed'.

Abuse

Some people with learning disabilities and challenging behaviour have been subject to abuse either through sins of omission or commission. Such abuse is often multifactorial and may take the form of physical, sexual, financial, psychological or institutional neglect. Beail & Warden (1995) discussed how a disproportionate number of people with learning disabilities have been sexually abused. Hames (1993) proposed that those abused can become abusers due to their having experienced inappropriate sexual behaviour.

Poor parenting

The parenting of a child with learning disabilities offers some unique and difficult challenges. Some approaches to parenting can lead to a child displaying symptoms of challenging behaviour. One such manifestation of this is the 'infantilisation' of some people with learning disabilities. McConachie (1986) suggested that due to over-protectiveness, it is not uncommon for parents of the learning disabled to fail to encourage their children to reach their maximum independence. An example of this is when people with learning disabilities continue to sleep in their parents' bed or bedroom when they are adults. When they are separated from their parents, due to illness for example, they may display inappropriate behaviour which would normally only occur within the first months of infancy. Other inappropriate behaviours developed in childhood may continue into adulthood because those displaying them have learned to use them to gain what they want from their environment. Sometimes these behaviours have been allowed to continue by over-indulgent parents who may have attempted to stop them and offer alternatives had their child not had learning disabilities. Vetere (1993) accounts for such examples by stating:

Parental overprotection may be a defensive manoeuvre against personal feelings of hostility, rejecting or guilt towards the child with disabilities. Such feelings can disrupt the earlier giving of affection and lead to a form of acceptance of the child's disabilities which results in infantilization (Vetere 1993, p. 123).

This 'infantilisation' can also be observed within a context of developing sexuality. Some parents do not imbue a person with learning disabilities with the same sexual needs as others. The sexual experimentation associated with adolescence can be denied to such people, resulting in their expressions of sexuality being demonstrated inappropriately, and perceived by others as deviant or, as

challenging behaviour. (It must also be noted that abuse can occur within families, with resulting inappropriate behaviours.)

Observability

Some people with learning disabilities and challenging behaviour are more 'visible' than most others, largely due to their dependency on care givers. Care givers can observe clients on an almost continuous basis. Their clients' private world is often in the public domain and therefore ordinary things that others do in different and/or private contexts are sometimes described as challenging. Examples of these ordinary things include losing one's temper, displaying sexuality and releasing aggression appropriately. People with learning disabilities, and particularly those with challenging behaviour, can be seen as deviant or aggressive if they display behaviour that deviates from a prescribed expectation. In many respects they are expected to display more appropriate standards of behaviour than those of the general population, for longer periods, and under the scrutiny of others. Often slight transgressions are used as evidence of the intractability of their challenging behaviour.

Psychological explanations

Chapter 12 discusses in depth issues relating to mental ill health, however it is necessary to discuss some facets of this here. Raghavan (1996) has stated that people with learning disabilities can experience the full range of psychotic disorders. Importantly, studies by Corbet (1979), Jacobson & Ackerman (1988), Lund (1985) and Rutter et al (1976) have all suggested that psychological disorders occur substantially more in this group than in the general population. However, much confusion exists around this issue due, in part, to the complexities of accurately identifying mental ill health in people with learning disabilities and challenging behaviour (Moss et al 1997). Murphy (1994) has stated that diagnosis of mental ill health in people with severe learning disabilities is particularly problematic as it is difficult for them to communicate the feelings on which any diagnosis may be based. Reiss et al (1982) have stated that any diagnosis is also subject to 'diagnostic overshadowing' which is a term used to describe when challenging behaviour is wrongly misinterpreted as the symptoms of mental ill health. Murphy & Holland (1993) have pointed out that a person may display challenging behaviour and not suffer from a psychiatric illness, however they have also suggested that an overlap can exist between challenging behaviour and psychiatric disorders. Borthwick-Duffy (1994b) and Menolascino & Fleisher (1993) have demonstrated that people with learning disabilities are at an increased risk of developing psychological disorders. It is plausible to suggest that these factors are manifestations of the effects of the way people with learning disabilities have been treated.

One important example of this is when people with learning disabilities periodically display outbursts of destructive and aggressive behaviour. Sometimes such people are diagnosed as having a personality disorder. Their behaviour can seem to lack explanation or causation because their destructiveness can appear arbitrary and result in negative consequences for them. An example of this is people who have been supported by care services and accommodated in supportive and appropriate surroundings. After brief periods of stability they will create disturbances and display destructive behaviours resulting in them being moved to often less appropriate, and more controlling environments; this pattern is regularly repeated. Although such behaviour seems to lack rational explanation, it can be understood in terms of low self-esteem, maintenance of role expectation and faulty cognition. It is proposed that some challenging behaviour, as described above, is displayed due to the people having such poor self-esteem that their cognition, or self-view is that they are irretrievably 'bad' people. Displaying destructive behaviour reinforces this deep-seated, and often subconscious belief that they are 'bad', expected to display such behaviour and are 'unworthy' of living in appropriate surroundings. The negative spiral that often follows such behaviour, involving moves to increasingly specialist and controlling environments, reaffirms the individual's designated role

and confirms the poor self-image. This concept is important as it will be discussed in a later section on cognitive therapy. Such scenarios, while not exclusive to people with learning disabilities, are common within this client group, and this may account for the prevalence of, and increased risk of developing psychological disturbances as discussed earlier.

APPROACHES TO MANAGING CHALLENGING BEHAVIOUR

The preceding sections of this chapter have suggested that causation of challenging behaviour is multifactoral. This section offers brief outlines of the widely accepted interventions used to manage and ameliorate challenging behaviour. It is recommended that an eclectic mix of interventions might be explored when offering support to a person with challenging behaviour in order to represent responses to multifactoral causations. It should be noted that each individual displaying challenging behaviour will have different reasons for doing so and therefore interventions should be chosen accordingly. Criticism has been made with regard to the efficacy of the approaches outlined. Some of this criticism is attributable to the fact that interventions have been used singularly, and in isolation from other techniques. It is also commonplace to find constructive interventions used within non-therapeutic and non-conducive environments, thus compromising their efficacy. A third common reason for the lack of success is that interventions are often practised by poorly prepared, unskilled staff. It is worth considering these problems with implementation when devising interventions, since not to do so would jeopardise their success or, in some instances, cause harm. Figure 10.1 adapted from Gear et al (2000) demonstrates how different interpretations of the causation of challenging behaviour lead to the choice of intervention.

Chemotherapeutic and physical interventions

The section outlining physical causation concluded that few challenging behaviours have a defini-

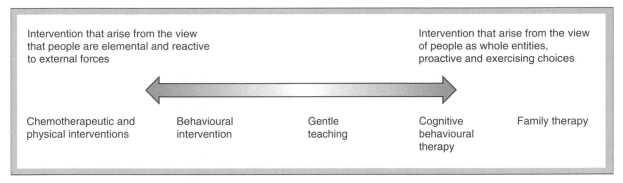

Intervention that arise from the view that people are elemental and reactive to external forces

Intervention that arise from the view of people as whole entities, proactive and exercising choices

Chemotherapeutic and physical interventions   Behavioural intervention   Gentle teaching   Cognitive behavioural therapy   Family therapy

Figure 10.1 Reproduced with permission from Gear (2000).

tive physical cause. If this assertion is true then it might be reasonable to assume that physical interventions are limited to dealing with a proportionally small amount of challenging behaviour. Historically this was not the case (see Ch. 3), with challenging behaviour being contained by physical means such as incarceration, physical punishment, strait-jackets, electroconvulsive therapy treatment, seclusion rooms, lobotomies and the use of aversive stimuli. Though many of these 'techniques' have rightly been discredited as being inhumane, challenging behaviour is still treated by chemotherapy. The disproportionate use of physical interventions is largely attributable to the medicalisation of challenging behaviour. In most instances those with learning disabilities and challenging behaviour are treated by psychiatric services that historically have sought to 'cure' and contain challenging behaviour. Whereas, more holistic and enlightened approaches have been introduced into contemporary services, a mainstay of clinical intervention remains the prescription of psychotropic/antipsychotic medications and the control of those displaying challenging behaviour in specialist units. The White Paper *Valuing people: a new strategy for learning disabilities for the 21st century* (DOH 2001) has acknowledged that: 'Psychotropic medication may be very effective when there is an underlying psychiatric disorder but there is concern that too often this medication is used as an alternative to adequate staffing' (DOH 2001, 8.43). This comment is supported by recent research conducted by Emerson et al (2000), which stated

that: ' . . . Findings indicate that residents with challenging behaviour are over three times more likely to receive psychotic medication than they are to receive behavioural support. Such an inequitable pattern of provision clearly violates the principle of evidence based practice' (Emerson et al 2000, p. 211).

It would be inaccurate to entirely portray the use of medication or specialist services as being without benefit. Rather, it is the case that such interventions can be of benefit if they are temporary, if specific conditions are targeted by appropriate medication, if the individual receiving them is compliant, if alternatives are sought and, most importantly, if they are used conjointly with other holistic therapeutic interventions. If these considerations are not taken into account then use of physical interventions remains an expedient and sometimes exclusive method of intervention. Their use may have some effect in managing challenging behaviour, but without the use of other measures, symptoms of challenging behaviour could be masked, and their causes remain undealt with.

Behavioural intervention

People with learning disabilities who present with challenging behaviour have been subject to many different approaches to modify their supposedly inappropriate behaviour through the use of behaviour modification. The section on causation has briefly dealt with how inappropriate behaviour can be learned. Behaviour modification offers strategies for 'unlearning' inappropriate behaviour, and for this to be replaced by the learning of new, acceptable behaviour. The principles of behaviour modification are based upon applying or withdrawing reinforcement systematically in order to manipulate behaviour; it should be noted that these can be either primary reinforcers, which meet an immediate physical need such as chocolate, sweets, food and drinks, or secondary reinforcers which can be used to meet primary needs. These include money or tokens, which can be used to exchange for primary reinforcers. Activities and spending time with significant others also have intrinsic rewards, which act as powerful reinforcers for appropriate behaviour. This is important as it incorporates elements of the gentle teaching approach to be discussed later. A vast array of literature (see further reading), for example Yule & Carr (1990), has supported the use of behaviour modification; however this approach fell from general usage in the 1980s and early 1990s for reasons to be discussed later. Oliver (1993) and McCue (2000) have suggested that the concept has undergone a renaissance in recent years and it is now less mechanical and more holistic than was the case previously. A further element of behaviour modification is that of functional analysis which focuses on the premise that all behaviour has meaning and serves a function for the person displaying it. Functional analysis is crucial in understanding and offering solutions for inappropriate behaviours, as it focuses the assessment on the reasons why someone may display seemingly inexplicable behaviours, rather than attempting to merely eliminate symptoms.

When the function(s) of an inappropriate behaviour have been ascertained, then appropriate behaviours can be encouraged which achieve the same function for the individual. To understand this more clearly it is helpful to consider the antecedent, behaviour and consequences when looking at behaviours. This approach is usually adopted during the assessment of challenging behaviour, by using an antecedent–behaviour–consequence (ABC) chart as shown in Table 10.1.

This is an example of an extract from an ABC chart. It is typical in that while it may offer some insight into the function of John's behaviour, it should be more detailed. The chart serves to demonstrate that:

1. John's inappropriate behaviours serve a communicative function in that by displaying them he is communicating his wish to receive a drink and attention.

2. John may be compelled to display inappropriate behaviour, the function of which is misunderstood by care staff. This can happen when his needs are not met if he is either sitting passively or displaying challenging behaviour.

3. It is possible to infer from the chart that John's inappropriate behaviour is likely to be repeated as it was reinforced by the primary reinforcer of a drink and the secondary reinforcer of attention.

The chart could have been improved by including more information. Gates (1997), for example, suggests that this could be done by using the ABC chart as follows:

Antecedents – Information should record the behaviour(s) immediately prior to the behaviour

Table 10.1 Example of an antecedent–behaviour–consequence (ABC) recording chart

Time	Antecedents	Behaviour	Consequence
10 a.m.	John was sitting watching television in the lounge	John ran towards member of staff and kicked their chair. John was also screaming loudly	John was taken back to the lounge by members of staff and asked to calm down
10 30 a.m.	John was sitting watching television in the lounge	John ran to the window and kicked it	Staff requested John sit down
11 a.m.	Sitting reading magazines in the lounge	John ran to the kitchen and banged loudly on the door	The housekeeper gave John a drink of tea and he returned to the lounge where he calmed down

manifested. Variables such as who was present, and any difference to routine, should be mentioned. Contextual information such as a recent family visit, or an event that created emotional upset could also be included. Conjecture should be avoided, as in the example where it was stated that John was 'watching' television. This may only be an assumption because he was in the lounge. Similarly, 'reading' magazines could be subject to the same misinterpretation. An equally valid interpretation could well be that John was sitting passively or bored in the lounge.

Behaviour – Descriptions of behaviour must be as precise as possible. Importantly, reference should be made to frequency, intensity and duration of the behaviour. Gates (1997) has pointed out the difficulties associated with accurate recording. The reader should consult McBrien & Felce (1995) for a comprehensive account of best practice in behavioural recording. Attention should be paid to recording behaviours in as exact a way as possible, for example exactly how long a behaviour lasted, or how many times a behaviour such as kicking occurred. The 'intensity' of a behaviour can be recorded by using a scale of intensity from 0 to 10, for example.

Consequences – Once again accurate recording is vitally important, as it potentially provides valid and reliable data from which to make hypotheses as to the function(s) of that behaviour. In the example of Box 10.5 it would have been useful to name staff involved, as John may only seek attention and/or only display inappropriate behaviour when certain staff members are present.

Thus, ABC recording is a fundamental tool of behavioural intervention approaches and part of a process elaborated on by McCue (2000), who has proposed that behaviour modification needs an understanding of the following ideas to ensure successful outcomes:

1. Challenging behaviour serves a function for the individual.
2. Some behaviours may serve more than one function and operate in a variety of contexts.
3. Intervention cannot proceed without a detailed functional assessment.
4. Interventions should use functional alternatives to replace challenging behaviour(s).

5. Interventions should seek to alter systems rather than individuals.
6. Results should be of a qualitative nature and result in beneficial life changes and not simply the elimination of inappropriate behaviours.

Case illustration 10.1 presents a case study that incorporates a well-planned and implemented systematic behavioural approach.

Although some of David's behaviour remains inappropriate, this behaviour modification programme seemingly has produced significant

Case illustration 10.1   Behavioural intervention

David is 40 years of age. He has severe learning disabilities and has lived in institutional settings from the age of 7. David exhibits ritualised, stereotypical behaviours associated with institutionalisation, and these include head slapping, screaming, hitting staff and peers and throwing objects. Many carers, while attending to David's physical needs, have given up hope of ameliorating this challenging behaviour. One particularly worrying behaviour was his extremely frequent attempts to scratch and pull the hair of staff and peers. David would do this around eighty times a day, resulting in a poor quality of life for himself, frequent minor injury to others and a detrimental impact on his peers. Functional analysis and thorough ABC recording seemed to indicate that David exhibited these behaviours to a) gain staff attention and b) be given a drink which would calm him down. David's behaviour could not be ignored (withdrawing positive reinforcement) as it was potentially dangerous and nor could he be denied drinks for any length of time. It was therefore decided that a well devised and thoroughly monitored time out programme be implemented (see Box 10.5 for an outline of good practice relating to time out). When David attempted to scratch or pull hair he was escorted to one of four areas within his home where he could be observed closely by staff while not receiving positive reinforcement. This plan was agreed by a multidisciplinary team, David's safety was ensured and the programme was time limited. Thorough recording indicated a significant reduction in his inappropriate behaviour. The next step for this particular behaviour modification plan involved offering David new behaviours and communication skills, to serve the same function as his previously inappropriate behaviours. The multidisciplinary team therefore took photographs of David sitting in the company of staff receiving attention while displaying appropriate behaviour, and also one of David with a drink. David has learned to use these photographs to communicate his wishes, as he now points to these when wishing to be in company, and have a drink.

Box 10.5 The principles underpinning time out from reinforcement

Time out can be an effective way of reducing behavioural excess. It is based on an assumption that challenging behaviour is maintained by the reinforcement it receives, and therefore by removing reinforcement, the behaviour will be reduced. It is an abbreviation for 'time out from positive social reinforcement'. Clearly, such an approach could be subject to misuse and abuse. Any time out programme must therefore:

• Clearly define the behaviour to be reduced
• Clearly define the time out contingency, i.e. exactly what behaviour will result from time out
• Clearly define where time out will be conducted and the place decided on must allow the client to be observed at all times. Any locked doors must be prohibited

Time out must be thoroughly recorded and records must state:

• The reason for implementing it
• When it commenced and how long it lasted for (it should not exceed 10 minutes)
• The effect of using it

Time out should be discussed and implementation decided on by a multidisciplinary team including the consultant psychiatrist. The multidisciplinary team must undertake regular evaluations of time out, preferably on a weekly basis. Appropriate guidance must be available on 'how to move' a person to the time out area.
Underpinning principles of time out are that:

• It is last resort after all other therapeutic alternatives have been tested
• It forms part of a programme, which will enable the client to achieve positive goals and a better quality of life while simultaneously reducing undesirable behaviours.

1. It is too simplistic
2. It is too mechanical
3. It is inconsistently applied
4. Care givers do not understand it adequately
5. It can only work in appropriate contexts
6. It often takes precedence over other more therapeutic and holistic interventions
7. ABC assessments lack accuracy
8. It is too controlling
9. Rewards and reinforcers can be meaningless
10. It has elements that are ethically questionable.

Systematic approaches mitigate some of these criticisms as they incorporate quality of life issues and system changes (McCue 2000). It is one approach that can be used to help those with challenging behaviour, and arguably it should be used in conjunction with other therapeutic approaches, and in environments conducive to raising the quality of life and self-esteem of those with challenging behaviour.

Gentle teaching

Criticisms of behavioural interventions such as its perceived controlling, simplistic, cold and mechanistic nature have been presented earlier in this chapter. From these criticisms it is reasonable to infer that behaviour modification is perceived to lack regard for equality, valuing, mutuality and the belief that each individual's intrinsic 'humanness' and worth are central to all else.

The approach offered by gentle teaching embraces concepts that include mechanisms for limiting some of the criticisms levelled at behaviour modification. First proposed and elaborated on by McGee (McGee et al 1987, McGee 1990 and 1992), gentle teaching is a therapeutic concept based on the unconditional valuing of people with challenging behaviour, and it places relationship at the centre of development. Gentle teaching not only attempts to eliminate the symptoms of challenging behaviour, it is also a philosophy designed to offer a pathway to valued, meaningful and purposeful lives. The main route to achieving this is through the mutual growth inherent in meaningful client–carer relationships.

improvement in David's quality of life and social acceptance. It has also demonstrated to sceptical care givers that challenging behaviour need not be a static and permanent part of a person's make-up, and that it can be altered.

Criticisms of behaviour modification

It should be understood that behaviour modification is not a panacea and that it has been criticised as being ineffective. Critics of behaviour modification such as Lovett (1996) offer the following criticisms:

McGee et al (1987) have described this philosophy thus:

Gentle teaching is based upon a posture that centres itself on the mutual liberation and humanisation of all persons, a posture that strives for human solidarity and one that leads care givers to teach bonding to those who attempt to distance themselves from meaningful human interactions. It is a pedagogical process that rejects cruel and cold practices and focuses on teaching the value inherent in human presence, human interactions and human reward. (McGee et al 1987, p. 11)

This statement serves to demonstrate that, whereas behaviour modification proposes the use of token and/or physical rewards for the development of appropriate behaviour, gentle teaching advocates that meaningful human interaction is a more powerful reinforcer.

Before elaborating on the value system underpinning gentle teaching, it is necessary to briefly outline what have become known as maladaptive postures. These postures are reflections of often unfair and controlling relationships between client and carer. O'Rourke & Wray (2000) have postulated that maladaptive postures preclude the development of reciprocity and compromise the warmth, mutuality, shared humanness and equality associated with gentle teaching. These maladaptive postures are shown in Box 10.6.

The humanistic philosophy of gentle teaching offers an antithesis of maladaptive postures by use of the following values:

1. Unconditional regard

Gentle teaching emphasises the importance of demonstrating unconditional regard for people even when they are displaying challenging behaviour. The labelling theory associated with stigma, discussed earlier, indicated that sometimes people with learning disabilities and challenging behaviour can be seen as not being human. Gentle teaching places huge importance on the belief that all people are self-conscious, complete and whole human beings. There is an existential element to this philosophy ,i.e. the compelling awareness that people with challenging behaviour are attempting to cope with problems and distress in their existence, just as all others do.

2. Equity

The establishment of a truly equal relationship is an ideal that is difficult to achieve due to people's differing skills, ability and maturity. Gentle teaching acknowledges this point but emphasises that it is the equal worth of an individual's contribution to a relationship that is important, regardless of skills. Caldwell (1999) in her book *Person to Person* has provided many interesting examples of this, and the reader should consult this for a fuller explanation.

3. Mutual change

The life of a person with challenging behaviour is often a narrow and static one. The individual's life is prescribed by behaviours which rarely change. The relationship of professionals and care givers with an individual can equally be driven by the challenging behaviour displayed by that person. This static relationship, made permanent by maladaptive postures, offers little hope for growth and development. The onus is on the care giver to initiate change. Such change will

---

Box 10.6 Maladaptive postures

The authoritarian posture

This is characterised by a paternalistic attitude, which has an underlying assumption that the care giver knows best. It also includes the central notion that change can only occur if the person with challenging behaviour complies with the interventions designed for them by the carer/professional. This posture can involve punishment and reward and therefore positive regard is contingent on compliance.

The over protective posture

This posture 'stifles' opportunity for development of the person with challenging behaviour. The carer seeks to control the client by attempting to maintain a static carer–client relationship. The carer may do this by declining to encourage the client to participate to avoid provoking inappropriate behaviour. This posture maintains challenging behaviour and creates dependency.

The cold and distant posture

This posture is an abdication of responsibility in the carer–client relationship, and is typically characterised by a cold indifference to behavioural distress. Carers 'trapped' in this posture will unquestioningly follow prescribed care plans without concern for their appropriateness, ethics or efficacy.

necessarily involve a repudiation of maladaptive postures and an acceptance of the valuing, equality and unconditional positive regard associated with gentle teaching. Thus gentle teaching offers a non-aversive framework for encouraging person centred approaches to working. These methods have been thoroughly discussed in other texts and it is suggested that the reader refers to O'Rourke & Wray (2000) for an excellent theoretical exploration, and Caldwell (1999) for practical case study examples.

Although gentle teaching proclaims a number of positive values, it should be noted that it is not a panacea, and it has well founded criticisms. These are reproduced in Box 10.7. Practitioners need to be aware of these criticisms before embarking on a potentially evangelical attempt to practice gentle teaching. Gentle teaching should be valued as an underpinning philosophy for carers and services involved in working with people who have challenging behaviour. Its basic tenets of empathy, warmth, reciprocity, unconditional regard and mutual growth should be prerequisites for all human services, and they should be an integral part of all care givers' practice. Gentle teaching is best used when seen to be an underpinning philosophy, rather than something care givers can engage in on a time-limited 'sessional' basis, as is sometimes the case. If gentle teaching is allowed to form a philosophical bedrock, then other therapies and practical interventions can be used in conjunction with it, and with an increased probability of success.

Cognitive behavioural therapy

Cognitive behavioural therapy (CBT) is currently a popular intervention in mental health services. Its use in learning disability services is limited but increasing. Cognitive behavioural therapy is based on the premise that individuals construct a self-view and a world view which may be at variance from reality. These personal constructs are developed through everyday experiences and they help individuals to function by enabling them to understand their own behaviour, and that of others. Should events and behaviours be persistently negative then the individual can develop profoundly negative constructs (Kelly 1955). The original theory of negative 'constructs' was elaborated by Ellis (1962), who proposed that reactions to negative events, rather than negative events in themselves, create emotional distress. Ellis has described these reactions as self-defeating beliefs or errors in thinking. Beck (1976) used the term *schemata* to describe cognitions or constructs based on the negative assumptions people make about themselves and their environment. Beck suggests that people can misinterpret events in a way that deepens their already negative self-view. Turnbull (2000) has commented that:

> Through our experiences, we develop constructs both to understand what has happened in the past and to anticipate and predict the outcome of future events. This does not mean that constructs are consciously developed. Very often we are only made aware of our beliefs when we either experience problems and crises or are directly asked to explain our behaviour. (Turnbull 2000, p. 261)

That constructs are often a subconscious entity indicates the necessity for skilled therapeutic intervention to be used to bring them to a conscious, self-aware level. The benefits of cognitive behavioural therapy are that negative self-constructs can be deconstructed; it is humanistic; it is holistic; and it pursues personal growth. It also offers an understanding of seemingly irrational behaviour by shifting the focus from symptomol-

---

Box 10.7 Criticisms of gentle teaching

- It lacks a comprehensive research base (O'Rourke & Wray 2000)
- It can be aversive and increase, rather than decrease self-injurious behaviour. Barrera & Teodoro (1990) have suggested that some people will display challenging behaviour to communicate their desire not to be with the person attempting to bond with them, and it is therefore aversive. Emerson (1990) also believes that some people will self-injure to escape the presence of others
- The suggested ways of engaging in gentle teaching are ill defined, vague and difficult to implement operationally. These factors prohibit the development of clear outcomes that would indicate success
- Gentle teaching is no more than a redefinition of behaviourism, and therefore as controlling as behaviour modification.

ogy to understanding the damaging nature of causative factors.

Case illustration 10.2 demonstrates how negative self-constructs dictated Joe's chaotic and inappropriate behaviour.

Although this case illustration demonstrates the effective use of cognitive behavioural therapy, it is necessary to be aware of criticisms of this approach, which are as follows:

1. It presupposes that a person engaging in it will have the cognitive ability to do so, thus potentially precluding some people in this client group.
2. It requires the client to be actively committed to the process.
3. It requires compliance with a 'normal' world view rather than an exploration of how people

with cognitive impairments can make sense of their 'world' (Clements 1997).

Family therapy

As with cognitive behavioural therapy, family therapy attempts to deal with causation rather than symptomology. Burnham (1986) has stated that: 'This approach looks at problems within the system of relationships in which they occur and aims to promote change by intervening in the broader system rather than in the individual alone' (Burnham 1986, p. 1). In family therapy the combination of a therapeutic approach with practical methods can have a beneficial effect on the individual with challenging behaviour within the family unit. Steven's story (Case illustration 10.3)

Case illustration 10.2   Cognitive behaviour therapy

Joe is 21 years of age and has been described as having borderline or mild learning disabilities. His childhood was characterised by a mixture of abuse and uncertainty. Joe was sexually abused by his family, and by older boys at one of his schools. Joe's family also exaggerated his level of disability to gain a range of state benefits. His family life involved violence, which was used as a first response if family members could not get what they wanted. Joe's father had spells away from the family, spent either in jail or with partners other than his mother. During these periods Joe's mother had relationships with a succession of violent men who physically abused Joe. The 'family' also moved regularly due to neighbourhood disputes and non-payment of rent. Joe's childhood and adolescence were also characterised by volatility, impetuosity, self-harm and aggression. He had been known to services for many years, however intervention became inevitable when he was admitted to a treatment and assessment unit for people with challenging behaviour from a Court on Section 37/41 of the Mental Health Act (1983).

Joe had appeared in Court after a series of offences including assault, theft, demanding money with menaces and arson. These offences had occurred when Joe was homeless after being evicted from his family home by an abusive partner of his mother.

Joe at 21 was the product of his environment. The causative factors discussed earlier in this chapter such as the deviancy cycle, poor parenting, abuse and stigma all contributed to his current position. Alongside these factors was the evident negative self-view that Joe held. His life events had obviously contributed to a profoundly negative set of personal constructs. Joe perceived himself to be a bad person, had a poor self-esteem and he expected to be

treated badly. Joe would refer to himself as being 'mentally handicapped' and as having a personality disorder. He would insist that he was incapable of some self-help skills when this was patently untrue. Joe would misinterpret events in a negative way, which would reinforce his self-construct. Examples of this included when a therapist was off sick and could not see him he would claim that this person hated him, was scared of him or couldn't help him. Similarly, if a person was moved from the unit, he perceived this to be because if that person had not been discharged they would have attempted to harm him.

Joe's thought processes were partially due to the constructs or 'schemata' discussed by Kelly (1955), Ellis (1962) and Beck (1976). Attempts have therefore been made to engage Joe in cognitive therapy. Therapists have offered Joe the opportunity to examine his beliefs and feelings of being eternally bad by offering rational explanations for events that he has misinterpreted. Joe's aggression and impetuosity have subsided in frequency and intensity. Although he remains an extremely damaged person who displays challenging behaviour, he is gradually gaining insight and a more accepting self-image. His constructs have shifted as a direct result of positive environmental factors. Through learning self-help skills he is gaining confidence in himself. The long abiding self-view of being inherently bad has also shifted due to Joe helping less able people within the unit; in so doing, Joe now feels some worth. One crucial factor has been the permanency of care staff. Joe once expected that significant others would both desert and harm him. Skilled care staff have demonstrated that this is not always so and Joe's self-construct has been positively altered.

Case illustration 10.3   Family therapy

Steven is 18 years of age and has been described as having a mild learning disability and epilepsy. He currently attends a local agricultural college during the day where he is well liked and displays appropriate behaviour. Steven has been referred to a local community learning disabilities team by his mother. His mother's concerns are that at meal times Steven throws utensils and pots, upturns the table and chairs and makes threats to harm family members, notably his father. He will also feign tonic–clonic seizures. Consultations with the local GP and consultant psychiatrists have resulted in the prescription of psychotropic drugs which have made Steven drowsy but have resulted in no behavioural change.

A community nurse and psychologist having completed an assessment of behaviour involving ABC charts, family interviews and liaison with college, have decided that family interactions precipitate Steven's display of challenging behaviour. It is evident that Steven's behaviour is 'situational' in that it only occurs within the family home, and only at meal times. Currently all family members blame Steven for the behavioural problems and the resulting family conflict. The community nurse and clinical psychologist had undertaken an accredited course in family therapy and therefore, with the consent of the family, offered support to the family. It was arranged for meal times to be filmed on video tape so that family interventions could be analysed. These tapes indicated that Steven had become a 'lightning conductor' for family discord, which was channelled through him. As Byng-Hall (1986) has suggested, the meal time altercations had become the family script and currently the family lacked the insight and commitment to alter it.

Drawing on the elements of family therapy, certain relationships existed within the family unit which lead to Steven, almost inevitably, displaying challenging behaviour. It would appear that 'enmeshment' existed between mother and Steven in that, maybe due to his learning disability, she had tended to over protect her son and this had led to other family members, in particular Steven's father, feeling excluded. Due to this, 'disengagement' existed between father and Steven, resulting in the father having a disregard for Steven's emotional distress. Steven would avoid his father but at meal times Steven was made to come to the table where his father would constantly point out Steven's perceived failings such as poor table manners. The father also had until recently attempted to impose a 'rigid' hierarchy on the family. Steven and his younger sibling Ruth (16) had begun to challenge this 'rigidity'. Steven had begun to refuse to come to the table but when coerced there by his father would demonstrate his anger at this by creating a disturbance. Rebellious behaviour is an expected part of adolescence as in this case. The prescription of psychotropic drugs could be seen as a medicalisation of both adolescence and challenging behaviour. Steven's challenging behaviour had a communicative function and perhaps his learning disability contributed to him being unable to communicate his distress appropriately. Ruth also disapproved of her father's conduct and while not usually engaging in open conflict with him, formed an 'alliance' and 'coalition' with her brother and used him to bear the brunt of the conflict. When this conflict became too distressing for Steven he would feign tonic–clonic seizures in an attempt to isolate himself and avoid further distress.

This interpretation was made relatively easy to arrive at by having an elementary understanding of family therapy. The objectivity of the nurse and psychologist also enabled this analysis to be made. That the family has not perceived these factors before can be attributed to them being unable to objectively account for factors which had contributed to this daily repetition of conflict, including lacking the awareness that the 'family system' and each member of it, rather than Steven's learning disability, were responsible for it. This understanding enables adjustments to be made to family relationships and routines, resulting in reduced conflict.

---

demonstrates this. This section presents only a brief outline of family therapy; the reader should consult *An Introduction to Family Therapy* (Dallos & Draper 2000) for a fuller explanation of this subject.

Therapeutic content

The therapeutic nature of family therapy is based on psychological interpretations of behavioural manifestations. When assessing an individual with challenging behaviour within a family unit, the following terms may be used:

- *Enmeshment* This term is used to explain relationships that are so close that they can exclude all others. The 'infantilisation' of people with learning disabilities can develop due to the 'enmeshment' and exclusive closeness that develops between the individual and an overprotective parent.

- *Disengagement* This is the converse of enmeshment and describes the coldness associated with under involvement in relationships. In extreme cases it can result in callous disregard for the emotional distress of others. It can be typified by the rejection of the person with challenging behaviour by their family.

- *Triads* These are very important when considering the person with challenging behaviour within a family unit. Triad is a term used to describe relationships involving three parties. Sub divisions of this include:

—*Alliance* This indicates two family members making an agreement and can importantly lead to

—*Coalitions* This indicates when family members join forces, often covertly, against another member. Challenging behaviour may be attributable in some instances to the often well-intentioned decisions taken by care givers that exclude the person with behavioural difficulties.

—*Hierarchy* This is used to describe how family decisions are made by the use of an executive function which may be the responsibility of one or more powerful family members. Some theorists such as Minuchin & Fishman (1981) and Haley (1980) have attributed the majority of problems that occur in families to the laxity or over-rigidity of hierarchical boundaries. Challenging behaviours can result due to laxity if attempts have never been made to rectify them or in response to inappropriately rigid boundaries.

It should be noted that only the terms used in Case illustration 10.3 are offered here. The reader should consult Burnham (1986) for a comprehensive analysis.

Belief systems

These are conceptual frameworks which families use as a way of knowing and understanding their world. Dallos & Draper (2000) state that:

... families do not simply absorb ideologies and discourses but translate them within their own 'family culture' and the traditions and current dynamics in their own families. Between society and the individual is a set of shared premises, explanations and expectations – in short a family's own belief system. (Dallos & Draper 2000, pp 7–8)

This is important when discussing challenging behaviour as those displaying it within a family unit can be expected to do so as part of their prescribed role. Byng-Hall (1986) has used the term 'family script' to describe how family members often repeat sequences of behaviour as actors fol-low the script of a play. Challenging behaviour may be both expected by the family unit, and perceived to be the designated role of the person displaying it.

An understanding of these concepts associated with family therapy predicts the nature of any resulting family therapy intervention.

Practical application

Family therapists can be influential in assessing a family's needs and recommending practical support as a result. Vetere (1993) has commented that many studies have demonstrated that practical support is associated with improvement in a family's ability to cope with a child with learning disabilities. Such practical support includes:

- access to appropriate financial benefits
- aids and adaptations
- support networks both formal and informal
- specific professional input such as portage
- support and instruction relating to parenting skills
- access to respite care / specialist care.

Family therapy involves observation of family interactions followed by a series of recommendations as to how to evolve interactions that limit the maintenance of inappropriate behaviour. Case illustration 10.3 exemplifies its uses.

Criticisms of family therapy

Family therapy helped Steven's family understand the causation of the behaviour, and offered ways of dealing with it, however critics of family therapy maintain that its success depends on:

- the family engaging actively in the process
- the family being willing to accept some sometimes unpalatable truths
- the ability of families to make meaningful changes to deeply entrenched belief systems.

QUALITY SERVICES AND ENVIRONMENTAL MANAGEMENT

Therapeutic techniques, such as gentle teaching, cognitive therapy and behaviour modification can all offer constructive ways of working with people who have challenging behaviours. The extent of their success is largely dependent on the environments in which an individual lives. The impact of the environment on a person with challenging behaviour has a huge influence on whether or not a person's behaviour will be maintained or altered. The environment encompasses both its physical characteristics and, more importantly, the management of it.

Staff skills

The most important environmental aspect to consider is the values, knowledge and skill base of direct care staff involved in working with people with challenging behaviour. Emerson et al (1988b), Harris & Oliver (1992) and Pougher (1997) have offered discussion around the importance of skilled staff. Staff working with clients who have challenging behaviour should be expected to:

- understand the possible causation(s) of challenging behaviour
- value the people for whom they care
- be aware of techniques for managing challenging behaviour
- clearly understand their role
- embrace the concepts of normalisation and encourage O'Brien's (1987) accomplishments (see Box 10.8)
- be able to contribute to assessment processes
- have the ability to work in a multidisciplinary way and across multi-agency boundaries
- seek to improve on their knowledge and skills base
- work flexibly.

Box 10.8   O'Brien's accomplishments

People with learning disabilities and challenging behaviour have a right to and should be encouraged to attain O'Brien's accomplishments which are briefly:

- Respect
- Community presence
- Meaningful relationships
- Choice
- Competence – The right to be allowed opportunities to reach full potential

In order to achieve these standards, services will need to support staff by developing systems that offer and monitor:

- supervision
- performance review
- training opportunities
- networking opportunities
- 'whistle blowing' procedures
- team-building mechanisms
- channels for effective communication
- stress management
- staff empowerment.

Client empowerment

Quality services for people with challenging behaviour necessarily should embrace and encourage client empowerment (Harris & Oliver 1992). Previously, through institutionalisation and maladaptive postures, people with learning disabilities have been denied control over their lives. Simons (1995) has suggested that empowerment is about people actively taking control of aspects of their lives. A well accepted and increasingly well developed mechanism for enabling people to become more empowered is the concept of advocacy, which can be best understood by looking at the areas of advocacy, self advocacy and citizen advocacy.

Advocacy

Teasdale (1998) has stated that advocacy is concerned with a person or organisation that will speak for those who lack the power to do so, and intercede on their behalf. People with learning disabilities have historically been unable to speak for (advocate) themselves, therefore advocacy has developed as a way of 'speaking up' for those people with learning disabilities who would be otherwise disempowered, and supporting decisions they have made. Tyne (1991) has asserted that an advocate must have a genuine commitment to represent a client's best interests.

Self advocacy

This involves speaking for oneself or as a group who share the same views. Gates (1994) has asserted that: 'In self-advocacy, people are encouraged to speak up for themselves, thus bringing about an element of self-empowerment, that is, people speaking for themselves rather than having an advocate speak for them' (Gates 1994, p. 4).

Citizen advocacy

This involves voluntary or paid groups working in partnership with clients to represent their concerns. It has been proposed that four principles underpin citizen advocacy and these are listed in Box 10.9.

Quality environments may well use these sources to encourage client empowerment. They are often used when major life decisions are being planned, such as the discharge or admission of a client from or to specialist services. Notwithstanding that such issues are extremely important, empowerment needs to pervade all aspects of an environment, and this can be achieved by staff encouraging clients to make seemingly very limited choices, for example whether to have brown or white bread. Services should encourage client participation in decisions such as when to go to bed, what to wear, or what to watch on television. Importantly, advocacy should be used to support attempts by people with learning disabilities and challenging behaviour, and by the services that provide care for them, to reach O'Brien's accomplishments (see Box 10.8).

Box 10.9   The principles of citizen advocacy. Adapted from Gates 1994

- Relationships should be formed that support and represent the best interests of those who need an advocate
- The advocate should enter into the relationship freely and have a desire to support the individual through difficult times
- The advocate should positively promote positive interactions and images of all people, irrespective of their disability
- Citizen advocacy schemes should be clearly defined within the communities they serve. They should also function independently from statutory organisations.

Risk taking

Adams (1995) has defined risk as: 'The probability of an adverse future event manipulated by its magnitude' (Adams 1995, p. 69). Adams has also postulated that risk is not an objective phenomenon but one that is culturally constructed. This factor has a huge impact on the lives of people with challenging behaviour as their care is characterised by services that are driven by minimising risk. Gabe (1995) suggested that when people perceive they have little control over events they tend to be more concerned than if they had some control. This argument extends to the care of people with challenging behaviour as care givers often feel unable to control behaviour. Adams (1995) has suggested that this channels them into seeking hierarchies within organisations that minimise and control any risk. Services therefore have historically, through institutionalisation, sought to contain and minimise risk, and by so doing have often intensified and maintained any pre-existing challenging behaviour. The Blom-Cooper Report (Blom-Cooper et al 1995), clinical governance agendas and localised service policies have all served to highlight risk, identify it and then manage it, with the result that services are increasingly adverse to risk taking. There exists, therefore, an institutionalised reluctance to allow people with challenging behaviour to take risks. Individual care givers are also influenced by notions of paternalism and attempts to act in the clients' best interests, and do so by 'erring on the side of caution'. Obviously some major risks need to be managed to safeguard client and public safety, however aversion to risk taking has permeated services to such an extent that minor risks are also avoided. Clients with challenging behaviour are frequently prevented from smoking where and when they want, drinking alcohol, engaging in sexual relationships, eating unhealthy foods, having electrical appliances in their rooms, spending money as they wish etc. Aversion to risk taking also limits their ability to achieve O'Brien's accomplishments (Box 10.8) as social trips into the community may be curtailed in case an individual displays anti-social behaviour. Denying clients the right to take risks impinges on their quality of life and the

Reader activity 10.1   Risk taking

Organise a sheet along the lines suggested below and simply jot down the things you do for enjoyment that involve taking risks. Do the same for someone you know with challenging behaviour.

Risk-taking activities that you engage in

examples – horse riding, cycling, hang gliding, climbing etc.

Now do the same for things you do to relieve stress.

Things you do to relieve stress

Risk-taking activities engaged in by a person with challenging behaviour

Things a person with challenging behaviour does to relieve stress

examples – drink alcohol, shout and scream, play squash etc.

It is not uncommon for the client's side to be entirely blank!

antagonism created by staff attempting to limit risk can result in more rather than less challenging behaviour.

Services need to embrace the concept that well-informed risk taking can dramatically improve the self-worth of the people they care for by offering opportunities for empowerment and access to social learning environments. Risk taking is a normal part of everyone's life but the opportunity to take risks is often denied those with chal-

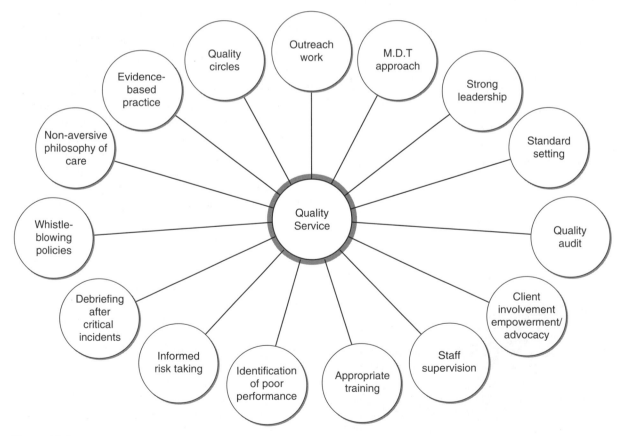

Figure 10.2

lenging behaviour due to institutionalised paternalism.

This brief overview of some aspects of service development has focused on key areas expected of a high quality service designed to produce environments in which challenging behaviour can be ameliorated. Figure 10.2 identifies a range of other relevant issues.

CONCLUSION

This chapter has outlined a number of issues concerning people with learning disabilities and challenging behaviour. It has been suggested that the definition of challenging behaviour is open to misinterpretation and that through labelling it can have a negative impact on those labelled. It has been suggested that often the symptomology associated with challenging behaviour is the focus of intervention and that causative factors may not be adequately identified and ameliorated. It has been identified that the causation of challenging behaviour is multifactorial and that its aetiology may be attributable to one or, more probably, several causative factors that could have a biological, behavioural, sociological or psychological basis. It has been suggested that an eclectic range of interventions be explored, dependent on the identified causations of the individual's challenging behaviour. Proposed interventions included chemotherapeutic, behavioural, gentle teaching, cognitive behavioural therapy and family therapy. Both the theoretical underpinnings and the criticisms of each of these approaches have been discussed. Finally, it was suggested that any interventions offered with the intention of ameliorating challenging behaviour will have a better chance of success if they are conducted in the conducive milieu provided by high quality, empowering services.

REFERENCES

Adams J 1995 Risk. University College Press, London

Alyward E H, Burt D B, Thorpe L U et al 1997 Diagnosis of dementia in individuals with intellectual disability. Journal of Intellectual Disability Research 41(2): 152–164

Bandura A 1977 Social learning theory. Prentice Hall, Englewood Cliffs, New Jersey

Barrera F J, Teodoro G M 1990 Flash bonding or cold fusion? A case analysis of gentle teaching. In: Repp A C, Singh N N (eds) Perspectives on the use of non aversive and aversive interventions for persons with developmental disabilities. Sycamore Publishing, Sycamore, Illinois

Barton R 1960 Institutional neurosis. Stonebridge Press, Bristol

Beail N, Warden S 1995 Sexual abuse of adults with learning disabilities. Journal of Intellectual Disability Research 39(5): 382–387

Beck A T 1976 Cognitive therapy and emotional disorders. International University Press, New York

Bicknell J, Conboy-Hill S 1992 The deviancy career and people with mental handicap. In: Waitman A, Conboy-Hill S (eds) 1992 Psychotherapy and mental handicap. Sage Publications, London

Blom-Cooper L, Hally H, Murphy E 1995 The falling shadow, one patient's mental health care 1978–1993. The report of the committee of inquiry into events leading up to and surrounding the fatal incident at the Edith Morgan Centre, Torbay on 1st September 1993. Duckworth, London

Blunden R, Allen D 1987 Facing the challenge: an ordinary life for people with learning disabilities and challenging behaviour. Kings Fund paper no. 74, Kings Fund Centre, London

Borthwick-Duffy S A 1994a Prevalence of destructive behaviours: a study of self-injury and property destruction. In: Thompson T, Gray B (eds) 1994 Destructive behaviour in developmental disabilities: diagnosis and treatments. Sage Publications, London

Borthwick-Duffy S A 1994b Epidemiology and prevalence of psychopathology in people with mental retardation. Journal of Consulting and Clinical Psychology 62: 17–27

Burnham J 1986 Family therapy: first steps towards a systemic approach. Tavistock Publications, London

Byng-Hall J 1986 Family scripts, the concept which can bridge child psychotherapy and family thinking. Journal of Child Psychotherapy 12: 3–13

Caldwell P 1999 Person to person: establishing contact and communication with people with profound learning disabilities and extra special needs. Pavilion Publishing, Brighton

Christie R, Bay C, Kaufman I A et al 1982 Lesch–Nyhan disease: clinical experience with nineteen patients. Developmental Medicine and Child Neurology 24: 293–306

Clements J 1997 Sustaining a cognitive psychology for people with learning disabilities. In: Stenfert-Kroese B, Dagnan D, Loumidis K (eds) 1997 Cognitive behaviour for people with learning disabilities. Routledge, London

Corbet J A 1979 Psychiatric morbidity and mental retardation. In: Snaith P, Jones F E (eds) 1980 Mental illness and mental retardation. Gaskell, London

Craft M 1984 Genetic endowment and the XYY syndrome. In: Craft M (ed) Mentally abnormal offenders. Baillière Tindall, London

Dallos R, Draper R 2000 An introduction to family therapy: systemic theory and practice. Open University Press, Buckingham

Department of Health 1992 Mansell report on services for people with learning disabilities and challenging behaviour or mental health needs. HMSO, London

Department of Health 2001 Valuing people: a new strategy for learning disability for the 21st century. Available via the internet at: www.doh.gov.uk/learning disabilities

Ellis A 1962 Reason and emotion in psychotherapy. Lyle Stuart, New York

Emerson E 1990 Some challenges presented by severe self injurious behaviour. Mental Handicap 17: 92–98

Emerson E, Cummings R, Barrett S et al 1988a Challenging behaviour and community services: 2. Who are the people who challenge services? Mental Handicap 16: 16–19

Emerson E, Toogood A, Barrett S et al 1988b Challenging behaviour and community services: 3. Planning individual services. Mental Handicap 16: 70–74

Emerson E, Robertson J, Gregory N et al 2000 Treatment and management of challenging behaviours in residential settings. Journal of Applied Research in Intellectual Disabilities. 13: 197–215

Gabe J 1995 (ed) Medicine, health and risk: sociological approaches. Blackwell Scientific Publications, Oxford

Gates B 1994 Advocacy: a nurse's guide. Scutari Press, Middlesex

Gates B 1996 Issues of reliability and validity in measurement of challenging behaviour (behavioural difficulties) in learning disability: a discussion of implications for nursing research and practice. Journal of Clinical Nursing 5: 7–12

Gates B 1997 Behavioural difficulties. In: Gates B (ed) 1997 Learning Disabilities. Churchill Livingstone, Glasgow

Gear J, Gates B, Wray J 2000 Towards understanding behaviour. In: Gates B, Gear J, Wray J (eds) Behavioural distress, concepts and strategies. Baillière Tindall, London

Goffman E 1961 Asylums, essays on the social situations of mental patients and other patients. Pelican, Bungay

Goffman E 1963 Stigma: notes on the management of spoiled identity. Prentice Hall, Englewood Cliffs, New Jersey

Haley J 1980 Leaving home. McGraw-Hill, New York

Hames A 1993 People with learning disabilities who commit sexual offences: assessment and treatment. NAPSAC Newsletter 6: 3–6

Harris P, Oliver R 1992 How to meet the challenge. Health Service Journal. 8th October 1991, 28–29

Jacobson J W, Ackerman L J 1988 An appraisal of services for persons with mental retardation and psychiatric impairments. Mental Retardation 26(6): 377–380

Kelly G 1955 The psychology of personal construct theory. Norton, New York

Lovett M 1996 Learning to listen: positive approaches and people with difficult behaviour. Jessica Kingsley, London

Lund J 1985 The prevalence of psychiatric morbidity in mentally retarded adults. Acta Psychiatrica Scandinavia 72: 563–570

McBrien J, Felce D 1995 Working with people who have severe learning difficulty and challenging behaviour: a practical handbook on the behavioural approach. BILD Publications, Kidderminster

McConachie H 1986 Parents and young mentally handicapped children: a review of research issues. Croom Helm, Beckenham

McCue M 2000 Behavioural interventions. In: Gates B, Gear J, Wray J (eds) Behavioural distress, concepts and strategies. Baillière Tindall, London

McGee J 1990 Gentle teaching: the basic tenet. Nursing Times 86: 68–72

McGee J 1992 Gentle teaching: assumptions and paradigm. Journal of Applied Behaviour Analysis 25: 869–872

McGee J, Menolascino M D, Hobbs D, Menousek P 1987 Gentle teaching: a non-aversive approach to helping persons with mental retardation. Human Sciences Press, New York

Menolascino F J, Fleisher M H 1993 Mental health care in persons with mental retardation. Past, present and future. In: Fletcher R, Dosen A (eds) Mental health aspects of mental retardation. Lexington Books, New York

Mental Health Act 1983 HMSO, London

Minuchin S, Fishman C 1981 Family therapy techniques. Harvard University Press, Cambridge, Mass.

Moss S, Emerson E, Bouras N, Holland A 1997 Mental disorders and problematic behaviours in people with intellectual disability: future directions for research. Journal of Intellectual Disability Research 43: 440–447

Murphy G 1994 Understanding challenging behaviour. In: Emerson E, McGill P, Mansell J (eds) Severe learning disabilities and challenging behaviour: designing high quality services. Chapman and Hall, London

Murphy G 1999 Self-injurious behaviour: what do we know and where are we going? Tizard Learning Disability Review 4(1): 5–12

Murphy G, Holland T 1993 Challenging behaviour, psychiatric disorders and the law. In: Jones S P, Eayrs B (eds) Challenging behaviour and intellectual disability: a psychological perspective. BILD Publications, Kidderminster

Nihira K, Leland H, Lambert N 1993 AAMR Adaptive Behaviour Scale-residential and community examiners manual, 2nd edn. Pro.Ed. Texas, USA

O'Brien J 1987 A guide to life planning: using the activities catalogue to integrate services and natural support systems. In: Wilcox B W, Bellamy G T (eds) The activities catalogue: an alternative curriculum for youth and adults with severe disabilities. Brookes, Baltimore

Oliver C 1993 Self injurious behaviour from response to strategy. In: Kiernan C (ed) Research to practice? Implications of research on the challenging behaviour of people with learning disability. BILD Publications, Clevedon, pp 135–188

O'Rourke S, Wray J 2000 Gentle teaching. In: Gates B, Gear J, Wray J (eds) Behavioural distress, concepts and strategies. Baillière Tindall, London

Pavlov I P 1927 Conditioned reflexes. Oxford University Press, London

Pilgrim D, Rogers A 1999 A sociology of mental health and illness, 2nd edn. Oxford University Press, Trowbridge, UK

Pougher J 1997 Providing quality care. In: Gates B (ed) Learning disabilities, 3rd edn. Churchill Livingstone, Glasgow

Qureshi H 1994 The size of the problem. In: Emerson E, McGill P, Mansell J (eds) Severe learning disabilities and challenging behaviour: designing high quality services. Chapman and Hall, London

Raghavan R 1996 Contrasting diagnosis. Nursing Times 92 (23): 59–62

Reeves S 1997 Behavioural misdiagnosis. Nursing Times 93 (19): 44–45

Reiss S, Levitan G W, Szyzo J 1982 Emotional disturbance and mental retardation: diagnostic overshadowing. American Journal of Mental Deficiency 86: 567–574

Rutter M, Tizzard J, Graham P et al 1976 Isle of Wight studies 1964–74. Psychological Medicine 6: 313–332

Simons K 1995 Empowerment and advocacy. In: Malin N (ed) Services for people with learning disabilities. Routledge, London

Skinner B F 1953 Science and human behaviour. MacMillan, New York

Slee R 1996 Clauses of conditionality: the reasonable accommodation of language. In: Barton L (ed) Disability and society: emerging issues and insights. Longman, London

Teasdale K 1998 Advocacy in health care. Blackwell Science, Oxford

Turnbull J 2000 Cognitive behavioural interventions. In: Gates B, Gear J, Wray J (eds) Behavioural distress, concepts and strategies. Baillière Tindall, London

Tyne A 1991 A report on an evaluation of Sheffield citizen advocacy. National Development Team, Manchester

Verri A, Vggetti C, Vallero E et al 2000 Oral self-mutilation in a patient with rhombencephalosynapsys. Journal of Intellectual Disabilities 44(1): 86–90

Vetere A 1993 Using family therapy in services for people with learning disabilities. In: Carpenter J, Treacher A (eds) Using family therapy in the 90's. Blackwell, Oxford

Yule W, Carr J 1990 Behaviour modification for people with mental handicaps. Chapman and Hall, London

FURTHER READING

Caldwell P 1999 Person to person: establishing contact and communication with people with profound learning disabilities and extra special needs. Pavilion, Brighton

Emerson E 1995 Challenging behaviour: analysis and intervention in people with learning difficulties. Cambridge University Press, Cambridge

Gates B, Gear J, Wray J (eds) 2000 Behavioural distress, concepts and strategies. Baillière Tindall, London

Ryan J, Thomas F 1987 The politics of mental handicap. Free Associated Press, London

Swain J, Finkelstein V, French S, Oliver M (eds) 1996 Disabling barriers – enabling environments. Sage, London

Waitman A, Conboy-Hill S 1992 Psychotherapy and mental handicap. Sage, London

USEFUL ADDRESSES

The information below includes internet web-sites and addresses of providers of information and training, which may be of interest to people wishing to explore issues relating to challenging behaviour.

The British Institute of Learning Disabilities (BILD)
Wolverhampton Road
Kidderminster
Worcestershire
DY10 3PP
Tel 01562 850251 Fax 01562 851970 www.bild.org.uk
BILD provides a range of well regarded training and education opportunities.

The Tizard Centre
Beverley Farm
University of Kent at Canterbury
Canterbury
Kent
CT2 7LZ
Tel 01227 764000 (ext 7771) Fax 01227 763674
http://www.speke.ukc.ac.uk/tizard/index.htm/

The Tizard Centre have developed useful training packs for those wishing to educate others about how to understand challenging behaviour.

Pavilion Publishing and Conference Services
Pavilion Publishing
8 St George's Place
Brighton
Sussex
BN1 4GB
Tel 01273 623222 Fax 01273 625526 http://www.pavpub.com

Pavilion Publishing provide useful information and training packs relating to challenging behaviour.

The East Yorkshire Learning Disability Institute (EYLDI)
The University of Hull
Hull
HU6 7RX
Tel 01482 465241 Fax 01482 466699
www.hull.ac.uk/Hull/health.ps/ld/eyld.htm

EYLDI offers consultancy and training on the subject of challenging behaviour.

11 Autistic spectrum disorder

Maggie Anderson

CHAPTER CONTENTS

KEY ISSUES

- The apparent recent growth in the number of children and adults diagnosed with autistic spectrum disorder has led to increased interest in the causes of autism and to renewed efforts to provide appropriate services.
- This chapter considers the causation of autistic spectrum disorder, currently being studied by many different disciplines, which is adding to an unfolding picture of autism.
- Currently, autism is addressed largely through educational means at pre-school and school age and the options open to parents will be presented.
- The problems faced by adolescents and adults on the spectrum will be considered, concluding that few services currently exist for more able adults on the spectrum whose difficulties lie in the realms of social and emotional knowledge and skills. Those whose autism is compounded by other learning disabilities fall within the broader disability services.
- It is suggested that the broader perspective on the issues, raised by the growth of autobiographical work, both on the internet and through publication, can help to shape future services.

INTRODUCTION

30 years ago, autism was considered to be a rare disorder. The causes of autistic behaviour in children and adults were poorly understood and confusion over the diagnosis of the disorder blurred the boundaries between cognitive disorders and mental health problems (Waterhouse 2000). Within the intervening years, a greater understanding of autism has resulted from ongoing research internationally, and publicity around the disorder has made it much more visible. Figures from the National Autistic Society and other sources (Mental Health Foundation 2000) indicate an apparently phenomenal increase in the numbers of adults and children who are diagnosed as on the autistic spectrum. This poses the interesting question of whether this is a real or apparent increase in the prevalence of the cluster of difficulties identified as autistic spectrum disorder.

PREVALENCE

Currently, the estimated prevalence of the disorder varies considerably. The Mental Health Foundation (2000) puts figures at between 31 and 47 per 10 000, although some estimates are considerably higher – up to 56 per 10 000 (The National Autistic Society 1997) – and some much lower – 10–14 per 10 000 (Trevarthan et al 1998). In this population, males far outnumber females. The estimates vary from 2:1 (Jordan 1999) to 13:1 (Gillberg et al 1991) with sources agreeing that the ratio is more balanced amongst those with profound and multiple disabilities. Despite the concern that parents have about the delay in the recognition of the child's difficulties and the receipt of a diagnosis, autism is being diagnosed earlier and at an alarming rate. In order to account for the huge increase in numbers of this population, we need to consider not only the causes of autism, which are discussed in this chapter, but also the cultural changes in social, educational and personal life patterns that provide a context for this increase. Children are expected to be participants in rather than recipients of education, learning skills in order to access the knowledge they need. This requires them to be much more active within the learning process, demanding in turn greater communication and interpersonal ability than in previous generations. Expectations about emotional relationships within families have changed, with much greater equality and freedom within family groupings. The era of children being 'seen and not heard' is gone: children are expected to be articulate, both linguistically and emotionally. The changing nature of the economy, with growth in service industries, requires better interpersonal and communication skills than in a primarily industrial work environment. Thus through these societal changes, emphasis is thrown on to the very areas in which people on the autistic spectrum have difficulties.

AWARENESS

Accounts of the lives of people on the autistic spectrum are seen on the television and, most famously, in the film *Rain Man*. This sympathetic portrayal of an autistic man's difficulties with the demands of everyday interaction spurred great interest in the condition. Similarly, Dr Oliver Sacks' work (Sacks 1995) with two autistic individuals – Temple Grandin and Jessie Park – also led to an increased understanding of the cognitive and emotional differences in the autistic population. The autobiographical material currently available from people on the spectrum (Grandin 1996, Kolinski 2001, Miedzianik 1997, Williams 1992) gives a unique insight into the cognitive and emotional worlds of these individuals. A cautionary note must be sounded here, as any one individual's autism will be a contributory factor (possibly a major one) in the composition of their perceptual and emotional set, but will not be the only factor. Each individual is greater than just his cognitive functioning, and many other life events and habits will have contributed to the evolution of a particular personality. Thus, one should value the contribution of autobiographical writing to the sum of knowledge about autism whilst acknowledging the limitations contained by default within it (Frith 1991).

Many people on the autistic spectrum feel positively about their condition: 'I enjoy being autistic rather than not, because it's me, it's what's natural. It's easy so I don't have to make any effort . . . ' (National Autistic Society 1997, p. 33). Temple

Grandin also offers great insight into the impact that autism has had on her perceptual system and how this has shaped her relationship with the world. Whilst she values the abilities her autism brings, many autistic children and adults are distressed and depressed by their condition: 'It's the fear, with autism, I think, that gets most of them down, and we do use our obsessions and our rituals or whatever it might be or preservation of sameness as reassurance, I think . . . ' (National Autistic Society 1997, p. 32). Ms Grandin recognises the differences in reaction to the condition and contrasts her own view of her autism – 'part of what I am' (Grandin 1996, p. 60) – with Donna Williams' view – 'Autism is just an information processing problem that controls who I am . . . ' (Grandin 1996, p. 61).

This increasing access to information and feelings about autistic spectrum disorder has raised the profile of this condition and has evidenced major changes in the way that it is perceived by those with the condition as well as professionals and the public.

BACKGROUND TO CURRENT KNOWLEDGE AND ATTITUDES

Later sections of this chapter will explore the issues of cause and presentation of autistic spectrum disorder in some detail and reflect the many 'unknowns' that still typify the disorder. As diagnostic systems become more complex and our ability to pinpoint cognitive and biological anomalies becomes more refined, it is easy to lose sight of the basics of the condition. Kanner described a group of children in 1943 who shared many unusual behaviours and characteristics. Kanner & Eisenberg (1956) selected five characteristics for diagnosis:

- Lack of affective contact with others
- Need for the preservation of sameness
- Fascination with and skill in manipulating objects
- Mutism, or non-communicative language
- Intelligent aspect and good cognitive potential.

At much the same time that Kanner's work was taking place in the U.S, Hans Asperger was identifying a group of children in Germany with specific learning difficulties (Trevarthen et al 1998). The

difficulties encountered by the children described by Asperger are very close to those suggested by Kanner. It is thought that Asperger's work received much less attention than that of Kanner due to the cultural prejudice engendered by the Second World War, and indeed Asperger's original papers have only fairly recently been translated. Some debate continues around whether Kanner and Asperger were describing children with the same difficulties or whether the two groups could be differentiated (see Frith 1991) and this debate continues to echo in the complex issues surrounding the diagnosis of Asperger's syndrome discussed below.

Autism attracted very little attention in the UK until Lorna Wing's seminal study (Wing & Gould 1979), which focused on a group of children in Camberwell. From this Wing identified the 'triad of impairments': this is the suggestion that people on the autistic spectrum have difficulties in the areas of communication, social interaction and flexibility of behaviour and thought. Case illustration 11.1 below provides a typical example. As outlined below, these difficulties vary enormously in individuals, ranging from people who are rule-governed, socially awkward and inflexible in routine, through to others whose autism has prevented the acquisition of even basic communication and socialisation skills. From the wide range of abilities found within this population has sprung the concept of a spectrum of disorder; all of the people on the spectrum have difficulties within the triad of impairments, but in different presentation. It is this very breadth of presentation that can cause confusion for all involved with an individual on the autistic spectrum.

LIFE PATTERNS

From around the time of Kanner's work in the 1940s onward, autistic people in the UK, in common with many other groups of children and adults with learning disabilities, found themselves caught up in health service provision for the 'mentally subnormal' (Sandu & Carruthers 1999). Based on the medical model (Maggs 1987), these services offered accommodation and intervention as one package, the emphasis usually being on the former. Thus, many adults on the

Case illustration 11.1

Jake is described by his parents as a very stubborn child. He is the second child in the family and has a typically developing sister. Jake's Mum, Pat, describes him as a 'good' baby, as long as he got his own way: as long as he slept in his parents' bed, he would sleep through the night; he would eat only a limited range of foods; he would only play alone; he would only use the toilet in his own home and needed nappies when out. Pat describes Jake's play and language development as very different from his sister's. He played almost exclusively with a toy train set, putting the tracks and trains in the same positions and running through the same 'routine' with them. To communicate his needs, he relied on physically pushing people toward what he wanted; he did not point and he did not take his parents by the hand, but rather by the wrist.

On beginning nursery, Jake appeared to be very distressed at being left and this did not resolve itself as with the other children. He would cry and tantrum for extended periods of time and, when he did settle in the nursery environment, he would not follow the routine along with the other children. He appeared not to respond when asked to do something and found it very difficult to fit into the flow of nursery activity.

Jake preferred to play alone and actively resisted any attempts by the other children to engage him in group activities. He also found structured one-to-one play with adults or children difficult. However, the major problem from the nursery's viewpoint was Jake's refusal to comply with requests, the situation often escalating to a full blown temper tantrum. On referral by the health visitor to a psychologist and speech and language therapist, testing revealed that Jake had very little language comprehension and thus had great difficulty in the language-dependent environment at nursery.

A speech and language therapist worked at home and with the nursery to introduce a pictorial communication system for Jake, which has eased his frustration considerably and he is now beginning to vocalise in addition to using his communication cards.

spectrum spent their lives in institutions, receiving little or no help to overcome the difficulties presented by their condition. Currently, it is felt that an educational framework is more appropriate and children and adults are helped to access ordinary life experiences and opportunities through careful teaching. A recent review of the research underpinning educational approaches to working with children on the autistic spectrum (Jordan et al 1998) suggests that whatever the philosophical stance of the educational intervention, working with children early and intensively is the key to a positive outcome.

Once the child reaches school age, focus shifts to the educational arena and children will access the mainstream or specialist services available to them. Many young adults on the autistic spectrum will follow regular life patterns, maintaining employment and entering into friendships and partnerships. However, for the less able, services within the health, social and voluntary spheres seek to find appropriate employment and living styles to promote optimum independence in adults (Waterhouse 2000).

Early intervention

Recently, the Mental Health Foundation has published a study, *The Cost of Autistic Spectrum Disorder* (Mental Health Foundation 2000), which reports on the estimated cost of supporting people with autism over their lifespan. At publication in 2000, it was estimated that the costs for supporting an individual on the autistic spectrum throughout his lifetime would vary between £525 070 for a very able person and £2 940 538 for an individual with autism and additional learning disabilities. Thus it is clear that early intervention to maximise the child's learning and ongoing education is not only important for the physical, emotional and social wellbeing of the individual but also makes economic good sense.

The next part of this chapter gives a sketch of the complex question of the causes of autistic spectrum disorder, considering research from several schools of thought. The very varied ways in which autistic spectrum disorder presents within individuals is then considered, and this leads to an outline of the services available to children and families within the UK. The final section of the chapter addresses the life course in autism, reflecting on the relatively 'new' knowledge we have about adolescence and adulthood experiences of people with this disorder.

AETIOLOGY
Background

As the prevalence of autistic spectrum disorder is increasing, so is the work focused on finding the causes of autism. Research in many fields is revealing a complex picture, highlighting disparate features which, within one individual, can lead to the presentation of behaviours which might lead to a diagnosis of autism. The different models of conceptualising autism – as a cognitive deficit, a biological reaction, an emotional disability – have led to a wide range of research approaches, all of which appear to add different light to the causation picture.

It is important to state that it is a combination of factors in any one individual that will ultimately lead to autism. Each of the features described below may not be sufficient alone to account for autism within the child or adult, but the aggregation of these factors in a particular fashion in particular people will do so (Seroussi 2000). Thus, one may come across families with two or three children, just one of whom may be autistic, although the other children may have some cognitive difficulties – delayed language, for example. Indeed, one of the more interesting new aspects of the work is the attempt to elicit the nature of the links in terms of cause between frank autism and the range of other difficulties within the perceptual/social/communication realms which seem to coincide within families.

For ease of explanation, the factors that are implicated in the aetiology of autistic spectrum disorder are presented as pre-, peri- or post-natal. Clearly, some of these factors run across these artificial time divisions, but the clarity offered by this framework outweighs the loss of sophistication of this explanation.

Causative factors

Prenatal

Genetics Some of the early work in the field (Bettelheim 1967) identified behaviours in the parents of autistic children that were characterised as cold or unemotional. The early interpretation of these observations was that these behaviours in parents caused autism in children, i.e. the child's language delay, lack of social motivation and rigidity of behaviour was a direct result of what we would now call parenting style. The impact of this assumption on parents can only

be imagined and, fortunately, this interpretation of the phenomenon is now relegated to historical accounts. However, the observation stands and a contemporary interpretation lies within the genetic component of autistic spectrum disorder.

Recent work (Piven & Folstein 1994) indicates that the higher the level of genetic similarity between individuals, the more likely they are to share autistic characteristics. The authors state that prevalence of autism in siblings of autistic children is 2.7% – 50–100 times greater than their prevalence figures would ordinarily suggest. Further, these authors report work by LeCouteur (LeCouteur et al 1989) which indicates that non-autistic siblings of autistic children may develop some social difficulties as adults that were not apparent in childhood. Indeed, these social difficulties may be observed in the parents of children on the autistic spectrum at a higher prevalence than in the non-autistic population (Wolff et al 1988). Case illustration 11.2 provides an example of this. Thus, whilst the observation of similar behaviours between parents and children was a sound one, the current state of knowledge has changed the interpretation of this observation profoundly.

X-linked autism? The disparity in the number of males to females on the spectrum invites speculation and research around the role played by the X chromosome. Szatmari & Jones (1991) have suggested that autism is, in some way, carried on the X chromosome. Thus, if a female has one X chromosome affected and the other not, then the effects would not be apparent. However, males would present with autism as a result of the X chromosome, as their Y chromosome would not balance out the effect. Should a female inherit two affected chromosomes, the effect would be to present with much more profound autism, which appears to be the case (Trevarthen et al 1998). The genetic mechanisms involved in this inheritance of (at least) predisposition to autistic spectrum disorder are unclear and present a field ripe for further research.

Links with other genetic difficulties The relationship between autism and more general learning disabilities as demonstrated by performance on tests of cognitive ability is discussed later in this

Case illustration 11.2

Harry's health visitor was rather concerned about his development. Whilst his motor development was at an age appropriate level and his speech advanced, his play was very atypical – he lined up and manipulated sticks, pens and cutlery and liked to run sand and gravel through his fingers. At 3 years old, Harry did not have any pretend play, showing no interest in cars, playing house or using construction or art materials. Harry was an only child, received a lot of adult attention and seemed disinterested in the other children at nursery, positively avoiding them when possible. His speech was rather pedantic and almost adult. The health visitor had expressed her concerns to Harry's mother, who responded that Harry's dad, Philip, was 'just the same'.

The health visitor then arranged a meeting with both parents and was, indeed, struck by the similarities in behaviour. Philip, Harry's dad, arranged his diary, pens and phone very precisely in front of him, was anxious that the meeting begin and finish exactly on time and he also had a pedantic manner of speaking. In what proved to be a difficult conversation, it emerged that Philip had also begun to speak late and that his parents had worried that he might be 'retarded'. He was miserable at school, having been teased, particularly at secondary school, for his odd mannerisms and idiosyncratic personal style. He found university frightening as he did not understand complex interpersonal behaviours and relationships. He became very depressed by his 'differentness' and had some time out following a suicide attempt. His life improved considerably when he found work as a bookkeeper and met Harry's mother, who has always been tolerant of and amused by Philip's 'oddities'. Both parents were keen, however, that Harry should have some intervention to prevent the pattern of isolation and depression recurring for him.

Reader activity 11.1

Make a list of the difficulties that may be presented by differentially diagnosing autism when it occurs with more global learning disabilities. It may help to consider what other factors may account for the diagnostic criteria outlined within the triad of impairments.
Then consider the following questions:

- What types of assessment might be used to make this differentiation?
- What difference would a diagnosis of coexisting ASD make to the intervention received by the individual?

chapter. However, the question raised in the context of autism accompanying other disorders is that of differential diagnosis, particularly when global delay clouds the clinical picture. With this caution in mind, autism appears to form part of a number of conditions and syndromes some of which spring from genetic and chromosomal causes. Fragile X is a very common cause of learning disabilities which is associated with autism, and for which children presenting with delays should be tested (Gillberg & Coleman 1992). Similarly phenylketonuria, neurofibromatosis and tuberous sclerosis have also been associated with autism. This is not to say that children with difficulties other than these may not also have concomitant autism – for example, there have been several reports of autism in children with Down syndrome (Ghaziuddin 1997). However, these conditions appear to carry a much greater than usual risk of autism as part of their presentation.

The uterine environment Some evidence appears to be emerging that factors related to the interuterine environment may play a part in the appearance of autism in children. For example, Szatmari & Jones (1991) suggest that maternal infection may be a factor in the causation of autism, but difficulties in diagnosis persist if the child's difficulties are more widespread. A charitable group that is particularly concerned with allergies and autism (Allergy Induced Autism) is also interested in the links between maternal vaccination and autism in children. This possibility is raised by Seroussi (2000) in relation to atypical development in children.

Brain structure A more established area of research considers differences in the brain structure of people with autism. The cerebellum has attracted much research attention as a possible site for the cause of behavioural and cognitive anomalies (Piven & Folstein 1994), although this work is inconclusive. Trevarthen et al (1998) provide an overview of the work on brain functioning and conclude that the evidence is, again, inconclusive.

Perinatal factors

Birth trauma Twin studies raise some questions around the part played by birth trauma. It would appear (see Brazelton 1993, Piven & Folstein, 1994) that difficulties during birth are associated with autism, although the question of the relationship between the two phenomena is not a clear cut one.

Postnatal factors

Vaccination The whole question of whether the link between the MMR vaccination and the appearance of autistic spectrum disorders in children is a proven one continues to attract much attention. It is suggested (Shattock 2001) that the current policy of administering the measles, mumps and rubella vaccination as one injection triggers such an intensive reaction in the child that it may contribute to the appearance of autism. The path linking these two events – the vaccination and the autism – is unclear. It may involve a process of damage to the membranes lining the gut, and consequently increased levels of opioid peptides in the central nervous system. Many children react to the vaccination with spiking temperatures, vomiting and crying (Seroussi 2000), whilst others appear to react very little. The timing of the vaccination, currently at around 12–18 months in the UK, appears to be a crucial factor and some authorities feel that postponing the vaccination or the delivery of single vaccines (see Fletcher 2001, Waterhouse 2000) may avoid these issues whilst still protecting children against disease. The timing of the MMR vaccination also coincides with many changes in the child's skill levels and this may be crucial in apportioning causal links.

Reader activity 11.2

Consider the general development of a child of around 12 months old. What are the major skills gains one would expect to see in the realms of:

* communication
* socialisation
* play

at this stage. Why might the MMR vaccination be seen, in retrospect, as a key point in the realisation of skills deficits?

Families whose history indicates a predisposition to autistic spectrum disorder will need to weigh up the vaccination issue very carefully and take advice from their paediatricians. Whilst it would appear that vaccinating presents a higher than usual risk for these children of developing autism, measles, mumps and rubella are childhood diseases whose dangers are currently grossly underestimated precisely due to the successful immunisation programme of the last 30 years.

Antibiotic use Another suspected mechanism through which damage can occur to the gut wall is the over-use of antibiotics in infants (Seroussi 2000). The lack of response to social (often vocal) interaction seen in many infants on the autistic spectrum leads to questions about their ability to hear. Repeated visits to doctors to explore the issue and repeated ear examinations may lead, in turn, to repeated doses of antibiotics. (See Case illustration 11.3). Again, the mechanics of how the antibiotics damage the gut wall are as yet not proven, but it is suspected that alteration of the intestinal microbiology occasioned by antibiotic therapy leaves the individual open to the effects of more hostile organisms (Shattock & Savery 1997).

Case illustration 11.3

As a baby and toddler, Jamie had almost constant coughs and colds, which were treated with antibiotics. From about 8 months onwards, Jamie's GP regularly diagnosed ear infections, and eventually 'glue ear'. Jamie's failure to respond to normal auditory cues in his environment led his parents and the professionals involved with him to suspect that he had some degree of hearing deficit. The infections were treated with antibiotics (of which Jamie had over 15 courses in 2 years) and eventually the insertion of grommets. However, as this therapy progressed, his parents began to suspect that Jamie could hear quite well (for instance, a favourite video being played elsewhere in the house) and that his problems were more about socialisation and communication. At the age of three and a half Jamie was diagnosed as autistic, which explained not only his failure to respond to speech but also idiosyncrasies in other areas of his development. Jamie's parents have had a series of shocks and resolutions within assessment and diagnosis processes but are relieved to have a 'label' for his difficulties at last.

Food intolerance Considerable contemporary research addresses the dietary challenges faced by some people on the autistic spectrum. The mechanisms outlined above, or an inherited disorder, result in a more permeable gut wall than is usual (Waterhouse 2000). It is suggested that an individual's 'leaky gut' allows incompletely digested protein molecules into the blood stream and thus to the central nervous system. These molecules are close in chemical structure to naturally occurring opioids and, it is argued, may cause some of the behaviours and cognitive deficits typical of autistic spectrum disorder. The foodstuffs that are implicated are largely wheat and dairy foods, which some parents remove from their autistic child's diet. Although not a proven link as yet, many parents report an amelioration in the child's condition once these opioid-like substances have been cleared from the child's system (Seroussi 2000); work continues in this field at the University of Sunderland.

This section of the chapter has highlighted the very complex picture around the causes of autistic spectrum disorder. All of the diagnostic systems that are to be discussed next indicate that the behaviours leading to a diagnosis of autism need

Case illustration 11.4

Christine describes her daughter Ella: 'I knew there was something wrong with Ella from the start. She felt really different to my son when I held her . . . sort of stiff and unhappy. She never seemed to want me . . . only for food . . . and preferred to be on her own, even as a tiny baby. Sometimes, she'd have these terrible screaming fits and I mean screaming, and there was nothing I could do to comfort her. When she was a baby I told the doctor, but he thought I was being neurotic or something.

She really wasn't interested in anything – she didn't look at you, she didn't play . . . When I weaned her, her nappies were terrible, she had constant diarrhoea and just wanted bottles all day. I kept going back to the doctor . . . Anyway, they started to take me seriously when she didn't speak by about two . . . Then we were backwards and forwards to the hospital and then they told us she's autistic.

She's a lovely little girl, but very serious. She hasn't started to talk yet and sometimes she laughs and laughs for no reason. She's starting playgroup soon, so I hope being with the other children will bring her on . . .'.

Case illustration 11.5

Martin is 6 years old and attends mainstream school for 3 full and 2 half days. As a baby he was very ill and required considerable surgical intervention in the first 6 months of his life. From then on, he appeared to progress normally, keeping up with his twin in most areas. Martin's speech, in fact, developed early and he has always had advanced speech for his age. His mum, Marian, describes Martin as always having been precocious in the way he interacts with adults: he speaks almost like an adult but can be very argumentative and bossy.

By the time Martin was about 4 years old, Marian realised that he had some fairly serious problems in coping with everyday life. He found playing with other children difficult, although he played beautifully on his own or with adults, and sharing toys or food with others was impossible for him. His self-care skills were age appropriate, but he was unwilling to initiate any of these activities without heavy prompting from his mother.

On starting school, Martin appeared to cope very well: he was able to keep up with his peers academically and play-time consisted of running around with a group of other boys, which presented few difficulties. However, his behaviour at home deteriorated progressively. Eventually, he was refusing to go to school, tantrumming quite severely most of the way there and again on return home. His tolerance of others also deteriorated over this period of time and life at home became very fraught. Acknowledgement of Martin's problems was hard to obtain, as he was indistinguishable from his peers whilst in school. He coped well with the academic work and at any evaluation always presented as the charming and personable little chap he was when not overwrought by the pressures of coping with his social and emotional challenges. Careful teaching at home has enabled Martin to begin to understand social interactions and his own and others' emotions and has given him the ability to make choices about his behaviour.

to be apparent before the age of three years: the appearance of these types of behaviours after that age should lead to a different diagnosis.

THE PRESENTATION OF AUTISTIC SPECTRUM DISORDER

As Case illustrations 11.4 and 11.5 indicate, the difficulties caused by autistic spectrum disorder can vary enormously within the population that attracts this diagnosis. Both of the children described have diagnoses of 'autism' but the intervention required is clearly very different. The variation in presentation has caused some confusion amongst professionals, parents and people with autism themselves, and a plethora of diagnoses has evolved: autism; autistic spectrum disorder; autistic traits; pervasive developmental disorder; pervasive developmental disorder not otherwise specified; and semantic- pragmatic disorder. Notwithstanding these diagnostic labels, people on the autistic spectrum have difficulties in three key areas:

- social interaction
- communication
- lack of flexibility in thinking and behaviour (Wing 1996).

The extent of the limitations placed upon the individual by these deficits will depend upon the profundity of the disorder. Some people may never attract a diagnosis, nor feel the need for intervention, whilst clearly having difficulties within the triad of impairments. Other people, like Philip, the father in Case illustration 11.2, will have experienced some negative consequences of their condition, and for yet others it will have meant a lifetime of dependence upon relatives and carers for the fundamental activities of life.

DIAGNOSIS

Whereas parents are usually the first people to notice that their child's development is not running along typical lines, the health visitor is well placed to follow up on any concerns parents may have. One tool that is available for use either by the health visitor or GP is CHAT (checklist for autism in toddlers, see Baron-Cohen et al 1992). This fairly simple checklist, designed to alert professionals to difficulties in the three areas mentioned above, is illustrated in Box 11.1.

Box 11.1   Checklist for autism in toddlers

This checklist considers the following areas:

- Pretend play
- Protodeclarative (communicative) pointing
- Joint attention
- Social interest

Children can then be referred to a paediatrician for further investigation to rule out other problems that may present in the scatter of skills observed in the child. Frequently children have extensive investigation for hearing loss, as their lack of responsiveness may lead to the conclusion that they are not receiving auditory stimulation from the environment. Testing for Fragile X is common and often an electroencephalogram (EEG) is performed if possible. The incidence of epilepsy in the autistic population is considerably higher, at 20–35%, (Trevarthen et al 1998) than in the 'normal' population (0.5%, Waterhouse 2000). Whilst the presence of more global brain damage in less able people on the spectrum may account in some part for these figures, it is important to rule out epilepsy as a cause of the periods of 'daydreaming' very often seen in children on the spectrum.

The Diagnostic and Statistical Manual IV (DSM) criteria (American Psychiatric Association 1994), widely regarded as the benchmark for diagnosis, are given in Box 11.2. As Jordan (1999) wisely points out, this does not constitute a 'checklist' for diagnosis but can serve as a useful reference point. More accessible diagnostic tools are being designed and used by psychologists and paediatricians. These include:

- Childhood Autism Rating Scale (Schopler et al 1980). This tool is divided into 15 categories of behaviour (for example, impairment in relationships, near receptor responsiveness) and the child is rated along seven scores, from normal to severely abnormal, on each.
- Autism Diagnostic Interview (LeCouteur et al 1989). This is a much more open interview approach which enables the diagnostician to build up a good picture of the child's developmental history.
- Autism Diagnostic Observation Schedule (Lord et al 1989). This schedule calls for standardised behaviour on the part of the examiner to try to elicit particular behaviour from the child in eight domains, for example, telling a story. Thus, whilst as Trevarthen et al (1998) point out, this is not a diagnostic tool per se, it can help to differentiate autism from other learning disabilities.

Box 11.2   The Diagnostic and Statistical Manual IV autistic disorder criteria

- Onset before the age of 3 years
- At least six of the following (at least two from category 1)

1. **Qualitative impairment in social interaction**
   - Marked impairment in the use of non-verbal behaviours such as eye contact, facial expression, body posture etc.
   - Failure to develop peer relationships appropriate to developmental level
   - Lack of spontaneous seeking to share enjoyment, interests or achievements with other people
   - Lack of social reciprocity

2. **Qualitative impairments in communication**
   - Delay or lack of spoken language with no compensatory non-verbal communication

- In people with speech, impairment in the ability to initiate or sustain conversation
- Stereotypical/repetitive /idiosyncratic language
- Lack of spontaneous and varied pretend play

3. **Restricted, repetitive and stereotyped patterns of behaviour, interests and activities**
   - Preoccupation with one or more restricted interest that is unusual in intensity or focus
   - Inflexible adherence to routines or rituals
   - Stereotyped and repetitive movements
   - Preoccupation with parts of objects
   - Social play

This checklist is completed by the health visitor or GP through interview with parents and also observation of the child at play

---

The acquisition of a diagnosis is an important marker. Parents report that having a name for the difficulties which beset the child's learning processes validates their experiences with and observations of the child. The sometimes inconsistent behaviours and abilities are given a framework by the diagnosis and parents now know 'what the problem is'. Stehli (1995) reports – and this is supported by personal experience – that the diagnosis gives a passport to a community of other families in the same situation who are an immediate source of expert help and advice.

Thus, a child may well be diagnosed as autistic within a health service which has very little to offer to the parent and child. The difficulties of autism are not currently perceived as amenable to either medical or surgical intervention, but as educational issues, requiring an early, intensive and prompt response. Unlike in other conditions the markers for autism are purely behavioural – we cannot search for a chromosome abnormality or the presence or absence of markers in the child's blood. Thus, in the absence of definitive 'proof' of the condition in any child, some grey areas continue to bedevil the processes of diagnosis. Once a diagnosis is secured, the child should then be referred to health and education authorities for intervention: the frequent response, however, is to monitor the child's progress, causing much frustration for parents and wasting irreplaceable time in the child's development.

Reader activity 11.3

Consider Case illustrations 11.4 and 11.5 and try to construct interpretations, other than a diagnosis of autism, that might explain the behaviours and skills presented by each child.

Autism and IQ

Another difficult area for both parents and professionals is that of the relationship between cognitive ability and autism. The research literature in this area suggests that many people on the autistic spectrum may have additional learning difficulties, and this has been touched on above. However, it is also fairly common to deal with children or adults whose measured IQ is normal, but whose autism prevents them from acquiring language and adaptive life skills. If we consider one of the world's most famous people with autism, Temple Grandin, we can see that her enormous intellectual ability has enabled her to function within the world of work and to acquire appropriate behaviours (Grandin 1996). Yet she remains very autistic in her thought, and in the way in which she knows the world and people within it. The temptation to equate levels of profundity of autism with lesser cognitive ability should be resisted. Although profound autism may make learning the types of skills valued by the majority of people very difficult, it does not necessarily indicate a lack of cognitive ability.

The individuals represented by the different lines on Figure 11.1 below will have very different strengths and needs. Whilst both on the autistic spectrum, one of them will have profound difficulties in understanding others, at the same time having considerable intellectual ability which will be of help in learning about others. The other person will have less cognitive ability but also more understanding of social processes and insight into other people's behaviour.

Autism and Asperger's syndrome

To complete this section of the chapter it may be useful to consider briefly the relationship between autism and Asperger's syndrome (see Howlin & Jordan 2000 for more information on this issue). The differential diagnosis of Asperger's syndrome in verbally able people who display behaviours typical of the autistic spectrum has been, and continues to be, an area subject to much debate. Popularly, the idea of a spectrum of disorder has led to the attribution of the label 'autistic'

to the less able and that of 'Asperger's' to the more able. However, the reader is referred back to the discussion on IQ and autism above and is advised that cognitive ability does not necessarily reflect in the acquisition of social and language at an expected age. In line with this thought, it is suggested (latterly in International Classification of Disease 10 (WHO 1993), and in DSM IV (American Psychiatric Association 1994)) that autism and Asperger's syndrome are related but distinct conditions that can be diagnosed adequately.

The main distinctions between the two conditions, it is argued, are that in Asperger's syndrome one sees:

- no clinically significant language delay
- no clinically significant cognitive delay
- some motor clumsiness, with typical stiff posture and gait.

However, other clinicians have argued that this differentiation is artificial (Wing 1996) and, further, that it is not helpful in designing intervention. More light may be shed on this area by the continuing research in the realms of both brain function and the outcomes of early intervention.

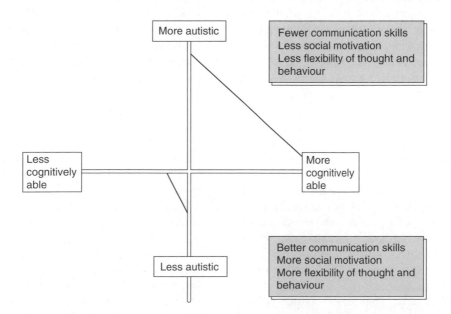

Figure 11.1

SERVICES FOR CHILDREN ON THE AUTISTIC SPECTRUM

The story of Ella's diagnosis (Case illustration 11.4) is typical of the struggle parents have in seeking recognition of their child's difficulties. However, this juncture, which should represent a starting point often brings a realisation that services for children on the autistic spectrum and their families can be patchy and poorly coordinated.

Pre-school provision

Diagnosis is, as has already been outlined, usually given by a paediatrician, but the response to the child's needs requires multidisciplinary input. Awareness of need is increasing within statutory services, and there are some good examples of multi-agency cooperation. An important factor here will be how autism is viewed by those involved with the child, i.e. parents and professionals. If autism is seen as a biological anomaly, the emphasis will be on identifying those facets of the child's physiology which require attention. If it is conceptualised as a difficulty/difference in cognitive functioning, minimally amenable to change, then the child will be taught within a modified environment, with the emphasis on routine and predictability. Attempting to enter into the child's perception of the world and moving through this together would be the preferred approach, if autism is conceived as a cognitive/emotional disorder.

However, the key to learning and using appropriate skills within the areas of difficulty appears to be early and intensive intervention (Leaf & McEachin 1999, Maurice 1996, Stehli 1995, Trevarthen et al 1998). The use of functional language before the age of 30 months is an important indicator of the child's likely progress and thus children on the spectrum require intervention to facilitate language and social skill development. Early intervention can prevent the evolution of stereotyped and repetitive behaviours by teaching more appropriate, useful and enjoyable alternatives. It is also important that parents are empowered to make choices about the services that they want and that their child needs. Catherine Maurice writes of this post-diagnosis–

pre-intervention period: 'Parents are often told that it is not only advisable but morally imperative to accept their child the way he is. Anything other than such acceptance is looked upon as a manifestation of a lack of love . . .' and 'there was a critical need for parents to gain access to science-based, accurate information . . .' (Maurice 1986, p. 5, p. 6). For many parents in the UK difficulties arise in accessing information about interventions, and in gaining support should they choose an intervention which lies outside that provided by their local health or education authority's provision.

Statutory provision

The quality and extent of services varies enormously throughout the UK, with some health and education authorities providing cohesive early support whilst others have a very scant response to the needs of this population. Services commonly provided by local education or health authorities are:

● Portage: This approach involves the allocation of a Portage worker, often a nursery nurse, who works with the family on a (usually) weekly basis for an hour or two. She initially observes the child's performance in six areas: infant stimulation; social development; communication; self-help; cognitive development; motor development. A set of goals is then agreed with the parent and written teaching activities set for the parent/s and child to follow, using a largely behavioural approach to skills building. The child's progress is recorded and evaluated and new goals set (Newman 1999, Portage 2000).
● Speech and language therapy: Clearly the area of speech and language development is one which, by definition, needs attention for all children on this spectrum. Despite recognition of this fact, the provision of speech and language intervention is very variable, due to an acute and chronic shortage of therapists, as can be seen by accessing the web sites of health authorities nationally. Thus, despite having speech and language therapy as part of their statement of special educational need, some children receive an assessment but no intervention.

• 'Special' nursery or playgroup: With the beginning of formal education comes the thorny question of inclusion in regular education of children with learning difficulties of all kinds. The aim of placing children on the autistic spectrum in a special playgroup or nursery is to enable intervention to meet the child's social and play needs (Trevarthen et al 1998). However, given a group of children with a variety of special needs, it is difficult to design and provide an environment appropriate for each of the children.

A statement of special educational need (see Ch. 7) is often useful in clarifying the services needed by and available to a child on the autistic spectrum.

Reader activity 11.4

Consider the typical difficulties which would need to be addressed in nursery for:

• a 3-year-old with Down syndrome
• a 3-year-old displaying the classic behaviours of autism.

Draw up a list of the design features (space, light, noise, materials, levels of support, type of grouping etc.) which would be ideal for each of these children within the nursery setting.

Whilst this exercise cannot take individual needs into account, you can attempt to work on the basis of 'typical' needs of someone with each of these conditions.

Non-statutory provision

Non-statutory intervention offers a wider range of approaches to working with pre-school children. Unfortunately, information about non-statutory intervention is not usually offered by health or education authorities and parents use other parents, support groups and the internet to discover what else may be available for their child's education. The NAS survey (National Autistic Society 1997) reflects that many families (83%) continue to have to fight even for statutory services and that the majority felt that it was difficult to get basic information about services and benefits. The internet is a very powerful tool in

disseminating information and is widely used by parents of children on the spectrum. Similarly, parent support groups are a valuable source of advice and information.

One of the dangers of moving away from statutory into private provision in the fields of health or education, is the danger of being exposed to poorly regulated services. Parents with a newly diagnosed child can be very vulnerable to promises of 'cures' or 'instant remediation' (Maurice 1996); this makes finding good information prior to choosing an intervention vital. Many interventions not offered through state services are not researched, and are based on testimonial alone. Whilst one would not wish to doubt the experiences of children and parents, sound empirical evaluation is imperative as a basis for any approach to working with children, and this is a premise which applies equally to all provision, whether within the statutory, private or voluntary sectors. The Department for Education and Employment commissioned the University of Birmingham to review the research available on the most commonly used educational approaches to autistic spectrum disorder. This was published in 1998 (Jordan et al 1998), and despite being over 3 years old, still serves as a useful starting point for parents and professionals. The major finding of the review is that all approaches to working with children on the autistic spectrum need further research: this is true for both statutory and non-statutory provision.

Details of three approaches rarely available through statutory support services are given below.

Option Parents who wish to use 'Option' ('SonRise' in the U.S.) will need to approach the organisation directly (The Option Institute) and arrange the programme themselves. The philosophy underpinning the work is that of complete acceptance of the child and his or her behaviour. Adults working with the children follow their lead, inviting them to extend their range of play and interaction. Clearly, this is a humanistic approach, placing emphasis on acceptance and understanding of the child's perspective of his environment. Adults work intensively with the child on a one-to-one basis for months or even years, encouraging him or her to develop. Although the programme has no set curriculum, and no outcome studies have been published (Jordan et al 1998), several case studies do report positive gains.

Early Bird The National Autistic Society is a widely known group serving the needs of children on the autistic spectrum and their parents. A scheme devised in 1997, called NAS EarlyBird Programme, provides parents with weekly training sessions over the course of 3 months, aimed at enabling them to work with their child. Parents are taught to gain an understanding of autism, to facilitate communication, and to manage their child's behaviour. This scheme is available through statutory providers in some areas, as professionals can be trained by the NAS to use the scheme under licence. This scheme has been well received by parents but is clearly not a long-term educational strategy.

The Lovaas approach Despite it being widely available within the US and indeed government-funded in some states, the onus for beginning Lovaas intervention with a child needs to come from parents within the UK. The programme comprises a curriculum designed to meet the needs and build on the strengths of children on the autistic spectrum (see Lovaas & Smith 1989). Teaching takes place in the child's home on a one-to-one basis and focuses on the skills a child will need to learn in a more regular educational environment, the aim of the programme being educational integration. Thus, parents are encouraged to use local playgroup/pre-school facilities alongside the programme. The Lovaas curriculum takes the child from early 'readiness' skills of being able to attend and imitate, through to school preparation. It accords well with the 'desirable outcomes' for nursery education (DfEE & SCAA 1996), and with Key Stage 1 of the National Curriculum. It is delivered through discrete trial teaching, enabling a high level of responsiveness to the child's learning style. The intervention has a broad and continuing research base (Lovaas 1987, McEachin et al 1993). Jordan et al's review (1998) acknowledges the extensive research base for this approach and current studies aim to fine tune earlier findings around the variables of successful outcome of discrete trial teaching. This work is continuing in a number of University bases around the UK, and involves short- and medium-term evaluation of children's learning.

Case illustration 11.6 shows some of the difficulties families can experience in trying to access services and support in the pre-school stage.

School provision

Many children on the spectrum are able to attend mainstream school without support or with minimal intervention within the school environment. However, children and young people with autistic

Case illustration 11.6

Natalie received a diagnosis of autism at 32 months. Her paternal uncle has Asperger's syndrome and there is a family history of dyslexia. Natalie's parents had felt fairly sure that she was autistic and had spent many hours researching how they might help her as early as possible. They decided to use a Lovaas approach to teaching Natalie at home. As soon as they received a diagnosis, they started this programme, even though they had to borrow money from their families and take out loans to do so.

They asked for an assessment of Natalie's educational needs, to which the local education authority agreed, although this took several weeks to complete. Despite her parents having made their wishes clear, the services offered to Natalie were a special nursery placement and speech and language therapy. After some weeks of negotiating with the local education authority, Natalie's parents felt they had no choice but to proceed to a special educational needs tribunal. This also took many months and cost the family several thousand pounds. The tribunal found in the family's favour and from this point on the education authority met the cost of Natalie's programme.

Natalie's parents feel that the emotional cost of the whole process has been 'horrendous'. They are bitter that, following the devastating blow of Natalie's diagnosis, they were then plunged into a system in which no-one seemed to be advocating for them, or for Natalie. Indeed, they felt that they had to 'battle' to obtain what they perceive as essential education for their daughter.

spectrum disorder often under-perform quite spectacularly at school (and later at work) due to the specific problems caused by their autism. Academic work alone may not offer particular difficulties to children of around average intelligence on the spectrum, but the dependence upon speech as a major teaching tool within education may lead to a poor performance (Powell & Jordan 1997). Similarly, children on the spectrum find the social environment of school challenging, the free flow of interaction appearing chaotic and unpredictable.

Unlike other countries within Europe, the UK retains a segregated education system for children with learning disabilities. A child on the autistic spectrum may be placed within any of the following:

- specialist autistic units within mainstream schools
- specialist schools for children on the autistic spectrum
- specialist units attached to schools for children with moderate or severe learning disabilities
- schools for children with generic learning disabilities
- schools for children with language disorders.

Within specialist units, the TEACCH (Treatment and Education of Autistic and related Communication Handicapped Children, Lord & Schopler 1994) approach is most widely used within the UK. This system was devised in North Carolina and remains the basis of educational and occupational provision in that State. The strategies taught during childhood are carried through to occupational and work placements and implemented within the home to promote independence (Mesibov 1998). The strengths in visual perception characteristic of people on the autistic spectrum are exploited through the use of visual timetabling and work systems, again to promote independence within the prosthetic environment. The philosophy underpinning the approach is that of a 'culture of autism', i.e. the way in which people with autism perceive the world (their cognitive style) is very different from that of the ordinary population, so rather than trying to teach 'more ordinary' means of perception and learning, the environment is altered to fit into these dif-

ferent cognitive patterns (Mesibov 1998). Jordan et al (1998) in their DfEE evaluation have a section on TEACCH from which, despite its wide use, they conclude, '. . . there has been surprisingly little done to evaluate the programme in terms of outcomes' (p. 90).

Secondary schooling

Many children on the autistic spectrum function well within the mainstream environment particularly during the infant and primary years. It is the realm of social and emotional functioning that presents the greatest challenges to these children, and to the educators providing for them. These areas of difficulty are thrown into sharper relief at the change from primary to secondary education (Morgan 1996). Whilst many children will continue to cope within the mainstream environment, the pressures brought about by increasing expectations of social and emotional independence and competence (Coleman & Hendry 1990) can bring about crises for the adolescent with autistic spectrum disorder. Young people can find these difficulties spilling over into school work and attendance, even resulting in mental and emotional health problems (Alvarez & Reid 1999). For those attending specialist educational provision, the inevitable question is raised concerning the individual's future. The tasks of adolescence and young adulthood – leaving home, entering the world of higher education or work, – are all the more difficult for young people with disabilities and leave the family with many uncertainties about the future of their child (National Autistic Society 1997).

THE LIFE COURSE IN AUTISM

The opportunity to understand, at least in part, about life as an autistic adolescent and adult has occurred only recently. Previously many factors may have played a part in keeping this group of people 'silent', but certainly either the extension of the parameters of diagnosis or the increase in the numbers of people on the spectrum has led to a louder voice being heard. Another factor that has facilitated learning about other people has been the acknowledgement of narrative as knowledge. Silverman (1993) has written: 'It is an increasingly accepted view that work becomes scientific by adopting methods of study appropriate to its subject matter' (p. 144). As the chapter has revealed thus far, there is much to learn from a variety of perspectives about autistic spectrum disorder, and learning about an issue from the 'inside' is a relatively recent epistemological shift (Van Maanen et al 1982) which brings pitfalls as well as insights. In this next section of the chapter we will consider the experiences of people on the autistic spectrum during adolescence and adulthood. The accounts of autistic adults will provide a major source of insight into the lived experience.

Adolescence

The onset of adolescence inevitably raises questions for young people about themselves in relation to the world and to other people. This is a difficult transitional stage for all young people, but particularly so for those on the autistic spectrum (Frith 1991). Many children who have coped quite well in junior schools, not attracting particular attention and certainly not a diagnosis, hit a crisis at this time of personal and school change. New and subtle rules around peer behaviour emerge; self-presentation assumes gargantuan importance; rebellious behaviour and peer dependency increase (Steinberg 1998) and all these serve to confuse the autistic youngster, who may appear immature and gauche to his or her peers (Grandin 1996). This can in turn lead to crises in friendships and in confidence, and subsequently performance at school may slip. Case illustration 11.7 gives an example of this. Unless addressed, the unhappy cycle can continue, with the person becoming more and more isolated and, eventually, depressed.

Unfortunately, very few services exist to address these needs. Academically, the young person may be managing reasonably well, and health may not be an issue until a clinical depression presents itself. Unless resources can be targeted to meet a teenager's social and emotional learning needs, difficulties will escalate and may

 Case illustration 11.7

Keith is 12 years old and has been increasingly unhappy in recent months. His transfer to a larger comprehensive school from a small junior school has led to an exacerbation of the problems he has always experienced, and these are now causing him real unhappiness. Whilst at one time his classmates were happy just to kick a ball around, games on the playground are becoming more dependent upon the social `pecking order' and this eludes Keith. The formation of groups and gangs also puzzles him and, although he knows that he is not welcome in any of these, he does not understand why.

Keith is now refusing to go to school at all, as he has been disciplined for getting into a fight. A teacher had asked whether he had set Keith's class any homework and Keith responded that he had not and, indeed, had not done so the previous week. This led to some rather unkind name-calling and, not knowing how to deal with his anger, Keith lashed out. He is so upset over what he sees as the injustice of the discipline that he says he wants to change schools.

result in school truanting, poor performance and great unhappiness.

Relationships in adolescence and adulthood

Friendship is frequently a topic that causes confusion for the autistic child and young adult (Frith 1991). In younger childhood, playing alongside others, running around with them and later engaging in joint activities will suffice to cover the role. However, as adolescence begins the emotional aspects of relationships become much more important (Steinberg 1998), and it is at this hurdle that the person with autism often fails. Whilst the concept of friendship may be grasped in an intellectual manner, the feelings of closeness and sharing are often not experienced and thus not understood by the autistic individual. Temple Grandin (1996) has written about the difference between an intellectual appreciation of issues and 'feeling' them, and this difference is acute in the area of relationships. Walker-Sperry has commented on this repeatedly in her account of the lives of 10 autistic people (Walker-Sperry 2001). She suggests that the lack of understanding of the nature of relationships can lead to very superficial friendships, based on frequency of contact rather than on any shared feeling. This is a theme echoed in Happe's (1991) account of the lives of autistic adults. Walker-Sperry relates a story which typifies the problem when writing about Tom, a young man with atypical autism: 'He took his parents to meet his friend, a 40-year-old woman with mental retardation with whom he had been bowling. After the introductions had been made, Tom ignored his parents and stood beside his friend most of the evening, neither one of them talking' (Walker-Sperry 2001, p. 40).

Intimate and sexual relationships can also be a minefield for the young adult with autism. The expectations around social and emotional behaviour here are even more subtle than in friendships and very often the 'rules' completely elude the autistic individual (see Walker-Sperry's (2001) account of Tom, pp 35–58). This area of interpersonal communication more than any other, perhaps, calls for the ability to 'read the mind', i.e. interpret the motivation and aspirations, of another person and people on the autistic spectrum, by default, have difficulties here. Thus, it is very easy for people on the spectrum to misread the intentions and desires of others.

However, many people on the spectrum do become involved in short- and longer-term relationships, having families and enjoying the benefits of sharing a home and commitment to another person. It is tempting to try to assess the difference that autism would make to the likely course of a relationship. However, it may be that the autism variable is just one of the many which exist within any relationship. For example, Donna Williams (1999) has written at length about her relationship with her partner and it is interesting to speculate how any of the issues she mentions could be reflective of any young couple's first months and years together. This is not to underestimate the difficulties raised for the couple by the constraints accompanying their disorder, but to place these within the context of the usual stresses and strains within any relationship.

Emotional and mental health

The mental health of adolescents and adults on the autistic spectrum appears to be less robust than that of the ordinary population (Morgan 1996). Anxiety is a feature that marks the condition throughout the life span. Clara Park has described her daughter Jessie's anxiety as a child (Park 1982) and other autistic adults can recall horrifying anxiety and fear as children (Williams 1992). Waterhouse (2000) has suggested that these patterns of reacting to the world established in childhood worsen as the child grows up. Autistic adults write about this anxiety with great clarity: 'I get very worried by having to deal with material things, like the heating, that sort of thing – my parents bought me a washing machine and I was really panicking the first time I put it on . . . ' (National Autistic Society 1997, p. 30). Whilst a degree of occasional anxiety is a usual state, Temple Grandin (1996) has written about the persistent and crippling anxiety that many people on the autistic spectrum suffer. She describes anxiety as having always been a feature of her life. Initially it acted as a motivator (an engine) but worsened considerably in adulthood: 'In my twenties, these severe attacks became more and more frequent. The jet engine was blowing up, exploding instead of propelling me . . . I could barely function. I remember one horrible day when I came home sweating and in a total state of fear for absolutely no reason' (Grandin 1996, pp 112–113). She has suggested that about half of high functioning autistic adults have this anxiety and fear. The difficulties in recognising and treating this extraordinarily distressing component of autism in those with additional learning disabilities is compounded by a lack of adequately sophisticated communication. The individual's behaviour in response to fear and anxiety may not be recognised as such and may lead to contrary conclusions.

Depression is also a feature of autistic spectrum disorder in adolescence and adulthood and Frith has estimated that this occurs in 15% of this population (Frith 1991). The variety of causes for this connection is interesting. An awareness of their situation may underlie this association in many

Reader activity 11.5

1. Make a list of the types of behaviour one might see as a response to anxiety in a person with autism and additional learning disabilities.
2. Consider the types of assessment one might use to try to find the cause of the behaviours exhibited.
3. Sketch out how one's intervention might differ when working with an individual whose self-injury sprang from fear as opposed to frustration.

high functioning adults with autism and those with Asperger's syndrome: 'I seemed to have a crisis of confidence in my mid-twenties – work wasn't going well, and I did feel rather useless . . . the message I was getting from the media that as I'm middle class and male I should have every advantage, but since life was turning out miserably I must be particularly useless at everything – I had some really terrible depressions . . . I even said suicide at one point . . .' (National Autistic Society 1997, p. 31).

Another approach to understanding this connection might be biological. Waterhouse (2000) has speculated that both serotonin and mono-amine-oxidase-inhibitors are implicated in the abnormal neurochemistry of autistic spectrum disorder. The effect upon mood of both of these agents is well known and the suggestion is that depression is a chemical 'side effect' of the condition and can be treated as a biological occurrence. By way of comparison, we do not seek emotional or social explanations for the chemical deficit in diabetes and perhaps depression in autistic spectrum disorder should be viewed in the same way.

Disorders along the obsessive-compulsive continuum are relatively common in this population. Again the question of how far that behaviour disorder may be seen as part of the autistic spectrum disorder, and how far it is a coexisting disorder is open to debate (Jordan 1999). Obsessive behaviour and insistence on sameness has been a fundamental marker for this condition since Kanner's original work, although whether the essential elements of distress accompanying the behaviour are sufficient to attribute a label of obsessive compulsive disorder is open to question (Baron-Cohen

1989). Frith (1991) quotes a young man with autism talking about his obsessional behaviour whose compulsive behaviour does appear to be accompanied by distress: 'I also had to do certain actions at certain times, I got so mixed up. Like if I didn't have a cup of coffee at 10am, something terrible would happen' (Frith 1991, p. 219).

The quotation used above suggests that for at least some people, rituals and obsessions are a means of exerting some control over a chaotic world and maintaining a degree of predictability. Whilst behaviours give some level of control they can quickly become maladaptive and add to rather than reduce the individual's ability to function adequately. Donna Williams has written of escaping from her rituals: 'I was going to run for help and real security by running to a real person and not some dominating bastard part of my own brain . . . All it had ever done was confuse me by painting its obsessional control as "caring" and its self denial as "protection" . . .' (Williams 1999, p. 132). Again, the perceived causes and nature of the obsessional behaviours will influence the intervention suggested for each individual.

Work

Of those individuals on the spectrum who attain educational or vocational qualifications, many move into jobs that do not reflect their ability level (Walker-Sperry 2001). All of the peripheral issues about work, which provide incentives for most people, serve as enormous hurdles for the person with autism. Thus, the social contact, camaraderie and shared humour marking out a workplace rich in reward for the typical worker, may cause confusion and distress for the autistic person. Positions that require the individual to make decisions quickly, use initiative or intuition and work closely with others may all prove beyond the skills of the autistic person and lead to job breakdown. Thus, the person may feel more comfortable in a job that is based on repetition and attention to detail. One autistic woman in the NAS survey described her work: 'It's so autistic-friendly . . . I sit there and I sort [the clothes] into size and colour . . . it's so methodical, and you've got to be obsessed to get it right . . .' (National Autistic Society 1997, p. 32).

Two studies (Kanner et al 1972 and Szatmari et al 1989) followed up on groups of high functioning autistic people and found a proportion of them were not in employment despite their obvious ability. However, once in employment, the character traits of reliability and honesty stand in favour of the person on the spectrum within the work environment (Grandin 1996).

This theme of transition leading to crisis is one that runs through the literature relating to living with autism. Changes of school, moving from school to higher education, leaving home, getting a job – all normal phases of adult development – can cause trauma for the person with autism.

CONCLUSION

Trevarthen et al have used the phrase 'different kinds of knowledge of autism' (Trevarthen et al 1998, p. 246) and this is a useful way of characterising the strands of research and literature within the field that have been reflected in this chapter. The knowledge we currently have about autism springs from widely varying perspectives: biology (anatomy, gastrointestinal anatomy and physiology, neuro-anatomy, physiology and chemistry); education; psychology (cognitive, behavioural); dietetics; first hand experience; art and literature. How are we to make sense of such disparate information?

Perhaps the first step here is to appreciate that knowledge is not generated in a vacuum; it is in fact a reflection of prevailing social and political ideology. Just as Galileo was branded a heretic for his ideas and theories, so today we castigate individuals for their apparently outlandish views, for example the way in which those who suggest a link between the MMR vaccination and autism are treated in the media. Thus, the way in which autistic spectrum disorder is perceived and researched (and, consequently, the way in which intervention approaches are adopted) is likely to be reflective of contemporary attitudes toward those factors which form a culture, i.e. science, education, individual rights etc. The somewhat depressing end to this line of reasoning is that autistic spectrum disorder does not rank very highly in our cultural consciousness, as very few (relatively speaking)

resources are available to researchers, families supporting autistic relatives or individuals with autism themselves. Whilst education for school age children is available, albeit of variable quality, services to enable ongoing education and support are few. Thus, for the young adult with autistic spectrum disorder, leaving home and entering either post-compulsory education or the work situation may not be a possibility due to the lack of support systems. Towbin (1997) has suggested that even supported independence would not be possible for the majority of autistic people, 60% of whom, he has suggested, remain severely impaired. For these individuals, the situation outlined back in 1991 by Jane Hubert, of continuing dependence on ageing and increasingly stressed (in all senses of the word) parents may persist (Hubert 1991).

Service provision

Many people on the autistic spectrum and their friends and relatives see autism as part of the person, but there remains a great danger in romanticising the disorder and underestimating the difficulties it can cause for affected individuals. For many (Grandin 1996, Williams 1999), the reality of autism is a lack of satisfactory communication, distorted perceptual systems, poor social understanding, inability to relax and the resultant anxiety and fear that springs from all of these. Thus in future, services will need to be able to respond flexibly, by placing the emphasis on individual needs, rather than providing a generic 'autism' response. Within services, practitioners will need to tread the balance of enforcing 'ordinary' life patterns and expectations on to individuals whose 'culture' of autism (Mesibov 1998) may conflict with those of the dominant culture. Karyn Seroussi (2000) has described the journey she made with her son in overcoming the worst effects of his autism and called this account *Unravelling the Mystery of Autism*. As research into the causes of autism continue in an attempt to do just this, educational, social and health services need to reflect the enormous range of strengths and deficits of people with autistic spectrum disorder in the provision of respectful and responsive support.

REFERENCES

Allergy Induced Autism. Online. Available: http://www.autismmedical.com

Alvarez A, Reid S 1999 Autism and personality – findings from the Tavistock autism workshop. Routledge, London

American Psychiatric Association 1994 Diagnostic and statistical manual of mental disorders, 4th edn. American Psychiatric Association, Washington DC

Baron-Cohen S 1989 Do autistic children have obsessions and compulsions? Journal of British Clinical Psychology 28: 193–200

Baron-Cohen S, Allen J, Gillberg C 1992 Can autism be detected at 18 months? The needle, the haystack and the CHAT. British Journal of Psychiatry 161: 839–843

Bauman M, Kemper T (eds) 1994 The neurobiology of autism. John Hopkins, Baltimore

Bettelheim B 1967 The empty fortress – infantile autism and the birth of the self. The Free Press, New York

Brazelton T B 1993 Touchpoints. Penguin, London

Coleman J, Hendry L 1990 The nature of adolescence. Routledge, London

Department for Education and Employment, School Curriculum and Assessment Authority 1996 Desirable outcomes for children's learning on entering compulsory education. DfEE and SCAA, London

Fletcher J 2001 The controversial MMR vaccination. Online. Available www.jabs.org.uk

Frith U 1991 Autism and Asperger syndrome. Cambridge University Press, London

Ghaziuddin M 1997 Autism in Down's Syndrome: family history correlates. Journal of Intellectual Disability Research 41(1): 87–91

Gillberg C, Steffenburg S, Schaumann H 1991 Autism: epidemiology: is autism more common now than 10 years ago? British Journal of Psychiatry 158: 403–409

Gillberg C, Coleman A 1992 The biology of autistic syndromes, 2nd edn. McKeith Press, London

Howlin P, Jordan R (eds) 2000 Autism 4(1) (March) Sage, London

Grandin T 1996 Thinking in pictures and other reports from my life with autism. Vintage Books, New York

Green G 1996 Evaluating claims about treatment for autism. In: Maurice C (ed) Behavioural intervention for young children with autism. PRO-ED, Texas

Happe F 1991 The autobiographical writings of three Asperger syndrome adults: problems of interpretation and implications for theory. In: Frith U (ed) 1991 Autism and Asperger syndrome. Cambridge University Press; London, pp 207–243

Hobson P 1993 Autism and the development of mind. Lawrence Erlbaum; Hove

Hubert J 1991 Home bound – crisis in the care of young people with severe learning difficulties: a story of twenty families. King's Fund, London

Jordan R, Jones G, Murray D 1998 Educational interventions for children with autism: a literature review of recent and current research. DfEE, London

Jordan R 1999 Autistic spectrum disorders – an introductory handbook for practitioners. David Fulton, London

Kanner L, Eisenberg L 1956 Early infantile autism 1943–1955. American Journal of Orthopsychiatry 26: 55–65

Kanner L, Rodriguez A, Ashender B 1972 How far can autistic children go in matters of social adaptation? Journal of Autism and Childhood Schizophrenia 2: 9–33

Kolinski B 2001 Growing in and out of an autistic mind. In: Walker-Sperry V (ed) Fragile success – ten autistic children, childhood to adulthood. Paul Brookes, Baltimore, pp 203–209

Leaf R, McEachin J (eds) 1999 A work in progress – behavioural management strategies and a curriculum for intensive behavioural treatment of autism. DRL Books, New York

LeCouteur A, Rutter M, Lord C et al 1989 Autism diagnostic interview: a standardised investigator-based instrument. Journal of Autism and Developmental Disorders 19: 363–387

Lord C, Rutter M, Goode S et al 1989 Autism diagnostic observation schedule: a standardised observation of communicative and social behaviour. Journal of Autism and Developmental Disorder 19: 185–212

Lord C, Schopler E 1994 TEACCH services for pre-school children. In: Harris J, Handleman J (eds) Pre-school programmes for children with autism. PRO-ED, Austin

Lovaas I 1987 Behavioural treatment and normal educational and intellectual functioning in young autistic children. Journal of Consulting and Clinical Psychology 55: 3–9

Lovaas I, Smith T 1989 A comprehensive behavioural theory of autistic children – paradigm for research and treatment. Journal of Behaviour Therapy and Experimental Psychiatry 20: 17–29

McEachin J, Smith T, Lovaas I 1993 Long term outcome for children who received early intensive behavioural treatment. American Journal of Mental Retardation 4: 359–372

Maggs C (ed) 1987 Nursing history – the state of the art. Croom Helm, Beckenham

Maurice C (ed) 1996 Behavioural intervention for young children with autism. PRO-ED, Texas

Mental Health Foundation 2000 The cost of autistic spectrum disorder. Updates 1(17)

Mesibov G 1998 The TEACCH approach to working with people with autism and their families. Spotlight on developmental disability 1(4): 6–10

Miedzianik D, Croskin S 1997 Autism: a life history approach. Journal of Learning Disabilities for Nursing, Health and Social Care 1(1): 4–9

Morgan H 1996 Adults with autism – a guide to theory and practice. Cambridge University Press, Cambridge

National Autistic Society 1997 Beyond Rain Man – experiences of and attitudes toward autism. National Autistic Society, London

Newman S 1999 Small steps forward – using games and activities to help your pre-school child with special needs. Jessica Kingsley, London

Option Institute . Online. Available: www.son-rise.org

Park C 1982 The siege, 2nd edn. Little Brown, New York

Piven J, Folstein S 1994 The genetics of autism. In: Bauman M, Kemper T L (eds) The neurobiology of autism. John Hopkins, Baltimore

Portage. Online. Available:http://www.portage.org.uk/

Powell S, Jordan R 1997 Autism and learning – a guide to good practice. David Fulton, London

Sacks O 1995 An anthropologist on Mars. Picador, London

Sandu J, Carruthers S 1999 Disability studies – a reader. Jessica Kingsley, London

Schopler E, Reichler R J, DeVellis R F, Kock K 1980 Toward objective classification of childhood autism: childhood rating scale (CARS). Journal of Autism and Developmental Disorders 10: 91–103

Seroussi K 2000 Unravelling the mystery of autism and pervasive developmental disorder. Simon and Schuster, New York

Shattock P, Savery 1997 The role of vaccines. Online. Available: http://osiris.sunderland.ac.uk/autism/vaccine.htm October 2001

Silverman D 1993 Interpreting qualitative data: methods for analysing text, talk and interaction. Sage, London

Steinberg L 1998 Adolescence. McGraw-Hill, New York

Stehli A (ed) 1995 Dancing in the rain. The Georgiana Organisation, USA

Szatmari P, Jones M B 1991 IQ and the genetics of autism. Journal of Child Psychology and Psychiatry 32: 897–908

Szatmari P, Bartelucci G, Bond S, Rich S 1989 A follow up study of high functioning autistic children. Journal of Autism and Developmental Disorders 19: 213–225

Towbin K 1997 Pervasive developmental disorder – not otherwise specified. In: Cohen D, Volkmar F (eds) Handbook for autism and pervasive developmental disorders. John Wiley, New York, pp 123–125

Trevarthan C, Aitken K, Papoudi D, Robarts J 1998 Children with autism – diagnosis and intervention to meet their needs, 2nd edn. Jessica Kingsley, London

Van Maanen J, Dabbs J, Faulkner R 1982 Varieties of qualitative research. Sage, Beverly Hills

Walker-Sperry V 2001 Fragile success – ten autistic children, childhood to adulthood. Paul Brooks, Baltimore

Waterhouse S 2000 A positive approach to autism. Jessica Kingsley, London

Williams D 1992 Nobody nowhere. Time Books, New York

Williams D 1999 Like colour to the blind. Jessica Kingsley, London

Wing L 1996 The autistic spectrum. Constable, London

Wing L, Gould J 1979 Severe impairments of social interaction and associated abnormalities in children: epidemiology and classification. Journal of Autism and Childhood Schizophrenia 9: 11–29

Wolff S, Narayan S, Moyes B 1988 Personality characteristics of parents of autistic children. Journal of Child Psychology and Psychiatry 29: 143–153

World Health Organisation 1993 The ICD–10 classification of mental and behavioural disorders: diagnostic criteria for research. WHO, Geneva

FURTHER READING

Baron-Cohen S 1995 Mindblindness: an essay on autism and theory of mind. MIT Press, London

Grandin T, Scariano M 1986 Emergence labelled autistic. Arena Press, New York

Howlin P 1997 Autism: preparing for adulthood. Routledge, London

Lovaas I 1992 The me book. PRO-ED, Texas

Shattock P, Savery D 1997 Autism as a metabolic disorder. Autism Research Unit, Sunderland

USEFUL ADDRESSES

Autism Network for Dietary Intervention.
www.AutismNDI.com
Gives useful information for those considering a dietary approach to helping a child with autistic spectrum disorder.

Lovaas Intervention. Available:
http://www.feat.org.autism/default.htm
The FEAT organisation is a really useful source of information on a whole variety of issues relating to autistic spectrum disorder. Their website publications have lasting value and are at the cutting edge of autism news.

National Autistic Society. Available:
www.oneworld.org/autism
The NAS is one of the older organisations supporting people with autistic spectrum disorder and their families. Sometimes criticised as being too conservative, the society provides a national network of support, internationally recognised research and sound advice.

The National Vaccine Information Centre. Available:
www.909shot.com
This website supports parental pressure for changes to the way in which vaccines are prescribed for children. The organisation promotes and reports on research and gathers data from parents about the perceived damage caused by the MMR vaccination and others.

Parents for the early intervention of autism. Available:
www.peach.uk.com
This website provides information and support for parents who wish to undertake early behavioural intervention with their children.

Paul Shattock at the University of Sunderland. Available: http://osiris.sunderland.ac.uk
Paul Shattock's work on the metabolic aspects of autistic spectrum disorder is outlined on this website. Advice for parents who feel that their child may be affected by diet is also available. The site is constantly updated.

Stephen Edelson at the Centre for Study of Autism (Oregon). Available: www.autism.com
This is a huge website which provides a link into many areas of autism news and research.

12 Mental ill health in learning disabilities

Ibrahim Turkistani

CHAPTER CONTENTS

KEY ISSUES

- People with learning disabilities are at least as vulnerable to the risk of psychiatric disorders as the general population. Additional and specific factors that contribute to this vulnerability are brain damage, epilepsy, repeated loss or separation, communication difficulties, poor coping mechanisms, family difficulties, deficient social skills leading to impaired relationships, low self-esteem, and other psychosocial factors.
- Presentation of mental illness in people with learning disabilities is often different from that of the general population, particularly in severe types because they may have difficulties in language and communication.
- The principles of treatment of mental illness in those with learning disabilities are generally similar to those for the non-learning disabled population.
- Anti-psychotic drugs have been used frequently and inappropriately in people with learning disabilities, particularly for controlling various behavioural problems, resulting in exposing them to various side effects of the drugs.

OVERVIEW

The chapter presents a brief history of mental illness in learning disabilities; this is followed by an account of its prevalence and the difficulties that are associated with this resulting in unreliable data. Then, various causes of mental illness in this population are discussed, and the factors that make them vulnerable and at a heightened risk for mental illness are outlined. The chapter will outline and discuss the importance of and ways of assessing clients with behavioural problems by taking full psychiatric, behavioural and medical histories.

Various treatments of mental illness and behavioural difficulties are discussed, including drugs, electroconvulsive therapy and psychological treatments. The chapter also includes a glossary of terms, further reading, a comprehensive reference section and a list of useful addresses that will provide additional information on various aspects of mental illness and its treatment.

HISTORY

Until the beginning of the nineteenth century, learning disability was conflated with mental illness. The guidelines for the management of disturbed and agitated learning-disabled clients were to isolate them from their communities and sometimes to chain them and/or use sedation.

On the other hand, some other authors, for example Schneider (1959), Gardner (1967) and Winokur (1974), had questioned whether people with learning disabilities could have mental illness. They claimed that they couldn't develop the psychological processes that lead to the development of mental illness.

However, the issue of mental health in people with learning disabilities has in general been neglected for quite a long time, but in the last few decades these issues have been given increasing attention and have become important areas of inquiry and interest for psychiatrists, psychologists, nurses, speech and language therapists, occupational therapists and other professionals. Now, it is accepted by professionals that learning disabilities is not a mental illness, but is a developmental state characterised by functioning below certain arbitrarily defined levels, and this population is thought to be more vulnerable to mental illness-

es (Fraser & Nolan 1995, Menolascino et al 1986, Sharav et al 1988).

EPIDEMIOLOGY

Until recently little attention was paid to the study of prevalence of mental illnesses in people with learning disabilities, but during recent decades, an increasing number of authors have studied this area, though reliable data is still lacking. The reasons for this could be the considerable difficulties in diagnosing mental illness in people with learning disabilities, as some of this group of people lack a verbal facility to describe their feelings and thoughts. Other reasons are that most researchers have also focused on selected populations, such as clients referred to clinics, or those in long stay hospitals, or focused only on major mental illnesses such as schizophrenia and affective disorder. For example Wright (1982) found on a survey of 1507 learning disabled adults in a long stay hospital, that 2.8% of them were diagnosed with affective disorder, 1.8% with schizophrenia and 2.7% with early childhood psychosis. Linaker & Nitter (1990) screened 164 people with learning disabilities in a long stay hospital for mental illnesses, using the Psychopathology Instrument for Mentally Retarded Adults (PIMRA is based on DSM-111 and consists of 56 items) (Senatore et al 1985), and they found that 29% of them were diagnosed with schizophrenia, 57% with anxiety disorder, 52% with personality disorder and no affective disorder was found among the sample. One of the major limitations of this study was that the authors had only reviewed case notes of the clients, and did not assess them clinically. Another study was conducted by Lund (1985), who randomly studied 302 learning disabled adult people using the MRC HBS-schedule. This is an assessment method for use in learning disabled populations. He found that 10.9% diagnosed with behaviour disorder, 5% with psychosis of uncertain type, autism and dementia each diagnosed with 3.6%, neurosis 2%, affective disorder 1.7% and schizophrenia diagnosed with 1.3%.

However, as will be discussed later, the prevalence of mental illness is arguably considerably greater in people with learning disabilities compared with the general population.

AETIOLOGY

Inexperienced professionals are often not mindful that people with learning disabilities are aware of their deficiencies and rejections, and that this makes them vulnerable and at a heightened risk for psychiatric disorders. Various studies have indicated that the psychiatric disorder is more common in people with learning disabilities than in the general population. Fraser & Nolan (1995) have described various factors that contribute to this vulnerability, such as brain damage, epilepsy, repeated loss or separation, communication difficulties, poor coping mechanisms, family difficulties, deficient social skills leading to impaired relationships, low self-esteem, and other psychosocial factors.

There are also various physical illnesses that may occur more often in people with learning disabilities than in the general population, such as thyroid gland disorders, particularly in those with Down syndrome (Sharav et al 1988), and these may lead to psychiatric disorders. Thyroid glands may be over or under functioning, and in these cases behavioural disorders simulating anxiety and depression, or dementia may occur respectively. Under functioning thyroid (hypothyroidism) in Down syndrome is common but underestimated clinically. Mani (1988) found in 50 clients with Down syndrome that 22% of them had biochemical evidence of hypothyroidism, but its clinical diagnosis can be difficult because of gross similarities in both conditions. Down syndrome is also one of the few well-established risk factors for Alzheimer's disease.

Some medications, such as phenobarbitone and the benzodiazepines, such as diazepam and lorazepam that are used for epilepsy and insomnia may have behavioural side effects, causing paradoxical excitement and impulsivity.

Another interesting factor is genetic causation, including a single gene defect. Thapar et al (1994) have emphasised the possibility that the new molecular genetic techniques will contribute to increased understanding of psychiatric and behavioural disorders in people with learning disabilities.

TYPES OF MENTAL ILLNESSES

Schizophrenia

Schizophrenia is a serious disorder and one of the major mental illnesses. It is characterised by fundamental and characteristic distortion of thinking and perception and by inappropriate or blunted affect. Its prevalence in learning disabilities is at least 3%, while in the general population it is approximately 1% (Kendell 1993). Other studies, for example Corbett 1979, Heaton-Ward 1977 and Menolascino et al 1986, found that the prevalence of schizophrenia in those with learning disabilities is higher (3%, 3.2% and 12% respectively).

According to the *International Classification of Mental and Behavioural Disorders, version 10* (ICD–10) (World Health Organisation 1992), to diagnose schizophrenia in the general population the following is reviewed:

- Presence of a minimum of one very clear symptom (or two or more if less clear-cut) belonging to any one of the groups listed as (a)–(d) below.
- Or symptoms from at least two of the groups (e)–(h) should be present.

This/these symptom(s) should be clearly present for most of the time during a period of 1 month or more and in the absence of organic causations such as state of concussion, delirium or dementia:

(a) Thought echo, thought insertion or withdrawal, and thought broadcasting.
(b) Delusions of control to body or limb movements or delusional perception.
(c) Hallucinatory voices; giving a running commentary on the patient's behaviour, or discussing the patient among themselves.
(d) Persistent delusions of other kinds that are culturally inappropriate and completely impossible, such as religious or political identity or superhuman powers and abilities, for example being able to control the weather, or being in communication with aliens from another world.
(e) Persistent hallucinations in any modality, accompanied either by fleeting or half-formed

delusions without clear affective content, or by persistent over-valued ideas.

(f) Breaks or interpolations in the train of thought, resulting in incoherence or irrelevant speech, or neologisms.

(g) Catatonic behaviour, such as excitement, posturing or waxy flexibility, negativism, autism and stupor.

(h) 'Negative' symptoms such as marked apathy, paucity of speech and blunting or incongruity of emotional responses. These usually cause social withdrawal and lowering of social performance.

(i) A significant and consistent change in the overall quality of some aspects of personal behaviour, manifest as loss of interest, aimlessness, idleness, a self-absorbed attitude, and social withdrawal.

The clinical presentations of schizophrenia depend on the severity of learning disabilities. The diagnosis is highly dependent on language communication, therefore depends on a certain level of intellectual development (Meadows et al 1991). In people with mild learning disabilities the presentation is very similar to that of the general population, because they often articulate their symptomology, while in those with severe learning disabilities the diagnosis of schizophrenia can be extremely difficult to make because of their limited language. However some authors, for example Tyrer & Dunstan 1997, believe that it is possible to diagnose schizophrenia in such clients when behavioural symptoms are taken into account; indications are flattened affect, fearfulness, and incongruity associated with withdrawal, deteriorating self-care, catatonic posturing, excitement and self-injury.

People with schizophrenia, particularly in the acute phase, present with florid symptoms as mentioned above with impaired insight into their condition. Their behaviour largely reflects the severity of the symptoms; they may present with odd, disruptive, suspicious or aggressive and violent behaviour, and this may possibly make them dangerous to themselves and/or to others.

Differential diagnosis

Differential diagnosis of schizophrenia, particularly in people with mild learning disabilities, includes the following:

- *Bipolar affective disorder*. Delusions and hallucinations are also associated with mania and severe depression, thus it may create confusion with schizophrenia. The main differences are that in mania the delusions are often of grandiose type, and the hallucinations are self-referential and concerning their special powers and abilities. Moreover, the course of bipolar affective disorder is characterised by repeated episodes of mood disturbance, i.e. mania/hypomania or depression, and characteristically the recovery is usually complete between episodes.

- *Drug induced psychosis*. Chronic amphetamine use may produce psychotic symptoms, which are very similar to those of schizophrenia, but the condition usually subsides within a week or so after stopping taking the illicit drug. Therefore it is important to enquire about drug abuse and to consider testing the urine for illicit drugs before prescribing antipsychotic medication.

- *Fantasy, poverty of thought and motor mannerisms* could be associated with learning disabilities, but they can also be linked with schizophrenia. Thus it is important to make a detailed history and undertake a careful examination of the mental state to differentiate between these two conditions.

Affective disorders

All forms of affective disorders can occur in people with learning disabilities, i.e. bipolar affective disorder (mania and depression), mania alone or depression alone, or depression with or without psychotic symptoms. The prevalence is approximately 1% of the general population while in those with learning disabilities it is higher, but underestimated. Lund (1985) has reported a prevalence rate of 1.7%, Wright (1982) has found 2.8%, and

Day (1985) has reported 5.3%. Most of these studies were inhibited by different factors such as lack of standardised case identification procedures, and the selection of the population groups.

The presentation of mania and depression in those with mild learning disabilities is similar to that of the general population.

In the case of depression, it is necessary to differentiate between depressive illness and simple unhappiness. A diagnosis of depressive illness is only made when the depressive symptoms continue for at least 2 weeks. These include: low mood, loss of interest in things, poor appetite with weight loss, fatigability, poor concentration, reduced self-esteem, broken sleep with early morning waking, ideas of guilt and suicidal ideation.

According to ICD–10 there are three types of depressive illnesses: mild, moderate and severe (World Health Organisation 1992). The difference between the three types lies in the severity and duration of the symptoms. The severe type may be associated with psychotic symptoms such as delusion of sin, nihilistic delusions and hallucinations. Another feature of severe depression is psychomotor retardation that may progress to stupor.

In people with severe learning disabilities, the presentation of depression is usually atypical. Meins (1995) has reported that about 50% of depressed clients exhibit irritable mood, aggressive and self-injurious behavior, screaming, temper tantrum, stereotypes, and incontinence. Reid (1972) has reported hypochondriacal symptoms such as headache, abdominal pain and vomiting. Deterioration in skills is another important feature of depression. Suicide is rare in those with learning disabilities and usually poorly planned.

The clinical features of mania, particularly in people with mild learning disabilities, are opposite to those of depression. Clients are usually euphoric, irritable, overactive, disinhibited with pressure of speech; they may present with flight of ideas and grandiose delusions. There is also a marked distractibility with almost uncontrollable excitement. These features do not last long and may shift rapidly to a depressive phase.

In people with severe learning disabilities, the presentation is usually different; several authors,

for example Reid 1972 and Heaton-Ward 1977, have reported that people with learning disabilities do not display the usual manic euphoria and flight of ideas. These groups of people usually present with a noisy, boisterous, and overactive outlook with aggressiveness in their behaviours.

Neuroses

Neuroses are a group of common disorders that include generalised anxiety disorder, panic disorder, phobic disorders, obsessive-compulsive disorder, post-traumatic stress disorder, adjustment disorders, dissociative (conversion) disorders, somatisation and hypochondriasis.

The presentation of neuroses in people with mild learning disabilities is similar to the presentation in general populations, but in those with severe learning disabilities, the presentation is often mixed with agitation, aggression, self-injurious and repetitive behaviours. Screaming or crying is another important feature. Thus close observation and proper detailed history taking from relatives or carers are essential. The neurotic disorders are usually precipitated by environmental circumstances, such as facing changes in the routine of their lives, for example following a loss, and this includes bereavement.

The clinical features of a range of neurotic disorders are briefly outlined:

- *Generalised anxiety disorder*. The clinical features here are generalised and not restricted to any particular environmental circumstance, i.e. they are free-floating. These include continuous feelings of nervousness, trembling, muscular tension, sweating, light-headedness, palpitation, dizziness, and epigastric discomfort. The course of this disorder tends to fluctuate and be chronic.
- *Panic disorder*. This is characterised by recurrent panic attacks that are unpredictable and not restricted to any particular situation. The clinical features of panic attacks are similar to those mentioned under generalised anxiety disorder, and it is associated with fear of dying, losing control and 'going mad'.
- *Phobic disorders*. All type of phobias (simple, social and agoraphobia) occur in this

population. Anxiety symptoms here are evoked only, or predominantly, by certain well-defined situations or objects that are not currently dangerous. In simple phobias, clients are restricted and will avoid particular animals, heights, thunders, darkness, urinating or defecating in public toilets, dentistry or the sight of blood. In social phobias, restrictions are centred on a fear of scrutiny by other people. In the case of agoraphobia, fear is not only of open spaces but may also include being in crowded places, travelling alone in trains and buses, and fear of leaving home. In addition to anxiety symptoms, clients usually cannot explain or reason the phobias away, and they are beyond voluntary control.

- *Obsessive-compulsive disorder*. Its prevalence in the general population is 1%, but it is thought to be as high as 3.5% in a sample of people with learning disabilities (Vitiello et al 1989). Generally it is characterised by recurrent obsessive thoughts or patterns of behaviours, such as repeated checking to ensure that doors and windows are closed, or repeated washing of hands for fear of contamination. Sometimes there is also fear of harm coming to one's self or loved one if certain things are not undertaken at certain times, for example counting in special ways or saying certain things. Clients recognise these features are coming from themselves, and are not implanted by outside forces. These symptoms usually occur against their will and the clients usually try to stop them from entering their minds but usually fail to do so. They describe these features as silly and nonsensical but cannot ignore them, otherwise they become increasingly anxious.

- *Post-traumatic stress disorder*. This is characterised by repeated episodes of re-experiencing a traumatic incident. These episodes manifest themselves as intrusive memories or dreams, which are accompanied by anxiety and depressive symptoms. This disorder is caused by extraordinary and major life stressors. The onset is usually delayed and may take months before being manifested. Clients with learning disabilities are at risk of abuse, which may put them at greater risk of post-traumatic stress disorder.

- *Adjustment disorders*. The prevalence of this disorder among people with learning disabilities is higher than in the general population. Eaton & Menolascino (1982) found that 21% of the total sample of 115 clients with learning disability had adjustment disorder, and this is mainly due to the limited understanding of social-interpersonal expectations. In general, clinical features include anxiety, worry, depression and feeling unable to cope or continue in the present situation. It is caused by significant life changes or by the consequences of a stressful life event. The onset of this disorder is usually within 1 month of the occurrence of a stressful event, and the duration of the symptoms does not usually exceed 6 months.

- *Dissociative (conversion) disorders*. Although these disorders are not common in the general population, they seem not uncommon among people with learning disabilities (Fraser & Nolan 1995). The term dissociative is used to indicate dissociation between different mental activities such as fugue, amnesia, somnambulism and multiple personalities. The term conversion is used to indicate that mental energy is converted into certain physical symptoms such as paralysis, fits, aphonia, disorder of gait and blindness. These symptoms may occur as a response to stress and are not produced deliberately. These features have also been viewed as a form of non-verbal communication in the doctor–patient relationship (this may particularly apply to those perceiving themselves in a dependent inferior role).

- *Somatisation*. This is a condition characterised by having multiple physical symptoms in the absence of physical pathology, i.e. nausea, vomiting, dizziness, shortness of breath and pains in different parts of the body. In people with learning disabilities these features are often copies of a particular disability such as convulsions or hemiplegia, or may take any other form such as aches and pains (Bicknell 1995).

- *Hypochondriasis*. In this disorder, clients fear illness and they have an excessive concern with their health in general. This leads them to think that they suffer from a serious disease. Hypochondriasis may coexist with actual physical disorders, but in this case clients concern is out of proportion and not justified. Hypochondriacal symptoms are common with depressive illness and anxiety but primary hypochondriasis is rare.

Organic psychiatric disorders

These can be divided into acute and chronic:

- *Acute organic psychiatric disorder.* This is common in people with learning disabilities. Eaton & Menolascino (1982) reported that transient behaviour, with or without psychotic symptoms, occurs in 30% of people with learning disabilities. The full syndrome is characterised by acute onset of cloudiness of consciousness, which is usually worse at night, with disorientation in time (but this may also be with place and person in severe cases), poor attention, agitation, delusions and visual hallucinations. Causes are numerous, and the most common is drug side effects; people with learning disability are more susceptible to adverse effects of psychotropic, antimuscarenic and anticonvulsant drugs. Other causes are infections, epilepsy, hypoglycaemia, electrolyte disturbances and hepatic, renal and cardiorespiratory disorders.
- *Chronic organic psychiatric disorder.* The most common condition is dementia, which is progressive in nature, and is characterised by insidious onset and deterioration in recent memory and cognitive abilities. The client becomes irritable and suspicious with personality changes and inappropriate behaviour.

An association between Down syndrome and Alzheimer's dementia has been reported. Wisniewski & Rabe (1986) found that between 15 and 30% of people with Down syndrome develop Alzheimer's dementia. Moreover, demented clients are prone to develop depression, psychoses and epilepsy.

Sexual disorder

Sexual offence is one of the most contentious problems to the general public, the authorities and to professionals who care for learning disabled clients. The majority of sex offenders are among the young learning disabled population and usually have mild learning disability, with a lifetime risk of 3–5% of offending (Day 1993).

Offenders among the general population are different from those with learning disabilities. The features of the latter's offences are listed below:

- The majority of sex offences are minor, such as public masturbation, and rarely involve physical violence.
- They show less specificity to age or sex of victims.
- The majority of the victims are under the age of 16 years, and are unknown to the offenders.

Sex offenders are usually associated with brain damage, family psychopathology, personality and psychiatric disorders, psychosocial deprivation, and deficiencies in sociosexual knowledge. Reduced supervision is also an important factor, such as the client having the opportunity to have access to children, for example in baby-sitting. It was also found that people who have been sexually abused during their childhood life might become sex offenders later on in their lives (Day 1994, Gilby et al 1989). The reader should refer to Chapter 14 for further details concerning sexual disorders.

Eating disorders

Little research has been carried out to study the prevalence of eating disorders in people with learning disabilities because it is extremely difficult to identify distortion in body image, or guilt feelings that are associated with bingeing, particularly in people with severe learning disability. Clients who refuse food and/or induce vomiting should raise the possibility of eating disorder, after other causes such as depression are excluded.

Pica is the persistent eating of inedible things, for example soil, paper, grass etc. Pica is commonly associated with learning disabilities, but may also be associated with nutritional deficiencies such as iron, zinc and calcium. These clients need to be under close supervision to help them not to eat harmful or toxic materials.

Personality disorders

Personality disorder is neither a mental illness, nor is it caused by a mental disorder or brain disease. It is mentioned here because its features occasionally mimic mental illness.

It is defined as a condition that is represented by a significant disturbance in the characterological constitution and behavioural tendencies of an individual, and usually involves several areas of the personality. It is frequently associated with subjective distress and difficulties in social functioning and performance. Personality disorder tends to appear in late childhood or adolescence, and continues into adulthood. In contrast to personality disorder, personality change is acquired, usually during adult life and following severe or prolonged stress, or serious psychiatric disorder.

Personality disorder is common in people with learning disabilities, with a prevalence of approximately 25.4% (Corbett 1979). The presentation of this disorder in clients with mild learning disabilities is usually the same as in the general population; but in people with severe learning disabilities, there are difficulties in establishing accurate diagnostic criteria.

According to the ICD–10 classification, personality disorders in the general population (non-disabled people) are classified as follows:

- *Paranoid personality disorder* is characterised by suspiciousness and hypersensitivity, with excessive self-reference and self-importance, and the person does not make friendships easily.
- *Schizoid personality disorder* manifests in social withdrawal, emotional coldness, aloofness, insensitivity and preoccupation with fantasies.
- *Dissocial personality disorder* involves lack of feeling for others, disregard for social norms and rules, incapacity to experience guilt and a tendency to blame others.
- *Histrionic personality disorder* is characterised by self-dramatisation with exaggerated expression of emotion and persistent manipulation with labile affect.
- *Anankastic personality disorder (obsessional)* involves indecisiveness, doubt, excessive attention to detail, perfectionism, stubbornness and rigidity with excessive conscientiousness.
- *Impulsive personality disorder* is manifested in emotional instability, lack of impulse control and outbursts of violence, particularly in response to criticism by others.

ASSESSMENT AND DIAGNOSIS OF MENTAL ILLNESSES

Doctors and nurses who are untrained in the field of learning disabilities are likely to miss psychiatric disorders in this population. Most of these doctors and nurses ascribe any unwanted behavioural symptoms in these populations to their learning disabilities. Many studies, for example Reiss 1990, suggest that there may be a tendency to under-diagnose psychiatric disorders in this population. In fact, people with learning disabilities exhibit all the varieties of psychiatric disorders found in the general population, but the presentation is often modified by their intellectual capacity, which makes the diagnosis of psychiatric disorders difficult (Reid 1972). Some clients with schizophrenia over-interpret innocent events as personal insults and counter-attack, while other clients with depressive illness may behave aggressively out of frustration and anger, and so on.

Many possible explanations have been proposed for the difficulties in diagnosing psychiatric disorders in people with learning disabilities:

- Behavioural difficulties in people with learning disabilities are common and can easily be mistaken for psychiatric illnesses. The causes of behavioural difficulties are numerous and include environmental changes, psychiatric disorders and physical pain or discomfort, which may then lead to behavioural distress (refer to Ch. 10).
- Some clients may be unable to communicate their feelings owing to impaired language ability. Thus, there is decreased effectiveness of the clinical interview, and this may consequently lead to incorrect diagnosis.
- Presentation of psychiatric illness in people with learning disabilities is not always typical. It may present with aggressive or self-injurious behaviour or with physical symptoms.
- Physical illnesses can produce behavioural difficulties directly by pain and discomfort, or

indirectly through systemic illnesses, such as hypo- or hyperthyroidism and electrolytes imbalance.

- Medication such as phenobarbital and benzodiazepines (diazepam and lorazepam) can cause paradoxical excitement and restlessness, as mentioned earlier.

Reiss (1992) has suggested four principles to differentiate behavioural difficulties that are caused by psychiatric disorder from other causes:

1. Evaluate the significance of unwanted behaviours by looking for psychiatric symptoms associated with those behaviours.
2. Note the changes in the behaviours; the behavioural difficulties due to psychiatric disorders usually have periods of onset and deterioration from the premorbid state.
3. Make allowances for low intellectual capacity on the presentation of symptoms; people with learning disabilities sometimes express their symptoms in different ways, for example some clients use physical complaints to obtain sympathy and support from others.
4. Admit limitations of knowledge; sometimes it is difficult to reach a diagnosis and in such cases no diagnosis should be made, acknowledging the diagnostic difficulty.

Thus it is very important to assess every client thoroughly by taking a full history of the psychiatric symptoms including a clear description of each symptom, its duration and the circumstances associated with its occurrence, and the effect of these features on the client and/or on his carer. Taking a full medical history is also important, especially in the case of epilepsy, head injuries, thyroid gland disorders and history of drug or alcohol abuse. Several brief interviews may allow a more accurate assessment than one long one. A careful physical examination should also be undertaken. Laboratory investigations should include full blood count (FBC) with differential erythrocyte sedimentation rate (ESR), vitamin B_{12} and red cell folate, thyroid function tests, urea and electrolytes. Urine test and electroencephalogram (EEG) should also be undertaken if indicated.

Reiss has developed a standardised psychometric instrument (the Reiss screen for maladaptive behaviour, Reiss 1988), to help formulate a decision whether behaviour is a symptom of learning disability, or due to psychiatric disorders. It has 36 items; carers who know the client well should personally complete the ratings.

MANAGEMENT

The principles of treatment of mental illness in people with learning disabilities are generally similar to those for the non-learning disabled population, and include:

- pharmacological treatment
- electroconvulsive therapy (ECT)
- psychological treatment
- other treatments.

Before commencing any treatment it is important to assess each client thoroughly; they and their carers need to be counselled and have explained to them briefly the nature of the illness, its prognosis, and how it can affect them and the people around them. It is also important to explain to them about the treatment (pharmacological and/or psychological) that they are going to have. In the case of drugs, they should be told about effect, duration of use and the side effects. This is also applicable to psychological treatments; clients and their carers should know about the nature and type of the psychological treatment, the number of sessions that they require, and how long each session will last.

Before being prescribed any drugs, the client should be asked if he is taking other medications, in order to avoid any serious drug interactions. It is also important to avoid prescribing multiple medications with different doses and different frequencies of use, in order to prevent confusion and improve compliance of treatment. Before medical practitioners prescribe, they should always check the latest edition of the *British National Formulary* (BMA & RPS (43)2002) for side effects, doses, drug interactions and any other information that may be pertinent.

Pharmacological treatment

Pharmacological treatment comprises two groups: psychotropic and non-psychotropic drugs.

Psychotropic drugs

Psychotropic drugs include the following:

- anxiolytics and hypnotics, including
  —benzodiazepines
  —barbiturates
  —buspirone
  —zopiclone and zolpidem
- antipsychotics
- antidepressants
- mood stabilisers
- stimulants

Benzodiazepines There are approximately 14 benzodiazepine drugs available for clinical use in the UK. They are divided into hypnotics such as nitrazepam and temazepam, and anxiolytics such as diazepam, chlordiazepoxide and lorazepam. Generally, anxiolytics have hypnotic effects when given in a large dose at night and equally the hypnotic drugs work as anxiolytics when given in small dose during the day.

All types of benzodiazepines have similar pharmacological properties. The most important distinction between them is in their elimination half-life, and in their potency.

Elimination half-life refers to the relative rate of drug excretion, i.e. the longer the half-life, the less frequently the drug is given, for example, the elimination half-life for diazepam and chlordiazepoxide is about 3 days. The elimination half-life of oxazepam and lorazepam is a few hours.

The advantage of a long half-life benzodiazepine is that it can be given once daily; while its disadvantages are that the next day there may be a hangover feeling and daytime sedation. In contrast, the advantages of short half-life benzodiazepines are that they produce much less hangover and day time sedation, while their disadvantage is the production of more severe withdrawal symptoms.

Benzodiazepines differ in potency, i.e. the amount in milligrams (mg) required to achieve comparable clinical effects. For example, 5 mg of diazepam is approximately equal to 0.5–1 mg of lorazepam, 15 mg of chlordiazepoxide and 10 mg of temazepam (BMA & RPS (43)2002).

Generally, all benzodiazepines are well and rapidly absorbed following oral administration, but the time of response differs between them; for instance, diazepam has rapid onset while oxazepam and chlordiazepoxide work more slowly. All of them are poorly absorbed if administered by intramuscular injection, except midazolam and lorazepam; thus it is inappropriate to give diazepam intramuscularly in status epilepticus, but it is more effective if it is given intravenously or rectally.

Indications Although benzodiazepines represent an effective treatment for all types of neuroses, they are seldom used among people with learning disabilities in the UK (Clarke 1997). These drugs should only be used in cases of emergency treatment of anxiety and insomnia because the relapse rate of anxiety following discontinuation of the drug is high.

Other uses of benzodiazepines include:

- *Psychosis.* Benzodiazepines can be helpful when combined with antipsychotic drugs in treating acutely disturbed clients who are not responding to antipsychotics alone.
- Detoxification of alcohol dependence: Chlordiazepoxide, for example, can be given to prevent or minimise serious withdrawal symptoms such as delirium tremens.
- *Status epilepticus.* Diazepam has well proven efficacy in many types of status epilepticus. It has rapid onset of action, but that effect does not last long after a single intravenous (IV) injection, with a strong tendency for seizures to relapse after initial control. Another disadvantage is that diazepam can cause a high risk of sudden respiratory depression, if given quickly by intravenous route. Midazolam, another benzodiazepine, is rapidly absorbed by intramuscular route and therefore it is useful in situations in which intravenous administration is difficult.
- *Epilepsy.* Clobazam and clonazepam are effective in treating almost all forms of epilepsy, but the majority of clients develop tolerance to its effects; thus benzodiazepines should only be used when all other treatments fail to control seizures.

Side effects Benzodiazepines are well tolerated by the majority of people when taken in therapeutic doses and generally have no serious side effects. They are reasonably safe even on overdose, especially if taken alone. These medications have no serious drug interactions; the common ones are potentiation of sedative effects of other psychotropic medicines and alcohol.

The most common undesirable effects include:

- A tendency to accumulate with repeated doses, causing excessive daytime sedation, slurring of speech, difficulties with attention and concentration, and increased risk of falls particularly in the elderly.
- Sedation, next day hangover and light-headedness, particularly with benzodiazepines of the long half-life type.
- Development of tolerance to its sedative and anxiolytic effect, which may lead to psychological and physical dependence.
- Paradoxical effects, including an increase in anxiety, hostility and excitement.
- Withdrawal symptoms. Sudden discontinuation of the benzodiazepine, particularly after prolonged use, may cause anxiety, insomnia, tremors, irritability, sweating, depression and occasionally seizures.

Other anxiolytic and hypnotic drugs

- *Barbiturates.* There are different types of barbiturates available, and many are not commonly used nowadays in people with learning disabilities, because of their unacceptable side effects. The ones that are used in those with learning disabilities are phenobarbitone and sodium amytal. Phenobarbital is one of the long-acting barbiturates; it is an effective hypnotic and antiepileptic. Sodium amytal is a short-acting drug, which is still used in some places to sedate people who are agitated before going for dental check ups. Barbiturates have many side effects, the most troublesome being behavioural problems and respiratory depression with high dosage; therefore, if sedation is required, it is better to avoid such drugs and to use one of the short-acting benzodiazepines such as lorazepam.
- *Buspirone.* This is a non-sedative anti-anxiety drug, but it does not alleviate the anxiety symptoms of benzodiazepine withdrawal. This drug requires a continuous use and takes about 2–3 weeks to have its therapeutic effect, therefore it cannot be used on a 'prescribed when needed basis'. It is generally a safe drug, and is less likely to cause dependence. This drug is well tolerated by clients, and the side effects are mild and include nausea, dizziness, headaches, light-headedness and excitement.
- *Zopiclone and zolpidem.* These hypnotic drugs are as effective as benzodiazepines, and can be tolerated by most people. Both have short half-lives, with little or no next day hangover effects. These drugs are less likely to cause dependence.

Antipsychotics These drugs are divided into groups that are based on their chemical structure. These groups include: phenothiazines, thioxanthenes, butyrophenones and butylpiperidines (see Box 12.1). In addition to these groups, there is a range of new generation drugs called atypical antipsychotics, which include risperidone, olanzapine, amisulpride, sertindole, quetiapine, zotepine and clozapine. All these groups of antipsychotics are equivalent in overall efficacy, with exception of clozapine, which is more effective in treating resistant schizophrenia. The difference between these groups lies mainly in their relative side effects and costs. Atypical antipsychotics have fewer side effects but are much more expensive than the typical ones.

Box 12.1 Groupings of antipsychotic drugs

Old generation (typical) antipsychotics

phenothiazine with:

aliphatic side-chain	i.e. chlorpromazine
piperidine side-chain	i.e. thioridazine
piperazine side-chain	i.e. trifluoperazine
thioxanthenes	i.e. flupentixol
butyrophenones	i.e. haloperidol and droperidol
butypiperidines	i.e. pimozide

New generation (atypical) antipsychotics
olanzapine
amisulpride
sertindole
quetiapine
zotepine
clozapine

Antipsychotic drugs have been used frequently in people with learning disabilities, particularly for controlling various behavioural problems (Deb & Fraser 1994). Bates et al (1986) have reported that 55% of people with learning disabilities in one hospital were inappropriately treated with these drugs, and that behavioural therapy would have been more appropriate. Generally there is a disagreement about drug use and how often drugs are appropriate. Crabbe (1994), for example, has pointed out that drug intervention is not a treatment, but a chemical restraint. James (1983) and Edwards & Kumar (1984) have suggested criteria for determining when drug use can be justified. They recommended that a regular review of prescribing practices might reduce the amount of inappropriate drugs given and, in particular, undesirable combinations of drugs.

Indications The uses of anti-psychotic drugs in people with learning disabilities are similar to those in the general population, and these include:

- The whole range of psychotic illnesses, such as schizophrenia (particularly in acute phase), mania, severe psychotic depression and organic psychosis.
- In the short-term (a few days to a few weeks), antipsychotics may be used to calm disturbed clients whatever the psychopathological cause, e.g. acute and severe anxiety, toxic delirium, and brain damage.
- Severe self-injurious behaviours, and other behavioural difficulties (short-term use).

Antipsychotics are well absorbed through oral or intramuscular routes. They are largely metabolised in the liver and most of them are excreted through the kidneys. These drugs can be given once daily because of their long half-lives.

Side effects All the recognised side effects of antipsychotics that occur in the general population also occur in people with learning disabilities. Reid (1982) has reported that people with learning disabilities may be more at risk than others of the deleterious neurological side effects of these medications. Moreover, Deb & Fraser (1994) have reported that this population are more at risk of side effects than the general population because of

their biological and psychological vulnerability. They found in their study that 69% of this population have parkinsonian side effects, 48% dyskinesia, 29% dystonia, 13% akathesia and 20–34% tardive dyskinesia.

Side effects of antipsychotic drugs can be summarised as follows:

1. *Extrapyramidal symptoms*. These are the most common and troublesome side effects that are associated particularly with typical antipsychotics, i.e. haloperidol, droperidol, trifluoperazine and depot injections, but are less frequent with the atypical type. The extrapyramidal symptoms include:

a. *Dystonias*. They constitute some of the most frightening side effects of the antipsychotic drugs. These include, for example, torticollis and oculogyric crisis. Torticollis is a contraction of neck muscles, causing twisting of the head to one side. Oculogyric crisis is spasms, causing maximal turning of the eyes in one direction, usually upwards, that persist for periods of minutes or hours.

b. *Akathesia*. This is an unpleasant feeling of being unable to keep still.

c. *Parkinsonian syndrome*. The clinical features of this syndrome are indistinguishable from the idiopathic parkinsonism and these include:

(i) *Akinesia*. This is a generalised slowing of volitional movements, expressionless face and reduction in the arm movements when walking. These symptoms may resemble features of depressive illness and chronic schizophrenia.

(ii) *Coarse tremors, cogwheel rigidity and shuffling gait.*

(iii) *Tardive dyskinesia*. This is characterised by chewing and sucking movements, which are repetitive, painless and involuntary.

2. *Antimuscarinic symptoms*. These include dryness of the mouth, constipation, blurring of vision and retention of urine in men. They are common with typical antipsychotics such as thioridazine and chlorpromazine, but much less so with the atypical type.

3. *Neuroleptic malignant syndrome*. This is a rare but serious side effect, particularly with potent and high dose antipsychotics. Its characteristic

features are hyperthermia, muscular rigidity, confusion and autonomic changes, i.e. increase in pulse, blood pressure and respiration. Its early diagnosis and treatment can be life saving. Testing for high creatinine phosphokinase is a useful diagnostic aid for this syndrome.

Other side effects include a benign drop of white blood cell count (WBC) which may occur with any antipsychotic drugs, but agranulocytosis (virtual absence of white cells) is not common with antipsychotic drugs, except clozapine, affecting about 1–2% of clients (this is a serious condition and can be fatal). Therefore, leucocyte and differential blood counts must be normal before commencing clozapine treatment and a complete blood count must be monitored weekly for the first 18 weeks, and thereafter at least once every 2 weeks. After 1 year of stable blood counts, blood monitoring may be reduced to every 4 weeks. Clozapine should be used with caution in clients with chronic constipation or those on drugs known to cause constipation, e.g. procyclidine, to prevent intestinal obstruction.

Sedation, weight gain and sexual dysfunctions are quite common side effects, while skin rash and seizures are less common.

Drug interactions Antipsychotics have a few drug interactions that include:

- Enhancement of hypotensive effects of antihypertensive drugs.
- Potentiate sedative effects of alcohol and other sedative medications.
- Clozapine should not be administered with drugs that potentially cause agranulocytosis, such as carbamazepine and trimethoprim, as there is a risk of developing this blood disorder.

Long acting depot injections These drugs can be administered once every 2–4 weeks, because the drug is slowly released from the injection site. The advantages of these drugs are that they offer some solution to clients with poor compliance, and they also increase contact between the client and the community team members. Disadvantages include extrapyramidal symptoms, which are more common and in general take longer to subside after stopping or reducing the dose, therefore every client should receive a test dose (small dose) initially, to check his tolerance of such drugs.

Antidepressants There are approximately 30 different antidepressants available in the UK and all are effective in the treatment of moderate and severe depressive illnesses. The Medical Research Council (1965) has reported that between one-half and two-thirds of clients with depressive illness improved with use of antidepressants.

The different antidepressants belong to different classes which include:

- Tricyclic antidepressants such as imipramine, amitriptyline, clomipramine and lofepramine
- Related antidepressants like mianserine and trazodone
- Monoamine oxidase inhibitors (MAOIs), for example phenalzine and isocarboxazid
- Reversible monoamine oxidase inhibitors (MAOIs) such as moclobemide
- Selective serotonin re uptake inhibitors SSRI, i.e. citalopram and fluoxetine
- Other antidepressants such as mirtazapine, nefazodone, venlafaxine and reboxetine.

All these classes of antidepressants carry equal efficacy, and the difference between them is largely in their side effects and cost. For instance MAOIs and tricyclic antidepressants are both quite cheap when compared with other antidepressants, but carry nasty side effects particularly for people with learning disabilities, because their brain damage and poor communication limit their ability to express their feelings.

Antidepressants are well absorbed from the gut, but poorly from muscle site. These drugs can be given once daily as they have long half-lives. They are not like benzodiazepines or barbiturates, they have little or no potential for abuse.

Indications Antidepressant drugs are not only effective in treating depressive illnesses but they are also reported to be effective in other conditions, including:

- Generalised anxiety disorders
- Phobic disorders
- Obsessive-compulsive disorder
- Panic disorder
- Post-traumatic stress disorder.

Some of the tricyclic antidepressants such as amitryptiline and imipramine have also been found to be effective in the treatment of nocturnal enuresis, and in some cases of chronic pain. Also some of the SSRIs, such as fluoxetine, have been used successfully in the treatment of bulimia nervosa.

MAOIs are used much less frequently than other antidepressants, because of their side effects and the dangerous interactions with certain drugs and foodstuffs.

Side effects Side effects depend on the class of the antidepressant:

- Tricyclic antidepressants commonly cause dry mouth, constipation, blurring of vision, retention of urine in men, postural hypotension, sweating, sedation and weight gain. This class of drug is very toxic in overdose and should be avoided for those clients with severe cardiac problems.
- MAOIs often cause postural hypotension, dizziness, headache, weakness, oedema and fatigue.
- SSRIs may cause nausea, vomiting, abdominal pain and dyspepsia. These side effects should subside within the first week or so. The advantages of the SSRIs over the old generation of antidepressants are that they do not cause sedation or weight gain, and are reasonably safe in overdose.

All these groups of antidepressants should be used with caution in people with epilepsy (except MAOIs and reversible MAOIs) as they lower the seizure threshold and precipitate convulsions.

Drug interactions The most serious drug interactions occur between MAOIs and drugs like barbiturates, other antidepressants, anaesthetic agents and sympathomimetic amines such as adrenaline (epinephrine), nor-adrenaline (norepinephrine) and ephedrine (which is present in drugs used for the common cold), some antihypertensives and antihistamines. MAOIs also interact with food and drinks containing tyramine like chicken liver, cheese, beer, and red wine. This interaction causes serious central nervous system excitation and a dangerous rise in blood pressure. Reversible MAOIs causes less drug interaction, but clients still need to avoid the drugs and foods already mentioned.

Mood stabilisers These drugs are used to maintain the mood of clients with affective disorders. These include lithium and antiepileptic drugs such as carbamazepine, sodium valporoate, lamotrigine and gabapentin.

Lithium This is the oldest mood stabiliser and comes in two main forms:

- Lithium carbonate, for example Priadel (Sanofi-Synthelabo), Camcolit (Norgine) and Liskonum (Smith Kline Beecham)
- Lithium citrate, for example Litarex (Dumex), Li-liquid (Rosemont) and Priadal (Delandale).

These preparations are equally effective, but the bioavailability of each preparation is different. Therefore, lithium should be prescribed by brand name.

Indications:
- Treatment and prophylaxis of mania alone, depression and bipolar affective disorders
- In acute cases of mania, a combination of an antipsychotic and lithium is often recommended to bring abnormal behaviour under rapid control
- May be used in severe cases of hyperactivity, aggression and self-injurious behaviour.

Starting and continuing lithium therapy Before commencing lithium it is important to note any history of renal, cardiac or thyroid diseases. Check creatinine, urea and electrolytes (U/E), full blood count (FBC), thyroid function tests (TFT), electrocardiogram (ECG) and pregnancy test as indicated.

After commencing lithium, the serum lithium should be checked weekly (blood should be tested 10–12 hours after the last dose) to adjust the daily dose, until the level is stabilised, then reduce the serum monitoring gradually to once every 6 months. Other tests such as TFT should be done once every 6 months, while CBC, U/E, creatinine, calcium levels and ECG should be done once a year.

Side effects There are early and late side effects. Early side effects are usually transient and include:

- Fine tremors
- Polyuria and thirst
- Nausea and diarrhoea.

Late side effects include:

- Weight gain
- Hyperparathyroidism and hypercalcaemia
- Impairment of the concentrating ability of kidneys occurs in 10% of causes, but this usually recovers when the lithium is discontinued
- Hypothyroidism can occur in 20%, while thyroid gland enlargement may develop in 5% of clients.

Toxicity This usually occurs at serum level of 2 mmol/l or more. Its clinical features are vomiting, diarrhoea, dehydration, coarse tremors, ataxia, slurred speech, muscle twitching and nystagmus. These features may progress, if not treated, to confusion, convulsions, coma and death.

The main precipitating factors for lithium toxicity are overdoses, and dehydration caused by vomiting, diarrhoea and excessive sweating particularly in summer.

Antiepileptics Drugs like carbamazepine, sodium valproate, lamotrigine and gabapentin are found to be as effective as lithium in prophylaxis and treatment of bipolar affective disorders. Each of these drugs can be used by itself or with lithium in clients not responding to lithium alone. These drugs do not require any regular blood testing. They are generally safe and are well tolerated by the majority of people.

Stimulant drugs The use of stimulant drugs like dexamfetamine and methylphenidate in psychiatry is limited. They have been recommended to treat only some cases of hyperkinetic disorder and narcolepsy. These drugs should not be used for other purposes because of their side effects, which include insomnia, anxiety, tremors, poor appetite and weight loss, and depression with psychological dependence and paranoid psychosis.

Non-psychotropic drugs

The most common ones used in psychiatry are beta-blockers and antimuscarinic drugs.

Beta-blockers There are many beta-blockers available on the market, and they all appear equally effective. Their main indication in psychiatry is anxiety dominated by physical symptoms such as tremors, sweating, palpitation and flushing. These drugs do not affect psychological symptoms such as worry and fear. Beta-blockers can be used with other anti-anxiety drugs in treating severe or chronic cases. Other indications include akathesia caused by antipsychotic drugs, and tremors induced by lithium.

Side effects These include bradycardia (slow heart rate) that may precipitate heart failure, sleep disturbances with nightmares, and fatigue. These drugs are contraindicated in clients with asthma, or having a history of obstructive airway disease, and uncontrolled heart failure. They should also be used with caution in diabetes as they interfere with autonomic responses to hypoglycaemia.

Antimuscarinic drugs These are also called anticholinergics and include procyclidine (Kamadrine), benzatropine (Cogentin), and biperiden (Akineton); they all appear equally effective. The main indication in psychiatry is to counteract the parkinsonian side effects of antipsychotic drugs (but this is not effective in akathesia and tardive dyskinesia). These drugs should not be given routinely with antipsychotics, particularly in people with learning disabilities who are more susceptible to develop acute organic reactions (delirium). They also potentiate the anticholinergic side effects of the antipsychotic drugs, i.e. blurring of vision, dryness of mouth, constipation and retention of urine in men.

Electroconvulsive therapy (ECT)

The treatment of some psychiatric disorders by inducing convulsions (seizures) has a long history. Initially, the seizures were produced by toxic drugs, but later Cerletti and Bini in the 1930s replaced this by the passage of an electrical current though the brain. In the past, it was recommended to treat all sorts of difficult psychiatric or behavioural disorders, and was given unmodified, i.e. without anaesthesia and muscle relaxants. As time has progressed, many changes have been applied: gradual modification of the use of anaesthesia, muscle relaxant, oxygenation and then using unilateral electrode placement and low energy stimuli.

ECT has an advantage over antidepressant drugs, in that it has more rapid onset of effect, but the experience of using it in people with learning disabilities is limited. However, the information available would suggest that ECT is a useful treatment for a minority of clients (McClelland 1995). Therefore, the main indication for its use in people with learning disabilities is in severe depression, with or without psychotic symptoms, particularly when it is associated with high suicidal risk and the client is refusing to eat or drink and not responding to pharmacotherapy and/or other treatments.

ECT is one of the good and relatively safe treatments used in the general population (individuals without learning disabilities), with a mortality rate of about 2 deaths per 100 000 treatments. (The complications arising from this treatment are due to the use of anaesthesia and muscle relaxant rather than the convulsions).

Psychological treatment

The term psychotherapy is applied to a wide range of psychological treatments which are only briefly outlined here. The therapy can be informal or formal. Informal psychological help simply means the help and support that anyone may get in a crisis, from friends or relatives; while formal therapy is administered by trained practitioners, to help clients with various psychological difficulties such as behavioural or thought patterns, self-awareness and self-esteem, or interpersonal relationships.

Two important psychological treatments are supportive therapy and cognitive-behaviour therapy.

Supportive therapy

This is the simplest and the most commonly practised and can be available from family, friends or a trained therapist. It is used to help a client through a time-limited crisis caused, for example, by social difficulties. Therefore, it is used to relieve the distress caused by various emotional or physical illnesses.

Clients are encouraged to talk about their feelings and difficulties, while the therapist listens sympathetically. In supportive therapy there are a number of components to consider, including:

- *Ventilation of emotions*. Talking out of problems and difficulties will relieve emotional tension; therefore listening by the therapist is an important part of this therapy.
- *Encouragement*. Clients should be encouraged to take responsibility and to work out solutions to their problems. Suggestion may be used sparingly.
- *Explanation*. It is important to explain to clients the issues relating to their circumstances and difficulties.
- *Advice*. This should take the form of open advice, particularly when facing an obstacle.
- *Reassurance*. This is valuable but must be truthful. Premature or untruthful reassurance may destroy the client's confidence in the therapist.

Cognitive behaviour therapy

Cognitive therapy was developed originally by Beck for treating depressive illness, but subsequently it has been applied, in conjunction with behavioural methods, in the treatment of various psychiatric disorders such as obsessive-compulsive disorder, eating disorder, panic attacks, phobias, and generalised anxiety disorder.

Here the therapist helps clients recognise patterns of negative thinking and encourages them to challenge and express alternatives. The emphasis of this type of therapy is on current difficulties rather than on the origins of a problem.

Other therapies

Other therapies such as group and family therapy have also been used successfully for people with learning disabilities. In group therapy, interactions among the people of the group are helpful and effective, as clients share their problems and are enabled to reassess their relationships. In family therapy the aim is to improve unhealthy interpersonal relations between family members. Such therapeutic approaches are dealt with more fully in Chapter 22.

CONCLUSION

Until recently there was considerable debate among scientists about the entity of learning disability. Some thought it was mental illness whereas others questioned whether people with learning disabilities could develop mental illness. Now, it is accepted by most professionals that learning disability is not a mental illness, but is a developmental state characterised by functioning below certain arbitrarily defined levels, and this population is thought to be more vulnerable to mental illnesses.

People with learning disabilities exhibit a variety of mental illnesses that are also found in non-disabled people. The prevalence of mental illness is argued by some to be higher than in the general population, though reliable data is still lacking. The reasons for this lack of data are numerous for example the considerable difficulty in diagnosing mental illness in those with learning disabilities, and the fact that this group of people lack the verbal facility to describe their feelings and thoughts. The factors that make this population vulnerable, and at heightened risk of mental illness include brain damage, epilepsy, repeated loss or separation, communication difficulties, poor coping mechanisms, family difficulties, deficient social skills leading to impaired relationships, low self-esteem, and other psychosocial factors.

Presentation of mental illness in people with learning disabilities is often different from that of the general population, particularly in severe types, because they have difficulty in expressing their feelings and complaints due to their poor language communication. Therefore many studies, for example Reiss 1990, have suggested that there may be a tendency to underdiagnose psychiatric disorders in this population.

The principles of treatment of mental illness in people with learning disabilities are generally similar to those for the non-learning disabled population, including pharmacotherapy, psychotherapy and electroconvulsive therapy (ECT). Medication has been used heavily in this population, particularly for controlling various behavioural problems, thus exposing them to various side effects of the drugs, as they are more at risk because of their biological and psychological vulnerability.

GLOSSARY OF TERMS

Bipolar affective disorder Disorder of mood characterised by recurrence of severe mood swings between elation and depression. Clients have remission between the attacks.

Blunted affect The normal response of emotion (happiness and sadness) is reduced.

Delusion Unshakeable false belief that is held despite evidence to the contrary and is culturally atypical. It is a characteristic feature of psychotic illness and present in many other forms. **Delusional perception** is a primary delusion that occurs suddenly with new meaning that cannot be understood as arising from the client's mood. For example, a schizophrenic client was asked by his friend if he wished to have a cup of tea. Immediately the client realised that his friend was accusing him of being a Mafia member and organising a gang to kill him. **Delusional control** is when a client believes that his thoughts and actions are controlled by outside forces. **Nihilistic delusion** is when the client denies the existence of his body, or part of his body, his loved ones and the world around him.

Emotional lability Frequent (minutes and hours), rapid and abrupt changes of emotion.

Hallucination False perception (absence of external stimulus) to the sense organs. It is a feature of psychotic illness, and includes auditory, visual, tactile (sensation of being touched), olfactory (sensation of unpleasant smell) and gustatory (sensation of unpleasant tastes) hallucination.

Hypomania A mild form of mania and usually not associated with delusions or hallucinations.

Mania A psychotic disorder characterised by elevation of mood, increased activity, rapid thought and speech, grandiose delusions, hallucinations and impaired insight.

Mannerisms Abnormal repetitive voluntary movements that appear to have some significance, e.g. saluting.

Negativism Clients' tendency to do the opposite of what they are asked to do, and usual resistance to comply.

Neologism New words or phrases created by the client; they are meaningful to them but not understandable to others.

Neuroses Psychiatric disorders, without any demonstrable physical cause and with the client retaining considerable insight. Examples are generalised anxiety, phobias, obsessive-compulsive disorder and panic attacks.

Over-valued idea Strongly held (but shakeable) false belief. It may occur in both healthy and psychiatrically disordered clients.

Poverty of thought An observed dullness, the client has few thoughts and lack of spontaneous ideas.

Psychomotor retardation Clients feel that all their actions have become difficult to initiate and carry out, including thought and speech. For example, there is a long delay before questions are answered.

Psychoses Psychiatric disorders such as schizophrenia, mania and organic psychoses characterised by delusion, hallucination, thought disorders and impairment of insight.

Stupor A condition in which the client is mute, immobile and not responsive. The client is conscious but there is some degree of clouding of awareness.

Thought broadcasting A delusion in which clients believe that their thoughts are withdrawn from their minds, and broadcasted publicly.

Thought echo A psychotic symptom that refers to clients hearing their own thoughts aloud.

Thought insertion A delusion where clients are convinced that their thoughts are not their own, but were inserted into the mind by other forces.

Thought withdrawal Clients strongly believe that their thoughts have been taken out of their minds. Clients often report that they have fewer thoughts left to use. It is one of the delusions of the control of thought.

REFERENCES

Bates W T, Smeltzer D J, Arnoczky S M 1986 Appropriate and inappropriate use of psychotherapeutic medication for institutionalised mentally retarded persons. American Journal of Mental Deficiency 90: 363–370

Bicknell J 1995 Psychological process: the inner world of people with mental retardation. In: Bouras N (ed) Mental health in mental retardation: recent advances and practices. Cambridge University Press, Cambridge, pp 46–56

British Medical Association and the Royal Pharmaceutical Society of Great Britain (BMA & RPS) 2002 British national formulary. BNF Number 43, London

Clarke D 1997 Physical treatments. In: Read S G (ed) Psychiatry in learning disability. Saunders, London, pp 350–379

Corbett J A 1979 Psychiatric morbidity and mental retardation. In: James F E, Snaith R P (eds) Psychiatric illness and mental handicap. Gaskell Press, London, pp 11–25

Crabbe H F 1994 Pharmacotherapy in mental retardation. In: Bouras N (ed) Mental health in mental retardation: recent advances and practices. Cambridge University Press, Cambridge, pp 187–204

Day K 1985 Psychiatric disorder in the middle-aged and elderly mentally handicapped. British Journal of Psychiatry 147: 660–667

Day K 1993 Crime and mental retardation. In: Howells K, Hollin C R (eds) Clinical approaches to the mentally disordered offender. John Wiley, Chichester, pp 111–144

Day K 1994 Male mentally handicapped sex offenders. British Journal of Psychiatry 165: 630–639

Deb S, Fraser W 1994 The use of psychotropic medication in people with learning disability: toward national prescribing. Human Psychopharmacology 9: 259–272

Eaton L F, Menolascino F J 1982 Psychiatric disorders in the mentally retarded: types, problems, and challenges. American Journal of Psychiatry 139(10): 1297–1303

Edwards S, Kumar V 1984 A survey of psychotropic drugs in a Birmingham psychiatric hospital. British Journal of Psychiatry 145: 502–507

Fraser W, Nolan M 1995 Psychiatric disorders in mental retardation. In: Bouras N (ed) Mental health in mental retardation: recent advances and practices. Cambridge University Press, Cambridge, pp 79–92

Gardner W I 1967 Occurrence of severe depressive reactions in the mentally retarded. American Journal of Psychiatry 124: 386–388

Gilby R, Wolfe L, Goldberg B 1989 Mentally retarded adolescent sex offenders. A survey and pilot study. Canadian Journal of Psychiatry 34: 542–548

Heaton-Ward A 1977 Psychosis in mental handicap. British Journal of Psychiatry 130: 525–533

James D H 1983 Monitoring drugs in hospital for the mentally handicapped. British Journal of Psychiatry 142: 163–165

Kendell R E 1993 Schizophrenia. In: Kendell R E, Zealley A K (eds) Companion to psychiatric studies, 5th edn. Churchill Livingstone, Edinburgh, pp 397–426

Linaker O M, Nitter R 1990 Psychopathology in institutionalised mentally retarded adults. British Journal of Psychiatry 156: 522–525

Lund J 1985 The prevalence of psychiatric morbidity in mentally retarded adults. Acta Psychiatrica Scandinavica 75: 563–570

McClelland R 1995 ECT in learning disability psychiatry. In: Freeman C P (ed) The ECT handbook, the second report of the Royal College of Psychiatrists Special Committee on ECT. Council Reports CR39, Royal College of Psychiatrists, London, pp 24–25

Mani C 1988 Hypothyroidism in Down's Syndrome. British Journal of Psychiatry 153: 102–104

Meadows G, Turner T, Campbell L, Lewis SW, Reveley MA, Murphy RM 1991 Assessing schizophrenia in adults with mental retardation. A comparative study. British Journal of Psychiatry 158: 103–105

Medical Research Council 1965 Clinical trial of the treatment of depressive illness. British Medical Journal 1: 881–886

Meins W 1995 Symptoms of major depression in mentally retarded adults. Journal of Intellectual Disability Research 39: 41–45

Menolascino F J, Gilson F S, Levitas A S 1986 Issues in the treatment of mentally retarded patients in the community mental health system. Community Mental Health Journal 22: 314–427

Reid A H 1972 A psychosis in adult mental defectives: 1. Manic-depressive psychosis. British Journal of Psychiatry 120: 205–212

Reid A H 1982 Psychiatry of mental handicap. Blackwell, Oxford

Reiss S 1988 Test manual for the Reiss screen for maladaptive behaviour. OH: international diagnostic system, Worthington

Reiss S 1990 Prevalence of dual diagnosis in community-based day programs in the Chicago metropolitan area. American Journal of Mental Deficiency 49: 570–585

Reiss S 1992 Assessment of man with dual diagnosis. Mental Retardation 30: 1–16

Schneider K 1959 Clinical psychopathology. Grune and Stratton, New York

Senatore V, Matson J L, Kazdin A E 1985 An inventory to assess psychopathology of mentally retarded adults. American Journal of Mental Deficiency 89: 459–466

Sharav T, Collins R, Baab P J 1988 Growth studies in infants and children with Down's syndrome and elevated levels of thyrotropin. American Journal of Disease of Children 142: 1302–1306

Thaper A, Gottesman I I, Owen M J, O'Donovan M C, McGuffin P 1994 The genetics of mental retardation. British Journal of Psychiatry 164: 747–758

Tyrer S P, Dunstan J A 1997 Schizophrenia. In: Read S G (ed) Psychiatry in learning disability. W B Saunders, London, pp 185–215

Vitiello B, Spreat S, Behar D 1989 Obsessive-compulsive disorder in mentally retarded patients. Journal of Nervous and Mental Disease 17(4): 232–236

Winokur B 1974 Subnormality and its relation to psychiatry. Lancet 2: 270–273

Wisniewski H M, Rabe A 1986 Discrepancy between Alzheimer type neuropathology and dementia in person with Down's syndrome. New York Academy of Sciences 477: 247–260

World Health Organisation 1992 International classification of mental and behavioural disorders ICD-10. WHO, Geneva

Wright E C 1982 The presentation of mental illness in mentally retarded adults. British Journal of Psychiatry 141: 496–502

FURTHER READING

Bouras N 1994 Mental health in mental retardation, recent advances and practices. Cambridge University Press, Cambridge

British Medical Association and the Royal Pharmaceutical Society of Great Britain 2002 The British national formulary.

BNF Number 43. British Medical Association and the Royal Pharmaceutical Society of Great Britain, London

Read S G 1997 Psychiatry in learning disability. Saunders, London

USEFUL ADDRESSES

American Association on Mental Retardation
444 North Capitol Street NW
Suite 846
Washington DC 20001–1512
USA
Tel: +1 202 387 1968
http://www.aamr.org

British Institute of Learning Disabilities
Wolverhampton Road
Kidderminster

Worcs.
Tel: 01562 850251
www.bild.org.uk

The Royal College of Psychiatrists
17 Belgrave Square
London
SW1 8PG
Tel: 020 723 52351
www.rcpsych.ac.uk

Self-injurious behaviour

Bob Gates

KEY ISSUES

- In the last 15 years there have been significant developments in our knowledge and the subsequent management of people with learning disabilities who engage in self-injurious behaviour.
- In the context of seeking evidence for best practice direct carers must familiarise themselves with contemporary research that is capable of directing their interventions with efficacy.
- Direct carers and particularly learning disability nurses must further develop specialist skills following pre-registration nurse education to work with individuals who self injure.

INTRODUCTION

This chapter brings together some of the research literature from the last 15 years concerning self-injurious behaviour in people with learning disabilities. The chapter will primarily focus on the contribution of medical, biological and psychological research literature because of the important insights these disciplines have made to our understanding of such behaviours. The chapter will also explore contemporary evidence for the management of people with learning disabilities who present with self-injurious behaviour. This group of people present parents and direct care staff with distinctively distressing challenges as to their care and management. Within the chapter definition, prevalence, topography, causation and evidence for best practice will be outlined. The chapter will conclude with a brief exploration of the role of learning disability nurses in contributing to the health and wellbeing of this group of people, and it is suggested that other carers might wish to adopt a similar role.

BACKGROUND

It is suggested that self-injurious behaviour falls within that spectrum of manifestations of distressed behaviour generally referred to as challenging behaviour. Understanding this spectrum of disorders is problematic, and this is for many reasons. First, there is a range of definitional issues to consider. Historically, during the 1980s, to avoid inappropriate or negative labelling, the terms behaviour problems or difficulties were replaced by the term challenging behaviour. However, this term has over time become over inclusive and has come to encapsulate a wide range of disorder, distress and complexity (Clifton et al 1993, Gates 1996, Slevin 1995) making the term opaque, and in some senses meaningless. A consequence of such imprecise terminology, whilst supposedly having the potential to avoid inappropriate or negative labelling, is that the complexity of some distressed behaviours of people with learning disabilities can be to some extent trivialised. By this, it is meant that some carers and professionals have a tendency to conflate self-injurious behaviour with other manifestations of challenging behaviour. Secondly, there are differing, and competing theoretical and professional explanations for such behaviour. This has resulted in those working with or caring for this group of people seeking professional and/or theoretical resolutions that are simplistic, perhaps even reductionist in nature. For example, the contribution of medicine along with research from the biological sciences has in recent years received poor reception, in preference of other explanations, for example contributors from the social model of disability. Rejection of knowledge, either from an ideological or a purely theoretical stance, results in a failure to comprehend the importance of differing theoretical explanations, and the need

for practitioners from diverse academic backgrounds and professional disciplines to research and work together in partnership. Finally, there are problems in determining the most appropriate and effective therapeutic interventions, and then translating these into sustained practice to assist in the amelioration of self-injurious behaviour.

DEFINING SELF-INJURIOUS BEHAVIOUR

Within this chapter the term self-injurious behaviour will refer to that range of distressing behaviours directed toward self that includes, for example, head slapping or punching, repeatedly biting oneself, scratching, hand biting, picking, eye gouging, rumination, pica, hair pulling or insertion of hands into body orifices. In particular Favell et al (1982) have identified a range of self-injurious behaviours that have been reported in the research literature and these are shown in Box 13.1.

More recently Symons et al (1998) have identified similar behaviours to be demonstrative of self-injurious behaviour: 'Head banging, biting, scratching, pinching, rubbing and other forms of self destructive behaviour' (Symons et al 1998, p. 273). Evidently, self-injurious behaviour comprises a range of self-destructive behaviours and has been defined as: 'A term referring to a broad array of responses which result in physical damage to the individual displaying the behaviour' (Favell et al 1982, p. 531).

Evidently, people who engage in self-injurious behaviour must not be conflated with others who present with aggressive behaviour or with

---

Box 13.1   Different manifestations of self-injurious behaviour (SIB)

- Self-striking (e.g. face slapping, head banging)
- Biting various body parts
- Pinching, scratching, poking or pulling various body parts (e.g. eye poking, hair pulling)
- Repeated vomiting or vomiting and reingesting food (i.e. rumination)
- Consuming non-edible substances (e.g. eating objects such as cigarettes, pica, eating feces, coprohagia)

specific degenerative neurological manifestations and/or behavioural difficulties. People who engage in self-injurious behaviour require the special attention of clinicians, researchers and carers because of the very different and unique challenges that they present. For example, it is known from a relatively recent study that the mortality rate of this group of people is higher than the expected mortality rate for the population of people with learning disabilities. A recent study undertaken in the Netherlands by Nissen & Haveman (1997) has estimated that 12% of deaths of the total population of people with learning disabilities, who had died over a 5-year period, could be attributed to their self-injurious behaviour.

PREVALENCE AND TOPOGRAPHY

Oliver et al (1987) undertook a survey of self-injurious behaviour in people with learning disabilities in one health region. They identified that 616 adults and children had engaged in self-injurious behaviour of sufficient magnitude to have caused damage to tissue. Of the 596 who were screened 50% resided in hospital, 28% resided in non-hospital care, and 21% lived at home. Emerson (1990, 1992), Chung et al (1996) and more recently Murphy (1999) have stated that self-injurious behaviour in people with learning disabilities has been variously estimated. These estimates would suggest that between 8 and 15% of people with learning disabilities who resided in hospital settings engaged in this type of behaviour. Although the ecological validity of these claims to newer community settings is not yet really known or understood, Schroeder et al (1978) have suggested that simply moving people from institutional to non-institutional locations will not necessarily reduce challenging behaviour, although the evidence is equivocal (Leudar et al 1984). Table 13.1 identifies the occurrence rate of self-injurious behaviour, and matches this with the type of environment that these people were located in. It is also known that people who engage in self-injurious behaviour tend to inflict injury to fairly well defined areas of the body, i.e. hands, wrists and head (Symons & Thompson 1995). More recently, in a study undertaken by Hare et al (2002), it has

Table 13.1 Percentage of learning disabled people in different environmental locations who are estimated to engage in self-injurious behaviour. After Emerson 1990

Type of Service	Occurrence rate (%)
Large institutions and hospitals	15
Special schools	3–12
Group homes	3–10
Segregated day centres	3–7
People living at home	1–4
10–20 year olds living in institutions (Murphy et al 1993)	40

been noted that self-injury sites were non-randomly distributed on the body and that self-injury may overlap with acupuncture sites associated with analgesia effects. The major sites identified were front of head 52.8%, back of hand 35.8%, outer arm 18.9%, with front of torso and front of legs 17%.

CAUSATION

This chapter now briefly considers biological and environmental factors that may explain, at least in part, why an individual might be driven to engage in self-injurious behaviour. Consideration of causation is important because it enables learning disability nurses and other carers to better understand the differing approaches that are adopted and/or advocated in the management of such behaviour.

Biological factors

It is well known that some genetic aberrations will result in individuals engaging in self-injurious behaviour, examples being Lesch–Nyhan, Cornelia de Lange, Prader–Willi and Fragile X syndromes. There is considerable literature and research to support such a proposition (Clarke 1997a, pp 350–379). However, nurses should not assume that a syndrome (genotype) will always result in an individual (phenotype) engaging in self-injurious behaviour. For example, in a recent keynote review Berney (1998) has stated that in the case of Cornelia de Lange syndrome it is now known that if underlying physical disorders such as gastric reflux are treated, then self-injurious behaviour is likely to diminish. Apart from an indisputable relationship of some, albeit rare, medical disorders with self-injurious behaviour, it is also the case that self-injurious behaviour may well be linked to faulty biological mechanisms (Clarke 1997a). It is the case that endorphins (opiate-like substances) are released into the bloodstream after an individual engages in self-injurious behaviour (Clarke 1997a). There are two possible hypotheses that have been put forward to advance our understanding of this. The first is that the release of opiates brings about analgesia to self-injurious behaviour and the second is that the euphoric effect of their release reinforces the self-injurious behaviour. Clarke (1997a) has described the relationship between self-injurious behaviour, dopamine and serotonin. For example, it is known that low levels of dopamine are a determinant of self-injury. Evidence for this initially emerged from studying rats and this suggested that dopaminergic agonists brought about self-biting (Oliver 1995). Therefore, there have been studies that have looked at the Lesch–Nyhan syndrome, and the reduction of self-injurious behaviour following the administration of dopaminergic drugs (Clarke 1997a). Symons & Thompson (1997) have provided a most useful review of the neurochemistry of pain and analgesia as it relates to self-injurious behaviour. This review provides learning disability nurses with a sound theoretical framework from which to understand the complex area of neurochemistry and its relationship to self-injurious behaviour.

Environmental factors

Emerson & Bromley (1995) have noted that self-stimulation is an important factor in understanding why people engage in self-injurious behaviour. It is the case that for some people the environment in which they are located in is simply not stimulating enough. Environment in this context refers to more than just the physical entity in which a person is located, but rather refers to the richness of relationship and stimulation that they are afforded. Emerson & Bromley (1995) have reported that when 'Motivation Assessment Scales' are used with this group a common function

of self-injury appears to be for self-stimulation. It is perhaps not unreasonable to hypothesise that an absence of external stimuli may create a need within an individual to engage in self-injurious behaviour for self-stimulation. It is likely that self-injurious behaviour is adopted, rather than other types of behaviour, because such individuals have such a limited repertoire of behaviours at their disposal. Ecological factors are indeed important in understanding self-injurious behaviour. Learning disability nurses have at their disposal evidence that unequivocally demonstrates environment to be an important predictor to intellectual development and the development of behaviour difficulties (Bradley and Caldwell 1976, Elardo et al 1975, Nihira et al 1985 and Richardson et al 1985). It is evident that self-injurious behaviour may be learnt, and that once learnt such behaviour may be reinforced either intentionally or unintentionally. A recent and interesting study has identified that self-injurious behaviour may be reinforced incidentally especially where there is a high number of unskilled carers (Nøottestad & Linaker 2001).

In an impoverished environment such reinforcement is likely to be unscheduled, and this may result in inadvertent reinforcement occurring for self-injurious behaviour (Emerson & Bromley 1995). Therefore, given the preceding comments concerning the poverty of some environments in which some people with learning disabilities have been forced to live out their days, it is not only possible, but also probable that self-injurious behaviour is likely to occur.

Finally, some people with learning disabilities present nurses with particular challenges. There are those, for example, who lie within the spectrum of autistic disorders, who may not wish their environment to be infiltrated, wishing instead to sustain a sameness that brings to them their own level of harmony. Strangers intruding into that environment will often generate catastrophic reactions, one of which might be an individual engaging in self-injurious behaviour (Wing & Gould 1979). A recent review of the literature in this area (Hare & Leadbeater 1998), has presented a range of autism-specific factors that should be considered when analysing and/or intervening for self-injurious behaviour for this group of people. These include:

- Lowered threshold for pain – it has long been known that some people with autistic conditions have a lower sensitivity for physical pain.
- Abnormalities of kinaesthetic and proprioceptive feedback – some people with autistic conditions very much rely upon existing motor programmes and this makes them prefer and over rely upon self-stimulatory sensations, such as rocking.
- Curiosity and special interest – once again some people with autistic conditions will engage in seemingly bizarre behaviour such as cutting skin to see what is underneath, or eye gouging. This may be due to an inability to separate themselves from the consequences of their actions or alternatively it may represent a psychotic state.
- Obsessionality and need for order – many people with autistic conditions will engage in patterns of behaviour that reinforce and sustain sameness.

Thus far this chapter has presented an outline of some of the causative mechanisms and explanations that are said to account for self-injurious behaviour. Consequently, it is advised that the reader explores other theoretical explanations for such behaviour. For example, the value of sociological, anthropological and psychodynamic approaches can greatly enhance our understanding of self-injurious behaviour. A recent paper by Harker-Longton & Fish (2002), for example, has adopted a phenomenological approach to understanding the nature of self-injurious behaviour in young women with mild learning disabilities. Such work, whilst in its infancy and not seeking to understand causation, does provide valuable insights into the lived experience of those engaged in self-injurious behaviour, and assists us in understanding the extent of the distress that such individuals endure.

BEFORE INTERVENTION

Understanding why an individual engages in self-injurious behaviour is often difficult. Attention

has already been drawn to the complex causative factors associated with such behaviour. This makes it imperative that any individual engaging in such behaviour is provided with a detailed physical and psychological assessment. It is necessary for the nurse to refer any clients who engage in self-injurious behaviour to their GPs in order to rule out underlying physical factors, for example sore throat, otitis media, toothache or headache. Assuming that no underlying physical cause, including ruling out specific genotypes, can be found for the self-injurious behaviour, then behavioural assessment may be required to identify the function of the self-injurious behaviour. This may be undertaken in a number of ways, for example using the ABC approach reported by McCue (2000). Alternatively use may be made of the Motivation Assessment Scale. This is a 16-item, seven point Likert scale where informants rate the probability of an individual's behaviour occurring in differing contexts. The scale comprises four sub-scales designed to identify behaviours that are maintained by either positive or negative reinforcement. This is a useful tool that enables clinicians to more readily understand the function/s of behaviour. Perhaps learning disability nurses should exercise some caution here concerning the reliability of this tool. Replication studies seem to present us with conflicting evidence concerning its reliability, although criterion validity seems more acceptable (see, for example, Zarcone et al 1991).

REVIEWING EVIDENCE FOR BEST PRACTICE IN THE MANAGEMENT OF SELF-INJURIOUS BEHAVIOUR

Given the prevalence, topography and causation of self-injurious behaviour, nurses and carers need to consider a range of evidence for best practice that they have at their disposal concerning the efficacy of differing approaches and/or interventions in the management of such behaviours. Appleby et al (1995) have defined evidence-based medicine as: 'A shift in the culture of healthcare provision away from basing decisions on opinion, past practice and precedent toward making more use of science, research and evidence to guide clinical decision making' (Appleby et al 1995). It is in the spirit of such a definition that this chapter reports on some of the research literature from different approaches adopted in the management of such behaviour for the purpose of guiding learning disability nursing practice.

Chemotherapeutic management

Many clinicians have called for a reduction in the overall use of chemotherapy to manage challenging behaviours, and this is especially so concerning the use of psychotropic drugs; therefore their use today is more limited than in the past. Clarke (1997b) has provided clinicians with a comprehensive paper on the use of psychotropic drugs that should assist in evidence-led practice. Concerning other chemotherapeutic approaches, endogenous opiates, serotonin and dopamine have all been implicated in some part in an explanation as to why an individual might engage in self-injurious behaviour. Consequently opiate blockers, such as naxolone and naltrexone, have produced results indicating that their use for some individuals will reduce self-injurious behaviour. There is also evidence to suggest that the use of serotonin and dopamine may assist some individuals in the reduction of self-injurious behaviour, and this is sometimes achieved by complex prescribing. For example, the combination of naltrexone and fluoxetine has been found to reduce skin picking in Prader–Willi syndrome (Benjamin & Buot-Smith 1993, Dech & Budow 1991). In addition, Winchel & Stanley (1991) have found that serious self-injurious behaviour was found to improve in subjects following the administration of a serotonin precursor.

Behavioural management

Psychology has offered us important knowledge as to how to assess self-injurious behaviour to form a hypothesis-driven form of intervention. It is now widely accepted that behaviour is manifested because it serves a function, but understanding that function in some people is very clearly difficult. Oliver (1995) has pointed out that in the last decade the most influential development has been in the area of 'functional equivalence'. At its simplest, functional equivalence is concerned with establishing the function of behaviour then teaching an individual alternative (less damaging) behaviour that has the same function. This approach is variously reported as 'functional equivalence training' or 'differential reinforcement of alternative or communicative behaviour'. Examples of strategies that may be employed include the use of tokens, simple singing, vocalisations, or the use of micro-switches (Bird et al 1989, Durand and Carr 1991, Steege et al 1990, Wacker et al 1990).

Newer and alternative interventions

Newer approaches such as gentle teaching have presented learning disability nurses with professional dilemmas. Research on the effectiveness of such strategies is certainly equivocal. In a recent study the comparative efficacy of two different therapeutic interventions was evaluated: behavioural intervention and gentle teaching (Gates et al 2001). Either one of these interventions was used by parents in the management of 77 children (subjects) who presented with learning disabilities and challenging behaviour (behaviour difficulties): a significant number of this sample presented with self-injurious behaviour. Using a workshop approach, parents were taught the principles and practice of one of these two interventions, to enable them to better manage their child's behaviour. A range of measures was taken to plot the subject's progress. These were taken before parents were taught the intervention, and then at assessment points up until 12 months following intervention. The results of these measurements were analysed and compared with a control group of 26 subjects whose parents did not receive any training. Few statistically significant differences were found between teaching parents behavioural intervention or gentle teaching techniques, when compared with a control group. This study found that behavioural intervention appeared to offer greater efficacy, although statistical significance was only found in one sub scale measure and another measure 'contact with services' (Gates et al 2001). It would seem that the measurement of any experimental effect of the efficacy of gentle teaching has mainly been confined to case studies and other anecdotal accounts. Jordan et al (1989) undertook a study which found that visual screening and gentle teaching were more effective than task training and the no treatment condition in reducing stereotypical behaviour. In addition, visual screening was found to be more effective than gentle teaching. Barrera & Teodoro (1990) found that self-injury did not decrease significantly with the use of gentle teaching, and was reduced to its lowest levels only when restraints, edible reinforcers and isolation between sessions were used in one of the experimental conditions. By way of contrast, Jones & McCaughey (1992) have found that gentle teaching was the more successful intervention with one particular subject in their study. Emerson (1990) has noted that gentle teaching increased self-injurious behaviour in some clients, and stated it to be: 'highly aversive to people whose self-injury is motivated by a desire to escape others' (Emerson 1990, p. 94). The ambivalent nature of the experimental effect found in all of these studies perhaps supports a view that gentle teaching is not universally effective, as proponents of this approach have claimed.

Whereas there is considerable evidence of the benefit of training caregivers in the use of behavioural techniques, the literature on gentle teaching is equivocal in its conclusions, despite the widespread use of this intervention within learning disability settings. For example, Mudford (1995) has undertaken a review of the gentle teaching data. He has questioned the empirical basis for the claims made by proponents of gentle teaching. He has asserted that those who are 'favourably disposed' to gentle teaching should be aware that embracing its use might:

- increase or maintain levels of behaviour difficulty
- result in teachers using inappropriate alternatives when gentle teaching fails to work
- result in possible injury to therapists
- result in disillusionment amongst caregivers if or when gentle teaching fails to fulfil the promises it makes.

Clearly only limited approaches used in the management of self-injurious behaviour have been presented here and therefore they represent a highly selective account of some of the evidence learning disability nurses have at their disposal concerning self-injurious behaviour. In this sense there has been an emphasis placed upon medical, biological and psychological research. However, other approaches have only just begun to be evaluated; clinicians should therefore also consider the evidence base of other interventions, for example multisensory rooms (Ayer 1998), and complementary and/or alternative therapies (Wray 1997). More recently Liebmann (2000) has reported on the use of music therapy in a young man with learning disabilities and self-injurious behaviour. The improvement noted in the reduction in his self-injurious behaviour was significant, although in this instance evidence was anecdotal. Clearly, in the future, it will be important to subject the use of newer and alternative forms of intervention, such as music, dance, drama and complementary therapies, to further and more extensive empirical scrutiny.

THE ROLE OF THE LEARNING DISABILITY NURSE AND OTHER DIRECT CARERS

It is clear that learning disability nurses have to make sense of the preceding evidence highlighted in this chapter, and transform research literature into everyday practice. This requires considerable compromise and crafting in order that nursing interventions develop in line with the best evidence at their disposal. This chapter now concludes with a brief outline of the role of learning disability nurses, who often find themselves caring for this group of people. The Department of Health (DOH) report *Continuing the Commitment* (Kay et al 1996) has provided learning disability nurses with a clear professional framework from which to identify contemporary practice for this group of people to enable them to lead more valued and healthier lifestyles.

Earlier in this chapter evidence has been portrayed concerning the utility of functional analysis and Motivational Assessment Scales, a knowledge of biological mechanisms, and the role that environment plays in self-injurious behaviour. Clearly learning disability nurses need to ensure that they are both knowledgeable of these factors, and competent to intervene with and/or teach others about people who engage in self-injurious behaviour. Given the emphasis on the learning disability nurse as health facilitator, and the newly articulated role of the community learning disability teams in leading and training staff in residential services (DOH 2001), developing a high level of competence and expertise in this area will be extremely important.

Assessment

It is interesting to note the increase in the number of intensive support services that have developed in England over the past few years. Learning disability nurses have contributed enormously to the development of many of these services (see, for example, Roy et al 1994 and Simpson et al 1997). However, it must be remembered that without reliable and valid measurement of the many variables that may account for self-injurious behaviour, interventions, no matter what evidence we have for their efficacy, might be valueless without the precursor of accurate assessment (Emerson & Bromley 1995). This makes it imperative that nurses seek, if necessary, additional education for skill development in the use of particular psychological assessment scales.

Health surveillance

People who engage in self-injurious behaviour are at risk of developing serious health problems (Hyman et al 1990). These may include hearing and visual impairments, damage to internal structures or organs, as well as systemic infections caused by repeated injury. Nurses should be able not only to detect these and their early onset, but also to educate other carers, both professional and lay persons, of the possibility of such outcomes. Additionally, concerning the use of chemotherapy, nurses must educate their colleagues and other carers in the significant developments in this area. It is the case that chemotherapy may be an appropriate treatment for some people, and that its rejection on ideological grounds is unacceptable and unethical. Learning disability nurses should, where appropriate, support physician-prescribed treatment; this will sometimes be in a climate of care context where the use of medication may be rejected as inappropriate. In addition, based upon a sound knowledge of prescribed medication, the nurse should demonstrate skills of observation, monitoring for side effects and the clinical effect in improvement or otherwise. Given that people with learning disabilities will have health action plans by 2005 and that learning disability nurses in particular will act as health facilitators, there is a very real need for nurses to be aware of the contribution that they can make to the health and well-being of this section of the population of learning disabled people (DOH 2001).

Enhanced therapeutic skills

Given the complexity of self-injurious behaviour, learning disability nurses need to develop a range of additional skills. Given the very tentative nature of some evidence regarding interventions for some people who engage in self-injurious behaviour, perhaps early intervention (Murphy 1999) or other strategies should be explored. For example, we still know relatively little of the role of complementary and alternative therapies. It is known that a deficit of communication skills plays a central role in some forms of self-injurious behaviour, but do we know the extent of competence of the learning disability nurse to use alternative communication systems? Nurses also need to consider the importance of simply being with people, and the nature and form of therapeutic relationships. There is a need to establish what behavioural and other skills learning disability nurses already possess, and what additional skills are needed. It is clear that nurses can and do make a valuable contribution to the care of this group of people, and this contribution may be furthered by enhancing their skills.

Management, leadership and coordinating services

Despite the introduction of care management, it is often the case that learning disability nurses represent the only professionally qualified group of people present in sufficient numbers to both manage and coordinate care in service settings. The tasks of managing and coordinating services within multidisciplinary and multiagency contexts are extraordinarily complex. Maturity and flexibility, along with clear and determined leadership skills are very necessary attributes for the successful management and coordination of care for people who engage in self-injurious behaviour, and the complexity of providing integrated care for people with learning disabilities who engage in self-injurious behaviour is self-evident.

Enhancing quality services

Ensuring that this group of people receives high quality services must be the subject of audit and measurement not only of outcome, but equally, if not more importantly, of process. That is, it is the quality of life that this group of people experience that determines their health and wellbeing. Nurses must ensure that they are ready to enter into dialogue and debate and advocate, if necessary, with a range of key players to ensure that those who engage in self-injurious behaviour are located within ordinary environments, even if this means supporting them in extraordinary ways. This issue of environment is especially relevant in the light of recent work by Emerson et al (DOH 1999). Nurses should ensure that they involve themselves in the monitoring of services through the use of audit and in the context of national standards for services.

Enablement and empowerment

Ensuring that this group of people and their carers are able to access a wide range of services, and be treated as equal and valued citizens, is in itself a challenge. It is well known that people with learning disabilities are not always treated with equity, and that carers face many challenges. This has been illustrated in the recent Mental Health Foundation report *Don't Forget Us* (1997). Once again, learning disability nurses represent a force for enabling and empowering this group by using skills of negotiation and assertiveness as well as a detailed knowledge of the range of services available. Where services are not available, it is for learning disability nurses to ensure that this group of people, as citizens, are in receipt of the services that they are entitled to: this may well require lobbying at health authority level by supporting parents to prosecute the services they need. Here the contribution of learning disability nurses might be measured by the use of satisfaction scales. Such scales could measure the level of support provided to carers; it should be noted that there are numerous examples in the literature where such measurement has been successfully used before, especially for community learning disability teams.

Developing personal competence

It is known that developing the competence of people who engage in self-injurious behaviour enables them to express their thoughts and feelings without having to resort to such behaviour. Therefore learning disability nurses need to ensure that they are well grounded and competent in a range of teaching skills that will assist this group of people in the development of their competence. Perhaps this is best achieved through combining the experience of being with learning disabled people with educational programmes designed at post registration level that more sufficiently and expertly prepare a nurse to meet the very complex needs of some of the people they will work with.

CONCLUSION

Recent research concerning the unique contribution of learning disability nurses to the multidisciplinary team supports a view that their role has changed over recent years and that their educational preparation does not adequately prepare them (Alaszewski et al 2000). Learning disability nurse practitioners, along with other carers, should acknowledge the progress that has been made in the last 15 years or so in our collective understanding and treatment of people who engage in self-injurious behaviour. People who engage in self-injurious behaviour, like all citizens, are entitled to lead valued and healthy lifestyles, but achieving this may require the intervention of the learning disability nurse, either as health facilitator or in leading and/or training direct care staff in a range of residential and community settings. In responding to this challenge learning disability nurses will need to set priorities in their practice, research and education. It is clear that they must learn to work with colleagues from a range of professional and academic disciplines, in partnership, in order to continue to improve the care and the quality of life for this group of people.

REFERENCES

Alaszewski A, Gates B, Ayer S, Manthorpe J, Motherby E 2000 Education for diversity and change: final report of the ENB funded project on educational preparation for learning disability nursing. Schools of Nursing and Community and Health Studies. University of Hull, Hull

Appleby J, Walshe K, Ham C 1995 Acting on the evidence. Research paper 17. National Association of Health Authority Trusts, Birmingham

Ayer S 1998 Use of multi-sensory rooms for children with profound and multiple learning disabilities. Journal of Learning Disabilities for Nursing, Health and Social Care 2(2): 89–97

Barrera F J, Teodoro G M 1990 Flash bonding or cold fusion? A case analysis of gentle teaching. In: Repp A C, Singh N N (eds) Perspectives on the use of non-aversive and aversive interventions for people with developmental disabilities. Sycamore Publishing Company, De Kalb, Illinois, pp 199–214

Benjamin E, Buot-Smith T 1993 Naltrexone and fluoxetine in Prader–Willi syndrome. Journal of American Academy of Child and Adolescent Psychiatry 32: 870–873

Berney T 1998 Born to . . . -genetics and behaviour. British Journal of Learning Disabilities. 26(1): 4–8

Bird F, Dores P A, Moniz D, Robinson J 1989 Reducing severe aggressive and self-injurious behaviours with functional communication training. American Journal on Mental Retardation 94: 886–889

Bradley R, Caldwell B 1976 The relation of infants' home environment to mental test performance at fifty-four months: a follow-up study. Child Development 47: 1172–1174

Chung M, Cumella S, Bickerton W, Winchester C 1996 A preliminary study on the prevalence of challenging behaviours. Psychological Reports 79: 1427–1430

Clarke D 1997a Physical treatments. In: Read S (ed) Psychiatry in learning disability. Saunders, London, pp 350–379

Clarke D 1997b Towards rational psychotropic prescribing for people with learning disability. British Journal of Learning Disability 25: 46–52

Clifton M, Brown J, Taylor V 1993 Learning disabilities, challenging behaviour and mental illness. Research highlights. English National Board for Nursing, Midwifery and Health Visiting, London

Dech B, Budow L 1991 The use of fluoxetine in adolescents with Prader–Willi syndrome. Journal of American Academy of Child and Adolescent Psychiatry 30: 298–302

DOH 1999 Quality and costs of residential provision for people with learning disabilities. HSC 1999/162: LAC (99) 28, London

DOH 2001 Valuing people: a new strategy for learning disability for the 21st century. Cm 5086. Stationery Office, London

Durand V M, Carr E G 1991 Functional communication training to reduce challenging behaviour: maintenance and application in new settings. Journal of Applied Behaviour Analysis 24: 251–254

Elardo R, Bradley R, Caldwell B 1975 The relation of infants' home environment to mental test performance from six to thirty six months: a longitudinal study. Child Development 46: 71–76

Emerson E 1990 Severe self-injurious behaviour: some of the challenges it presents. Mental Handicap 18(3): 92–98

Emerson E 1992 Self-injurious behaviour: an overview of recent trends in epidemiological and behavioural research. Mental Handicap Research 5(1): 49–81

Emerson E, Bromley J 1995 The form and function of challenging behaviours. Journal of Intellectual Disability Research 39(5): 388–398

Favell J E, Azrin N H, Baumeister A A et al 1982 The treatment of self-injurious behaviour. Behaviour Therapy 13: 529–554

Gates B 1996 Issues of reliability and validity in the measurement of challenging behaviour (behaviour difficulties) in learning disability: a discussion of implications for nursing research and practice. Journal of Clinical Nursing 5: 7–12

Gates B, Newell R, Wray J 2001 Behaviour modification and gentle teaching workshops: management of children with learning disabilities exhibiting challenging behaviour and implications for learning disability nursing. Journal of Advanced Nursing 34(1): 86–95

Hare D J, Leadbeater C 1998 Specific factors in assessing and intervening in cases of self-injury by people with autistic conditions. Journal of Learning Disabilities for Nursing, Health and Social Care 2(2): 60–65

Hare D, Wisely J, Fernandez-Ford L 2002 A study of the topography and nature of self-injurious behaviour in people with learning disabilities. Journal of Learning Disabilities 6(2): 441–452

Harker-Longton W, Fish R, 2002 Cutting doesn't make you die: one woman's views on the treatment of her self-injurious behaviour. Journal of Learning Disabilities 6(2): 512–523

Hyman S I, Fisher W, Mercugliano M, Cataldo F 1990 Children with self-injurious behaviour. Paediatrics 85: 437–441

Jones R S P, McCaughey R E 1992 Gentle teaching and applied behaviour analysis: a critical review. Journal of Applied Behaviour Analysis 25(4): 853–867

Jordan J, Singh N N, Repp A C 1989 An evaluation of gentle teaching and visual screening in the reduction of stereotypy. Journal of Applied Behaviour Analysis 22(1): 9–22

Kay B, Rose S, Turnbull J 1996 Continuing the commitment: the report of the learning disability nursing project. HMSO, London

Leudar I, Fraser W, Jeeves M A 1984 Behaviour disturbance and mental handicap: typology and longitudinal trends. Psychological Medicine 14: 923–935

Liebmann M 2000 The arts therapies. In: Gates B, Gear J, Wray J (eds) Behavioural distress: concepts and strategies. Harcourt Brace, London, pp 124–125

McCue M 2000 Behavioural intervention. In: Gates B, Gear J, Wray J (eds) Behavioural distress: concepts and strategies. Harcourt Brace, London

Mental Health Foundation 1997 Don't forget us: children with learning disabilities and severe challenging behaviour. The Mental Health Foundation, London

Mudford O C 1995 Review of the gentle teaching data. American Journal on Mental Retardation 99(4): 345–355

Murphy G 1999 Self-injurious behaviour: what do we know and where are we going? Tizard Learning Disability Review 4(1): 5–12

Murphy G, Oliver C, Corbett J et al 1993 Epidemiology of self-injury, characteristics of people with severe self-injury and initial treatment outcome. In: Kiernan C (ed) Research to practice? Implications of research on challenging behaviour of people with learning disability. British Institute of Learning Disability, Kidderminster, pp 1–35

Nihira K, Mink I T, Meyers C E 1985 Home environment and the development of slow learning adolescents: reciprocal relationships. Developmental Psychology 21: 784–794

Nissen J, Haveman M 1997 Mortality and avoidable death in people with severe self-injurious behaviour: results of a Dutch study. Journal of Intellectual Disability Research 41(3): 252–257

Nøottestad J A, Linaker O M 2001 Self-injurious behaviour before and after deinstitutionalization. Journal of Intellectual Disability Research 45(2): 121–129

Oliver C 1995 Self-injurious behaviour in children with learning disabilities. Journal of Child Psychology and Psychiatry 30(6): 909–927

Oliver C, Murphy G H, Corbett J A 1987 Self-injurious behaviour in people with mental handicap: a total population study. Journal of Mental Deficiency Research 31: 147–162

Richardson S, Koller H, Katz M 1985 Relationship of upbringing to later behaviour disturbance of mildly mentally retarded young people. American Journal on Mental Deficiency 89: 1–8

Roy M, Abdalla M, Smee C et al 1994 Evaluation of a community facility for people with learning disabilities and behaviour disorder (challenging behaviour). British Journal of Learning Disabilities 22: 11–17

Schroeder S, Schroeder C, Smith B, Dalldorf J 1978 Prevalence of self-injurious behaviours in a large state facility for the retarded: a three-year follow-up study. Journal of Autism and Childhood Schizophrenia 8: 261–269

Simpson K, Campbell M, Ord P, Fairhurst A 1997 A brief report on the Wolverhampton Intensive Support Service (ISS): a retrospective and prospective study. Journal of Learning Disabilities for Nursing, Health and Social Care 1(4): 196–199

Slevin E 1995 A concept analysis of and proposed new term for, challenging behaviour. Journal of Advanced Nursing 21: 928–934

Steege M W, Wacker D P, Berg W K et al 1990 Use of negative reinforcement in the treatment of self injurious behaviour. Journal of Applied Behaviour Analysis 23: 459–467

Symons F J, Thompson T 1995 Implications for the analysis of social and non-social mechanisms in SIB: sleep disturbance and self-injury sites. Paper presented at the annual Association for Behaviour Analysis Conference, Washington DC

Symons F J, Thompson T 1997 A review of self-injurious behaviour and pain in persons with developmental disabilities. In: Bray N (ed) International review of research in mental retardation. Volume 21. Academic Press, London, pp 69–111

Symons F J, Fox N D, Thompson T 1998 Functional communication training and Naltrexone treatment of self-injurious behaviour. Journal of Applied Research in Intellectual Disabilities 11(3): 273–292

Wacker D, Steege M W, Northup J et al 1990 A component analysis of functional communication training across three topographies of severe behaviour problems. Journal of Applied Behaviour Analysis 23: 417–429

Winchel R M, Stanley M 1991 Self-injurious behaviour. A review of the behaviour and biology of self-mutilation. American Journal of Psychiatry 148: 306–317

Wing L, Gould J 1979 Severe impairments of social interaction and associated abnormalities in children; epidemiology and classification. Journal of Autism and Childhood Schizophrenia 97(1): 57–63

Wray J 1997 Complementary therapies in learning disabilities: examining the evidence. Journal of Learning Disabilities for Nursing, Health and Social Care 2(1): 10–15

Zarcone J R, Rodgers T A, Iwata B A et al 1991 Reliability analysis of the motivation assessment scale: a failure to replicate. Research in Developmental Disabilities 12: 349–360

14

People with learning disabilities who have offended in law

Dermot Rowe, Odete Lopes

CHAPTER CONTENTS

KEY ISSUES

- There is a strong association of cognitive impairment and offending in general. However, only a minority of offenders have a formal learning disability.
- Certain sexual offences, especially indecent exposure and arson, are over represented in people with learning disabilities.
- The full range of therapeutic options should be available to offenders with learning disabilities. It is important to note that pharmacological interventions need to be approached more cautiously in people with neurodevelopmental disorders. Also, psychosocial interventions should take account of the developmental level of the offender.
- Much more work is needed to establish evidence-based practice in this area and much current practice is informed by extrapolation from studies in the general population without learning disabilities.

INTRODUCTION

This chapter concerns people with learning disabilities who offend in law and present with problems which do or may legitimately involve the Courts. It does not address broader 'forensic' mental health concerns which relate to non-criminal aspects of the law such as testamentary capacity (the ability to make a reliable and valid will), the Court of Protection for finances, Guardianship Orders under the Mental Health

Act (1983) and so on. Readers interested in these areas may wish to consult the relevant legislation or a general review such as that provided by Gelder et al (1996).

This chapter starts with a brief discussion of how learning disabilities and associated mental health problems may be associated with crime. Secondly, there is an account of the specific types of offences most likely to be associated with learning disabilities and mental health problems. Thirdly, there is a description of the principles of assessment and treatment of people with learning disabilities who offend in law. A broad view of the scope of mental health is taken here, embracing behaviour disorders as well as mental illness. This reflects the totality of significant problems suffered by clients and also the rather difficult nature of the distinction, in that many people with mental illness display 'behavioural overlay'.

Searching major electronic databases, for example Medline, Embase and PsycLit, reveals few original data papers concerning people with learning disabilities who offend in law and so there is considerable scope for future research. However, where possible, the evidence base for statements made here is quoted; much of the rest relates to 'best professional opinion'.

In practice, there is considerable overlap between people with learning disabilities who offend in law and those whose behaviour is not containable in ordinary community and NHS settings. Such behaviour often involves aggression and violence, of a nature and also a degree that would normally result in contact with the police outside of specialist learning disability settings. However, such settings are well known for a high degree of tolerance of challenging behaviour and so the police tend not to be involved. Currently, there is some debate about the extent to which people with milder learning disabilities should be dealt with by the general criminal justice system. This relates to the extent to which such people may indeed be aware of, and culpable for, the nature of their actions. However, most learning disability specialists would interpret this with caution; people with learning disabilities tend to be vulnerable in prison, and treatment and rehabilitation options are likely to be optimised in health settings. Apart

from those who are dealt with by the Courts and those whose behaviour is not containable in ordinary settings, a third group is relevant here. This includes people who have a temporary need for 'intensive care' to prevent harm to self or others. Such care can often only be provided in relatively secure settings and so all three groups will be considered to some extent. Nevertheless, the principle of the 'least restrictive option' in the current Mental Health Act Code of Practice must be respected in that clients should 'step down' to less secure settings once their state has improved sufficiently. This will be focused on increasingly in future, now that the UK has formally adopted the European Union Human Rights Act.

This chapter describes some of the principal sections of the law in England and Wales relating to people with learning disabilities, but practitioners elsewhere in the UK and further afield will need to consult guides to their local legislation and its application in clinical and social practice. As well as compulsory 'regulations', practitioners should familiarise themselves with the advisory *Code of Practice*. There are three broad groups of compulsory order under the Mental Health Act: those facilitating assessment (Sections 2, 4, 5, 135, 136), those allowing assessment and treatment (Sections 3 and 7) and those concerned with the admission and transfer of clients concerned with criminal proceedings (Sections 35–37, 41, 47–49). The latter group is of special importance for this chapter.

The longer-term compulsory order sections of the Mental Heath Act require that the type of mental disorder involved is specified: mental illness, psychopathic disorder, mental impairment or severe mental impairment. The Mental Health Act does not define 'mental illness' but does state that no one should be 'treated as suffering from mental disorder by reason only of promiscuity, or other immoral conduct, sexual deviancy or dependence on alcohol or drugs'. Psychopathic disorder refers to a persistent disorder or disability of mind (whether or not including significant impairment of intelligence) which results in abnormally aggressive or seriously irresponsible conduct on the part of the person concerned. It can be seen that this definition is largely behaviourally-informed and can be interpreted in disparate ways. Indeed, there are a number of areas where differences exist between legal and clinical concepts. For example, the Act gives a rather different version of psychopathic or dissocial personality disorder to that provided by major classificatory schemes such as the *ICD-10 Classification of Mental and Behavioural Disorders* (World Health Organisation 1992) or the *DSM IV Diagnostic and Statistical Manual of Mental Disorders (4th edn)* (American Psychiatric Association 1995). In the Act, severe mental impairment refers to a state of arrested or incomplete development of mind, which includes severe impairment of intelligence and social functioning and is associated with abnormally aggressive or seriously irresponsible conduct on the part of the person concerned. Mental impairment is defined in a similar fashion, but the state of arrested or incomplete development of mind does not amount to severe mental impairment and is restricted to significant impairment of intelligence. No IQ cut-off is given to aid classification in the Act but most practitioners equate mental impairment to IQs of around 51–70 and severe mental impairment to IQs below this range. Of course, people with learning disabilities whose social functioning and performance on psychometry places them on the borderline of mental impairment should be assessed on an individual basis and agreement should be established between specialist learning disabilities and generic teams as to the best service for the individual and those on whom their behaviour may impact. As is the case for psychopathic disorder, the definition of risk to self and others is predominantly behaviourally informed.

Studies of the patterns of crime reveal strong associations of offending with male gender and youth. In England and Wales half of all indictable offences are committed by males of less than 21 years of age whilst a quarter are committed by males of less than 17 years of age. About thirty times as many men as women are imprisoned and this largely relates to genuinely higher rates of offending amongst them (Heidensohn 1994). Violent and non-violent crimes have increased in the UK over the past 50 years (see Wilson & Herrnstein (1985) and McGuire et al (1994) for reviews).

Study of the causes of offending in general has moved away from individual factors towards social factors. However, the former may include genetic factors in a subgroup of severe and persistent offenders, possibly mediated by physiological arousability, which is believed to be related to the speed of learning to inhibit antisocial behaviour (Brennan & Mednick 1993, Lange 1931, Raine et al 1990). The XYY and XXY chromosomal abnormalities have been incorrectly reported as being strongly associated with offending and even Special Hospital status in the past, but this was corrected by the careful study of Witkin et al (1976). These conditions are probably more common in the general population than was originally thought and any excess in custodial settings is likely to relate to enhanced vulnerability and suggestibility associated with mild or borderline learning disabilities. Social studies have addressed important causes of crime, including poverty, poor education and unemployment (Downes & Rock 1988). Of course, individual and social factors may interplay to account for the offending of some people with learning disabilities and mental health problems, and it is this group we are most concerned with here. Although aggression and severe non-compliance are common in people with moderate, severe and profound disabilities, these individuals can often draw on greater support systems than people with mild and borderline learning disabilities who may lead quite independent lives in settings which render them exploitable and vulnerable. Also, the conceptualisation of aggressive and violent behaviour by the police, the Crown Prosecution Service (which takes a view on the appropriateness of criminal proceedings), and health and social providers will differ in these two groups. Consequently, in practice, offenders in law tend to have more mild learning disabilities.

Assessment and treatment of people with learning disabilities who offend in law is a particularly multidisciplinary and multiagency area of work. Health needs are likely to require input from many workers in the community team for people with learning disabilities or in specialist inpatient teams. Similarly, the needs of these people tend to be complex such that inputs from the police and from social and educational providers are warranted.

SERVICE PROVISION FOR THOSE WHO OFFEND

In Chapter 3 a comprehensive account was provided concerning an historical overview of learning disabilities. However, since the indroduction of the Mental Deficiency Act 1913 considerable laterality was applied in the implementation of this Act and certain behaviours in the presence of intellectual disability, including that of a mild or borderline nature, were regarded as evidence of 'moral insanity'. This led to the compulsory long-term detention of many young women with illegitimate pregnancies and many people with minor offending such as petty theft. The unfortunate experience of many people with learning disabilities informed some of the changes to the law relating to mental health, such as the exclusion of spurious 'moral' criteria for compulsory detention, referred to above. The Mental Health Act of 1959 allowed greater provision for voluntary admission to learning disabilities and generic mental health facilities. The Mental Health Act of 1983 extended this and provided checks and balances in the system for those subject to compulsory orders, for example appeals to hospital managers and mental health review tribunals, access to second opinion doctors and independent inspection by the multidisciplinary Mental Health Act Commission.

Over the past 20 years or so there has been a major move away from long-term institutional care for people with learning disabilities towards community care. This includes those with offending behaviours in that the minimum safe level of security is preferred, as described above. Thus services have had to align themselves along a spectrum of security. At the top of this is the special hospital system whilst medium-secure units for people with learning disabilities tend to be provided on a regional basis. Step-down learning disability inpatient facilities, for example acute units and rehabilitation units, are usually provided in each district. Community placements may provide some level of 'situational security'. This refers not to the 'bricks-and-mortar' or high fence nature of units but to the quality of support and supervision afforded to the client. In many respects, learning disability services lead the way in this regard, particularly when good person-centred packages of support are provided to individuals based on their needs.

MENTAL HEALTH AND COGNITIVE DISORDERS AS CAUSES OF CRIME

In general, studies of mental health problems in offenders tend to address highly selected groups, especially those in prison. Gunn et al (1991) described the prevalence of mental disorders and treatment needs in the male sentenced prison population of England and Wales on the basis of a 5% sample. Standardised psychiatric diagnostic measures were used. Overall, 37% had a diagnosable mental disorder with more than one diagnosis in a minority. Psychosis was present in 2%, neurotic disorder in 6%, personality disorder in 10%, alcohol dependence in 12% and illicit drug dependence in 12%. Treatment options varied from inpatient admission to therapeutic community work within the prison system to integrated mental health input in general prison settings. Despite the claims of some authors that findings like these may be due to coincidence (Monahan & Steadman 1994), the numbers involved suggest a genuine excess of mental health burden amongst prisoners (Wessely & Taylor 1991).

The vast majority of epidemiological studies show that people with learning disabilities are about twice as likely to have mental illness as people without such disabilities (see Russell (1997) for helpful reviews of prevalence studies and pathogenetic mechanisms involved, also refer to Ch. 12). Therefore, it could be predicted that people with learning disabilities would be over-represented in the prison population, given that mental illness is more common in prison than in the general population. This is not true. Gunn et al (1991) found only 0.6% of sentenced male prisoners in the UK to have learning disabilities and a more recent study has arrived at a similar figure – approximately 0.5% (Fazel 2001). Studies in other countries, for example Denmark, report similar results. The most likely reason for this is the success of learning disability teams at diverting-offenders with learning disabilities away from the criminal justice system into health and social care settings. The specific mental disorders below are roughly in the order of their prevalence in offenders.

Substance abuse

There are close links between substance abuse and crime, which are well reviewed in each of the major texts in the further reading list at the end of this chapter. Little work has been done on this association in people with learning disabilities. Intoxication with alcohol may lead to charges related to public drunkenness or driving offences. Intoxication with alcohol or illicit drugs reduces inhibitions and this may precipitate violent, acquisitive and other crimes. The longer term neuropsychiatric consequences of substance dependence may also be linked with offending, for example through superadded cognitive impairment. Episodes of *palimpsest* or 'alcoholic blackouts' may last several hours or days and are not subsequently recalled by the heavy drinker. The relationship of offending to such episodes is complex and is likely to relate to psychosocial factors in the individual, as well as neuropsychiatric impairment (Lishman 1997). Illicit drug dependence, particularly that with heroin and cocaine, is strongly associated with persistent offending to gain money to pay for drugs.

Personality disorder

This is common in people with learning disabilities – probably because of difficulty in establishing a full range of mature coping mechanisms in the presence of developmental disorder. Dissocial personality traits are common, particularly in men. These include: aggressive behaviour, inability to delay gratification, failure to learn from previous adverse experiences, lack of empathy and inability to sustain stable relationships. It is important to remember that the phenomenology of dissocial personality disorder is different from that of mental impairment per se, for example the

latter may be associated with behavioural outbursts but empathy and affiliation with others is likely to be maintained. A minority of people with learning disabilities may show features of both categories. Emotionally unstable personality traits are more common in women and these may take an impulsive or borderline form. The latter includes chronic feelings of boredom, dramatic responses to minor stimuli, self-harm and sexuality difficulties. There may be an association with 'pseudo-psychotic' experiences when subjected to stressors and there is a definite association with having been the victim of abuse in childhood. The Mental Health Act (1983) definition of psychopathic disorder is given above. However, if a compulsory order is to be made on the grounds of psychopathic disorder, the Act requires there to be evidence that treatment 'is likely to alleviate or prevent a deterioration of [the patient's] condition'. Treatability criteria may be broadly interpreted as in containment within a safe setting to prevent future problems or a more specific approach may be adopted in that response to therapeutic work should be anticipated. There is also a requirement that such treatment 'is necessary for the health and safety of the patient, or the protection of other persons'. As is often the case where the Act is concerned, decisions are based on judgements of the balance of evidence; simple 'right or wrong' dichotomies are seldom encountered. This can lead to considerable debate and practitioners are well advised to discuss such matters with experienced colleagues and a social worker approved by the local authority as having appropriate experience in dealing with mentally disordered persons – an 'approved social worker'. When in doubt, ask.

Mood disorders

Depressive disorders are definitely over-represented in people with learning disabilities who have enhanced biological and psychosocial risk factors for these. The rate of bipolar affective disorder (manic-depressive illness) is probably about the same as that in the general population. Depressive disorder is sometimes associated with shoplifting (see below). More seriously, depressive disorder can be associated with aggression and some people with learning disabilities who find it difficult to describe symptoms may present in this way. Most serious of all, depressive disorder may be associated with homicide. In these rare circumstances the client will usually have mood-congruent delusions, for example that the world is too horrible a place for his or her family and friends to live in. Such homicides are very frequently followed by suicide of the client. Thus it is imperative to ask all clients with depressive disorders about thoughts of harm to others as well as to themselves. Puerperal (postpartum) psychosis with depressive symptomatology and postnatal depression are associated with mothers killing their children on rare occasions (see below).

Clients with mania or mixed affective states are often irritable which can lead to aggression. There is some clinical suspicion that this is a frequent presenting feature of mania in people with learning disabilities in whom cognitive symptoms such as elation and expansive and grandiose ideation may be less apparent. The general chaos that surrounds such mental states may be associated with rather impulsive offending. Most seriously, but quite rarely, serious sexual offences may be committed. This is usually the result of excited overactivity added to disinhibition and a failure to recognise the inappropriacy of the behaviour.

Learning disability

Despite the low prevalence of people with learning disabilities in prison in the UK, it is important to remember that offending behaviours, as opposed to convictions and criminal justice system disposals, are common in this client group. Hence,the full range of offending and alternative disposals must be considered. Offending behaviours may relate to a lack of appreciation of the implications or to susceptibility to exploitation by others. Alternatively, there may be a group of people with mild and borderline learning disabilities in whom offending parallels the general population in terms of the relevance of mental health issues or, indeed, straightforward culpability. In any case a formal diagnosis of learning disability usually militates strongly in favour of a health or social services disposal, for reasons described above. The strongest associations of offending with learning disabilities concern sexual offences, especially indecent exposure by males (Craft 1984), and arson, both of which are described in more detail below.

Two relatively recent and particularly thorough original data studies merit description here. First, a study undertaken in London compared clients admitted to a learning disability medium-secure unit to those on a generic medium-secure unit (Puri et al 2000). Sociodemographic, mental health, medical and legal data were recorded in a systematic fashion. Clients in the generic unit were more likely to be older at the time of conviction for the index offence and were more likely to have been admitted from penal settings such as prison. They were also more likely to have a psychiatric diagnosis of schizophrenia or bipolar affective disorder – of course, people with relatively 'pure' behaviour disorders would be excluded from such settings. The index offence was more likely to be homicide, attempted murder, manslaughter or grievous bodily harm. Those on the learning disability unit were more likely to have an index offence of a sexual nature. The authors concluded that differing psychiatric and behavioural requirements of the two client groups supported having separate units. There is general agreement that psychopharmacological, psychotherapeutic, systemic and social interventions for people with learning disabilities should meet their individual needs and should be informed by assessment with recognition of developmental principles (Gelder et al, in press).This is as true of offenders as anyone else and supports specialist work, although this can be organised in many different ways.

The second paper concerned potential aetiological factors for offending in adults with self-reported learning disabilities in Cambridge (Winter et al 1997). Adults held in custody at a police station were screened for possible learning disabilities using a four-item questionnaire (Lyall et al 1995). 21 participants were recruited in this way and comparisons were made with a control group of 17 adults, matched for age, gender and IQ.

Systematic interviews yielded information on medical, mental health and social histories. Offenders were more likely to have lost contact with their fathers, to come from families with forensic histories and to have experienced homelessness. They were also more likely to have had contact with the police in childhood and to be known to probation services. Current mental health risk factors for offending included illicit drug use or drug/alcohol dependence and an excess of recent adverse life events. Past mental health factors included self-reported behavioural problems at school, including truancy. All in the study group had a history of repeat offending. The authors concluded that social disadvantage may interact with individual factors such as childhood behaviour disorders and substance misuse in the genesis of offending amongst people with learning disabilities. Of course, it is difficult to be sure about causality from retrospective data and, although difficult to organise, prospective studies would be invaluable to test the independence or otherwise of such influences. Additional psychological assessments revealed that all of the study group had mild or borderline learning disabilities and, therefore, the similarity of some of their characteristics with offenders in general was not surprising.

Schizophrenia spectrum disorders

These include schizophrenia, and schizotypal and delusional disorders in ICD–10. The prevalence of such disorders in adults with learning disabilities is around 3–5% which is at least double that in the population without learning disabilities (Doody et al 1998). Most researchers in this field would agree that this is probably attributable to greater neurodevelopmental impairment in many people with learning disabilities, which may predispose to intellectual disability and schizophrenia if the developmental CNS damage occurs at strategic sites within the CNS – particularly the medial area of the dominant temporal lobe (Rowe et al 2000). However, a research group based in Edinburgh have elaborated a novel hypothesis concerning people with strong family histories of both learning disabilities and schizophrenia. Some of these clients seem to present with very severe schizophrenia and a surprisingly high number have been admitted to the Scottish special hospital system with extreme aggression. This raises the possibility that a *de novo* genetically determined condition exists which presents with features of both learning disabilities and schizophrenia. This hypothesis is difficult to test in the absence of identification and characterisation of the genes involved. An alternative explanation may be that schizophrenia in learning disability practice represents an extreme form of the disorder. This implies that social and cognitive impairment in childhood may result in the involvement of special educational providers and so on. Later, first rank symptoms of schizophrenia appear and the severity of the disorder may involve aggression and violence. Rates of offending are moderately increased in people with schizophrenia and this may relate to underlying psychosocial disadvantage or positive symptoms such as hallucinations and delusions (Buchanan et al 1993). The assessor should bear in mind certain risk factors for the occurrence of violence in people with schizophrenia spectrum disorders. These include great fear and loss of self-control associated with non-systematised delusions, systematised delusions of a paranoid-persecutory nature, some passivity phenomena, command hallucinations and inexplicable frenzy. Although such factors and threats of violence should be taken very seriously, it should be remembered that the vast majority of people with schizophrenia, with or without learning disabilities, are no more dangerous than other members of the general public.

Organic mental disorders

Acute brain syndrome (delirium) is occasionally associated with rather chaotic offending. Likewise, chronic brain syndrome (dementia). New and inexplicable offending in older adults, particularly of a sexual nature in men, should always raise the possibility of such disorders in the assessor's mind. Adults with learning disabilities are prone to such syndromes and this relates to the concept of diminished 'cognitive reserve'. This refers to structural and/or functional impairments of developmental origin at strategic sites within the CNS which may account for their learning disability. Thus intercurrent physical illness, such as a chest infection causing cerebral hypoxia, will result in delirium relatively rapidly. Furthermore, age-related neuronal loss will result in the threshold for clinical dementia being breached at a relatively young age for some people with learning disabilities. This is separate to the well known special association between Down syndrome and Alzheimer's disease, which probably rests upon a molecular genetic basis (see Berg et al (1995) for a review).

Some people with severe head injury sustained during the developmental period (usually taken to be up to 18 years of age) become known to learning disability providers. Aggressive and disinhibited behaviour may be occasioned by such injury and sites of particular relevance include the frontal lobes and the limbic system. Good neuropsychological assessment is necessary to pave the way for habilitation and rehabilitation.

The potential relationship between epilepsy and offending is very important for learning disability practitioners, especially as one-third of people known to such providers have epilepsy (Laidlaw et al 1993). Also, there is some evidence that epilepsy imposes an additional mental health burden for children and adults with learning disabilities (Rowe 1997). Surveys of prisons in the UK, USA and Scandinavia show that about twice as many inmates with epilepsy are encountered than would be predicted (Gunn & Fenton (1971) did the seminal work in this area). However, detailed video studies of thousands of epileptic seizures confirmed the widely held clinical opinion that violence is rare as part of the ictal phase, i.e. when the hypersynchronous epileptic electrical discharges are present in the brain (Delgado-Escueta et al 1981). Indeed, the few cases that were encountered related to chaotic epileptic automatisms, usually wheeling movements of the arms, as part of complex partial seizures, or post-ictal resistive violence, such as pushing away attendants at the end of a seizure whilst the person was still somewhat confused. However, it is important to remember that broader psychosocial factors may be relevant (Fenwick 1986); for example,

people with epilepsy are more likely to come from lower social class backgrounds, on a population basis, and they may have experienced poor antenatal and perinatal care, CNS infection or childhood head injury as the aetiology of their seizures. There is, of course, a strong association between socioeconomic disadvantage and offending. Furthermore, people with epilepsy are more likely to have mental health problems relating to CNS damage per se or understandable psychological reactions to chronic stressors (Reynolds & Trimble 1981). As described above, people with epilepsy are also more likely to have learning disabilities. Therefore, taken as a whole, these confounding variables probably account for any excess of offending seen in epilepsy – people with epilepsy who do not have mental health problems or learning disabilities and who do not come from socially disadvantaged backgrounds do not present with heightened levels of offending.

Occasionally, the 'episodic dyscontrol syndrome' is invoked as the cause of offending. This controversial diagnosis was first described by Bach-y-Rita et al (1971) in people with repeated, apparently unprovoked, episodes of violence. It was argued that subtle epileptiform discharges, not necessarily evident on the standard EEG, could be responsible. However, although all this is scientifically conceivable, the absence of any clear way of proving the diagnosis has led to considerable doubts, especially as subsequent studies have not supported this as a distinct syndrome (Fenton 1986).

SPECIFIC OFFENCES LIKELY TO BE ASSOCIATED WITH MENTAL HEALTH AND COGNITIVE DISORDERS

The main part of this section is taken up by sexual offences and arson as these have the closest link with learning disability. There is also some description of maternal infanticide as this is strongly associated with mental health problems. More generally, homicide is usually divided into 'normal' and 'abnormal' categories, according to the legal outcome. The former occurs when there is a conviction of murder or common law manslaughter; the latter if there is a finding of insane murder, suicide murder, diminished responsibility or infanticide. Abnormal homicide accounts for a third to a half of all homicides in the UK. The most common psychiatric diagnoses involved are depressive disorder, personality disorder, substance dependence and schizophrenia (Taylor 1993). The syndrome of pathological jealousy may be associated with any of these diagnoses as it is a disorder of 'content' and not 'form'. Learning disabilities may also be associated with any of these diagnoses. A subgroup of shoplifters have a strong association with depressive disorder. These are usually women and they may well have an excess of recent adverse life events and chronic background psychosocial stressors (Gudjonsson 1990). Treatment should address the underlying depressive disorder and promote prevention of relapse. Any Court report should differentiate depression predating the offence from that occurring following arrest.

Sexual offences

Although sexual offences account for less than 1% of all indictable offences recorded by the police in the UK, such offenders form a large proportion of forensic referrals to mental health and learning disability teams. This principally relates to concerns over potential mental health and cognitive problems in the offender and a desire to try to judge future risk. The vast majority of sexual offenders are men. Despite popular opinion, the reconviction rates are lower than for offenders in general. Most surveys indicate 25–33% reconviction rates within 5 years or so. However, such estimates should be interpreted with caution as there is considerable attrition with most sexual offences not being reported to the police in the first place and most of those reported not leading to successful convictions. The most common sexual offences are indecent assault, indecent exposure and unlawful intercourse with underage children. People with learning disabilities are probably over-represented in all three categories. The emotional and psychological consequences of having been the victim of serious sexual offences are invariably very severe and always indicate careful therapeutic support, once the offence has been recognised.

The majority of sexual offences against children do not involve violence but they are particularly likely to involve coercion and abuse of power. Such offenders are often referred to as paedophiles and they may have heterosexual, homosexual or mixed orientation. It is important to distinguish between two groups of offender. First, there are men who are often timid and sexually inexperienced – some of these may have significant learning disabilities. Their offences may relate to a lack of appreciation of the inappropriacy of their actions or to identification with children at a similar developmental level to themselves, in many respects. This is not to deny that some child sex offenders with learning disabilities do understand the nature of their actions and do share a considerable amount in common with more able offenders. These people probably simply represent the lower end of the ability spectrum in terms of offenders in general. The second main group of people who commit sexual offences against children are more likely to prefer such activity, rather than to indulge in it as a consequence of other limitations. Such men may have had normal consenting adult sexual relationships and, most worryingly, some of them are highly predatory and repeatedly seek out vulnerable children. This group are less likely to have learning disabilities and many of them are highly secretive and manipulative in their actions.

In trying to assess the risk of repetition of sexual offences against children, and the likelihood of progression to similar offences of a more serious nature, for example with greater degrees of violence, the literature identifies one factor as much the most important. This is the duration and strength of such sexual preferences and the associated frequency of offending. It is essential that this should always be looked into by the assessor (Becker & Quinsey 1993). Of course, many offenders deny their histories and it is mandatory to study the depositions, including previous convictions, and carefully evaluate the victim's statement (Kennedy & Grubin 1992). Other historical factors of relevance include the presence of major mental illness or personality disorder, in particular dissocial personality disorder. Relatively enduring psychological variables may be of importance, such as emotional loneliness and emotional congruity with children, by which it is meant that the offender reports a special understanding of children and the belief that they are drawn to him. Cognitive distortions may include overestimating the sexual knowledge of children, underestimating the coercion involved and playing down the distress and long-term problems caused by the offence. Various standardised questionnaires can be used to augment clinical interviewing here. More dynamic factors, closer to the time of the event may include access to children, recent adverse life events and intoxication with alcohol or drugs. Successful treatment is therefore likely to be complex and multimodal with attention paid to any underlying mental illness or personality disorder as well as psychological work, usually cognitive-behavioural in orientation, and social interventions to try to optimise the safety of the person's situation. There is increasing evidence that treatment can reduce undesirable psychological attitudes in child sex offenders but there has been little work on whether this translates to prevention of future offences – particularly in people with learning disabilities. Systematic reviews of the efficacy of such treatments are awaited from active Cochrane research groups based in Oxford. When published, the results will be available on the Cochrane database on the internet.

There is some controversy as to the prevalence of a history of having been the victim of childhood sexual abuse in such offenders. Some large number surveys in the USA indicate that less than 50% of offenders have such histories and, of course, the vast majority of victims do not go on to become offenders. Nonetheless, in clinical practice a subgroup of such offenders, often amongst the most disturbed and polymorphous in orientation, have suffered severe childhood sexual abuse. Currently there is something of a tendency to concentrate on the 'here-and-now' in treatment, so as to minimise future risks, rather than to place too much store on retrospective enquiry leading to greater understanding. This parallels cognitive-behaviour therapy principles in general. Group therapy is frequently advocated to minimise denial as well as to enhance the cost effectiveness

of what is often a lengthy and expensive endeavour. However, there has been little work on potential inadvertent reinforcement of offending and attitudes related to this in men with learning disabilities exposed to a more able peer group. It is also likely that future developments will include a public health dimension in that many people at high risk of repeated offending can be spotted relatively early and resources could be targeted at them in a preventive way. This is likely to be especially important for adolescents who offend.

Incest is almost certainly more common than conviction rates would suggest. Most reported cases involve a father and daughter but other first degree relative configurations, including mother and son, are probably more common than generally appreciated. Certain risk factors have long been advanced in the literature, such as marital breakdown leading to replacement of the mother by her daughter, social isolation, overcrowded living conditions and alcohol abuse and dissocial personality in the father. Most offenders offer a different psychological profile to child sex offenders in general, and most seem to prefer adult sexual relationships. However, there is increasing recognition of a minority of great importance to health and social providers as well as to the criminal justice system. These are men who superficially appear to have predominant problems along incestuous lines but who, on more detailed enquiry, closely resemble the profile of paedophiles per se described above. These men may enter into family relationships to gain access to child victims and, as such, their treatment and prognosis are more similar to those of child sex offenders in general.

The term indecent exposure is the legal name given to the offence of indecently exposing the genitals to other people. It is one of the few offences particularly strongly associated with learning disabilities. To put this in perspective, it is important to remember that indecent exposure is the term applied to quite a wide variety of offences. These vary from simple exhibitionism, which is very common, to exposure as a prelude to sexual assault. In some respects, offenders with learning disabilities occupy a middle ground here. Simple exhibitionism is predominantly the domain of rather timid men with broader sexual difficulties who generally have a flaccid penis at the time and enjoy the shock they cause to the victim. The reconviction rate is low and most offenders are between 25 and 35 years of age. Those who expose themselves as a prelude to sexual assault tend to have an erect penis at the time and go on to try to force sexual contact with the victim. Their reconviction rates are much higher. This dichotomy should not detract from the undoubted distress caused to victims in either case, but the management of these offenders differs as the latter group resemble those who commit indecent assault in general. People with learning disabilities may conform to either group in a minority of cases. However, most felt sexually driven at the time of the index offence and simply failed to recognise the significance of their actions or may have indulged in this kind of behaviour to try to engage a desired person in a gauche and highly inappropriate way. Cognitive-behavioural therapy approaches are preferred and victim empathy is promoted, in addition to appropriate sex education and 'situational security' interventions. In appraising the specific efficacy of these types of interventions, it is difficult to rule out certain potentially confounding factors. First, there may be a non-specific effect from the provision of a large amount of therapeutic input for a person who may be generally disadvantaged and disenfranchised. Secondly, there may be a 'halo' effect of the situational security being attached to ongoing supervision which motivates the offender to stay out of legal trouble, irrespective of the exact nature of therapeutic input.

Indecent assault is a very broad category in law, from attempts to touch the victim in a sexual manner to severe sexual assault without attempted penetration. There are associations with dissocial personality disorder and learning disabilities in a minority of offenders. There is also an association with physical stigmatisation in the offender who may find it difficult to establish mutually consenting adult relationships. This can be a problem for some people with learning disabilities whose cognitive impairments may be added to by a rather

syndromic appearance to render them at risk of such offending.

In England and Wales, the Sexual Offences Act (1956) states that a man commits rape if he has unlawful sexual intercourse with a woman who at the time of the intercourse does not consent to it and if at the time he knows that she does not consent to the intercourse or he is reckless as to whether she consents to it. The Act excludes male rape and forcible anal intercourse with a woman but these are extremely serious sexual offences and are dealt with as such by the Courts. Indeed, there is currently something of a debate in legal and legislative circles as to whether a more flexible approach should be taken in law such that a spectrum of indecent assault is considered and the narrower definition of rape would be superseded. The Act also excludes forced sexual intercourse within marriage but there is now considerable case law recognising rape within marriage. Hostile attitudes towards women or other victim groups are prevalent in rapists and may form a focus for cognitive-behavioural interventions.

Arson

This offence is generally regarded with the utmost seriousness by the Courts. This gives credence to its potential for loss of life and extensive damage to property. The relationship between arson and mental disorders in general has been carefully reviewed by Geller (1992). Attempts have been made to establish a behavioural classification of arsonists. One group includes people who are free of significant mental health problems and who start fires for financial or political reasons or for revenge; they are sometimes referred to as 'motivated' arsonists. The second group are referred to as 'pathological' arsonists. These people may have learning disabilities, mental illness (including psychosis) or substance misuse, as well as fragile personality traits such as sensation-seeking, associated in some cases with conspicuous attempts to join in the subsequent firefighting. Most dangerously of all, given the propensity for behavioural conditioning and repeated offending, a small minority of arsonists are sexually motivated and obtain intense satisfaction and tension reduction from firesetting.

Soothill & Pope (1973) reported on a follow-up study of convicted arsonists with an unusually long length of assessment – 20 years. The reconviction rate for arson was only 4% but approximately 50% were later charged with other criminal offences– this sort of generalisation of offending at follow-up is a common finding in forensic studies. It is essential to remember that a person who is convicted of arson for a second time is at extremely high risk of future recidivism and the appropriate security and therapeutic measures must be imposed. Other risk factors for recidivism include: dissocial personality disorder, learning disabilities, persistent psychosocial stressors, especially social isolation, and sexual motivation for the offending.

In assessment of arsonists, it is important not to be swayed by the extent of the damage caused by the fire. This is because other factors than intent will come into play here and subsequent fires may have different results. Risk assessment should include the possibility of other types of offences being committed. Treatment tends to be within secure settings with high levels of observation. Any underlying mental illness should receive appropriate assessment and treatment, as should any attendant personality disorder. Cognitive approaches may include education about the risks of future offending and victim empathy work. The evidence base for such interventions is yet to be established. On discharge to less secure settings and the community, situational security may well be required along the lines described above, particularly for more disabled offenders in whom major cognitive change might prove difficult to achieve.

Maternal infanticide

Although this is rare in people with learning disabilities, its association with mental health problems is particularly strong and urgent health input is essential. In the UK the vast majority of mothers who kill their children of less than 12 months of age are regarded as in need of some sort of health disposal. In practice, the Infanticide Act (1938) in England and Wales defined a category of offence which can be seen as a special case of the later and wider concept of diminished responsibility.

The seminal work of d'Orban (1979) described a classification of mothers who commit infanticide, which informs assessment and treatment. The categories included those who commit or attempt neonaticide in that the baby is killed or left to die within 24 hours of birth. Such mothers are often young and unprepared to care for the child. Some will have learning disabilities and some will have panicked at the time of the birth. Some will have concealed their pregnancy and all are in need of major mental health support as well as practical support in parenting for those whose children survive and are felt to be safe to return to maternal care. A very small minority of women with mental illness may kill their children and this is likely to relate to puerperal psychosis or postnatal depressive disorder, with the mother believing that she is saving the child from an unkind world and future suffering. Another group of so-called 'mercy-killers' do indeed kill their children on the grounds of genuine disease, suffering and pain. A more numerous group batter their children repeatedly and this ultimately leads to an unplanned death. Such mothers resemble batterers in general and they are often socially disadvantaged and unsupported. Some have learning disabilities and limited coping mechanisms to deal with stressors as well as diminished appreciation of the nature and consequences of their actions. Finally, there is a group with the 'Medea complex', named after the ancient Greek goddess who killed her children whowere fathered by Jason. This was essentially an act of revenge for his infidelity and the psychodynamic mechanism behind such killing is seen to be that of anger being displaced from the father on to his children as a way of punishing him.

PRINCIPLES OF ASSESSMENT AND TREATMENT OF OFFENDERS WITH LEARNING DISABILITIES

In many respects the assessment of people with learning disabilities who offend in law represents a mixture of the assessment of people with learning disabilities and potential mental health problems in general and the forensic assessment of offenders with potential mental health problems. The causes and effects of learning disabilities should be simultaneously evaluated with the causes and effects of any mental health problems. There is a dearth of reliable and valid instruments to aid this process for offenders but there are some notable exceptions, such as the treatment of dual diagnosis with underlying mental disorder which should be aimed specifically at that mental disorder. This gives credence to the recognition of the relevance of the illness to the offending. The treatment of people who present with specific types of offences is described in the section above. Below, there are three brief case illustrations that describe the assessment and treatment of three types of presentation. The first (Case illustration 14.1) relates to relatively straightforward offending in law. The second (Case illustration 14.2) to a client whose violent behaviour was not containable on

Case illustration 14.1

Graham R is a 21-year-old man with a moderate learning disability with the aetiology being arrested hydrocephalus. He also has generalised tonic–clonic epileptic seizures, which are under good control with the antiepileptic drug, sodium valproate. Graham, attended special education and his family originally had a travelling culture. He has some features of complicated grief following the deaths of his father and grandfather. By mid-adolescence he was subject to multiple exclusions from educational and social services providers owing to sexually inappropriate behaviours, especially grabbing others, aggression and severe non-compliance. From 16 years of age he spent time in private provider, rehabilitation and acute hospitals, initially under section 3 of the Mental Health Act on the grounds of severe mental impairment. Functional analysis of the nature of challenging behaviours, their antecedents and consequences paved the way for careful behavioural therapy, including differential reinforcement of more positive behaviours. After a period of relatively settled behaviour, Graham absconded from hospital and impulsively seriously indecently assaulted a young woman. The Court placed him on a hospital order with a Restriction Order, section 37/4, and he was entered on the Sex Offenders Register. He was admitted to a learning disability medium-secure unit. Ongoing impulsive aggression, especially punching and kicking, led to the use of anti-agitation drugs such as chlorpromazine, on a regular and 'as required' basis. Also, the selective-serotonin reuptake inhibitor citalopram was commenced to try to reduce impulsivity. Further severe sexual challenging behaviours resulted in a therapeutic trial of the anti-androgen drug cyproterone acetate. There is ongoing behavioural input and the care management team have been involved in strengthening the links with his family. Nursing input has also included grief therapy. He continues to challenge his systems of support.

Case illustration 14.2

Stephen L is a 22-year-old man with a mild learning disability of uncertain aetiology. He was the victim of sexual abuse in adolescence whilst attending a special education boarding school. He has the chronic stressor of his principal carer, his father, having a terminal illness and, in some respects, there is a reversal of roles as he assumes a more caring role himself. Stephen lived in a deprived area where he was subject to exploitation by rather delinquent local youths – for this reason, and repeated attacks on his own family, he became known to the local police. Following further deterioration in family relationships, Stephen agreed to come into the learning disability acute unit as a voluntary inpatient. Matters deteriorated and punching and headbutting resulted in the hospitalisation of two nurses. Attempted 'rapid tranquillisation' with sedative drugs was unsuccessful. A section 3 on the grounds of mental impairment was applied and he was transferred to the learning disabilities medium-secure unit. Stephen responded well to consistent behavioural boundaries and simple cognitive work along problem-solving lines. He also benefited from protective behaviours work to minimise future vulnerability, for example, by identifying early signs of problems and who he can go to safely for help. A diagnosis of complex partial epileptic seizures was also made and this may have been missed in the past. Treatment with the antiepileptic drug carbamazepine abolished clinical seizures. Positron emission tomographic (PET) brain scanning revealed perfusion deficits of the posterior dominant parietal lobe – an area likely to be implicated in his relatively slow information and language processing skills. This paved the way for speech and language therapy input to define the best means of communicating with Stephen. Return to the community after a 4 month admission was supported by care management arranging rehousing in a more suitable area where he would be less vulnerable. Also, Stephen has considerable occupational therapy input to enhance meaningful daytime occupation and supported working. There is a component of ongoing education for extended activities of daily living at a local college. A community nurse with a special interest in challenging behaviour monitors progress and acts as a key worker in coordinating the work of others. There have been no major problems since discharge over 12 months ago.

an open NHS unit. The third (Case illustration 14.3) describes the anticipated need for 'intensive care' in a client with a history of severe aggression.

In the assessment of dangerousness, in addition to some of the specific factors described above, certain general principles should be remembered with regard to the history, the index offence, the mental state and the general circumstances of the offender. Historical factors of relevance include: previous violence and offending, impulsivity, poor coping mechanisms, sadistic tendencies and dissocial personality traits. Factors associated with the offence indicative of high dangerousness include: bizarre violence, lack of provocation, absence of regret and continuing denial. Mental state factors of concern include: morbid jealousy, paranoid-persecutory delusions, ongoing aggressive ideation, deceptiveness, poor self-control and

Case illustration 14.3

Robert T is a 24-year-old man with mild learning disabilities and Asperger's syndrome. He was well known to specialist learning disability educational and then day services providers. Robert has a long history of problems with high levels of anxiety and agitation. He has not consistently complied with psychotropic medication and often refuses to see various therapists. At times of additional stress he has been admitted to the local acute learning disability unit to stabilise his mental and behavioural state. Such admissions were marred by sexual challenging behaviour directed at female staff, such as attempts to grab their breasts and severe verbal sexual threats to them. He also punched two nurses so hard that they required A&E treatment and he smashed up the contents of his room. Robert was re-referred following further psychodynamic tensions in the family and physical attacks on a younger sibling. Robert recognised his own need for a place of safety but the acute unit was understandably reluctant to admit him. Given the anticipated need for intensive behavioural care, a voluntary admission to the learning disability medium-secure unit was arranged. Supportive psychotherapy, problem-solving work and consistent behavioural boundaries resulted in rapid diminution of anxiety and agitation without psychotropic drugs being needed. Within 2 weeks, risk assessment informed the opinion that he was safe to move to a step-down unit before return to the community some 4 weeks after that. This sort of crisis work does not negate Robert's long-term risk of deterioration, especially as some of the psychosocial conditions he finds stressful in the community have not changed.

non-compliance with treatment. Dangerousness is also associated with social circumstances which place the offender in contact with ongoing precipitating factors, alcohol or drug abuse and general social disadvantage and lack of support.

It is sometimes helpful to conceptualise the involvement of an offender with the criminal justice system as a journey, at any point of which substantive clinical and social input may be appropriate. The first stage is at the time of arrest. Removal to a place of safety (under section 136 of the Mental Health Act 1983) allows for the assessment of some suspected offenders with potential mental disorder in a police station or mental health hospital. Assessment after arrest may involve psychiatrists and psychiatric or learning disability nurses, for example in Court diversion schemes to triage offenders towards health and social support, where appropriate. Even in the absence of such formal arrangements, it is important that people with major mental illness and/or learning disabilities are interviewed by the police only in the presence of an 'appropriate adult', according to the Police and Criminal Evidence Act 1984. This is usually a social worker who has received appropriate training. The key task for the appropriate adult is to ensure that, as far as possible, suspects understand their rights, the meaning of questions put to them and generally what is going on whilst in custody. They should also prevent the suspect from being subject to any undue pressure.

This last point is especially important for people with learning disabilities who may be very suggestible and admit to things they have not done. Gudjonsson (1992) examined the phenomenology of false confessions and arrived at three categories. First, there were 'voluntary' confessions made from a morbid desire for notoriety, major difficulty in differentiating fact from fantasy or an intention to protect another person. Secondly, there were 'coerced-compliant' confessions resulting from forceful interrogations, which were usually subsequently retracted. Thirdly, there were 'coerced-internalised' confessions which arose from an iterative process of undermining the suspects' recollections so that they came to believe they were responsible for the crime. Neuropsychological impairment is a risk factor for the latter and people with learning disabilities are at risk of making all three types of false confessions. Subsequently, Gudjonsson has devised a suggestibility scale which augments clinical assessment in terms of evaluating the propensity for embellishment in general and the propensity to acquiesce to suggestions made at interrogation. Clinical assessment of possible false confessions should also include a thorough review of the circumstances of the arrest, custody and interrogation as well as the personality and mental state of the suspect (this is helpfully reviewed in a Lancet editorial, Lancet 1994).

The second stage in the journey of criminal proceedings is pre-trial when a Court report may be required and this will usually include psychiatric, clinical psychology, social work and nursing input. Remand for inpatient assessment and/or treatment may be made and transfer from prison to hospital for assessment is appropriate for some people.

The third stage involves the trial when special problems may arise. These include the issue of fitness to plead, the assessment of which is usually undertaken by a psychiatrist. Relevant factors in this judgement are the defendant's ability to understand the nature of the charge, to understand the difference between pleading guilty and not guilty, to instruct counsel, to challenge jurors and to follow the currency of the case in Court. People with learning disabilities may not be fit to plead and they should not then be subjected to an unfair trial, the nature of which they do not comprehend. A 'trial of the facts' should take place in the absence of the suspect and, if the suspect is convicted, the judge has a broad range of options from the equivalent of a Restriction Order to absolute discharge. Another special problem worthy of mention is the issue of diminished responsibility. This plea may be entered as a defence to a charge of murder. If the defence is upheld, the accused is found guilty of manslaughter. The concept of diminished responsibility is based on a quite broad definition of mental abnormality of relevance to the person's responsibility for the acts connected with the killing. Learning disabilities are certainly a highly relevant factor here. If there is a conviction, the judge may pass whatever sentence he or she thinks necessary on the grounds of dangerousness and the best means for rehabilitation. Regarding the latter point, psychiatrists are frequently asked for an opinion as to the best disposal for a convicted person by the Court.

The fourth stage is after the trial. Treatment may take place under hospital orders or guardianship and some offenders are transferred from prison for assessment and/or treatment. Specialist mental health and learning disability teams have a key role to play in decisions about release and in the planning and provision of treatment in the community.

Readers may find it useful to undertake the 14.1 to 14.5 activities reader.

 Reader activities 14.1–14.5

- Spend some time recalling some principles of general criminology, for example the nature and causes of offending.
- How can it be that mental health problems contribute to people with learning disabilities offending?
- Discuss with a colleague the connection between some specific offences and mental health and cognitive problems.
- What are the major parts of the Mental Health Act that relate to offenders with learning disabilities?
- Why do you think that it is important to undertake a holistic assessment and treatment of people with learning disabilities who have offended in law?

REFERENCES

American Psychiatric Association 1995 Diagnostic and statistical manual of mental disorders, 4th edn. International version. American Psychiatric Press, Washington DC

Bach-y-Rita G, Lion J R, Climent C E, Ervin F R 1971 Episodic dyscontrol: a study of 130 violent patients. American Journal of Psychiatry 127: 1473–1478

Becker J, Quinsey V 1993 Assessing suspected child molesters. Child Abuse and Neglect 17: 169–174

Berg J M, Karlinsky H, Holland A J (eds) 1995 Alzheimer disease, Down syndrome and their relationship. Oxford University Press, Oxford

Brennan P A, Mednick S A 1993 Genetic perspectives on crime.Acta Psychiatrica Scandinavica 370 (Suppl): 19–36

Buchanan A, Reed A, Wessely S 1993 The phenomenological correlates of acting on delusions. British Journal of Psychiatry 163: 77–81

Craft M 1984 Low intelligence, mental handicap and crime. In: Craft M, Craft A (eds) Mentally abnormal offenders. Baillière Tindall, London

Delgado-Escueta A V, Mattson R H, King L et al 1981 The nature of aggression during epileptic seizures. New England Journal of Medicine 305: 711–716

Doody G A, Johnstone E C, Sanderson T L et al 1998 `Pfropschizophrenie' revisited: schizophrenia in people with mild learning disability. British Journal of Psychiatry 173: 145–153

D'Orban P T 1979 Women who kill their children. British Journal of Psychiatry 134: 560–571

Downes D, Rock P 1988 Understanding deviance, 2nd edn. Clarendon Press, Oxford

Fazel S 2001 Unpublished doctoral thesis, Edinburgh University

Fenton G W 1986 Epilepsy and hysteria. British Journal of Psychiatry 149: 28–37

Fenwick P 1986 Aggression and epilepsy. In: Trimble M R, Bolwig T G (eds) Aspects of epilepsy and psychiatry. Wiley, Chichester, Ch 4

Gelder M, Gath D, Mayou R, Cowen P (eds) 1996 Appendix: The law in England and Wales. In: The Oxford textbook of psychiatry, 3rd edn. Oxford University Press, Oxford, pp 781–787

Gelder M, Gath D, Mayou R, Cowen P (eds) In Press. Mental retardation. In: The Oxford textbook of psychiatry, 4th edn. Oxford University Press, Oxford

Geller J L 1992 Pathological firesetting in adults. International Journal of Law and Psychiatry 15: 283–302

Gudjonsson G H 1990 Psychological and psychiatric aspects of shoplifting. Medicine, Science and Law 30: 45–51

Gudjonsson G H 1992 The psychology of interrogations, confessions and testimony. Wiley, Chichester

Heidensohn F 1994 Women as perpetrators and victims of crime: a sociological perspective. British Journal of Psychiatry 158 (Suppl 10): 50–54

Kennedy H, Grubin D 1992 Patterns of denial in sex offenders. Psychological Medicine 22: 191–196

Laidlaw J, Richens A, Chadwick D 1993 A textbook of epilepsy, 4th edn. Churchill Livingstone, Edinburgh

Lancet 1994 Guilty innocents: the road to false confessions. Lancet 344: 1447–1450

Lange J 1931 Crime as destiny (transl. Haldane C). George Allen, London

Lishman W A 1997 Organic psychiatry, 3rd edn. Blackwell Scientific Publications, Oxford

Lund J 1990 Mentally retarded criminal offenders in Denmark. British Journal of Psychiatry 156: 726–731

Lyall I, Holland A J, Collins S, Styles P 1995 Incidence of persons with a learning disability detained in police custody: a needs assessment for service development. Medicine, Science and the Law 35: 61–71

Monahan J, Steadman H 1994 Crime and mental disorder: an epidemiological approach. In: Morris N, Tonry M (eds) Crime and justice: an annual review of research 3: 145–189

Puri B K, Lekh S K, Treasaden I H 2000 A comparison of patients admitted to two medium secure units, one for those of normal intelligence and one for those with learning disability. International Journal of Clinical Practice 54: 300–305

Raine A, Venables P H, Williams M 1990 Relationships between central and autonomic measures of arousal at age 15 years and criminality at age 24 years. Archives of General Psychiatry 47: 1003

Reynolds E H, Trimble M R (eds) 1981 Epilepsy and psychiatry. Churchill Livingstone, Edinburgh

Rowe D 1997 Psychiatric disorders in adults with learning disability and epilepsy. Proceedings of the Royal College of Psychiatrists. AGM p. 31

Rowe D, Rudkin A, Crawford L 2000 Cerebral dominance and schizophrenia-spectrum disorders in adults with intellectual disability. Journal of Intellectual Disability Research 44: 638–643

Russell O (ed) 1997 The psychiatry of learning disabilities. Gaskell, London

Soothill K L, Pope P J 1973 Arson: a twenty-year cohort study. Medicine, Science and the Law 13: 127–138

Taylor P J 1993 Violence in society. Royal College of Physicians, London

Wessely S, Taylor P 1991 Madness and crime: criminology versus psychiatry. Criminal Behaviour and Mental Health 1: 193–228

Wilson J Q, Herrnstein O 1985 Crime and human nature. Simon & Schuster, New York

Winter N, Holland A J, Collins S 1997 Factors predisposing to suspected offending by adults with self-reported learning disabilities. Psychological Medicine 27: 595–607

Witkin H A, Mednick S A, Schlusinger F 1976 Criminality and XYY and XXY man. Science 193: 547–548

World Health Organisation 1992 The ICD-10 classification of mental and behavioural disorders. World Health Organisation, Geneva

4

Helping people achieve independence and wellbeing

In this section, Rita Ferris-Taylor presents a chapter on communication that is followed by a comprehensive account of health and health promotion for people with learning disabilities. Eileen Wake, in Chapter 17, provides a very comprehensive and practical guide as to how to work with people with profound and complex needs. In Chapter 18, Ruth Northway, Robert Jenkins and Ian Mansell provide an excellent chapter on specialist learning disability services and personnel currently to be found in the UK. Finally, in Chapter 19, Helen Sanderson provides a helpful overview of person-centred planning, which is so pivotal to the modern construction of services for people with learning disabilities.

15

Communication

Rita Ferris-Taylor

KEY ISSUES

- This chapter defines the key components of communication, distinguishing between speech and language and discussing the possible discrepancies between comprehension of language and expressive language in people with learning disabilities.
- Recent legislation, such as the Disability Discrimination Act 1995 and the Human Rights Act 1998, is reviewed in relation to its possible impact in highlighting the importance of communicating with people in a range of ways, such as use of manual signs and pictorial symbol systems, and seeking people's view about the services they receive.
- The chapter adopts the approach of the social model of disability, which views the concept of disability as discrimination based on impairment. This implies that there is the need to change the way we communicate with and our attitudes towards people with communication impairments in society, rather than focusing purely on the individual with learning disabilities.
- A range of ways of adapting communication for people with differing needs is suggested. The importance of sensory abilities, race and culture and environmental influences on communication are highlighted, together with the need for active involvement with others and the opportunity to exercise choices.

- **Alternative and augmentative communication systems are described and discussed.**

INTRODUCTION

Communication is important to many of the things we do in our everyday lives. We communicate with one another for a wide range of reasons. Crystal (1992) has summarised the main functions of communication as the exchange of ideas and information, emotional expression, social interaction, control of reality, recording facts, thinking and expressing identity. In addition to speech we use a range of non-verbal means to communicate, for example gestures, tone of voice, eye contact, facial expression and body posture, and these vary culturally.

Communication is a two-way process, involving at least two people who alternate in sending and receiving messages.

The focus of this chapter is communication as a whole, not just speech and verbal communication. It takes the approach that all human beings use a variety of means of communication, and that all of these have a place, no one means being inherently superior. In working with people with learning disabilities we need to be prepared to learn to recognise a wide range of behaviours as possible communication, and to use a variety of methods in communicating back. Carers and professionals have an influential role in interacting with people with learning disabilities and seeking to reduce the impact of any communication difficulties. This is linked to the overall approach in this chapter of using a social rather than a medical model of disability.

In recent years there has been lively debate about ways of defining and understanding disability, in particular, whether the difficulty is located within the individual or in society as a whole (Campbell and Oliver 1996, Morris 1991, Oliver 1990, Reiser & Mason 1992, Shakespeare and Watson 1997). The social model of disability has defined disability as discrimination based on impairment and emphasises that our view of disability varies according to the physical, social and attitudinal barriers imposed within society. For example, someone who uses a wheelchair in central London is likely to be significantly restricted by the environmental barriers involved in using public transport, gaining access to buildings etc. Someone using a wheelchair in Milton Keynes is likely to be less restricted in moving about the town, owing to its layout. In relation to communication, those who use sign language as their first language will experience significant difficulties if others do not understand, use and value it; whereas in an environment where everyone uses sign language, non-sign users will be disadvantaged. Sacks (1990) described just such a situation in Martha's Vineyard in the USA.

Methods of speech and language therapy now concentrate more on interaction with others in everyday settings rather than on individual work away from real-life settings (Bartlett & Bunning 1997, Dobson et al 1999). Van der Gaag (1998) put forward the case for learning disability services to develop locally agreed strategies for communication (parallel to organisational strategies on issues such as housing and employment) if there is truly to be a more enabling environment.

The incidence of communication difficulties among people with learning disabilities is high. Depending upon definitions and the population involved (e.g. hospital or community), it has variously been estimated as 40–50% (Mansell 1992). This has led some to suggest that there is an almost open-ended need for speech and language therapy, although as discussed above, current approaches are moving towards trying to apply the social model of disability to bring about changes in the environment. Given that communication is a two-way process, it is important to avoid locating all the difficulty with the person with learning disabilities and rather to consider what the other party to the communication can do to maintain or extend communication. Certainly, communication will be a key consideration for all who come into contact with people with learning disabilities, especially those who do so on a regular basis. Dobson et al (2000) have highlighted the difficulties with role expectations of different professionals in multidisciplinary learning disability teams. There is a need to share detailed information about communication, for example to help one another guess what a non-verbal person wants and so respond consistently and effectively.

During the last decade, legislation such as the Children Act 1989 and the NHS and Community Care Act 1990 has emphasised the importance of involving disabled adults and children in their own assessments of need, planning for their own futures and taking account of their views about the services they receive. In particular, the Children Act asserted that 'Even children with severe learning disabilities or very limited expressive language can communicate preferences if they are asked in the right way by people who understand their needs and have the relevant skills to listen to them'. This should not be dependent on age or mode of communication and challenges professionals to find creative ways to enable this to take place. For example, Minkes et al (1994) have described the development of a range of tools, such as simplified questionnaires, photographs and pictures, to obtain the views of disabled children about the respite care they received. Millner et al (1991) have described creative approaches to involve adults with learning disabilities in quality action groups.

More recent government initiatives such as 'Best Value' emphasised that local authorities need to ensure that the views of those who receive services are considered closely when deciding how services should be delivered and reviewing them. This requires time, effort and commitment when people with learning and communication disabilities are involved, or consultation may be tokenistic (Ferris-Taylor1999, Grant 1997).

The Disability Discrimination Act 1995 placed an onus on providers of goods and services to make reasonable adjustments for disabled people. Although the definition of 'reasonable' is open to interpretation, it could be argued that it would be 'reasonable' for shops, museums, libraries and leisure services to provide information in alternative formats, e.g. plain English, large print, pictures and symbols. To some extent this is beginning to happen (see, for example, the Makaton symbol translations occurring later in this chapter) and although such translations are not widespread at the moment, the Disability Discrimination Act may serve as an impetus to service providers to develop more accessible printed materials. (People First have been involved in producing a guide to the Disability Discrimination Act for people with learning disabilities.)

The Human Rights Act 1998 could be used in the future in combination with the Disability Discrimination Act to strengthen the case for public information to be made available in a range of formats so as to be more accessible to people with learning disabilities, remembering that no one format will be accessible to all. In particular, Article 10, *The right to freedom of expression*, could be used in this way (Daw 2000, Hughes and Coombs 2001).

It is encouraging that *Valuing people: a new strategy for the 21st century* (DOH 2001) emphasises the importance of staff training and sets targets for services for staff to achieve NVQ based qualifications, based around standards which are specifically focused on working with people with learning disabilities. These include a mandatory unit on communication.

It is important to remember that the range of people described as having learning disabilities is very wide, from those with profound and multiple disabilities to those with mild difficulties. Correspondingly, and given the complexity of communication, the nature of communication difficulties can be very diverse. Accordingly, this chapter will discuss and put forward general principles (and there are always likely to be exceptions). It is important that people with learning disabilities and their carers have access to advice from speech and language therapists, in order to maximise their communication.

THE NATURE OF COMMUNICATION

Communication involves the transmission of meaning from one person to another, irrespective of the method. Thinking broadly, it may involve dance, music, Braille, pictures, telephones, the internet and sexual activity! Yet we generally tend to think mostly in terms of speech and language as our prime means of communication.

Using language to communicate involves understanding and producing the rules of grammar and word order (syntax), and formulating meaning (semantics) in a way that someone else can understand (pragmatics). This is complex because there is no reason why particular words should stand for particular objects or ideas. Whether the word *dog*, *Kalb* (Arabic) or *chien* (French) is used, there is no relationship between the chosen sound formation and the animal it represents. It is by convention that we learn to associate sound sequences in our first language with their referents. In addition, many words cannot be taught by easy reference to an object or event. For example, a word such as 'in' can be demonstrated by placing objects in boxes, drawers, cups etc. However, 'in the swimming pool' may be a little harder to understand, and other meanings of the same word, such as 'in time' or 'in the first place' cannot be demonstrated so readily.

Consider the complexity of grammatical rules and word order. For example, 'The dog chases the cat' has the same meaning as 'The cat is being chased by the dog'. Also, although there are various grammatical rules, many of these have exceptions. For example, English noun plurals are often formed by adding 's' to the end of the word, but some plurals, such as 'geese' and 'mice', are formed differently. Similarly, the past tense of verbs is often formed by adding '-ed' to the root of the verb, but there are exceptions, e.g. 'went', 'brought'.

Pragmatics is also a complex area. For example, language varies according to the social context, so that the spoken and body language used with friends is different from the more formal approach used at a job interview.

In addition, non-verbal communication, which can be conscious or unconscious, adds to the meaning of what we say, either to reinforce it or to give a contradictory message. Abercrombie (1968) suggests that 'We speak with our vocal organs but we converse with our whole bodies'. Morris (1987) contends that as much as 50% of our communication is accomplished non-verbally.

Argyle (1977) has suggested that non-verbal communication has three main functions:

1. Communicating interpersonal attitudes and emotions We tend to judge whether someone likes or dislikes us by subtle features of their non-verbal communication (although dislike is often deliberately concealed). In fact, when there is a mismatch between the verbal message and the non-verbal communication, the non-verbal communication often assumes more significance. For instance, a friendly message delivered with an unfriendly tone of voice and facial expression will usually be interpreted as unfriendly.

2. Supporting verbal communication The way something is said – the timing, pitch and stress patterns – provides punctuation and may change the meaning. Compare 'I *can't* wait for you' with 'I can't wait for *you*'. Gestures may also add to the meaning, for example pointing. Turntaking in conversation is regulated by a variety of non-verbal signals, such as gaze shifts, head nods and grunts. Non-verbal communication also enables us to obtain feedback about how others are responding to us. Are they in agreement, disagreement, bored, surprised etc.? This information is obtained chiefly from looking at others' faces, particularly the eyebrows and mouth. Attentiveness tends to be signalled by looking at the other person more when listening than when talking.

3. Replacing speech This may occur, for example, in a noisy environment such as a cafe or racecourse, or during a rescue action by the fire brigade. It may also be used where verbal communication is difficult because different languages are in use, e.g. the hand talk systems developed by native Indian peoples in America. It can also be a first language, as used by deaf people, such as the British Sign Language or Cantonese Sign Language.

Reader activity 15.1

Which methods of communication do you use most in your daily life? Which do you feel most at ease with and why? Many adults will have a preferred sensory modality, e.g. vision, hearing, touch: which is yours? How does this relate to people with learning disabilities whom you know?

DEVELOPMENT OF COMMUNICATION

Many studies have examined the fascinating process of how communication develops before speech (see, for example, Crystal (1984) for a general overview and Hewitt & Ephraim (1994) for a very detailed description of one mother–infant interaction and a framework for observations). In this section the aim is to highlight some of the crucial processes involved, rather than give a stage-by-stage account.

Babies' communication usually develops as a result of using all their senses and mental processes to make sense of environmental stimuli, and in the context of appropriate interaction with carers. The baby plays a very active role in this two-way process, to some extent controlling the interaction. To begin with, the baby's messages to his or her carers are unintentional, i.e. the result of physiological changes such as pain, hunger, boredom etc., but not deliberately intended to convey a given message. However, carers tend to respond as if the baby's cries or changes in facial expression do have a deliberate meaning. Gradually the baby learns that different behaviours result in different responses from the carers, and repeats them in anticipation of these responses. The baby is now beginning to send intentional messages, and to understand the nature of cause and effect and the sense of being a powerful and influential person. For instance, at around 9 months of age many babies begin to point to objects in order to draw attention to items and request them. This has an enormous impact on communication. Previously, carers could only guess at what the baby wanted, perhaps following his or her direction of gaze and trying to infer from that. Now, the baby is able to convey the object of intention very clearly and deliberately, and will often experiment by doing so repeatedly and imperiously! In many instances of early communication there is two-way turntaking, with the carer pausing to give the baby the opportunity to vocalise or gesture and being responsive to the baby, taking his or her lead and framing conversation around the baby's actions.

Non-verbal communication develops alongside and before the development of speech and language. It has been observed that new-born infants move in synchrony with the voices of people around them (Trevarthen 1977). These minute movements may not be readily observable or obvious to those around, but have been demonstrated by analysis of filmed sequences of interaction. Linked to this is the probability that hearing is the first sense to develop in utero, so that the baby is able to hear the sound of his or her mother's voice and environmental sounds, perhaps even before birth.

Young children continue to develop synchronous movements to their own speech and that of others, and this is particularly the case with hand movements. For example, first words are often accompanied by gestures, e.g. raised hand, palm facing upwards, accompanied by the word 'where?' The 'sign with your baby' system developed by Joseph Garcia (described by Crompton 2000) teaches sign language to parents of non-disabled babies in order to bridge the gap before speech develops, minimise frustration and accelerate language development. Research into sign use with children and adults with learning disabilities has similarly demonstrated that use of signs tends to facilitate, rather than inhibit, speech and language development (see Powell 1999 for a summary of current research findings).

Before speech develops an infant hears thousands and thousands of words a day, becoming very familiar with the sounds and speech patterns of his or her first language. Gradually, through familiar routines and activities, the infant begins to build up an understanding of familiar words in context; for example, he or she may appear to understand the word 'bath', but only in the context of the time of day, hearing and seeing the bathwater running and smelling the soap.

Understanding of words and concepts will continue to develop throughout the early years. Even when a child has developed a purely linguistic understanding of words independent of the overall context, there will be some situations where he or she will be continuing to work out the multiple meanings that words can have (for example the difference between a 'plug' in an electrical socket in the wall, as compared to the one in the sink). What appears to be a rapid acquisition of a first language is, in fact, underpinned by years of daily experience of being constantly exposed to that language before becoming a fully competent speaker.

These processes demonstrate the importance of two-way interaction in the development of communication, with each person being influenced by and taking their cues from the other. They are useful in considering how to facilitate communication with people with learning disabilities, although this should always be done in an age-appropriate way.

COMMUNICATING WITH PEOPLE WITH LEARNING DISABILITIES

This section highlights some of the general issues that are significant when devising strategies to communicate with people with learning disabilities.

Active involvement with others and the development of relationships

As outlined above, communication usually develops as part of a pleasurable, reciprocal, social process. For some people with learning disabilities, communication may not be enjoyable because they are ignored, bored or cannot see the value of or any results of their attempts to communicate. The process may also be too effortful or threatening: in some instances, for example, for some autistic people social interaction may be positively fear inducing.

Despite service aspirations towards community integration, most children and adults with learning disabilities are still segregated in special schools, day centres, special clubs and other organisations. Their experience of non-disabled people is usually in relation to receiving help and support, which can reinforce a sense of helplessness and power imbalance. Community participation is perhaps one of the most difficult of O'Brien's (1986) five service accomplishments to achieve.

A feature of many institutional settings is that service users may see themselves in a less active, less powerful role. For example, a study of non-disabled children in nurseries (Tizard et al 1972) found that staff speech to the children tended to be predominantly controlling (i.e. designed to begin, control or terminate activities) rather than conversational (designed to explain, give or ask for information). In a further study by Tizard & Hughes

(1984), it was noticeable that young children used a less complex language at school than at home. This seems to be related to the demands of a task-oriented situation (for example, utterances such as 'Where's the glue?' were typical at school, compared to more complex questioning at home, e.g. 'Why is the grass green?').

This preponderance of 'controlling speech' as compared to 'conversational speech' has similarly been demonstrated in settings for adults with learning disabilities (see, for example, Van der Gaag & Dormandy 1993).

Where children and adults are using sign or symbol systems to communicate, a repeated finding is that the non-disabled person tends to dominate the communication, initiating more frequently and taking more turns in the interaction (Basil 1992, Williams & Grove 1989).

For people who are dependent on others to meet their basic needs, routines may take over, so that there are few opportunities to communicate. Bruce (1993) gives examples of children with physical disabilities whose lack of opportunities for free-flow play contributed to reduced opportunities to learn and to communicate.

Children and adults with learning disabilities may inherently make fewer demands, either sending fewer messages or else messages which are not in a form carers can easily recognise, such as ambiguous gestures, or unintelligible sounds or words. If these attempts at communication meet with little success, they may decrease. The carer may attempt to compensate by speaking more, thus giving the person even less opportunity to communicate. This can become a vicious circle, with adverse effects on the person's motivation, confidence and use of skills. The effect on the person's self-esteem is thus likely to be very detrimental. This links to Wolfensberger's (1980) second core theme of normalisation: role expectancy and role circularity, i.e. low expectations tend to be self-fulfilling (see Ch. 3 for a fuller description and discussion).

In summary, in the reciprocal process of communication carers may dominate owing to the demands of the task, in an attempt to overcome communication difficulties or through devaluing the potential role of a person with learning disabilities in active communication. The person with learning disabilities may not behave in ways that are interesting to the carer, or readily understood. If communication is too fast (our average rate of speaking is around 250 words per minute) and there is insufficient time to respond, the person may give up. For example, if Leslie needs 80 seconds or so to begin to reply, but her carers typically repeat, rephrase or answer the question themselves after around 20 seconds, she will eventually conclude that there is little point in bothering.

So, what can be done? Some general principles are:

- Learn to take the person's lead. This may involve noticing small signals they make and acting upon them, e.g. eye movements in the direction of a desired item. Or it may involve picking up on what the person wants to talk about and finds important and interesting, such as a bereavement, someone else's epileptic fits, or aspects of family relationships.
- Monitor the amount of speech you use, compared to that of the children or adults you are communicating with. Do you dominate the conversation? Can the other person get a word in edgeways? The use of audiotape or video cassettes can be very helpful in encouraging you to be more objective about this, although sometimes painful to watch!
- Consider carefully the type of speech you use. Where does it come along the dimension 'control' as compared to 'conversational'? Once again, video or audio cassettes can be revealing. Try to make more use of comments that convey genuine information. Questions can be useful, particularly open-ended ones, if the person can understand them. Be aware, though, that too many questions can be controlling or confusing.
- Adapt the pace of your communication to suit the other person. Allow sufficient time for a response. This may feel uncomfortable if the person's pace is much slower than your own. However, it is possible to learn to do so and this method has been used to good effect in a structured way in 'expectant time delay' (see Kozleski 1991 for a fuller explanation).

- Try to create opportunities for the person to have contact with positive role models of other disabled people with communication difficulties, for example deaf people using sign language, images of Stephen Hawking, the book and film 'Annie's Coming Out' (Crossley & McDonald 1982), members of self-advocacy groups, videos/performances by theatre groups such as Strathcona, or the pop group Heart 'n' Soul, who are all people with learning disabilities.
- In community settings, try to ensure that the person with learning disabilities is included in conversation. For example, if members of the public address their questions and comments to you, re-direct them back to the person with learning disabilities. If the person does not use speech, explain to others how that person communicates. For example: 'This is Karen. She uses this book of pictures to say what she wants.'

Remember that out in the community, the way you communicate with someone with learning disabilities provides a role model for members of the public. They will take their lead from you!

Influencing the environment by exercising choice and being listened to

The range and type of daily choices, both large and small, is likely to be restricted for people with learning disabilities compared to others of a similar age. Given that a primary motivation to communicate is to make choices and influence what happens next, it is important to recognise nevertheless that exercising choice is a complex process. It involves the following:

- Awareness that choices are possible and available.
- The opportunity to make choices – this is easy to pre-empt because when someone has communication difficulties it may often be easier or quicker to choose for them, or to anticipate what they want. Halle et al (1981) described three levels of pre-empting:

1. Environmental: the desired item or activity is physically present or readily available, so there is no need to communicate in order to obtain it.
2. Non-verbal: the person's need is anticipated by others, who offer or provide it.
3. Verbal: that is, others notice the individual's likely need and verbally initiate or offer it before the person has a chance to express it themselves.

- Awareness or experience of what choice means. For instance, someone who has never been horse-riding or received a massage before may not be able to choose between the two, and is likely to need to experience the activities first.
- Understanding the consequences of choice, i.e. that if you make a choice, you may not like what you have chosen. For instance, if you choose 'four seasons' pizza in a restaurant, you're stuck with that choice, even if you don't like it! This element of learning by mistakes is important, and one that people with learning disabilities are often protected from.
- The constraints inherent in financial considerations or the impact of our choice on others. Given that people with learning disabilities are likely to be among the poorest people in society, their choices may be unduly constrained. Similarly, living in group settings with others may mean there are more rules and more compromises to be made.
- Assertiveness to carry through your choice and 'stick to your guns', even if others disagree with or dislike the choice you have made. This may be particularly difficult if choices are being suggested by a member of staff the person wants to please, and therefore they think they have to find the 'right' answer. This can also link to fluctuations in decision making.
- Having a means of expression to convey your choice. The person needs to have spoken, signed or symbol vocabulary which is understood by others and acted upon. With use of sign and symbol systems it is particularly important to try to select and teach initial vocabulary which corresponds to the individual's preferences. It can be very difficult to divorce yourself from your role in the person's

life and to consider what they might want to communicate about, rather than what would be helpful or convenient to you.
- Choosing from a range of alternatives that is within the person's memory and understanding, for example two or more concrete items which are physically present, rather than items or activities which are not present, or are more abstract.

Some strategies to facilitate choice making include:

- Consideration of the range and type of choices available: are there ways to extend this?
- Ensuring that the environment does not pre-empt the making of choices. The Intercom communication package developed by Jones (1990) provides an assessment and observation checklist together with a framework for planning to widen opportunities. It also provides useful suggestions to avoid pre-empting, based on the three levels mentioned by Halle et al (1981).
- Providing the person with spoken, signed or symbol vocabulary which is potentially reflective of their choices.
- Providing opportunities to develop assertiveness skills. This may be as basic as the opportunity to learn to use a sign or symbol for 'No', or it may be the chance to develop these skills through attendance at an assertiveness or self-advocacy group (see Crawley 1988, Downes 1996, Holland & Ward 1990, Weston & Went 1999 for examples of relevant approaches).

Knowing the person's current level of communication and starting from there

Careful observation will show that most people do communicate in some way, even if this is unintentional and their signals or messages are not readily understood by others. A key principle is to recognise that a person with learning and communication difficulties is often making his or her own best efforts to communicate, and to treat all behaviour as if meaningful.

For example, if the person enjoys flicking or twiddling string, one approach would be to sit some distance away and do similarly. Eventually the person may allow you to sit nearer and a possible dialogue may develop, with the pace, rhythm and timing of string flicking being influenced by one another. This is a type of mirroring, which is a key component of intensive interaction or augmented mothering (Hewitt & Ephraim 1994).

Another example is in a group movement to music activity, where each person is asked to contribute a movement for the others to copy. Someone who does not seem to understand or to deliberately suggest a movement may make one inadvertently, e.g. a knee jerk. This can then be copied by the others as if it was a genuine suggestion. Attention can also be drawn to what the individual has done and the fact that everyone is copying, so that over time the person may begin to gain more sense of cause and effect. Explicitly referring to what the person has done (e.g. 'Well done Kamal, you moved your knee') may be more useful in promoting this concept than generalised praise ('good, well done').

In situations where someone's behaviour is very ambiguous, it can be useful for carers to share their different perceptions about how the person is communicating. It may emerge that carers have very different views about a particular aspect of behaviour. For example, one may think a particular head movement indicates 'more', whereas another thinks it means 'no'. Viewed from the perspective of the person making the movement, the results can be very confusing because it is likely that different and potentially conflicting responses will be experienced. In this example, one carer is likely to give more food in response to this head movement, whereas the other is likely to remove it altogether.

As discussed earlier, given that communication usually develops intentionally through relatively consistent relationships and interaction with carers where consistent meaning is assigned to actions, it is important to try to establish this. If, in the absence of clear evidence of a particular meaning to a given signal, carers decide to treat it consistently as if it has one meaning, e.g. 'more', then over time it is possible that a degree of intentional communication may result. In effect, this method involves systematically over-interpreting the person's communication (Baumgart et al 1990, Campbell & Wilcox 1986).

It is important to consider that even difficult or challenging behaviour has a communicative function. There is a high incidence of communication difficulties among people regarded as having challenging behaviour (Mansell 1992, Bradshaw 1998). Challenging behaviour may be an attempt to communicate messages such as 'I'm hungry', 'I'd like a coke', 'My skin is itchy', 'I'm in pain', 'I don't want to do this'. The difficulty is that the form of the message may be very unclear, or it occurs in a form which is unacceptable or conflicts with the behaviour/tasks required in the context. Take, for example, Jyoti, who has no speech and does not use signs or symbols to communicate with. In the middle of a relaxation session she gets up and goes to the door. A member of staff walks after her, blocking the door and bringing her back to the main part of the room. Jyoti again gets up, this time grabbing the staff member's hand and putting it on the door handle. The staff member explains that it is time to relax and brings Jyoti back to her chair. This is repeated several times, until Jyoti scratches the worker's hand and slaps her on the side of the face. Jyoti's behaviour is now recorded in her file as being challenging and uncooperative in relaxation sessions. In fact, Jyoti might enjoy music but, because she has no way of drawing others' attention to anything other than items, which are physically present in the room, she has few means to indicate her needs. Her behaviour may be her best attempt to get her needs met, rather than a deliberate attempt to disrupt the relaxation session.

An alternative approach would be to allow Jyoti out of the room, accompanying her to see what she wants. For instance, she might want to go to the toilet, to get a drink or simply to walk up and down the corridor. The member of staff could then show Jyoti a sign for the desired object/activity, modelling it and prompting her to copy, if amenable. In this way, Jyoti might gradually begin to develop a small signed vocabulary for her everyday needs. Pictures or written symbols might facilitate this, as these rely on recognition rather than recall and so may be easier on the memory. Remember, in language development, how much repetition may be needed before someone can use a word or sign themselves. So, bear in mind that Jyoti will probably need to see the signs or symbols being used for quite some time before she can use them meaningfully herself.

Challenging behaviour may also be related to difficulties in understanding others' speech, and being confused by picking up only part of a message. Another contributory factor may be unrecognised hearing or visual difficulties or underestimation by carers of the impact of such additional difficulties (see later in the chapter).

Importance of culture and race

It is easy to overlook the cultural and racial background of someone with learning disabilities when it differs from that of the professionals involved.

There are likely to be misunderstandings and inaccuracies involved in assessing someone's speech and language in anything other than their first language. Assessments may use materials which are unfamiliar or offensive to someone on account of their religious or cultural background. The involvement of an interpreter and careful planning for how to work together is crucial to effective assessment. Although family members are frequently involved in this way, it is preferable to avoid this as there may be difficulties owing to family roles, status and conflicting interests. For instance, Amira was thought to have a severe communication difficulty. However, once an appropriate interpreter was found it emerged that she had much greater fluency in her first language and that the issue was more one of difficulty in learning a second language. She was also able to express strong ideas about the day and residential services she was receiving, in particular those aspects which conflicted with her religious and cultural views.

Some children and adults will have merged language development, i.e. through moving regularly between different cultures and communication systems, components from two languages may be used. For example, English words may be incorporated into Punjabi sentences, or the person may have some degree of fluency in both languages but the vocabulary in each may not overlap readily, so that interpretation or translation from one to the other is difficult. This is sometimes known as semilingualism.

It is both useful and courteous to learn to use a few words that occur frequently in the person's first language, and to encourage that person's peers to do so. Also, remember that non-verbal communication is linked to language and culture, and there may be different rules, for example about eye contact, and conventions about bodily proximity and touch. Gestures may have different meanings in different cultures. For instance, whereas in British culture a 'thumbs up' gesture is interpreted as having a positive meaning, for some Bengali-speaking people it may be interpreted as being quite rude.

Baxter et al (1990) have described in detail some issues connected to double discrimination for black people with learning disabilities, on account of both race and learning disability. They also provide some striking examples of some of the issues relating to communication.

General good practice guidelines include:

- Use materials which are appropriate to the person's culture, in both assessment and any subsequent work.
- Ensure that the environment contains a range of images which include people of different races in a variety of roles (this should be the case irrespective of the racial background of people using the service); this can encourage relaxed and relevant conversation.
- Learn some key words in the person's first language; encourage other colleagues and peers to do so.
- Use an interpreter for an assessment or other important meetings or appointments.
- Ensure that you understand some of the cultural and non-verbal rules of the person's first

 Reader activity 15.2

Imagine that you used a sign to convey something you wanted. You knew what it meant but no-one responded. How would you feel? How might you show these feelings?

language, to minimise misunderstandings. Avoid making assumptions about the person's preferences and customs based purely on culture. Find out from the person and their family, where possible.

Importance of sensory information

Information from all five senses is important in developing and maintaining communication skills. However, the main sensory channels related to communication are the distance senses of hearing and vision. Many people with learning disabilities have additional difficulties in communicating because of sensory disabilities. Clarke-Kehoe (1992) estimated that as many as 45% of people with severe and profound learning disabilities may have some kind of visual or hearing impairment. Sensory disabilities are also more common in elderly people. Approximately 34% of people aged over 60 have a significant hearing loss, which rises to approximately 74% in those aged over 70 (RNID 1990).

Screening tests of hearing among groups of people with learning disabilities reveal substantial underestimates of hearing loss by carers (Lavis et al 1997, Yeates 1995). So, there is a need generally to be aware of possible signs of hearing or visual impairment, and also to recognise that, as for the rest of the population, sensory disabilities may be more prevalent in people with learning disabilities as they age.

However, when someone has a learning disability, any other difficulties they experience can often be attributed by carers to the disability, rather than to any additional impairments. Heider (1958), in his attribution theory, described how we tend to explain people's behaviour in terms of one cause rather than multiple causes. If someone is described as having a learning disability, this will often take precedence over any other explanations of unusual behaviours or problems. For example, someone's lack of attention and concentration may be attributed to their learning disability rather than to the fact that they also have a hearing difficulty, or to the fact that they are becoming bored or irritable during mainly visual tasks because of a visual impairment. A person who

seems to be able to hear in some situations but not in others may be labelled as stubborn or unco-operative ('can hear when they want to'), but fluctuating hearing levels can be characteristic of some types of hearing loss. Someone who leans down to the table to eat may be regarded as having an unusual mannerism or poor posture, rather than a possible visual impairment.

In addition, some people with learning disabilities may spontaneously begin to compensate in ways which make a sensory disability less obvious to carers. For instance, someone with a hearing loss may attend more to the facial expressions, lip patterns and gestures of others. This may only become apparent if someone turns away or speaks to them from the next room. Someone with a visual impairment may avoid tasks involving small details, and may explore things more by touch.

Often, no allowances are made for sensory disability unless it has actually been diagnosed. This may mean that unrealistic expectations are placed on people. It is important not to assume that people with learning disabilities have good vision or hearing. Some conditions related to learning disabilities are so closely associated with sensory disability that extra vigilance is recommended on these grounds alone; for example, a great many people with Down syndrome have hearing loss, and there are strong links between rubella damage and hearing or visual loss, or both. It is important that nurses be aware of and vigilant for possible signs of sensory disability. (The Royal National Institute for Blind People produces very detailed fact sheets, containing checklists with possible signs to consider: see also Boxes 15.1 and 15.2.)

Thorough professional assessment is needed where there is any suspicion of sensory disability. Audiological or ophthalmological services for children are available through GPs or the school medical service. However, there are often difficulties in obtaining adequate assessment for adults. Staff in audiological or ophthalmological services for adults may not feel sufficiently skilled in assessing people with learning disabilities, or may be reluctant to see them at all, regarding the process as too time consuming or not beneficial for someone with learning disabilities. However, the learning disability makes it even more important to obtain an accurate idea about a person's sensory abilities. As mentioned earlier, some people with learning disabilities may spontaneously attempt to compensate by using their other senses more fully. However, others may have great difficulty in adapting and learning new skills, and so extra help is vital. In such situations, it may be that one of the roles of the nurse, social worker or other professional is to persist in asking

---

Box 15.1 Behaviour or features which may indicate a hearing impairment

- Pulling, poking or rubbing the ears
- Watching the speaker's face and lips constantly
- Tilting the head to one side, towards the speaker or source of sound
- Appearing to hear on some occasions but not others (this may be due to a fluctuating hearing loss, or the fact that some voices may be easier to hear than others; some acoustic conditions are also more favourable than others)
- Speaking very loudly (typical of a sensorineural hearing loss, where people raise the voice so it is audible to themselves)
- Speaking very softly (typical of a conductive hearing loss, where people may match their own voices to the level at which they hear others' voices)
- Dislike of loud sounds (this may be due to recruitment, where people have a reduced range between the point where they can just hear sounds and the point where sound is perceived as unbearably loud)
- Appearing startled when someone approaches
- Visible signs of discharge from the ears, or excessive wax

Box 15.2 Behaviour or features which may indicate a visual impairment

- Poking or rubbing the eyes
- Exploring items by touch
- Not appearing to notice people or things unless they are very close; needing to examine things at close quarters
- Reluctance to move around, especially when in new places
- Reluctance to look for/search for things visually
- Appearing startled when someone approaches
- Dislike of predominantly visual tasks/reluctance to engage in such tasks
- Visible signs of eye pathology, for example inflammation, swelling

---

for hearing or visual assessment, acting as an advocate on the person's behalf.

Most methods of visual and hearing assessment require a degree of cooperation, understanding and response from the individual. However, if materials are presented at an appropriate level and pace, many people with learning disabilities can respond reliably. Again, there is a role for someone who knows the person to give support by attending the appointment, reassuring the person and working with specialists in the clinic to ensure that the person understands what is required.

The effects of such impairment on the person will vary according to:

- Age of onset: If the person has had the experience of seeing and hearing this will have helped them learn to communicate. An acquired sensory loss means the person has to adjust to taking in information in new ways.
- Severity of impairment: In general, the more severe the impairment the more marked the probable impact on the person.
- The type of visual or hearing loss: Sensory impairments are not an all-or-nothing matter. Most people described as 'blind' or 'deaf' will have some usable vision (e.g. for light or dark perception) or hearing (e.g. for some sounds, for example bass tones). Some types of hearing loss, e.g. conductive (arising in the outer or middle ear) involve general distortion and loss of volume. Sensorineural hearing loss (arising in the cochlea or auditory nerve) involves distortion of particular pitches of sound.
- Whether one or both senses are involved: It will be more difficult to make sense of the world and to communicate if both vision and hearing are affected.
- The person's ability to compensate: This may be partly related to the person's level of cognitive ability. The more severe the learning disability, the more difficult it may be to adapt to learning new skills.

Assisting people with hearing impairment

If someone has had an audiological assessment and a hearing aid is recommended, nurses and

Reader activity 15.3

Consider how many of the people with learning disabilities you know have a visual or hearing impairment. If the numbers are very low and do not correspond to those mentioned in this chapter, could this be due to lack of assessment/awareness of possible signs of impaired hearing or vision? Are you aware of possible indicators of sensory impairment? What facilities exist in your locality for assessment?

Can you build up positive links with staff in audiological and ophthalmological services to facilitate cooperative working? This is especially important if you are undertaking a programme of study to become a learning disability nurse as you will more than likely be working as a health facilitator for people with learning disabilities.

carers will have a vital role to play in helping the person to use it. Unfortunately, a hearing aid does not restore hearing to 'normal', and so it may take a long time for the person to adjust to it. The hearing aid will amplify sounds non-selectively, not just speech, and all sounds may appear particularly distorted in noisy places, such as on public transport, in the canteen or in the street. Advances in technology mean that it is likely that there will be more digital hearing aids in the future. These can amplify sounds more effectively, reducing distortion and possibly making it more likely that individuals will be able to adjust to hearing aids more readily and therefore benefit from them.

It is important to introduce the hearing aid to the person gradually and, in order to do this, nurses and carers themselves need to be familiar with the components of the aid, how it works and basic maintenance.

There are three main types of hearing aid:

- body worn
- behind the ear, or postaural
- all in the ear.

Generally, body-worn hearing aids are used by people with severe hearing loss who need more powerful amplification. They are sometimes used by disabled or elderly people with arthritis, who may find the control switches of a behind-the-ear aid difficult to operate. All-in-the-ear aids are pre-

dominantly used by people with very mild hearing loss. The most frequently used are behind-the-ear aids (Fig. 15.1).

The main components of a hearing aid are:

- The microphone: This picks up the sound and therefore needs to be kept free from dirt or other debris.
- The control switch: This usually has three settings: O = off; T = transduction loop; M = microphone; this is the 'on' switch. The transduction loop setting can be used in environments which have an induction loop. By using this switch, the person will be able to hear the important sounds by radio link, without the interference of background noise. Induction loops are available in some public buildings, such as theatres, cinemas or churches. They can also be fitted in an individual's home, to assist with hearing the television.
- Volume control wheel: This will need to be adjusted to the optimum level for the person, as advised by the audiologist. However, it is likely to need adjusting in different circumstances, for example turned down in a noisy environment. Some volume control wheels are numbered, others are not, and it can be useful to mark the optimum level with a spot of Tippex for easy reference.

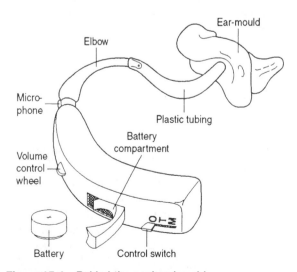

Figure 15.1 Behind-the-ear hearing aid.

- Battery compartment: This flicks open to allow easy changing of the batteries. It is essential that the battery is inserted the right way round, with the '+' side on the battery aligned with the '+' mark on the battery compartment. Batteries last a variable time, depending on the amount of use. They should be retained and returned for exchange to the audiology department or, in some cases, local health clinics maintain battery supplies.
- Plastic tubing: Amplified sound is relayed from the aid to the earmould via this tube. It needs to be cleaned regularly and replaced if distorted or cracked.
- Earmould: This relays sound to the person's ear and is individually made for him or her. Again, this needs to be cleaned regularly (after disconnection from the hearing aid) and inspected for obvious signs of damage. It is important that it is a good fit.

The person will need to be introduced to the aid gradually, as it may be difficult to explain the potential benefits beforehand. It may be useful to prepare the person for having something in or around the ears by using sunglasses or personal stereo earphones for a while. Initially the aid should be worn for short periods in a quiet room with good acoustics, preferably during an enjoyable activity. Tolerance to wearing the aid for longer periods and in a variety of settings can be developed gradually. It can be helpful to teach the person, early on, how to take the aid out, so that they have some feeling of control (Ferris-Taylor & Pinney 1994).

Tips for communication Irrespective of whether the person uses a hearing aid or not, the following points are important to remember when talking to someone with a hearing loss:

- Ensure that you have the person's attention, and that the person is looking at you before you start talking, so that lip-reading and your facial expression can help communication.
- Ensure your face can be seen clearly. If possible, face the window so the light is shining on your face and not in the eyes of the person you are talking to.
- Slow your speech – this generally makes it clearer.

- Use reasonable volume but do not shout.
- Avoid exaggerating your lip patterns – this will distort the natural rhythms and visible patterns of speech.
- As far as possible, cut out any background noise such as TV, running water etc.
- Get reasonably close to the person. If a hearing aid is used, the optimum distance apart is approximately 3 feet; beyond that, background noise will sound as loud as speech.
- Be aware that group settings will be more difficult for the person, particularly where there are rapid changes of topic or speaker.
- Ensure that the person has had a recent opthalmological assessment; when someone has a hearing impairment it is all the more important to know about that person's visual acuity. Encourage the use of spectacles, where appropriate.
- Use your facial expression, body language, and gestures and signs from the Makaton vocabulary to back up what you say.

Assisting people with visual impairment

As with hearing impairment, it is important to establish the degree and type of visual impairment. For instance, very few blind people have no useful vision at all. Types of visual impairment vary, for instance tunnel vision compared to peripheral vision. It is important to be aware that the nature of the visual impairment may mean that the person behaves in ways which can easily be misunderstood. For instance, people who have some peripheral vision may turn their heads to one side in order to maximise the vision they have. This can easily be incorrectly interpreted as ignoring or avoiding the other person. It may also, for similar reasons, be difficult to establish eye contact with the person.

It is crucial to help people with visual impairment make best use of whatever vision they have. If they wear spectacles these need to be cleaned regularly and checked for comfort, for example, do the spectacles rub the bridge of the nose or behind the ears? Lighting needs consideration, and the source should be from behind the person so that glare is avoided. Magnifying aids may be useful; advice may be obtained from the social services visual impairment team regarding such equipment and aids for the home, such as talking clocks.

Remember too that there are sometimes medical solutions. For example, in recent years some adults with learning disabilities have had successful cataract operations which previously may not have been readily available due to possible discrimination in allocation of resources within the health service. Some people with Down syndrome have keratoconus, a rare eye condition which makes the front of the eye bulge. This may be helped by contact lenses or a graft from a donated cornea. However, these options are rarely offered to people with learning disabilities. Such issues are now being debated more widely and openly with medical staff (Levy 2000).

There is a need to use more verbal cues to alert the person to what is happening and to explain what and who is present. The person will need more time to explore objects by touch. For example, a sighted person is able to gather information quickly by rapid visual scanning. A blind or partially sighted person will need much more time to become familiar with the location of objects in the room, and to explore them by touch. For a person with severe learning disabilities, understanding of everyday objects and the words used to denote them may be very difficult. Items such as cups may have very different properties, such as size, texture, shape, or the presence or absence of handles. Sighted people will have seen many, many examples of different cups, but blind people will only have experience of the ones they have actually touched. Some items may be very difficult to comprehend as a whole by touch; Rudyard Kipling wrote a poem about three blind men each touching different parts of an elephant, and each having a completely different idea of what the animal was.

It is not automatically the case that blind or partially sighted people will make maximum use of their other senses. Some people may be tactile defensive, i.e. fearful of touch and liable to avoid or withdraw from it. Tolerance will need to be built up gradually in predictable situations. The use of massage can be helpful and enjoyable, and the interactive massage sequence (Sanderson & Harrison 1992) can be used as a guide to progress, working from passive to more interactive communication.

Smells can be used systematically to alert the person to different activities and events in the day. Consistent use of the same toiletries can also help the person to identify different nurses or carers. Similarly, a tactile reference, such as encouraging the person to feel your ring, bracelet, watch or wristband, can assist with this.

It is important that carers know how to guide a blind person from one place to another. Useful leaflets are available on this topic from both the Royal National Institute for the Blind and Action for Blind People: see 'Useful Addresses' at the end of this chapter.

Tips for communication General points for communicating with a blind or partially sighted person include the following:

- Use your speech to supplement for non-verbal cues which the person will be missing out on. For example, use the person's name, especially when first beginning to talk. Indicate that you are listening by saying 'Yes', 'Mmmm', 'I agree' etc., rather as you do during a telephone conversation. In a group, encourage people to say who they are each time they talk. If others are pointing to something or using facial expressions which are particularly important, then describe what is happening. Tell the person who is coming into the room or leaving, or what is about to happen, e.g. 'I'm going to get your dinner'.
- Use language carefully where directional words are concerned, for example 'It's over there' is not very helpful, whereas 'The box is next to the table' may be. Words such as 'look' or 'see' do not necessarily need to be avoided, as the person may have residual vision, but it may be more appropriate to use alternatives such as 'touch' or 'find'.
- Try to help people understand the meaning of what you are saying by encouraging them to feel the object, or by demonstrating the appropriate action.
- If it is appropriate to use signs or symbols as a means of communication, these will need to be

adapted. For example, signs which are made out in space in front of the person's body will not be perceived or understood, but can be adapted so that they give more contact and feedback to the person. 'Hands-on' approaches to teaching signing are often used, i.e. taking the person's hand and physically guiding them through the sign. Symbols will need to be enlarged, presented in bold colour contrasts or using raised materials (Best 1987, Bradley & Snow, undated, Lee & MacWilliam 1996).

- Additional tactile means of conveying information should be considered if appropriate, for example, Braille or Moon.

Braille represents letters of the alphabet by a matrix of six raised dots, each composed in different configurations. It therefore requires good language and tactile skills. Moon is simpler, consisting of raised letters based on the written alphabet. For both systems the person will need existing literacy skills or the ability to develop them. Advice can be obtained from local services for blind and visually impaired people. Carers will need to learn the system too.

Dual sensory losses

Where the person has a dual sensory impairment, or a profound and multiple disability accompanied by visual or hearing impairment, then specialist advice should be sought from organisations such as Sense, the national deaf–blind organisation (see also Ch. 17).

SPECIFIC ISSUES REGARDING INDIVIDUAL COMMUNICATION

Gaining an accurate idea of the person's comprehension of language

It can be difficult to work out how much someone with learning disabilities can understand of what we say. Although in many instances we tend to assume that understanding and expression are on roughly equivalent levels, this is not always the case.

Judging people's understanding by their ability to express themselves may lead to jumping to false conclusions. Some people may have relatively good understanding but little or no speech. This could lead to underestimating their understanding (think of any experiences you have had of learning another language and being at the stage where you can understand more than you are able to say). Conversely, some people with learning disabilities appear to be able to express themselves fairly well. This may lead to overestimating their understanding. (Once again, think of learning a new skill, such as computing, where you may have begun to use some of the jargon but do not fully understand it.)

Sometimes it may be very obvious when people have not understood what we say. However, often they may understand the total situation rather than what is actually said, and so respond appropriately. To take a simple example, you might say 'Go and get your dinner', but an appropriate response might be caused by a variety of factors other than understanding the language used. Consider the other cues in the situation: the person may know from routine that it is dinnertime (and may be hungry), and may see others going towards the dining room. Possibly you are gesturing and propelling her towards the dining room, and maybe she can smell the food. On a verbal level, she only really has to grasp one word, 'dinner'. So a variety of cues are available – time related, visual and olfactory – and the verbal message is only one part of the situation. All these additional cues may be needed, but lack of clarity about how much language is understood may lead to unrealistic expectations and instructions later on.

It is important to try to find out how much language is understood independently of other cues, in order to consider:

- how to talk to someone appropriately in general conversation, when communicating important information and when teaching new skills
- whether someone needs additional cues, such as signs, pictures or symbols, to help in understanding others' communication. (Pictures, symbols or signs are not just a means for self-expression, but can also be aids to understanding, since they often have a more obvious link to the underlying idea than do words. For example,

the sign for 'tea' or a drawing of it has a more obvious link to this drink than the spoken word)

- why any inappropriate responses or challenging behaviour are occurring. Is it because of boredom or an uncooperative attitude etc., or is it because of lack of understanding of what is required?

There are various methods which speech and language therapists can use to assess a person's understanding of speech. Most of these involve structured ways to experiment with the amount of non-verbal cues used, and setting up situations that involve purely linguistic understanding. The Derbyshire Language Scheme provides a useful framework for assessing the number of information-carrying words a person can understand at a time. The assessment methods and suggested development activities can be adapted for use with adults. A recent study by Bartlett & Bunning (1997) found that it may be more difficult to adapt speech to the level of understanding of the person with learning disabilities in free conversation than in more structured activities, e.g. looking at pictures, where the topic is more concrete. Use of Makaton signs and symbols may be helpful in ensuring that conversation is understood.

Factors which may make language difficult to understand include:

- Vocabulary: there are many different words which can be used to say the same thing; for example the same drink could be referred to by various people as squash, pop, fizz, juice or a brand name. Tidying up could be referred to as clearing things up, cleaning up, or sorting out the mess! Conversely, some words may have a range of different meanings, for example 'my hand', compared to 'give me a hand' or 'hand me a cup'. Words may also be used metaphorically, in a way which may be confusing or taken literally by people with learning disabilities, for example 'skating on thin ice' or 'Don't fly off the handle!'
- Understanding of words may be linked to particular contexts or experiences. For instance, one disabled child who was asked if she would like to go to the theatre declined the offer and appeared quite fearful. It emerged that her main

experience of the theatre was the operating theatre, because of a persistent illness.

- Crystal (1987) has discussed how vocabulary is acquired according to its relevance to the individual. For example, it might be assumed that a child would learn vocabulary related to bodily parts in a fairly predictable sequence. However, if children have had unusual experiences or illness, they may have acquired some surprisingly complex or detailed vocabulary. Similarly, adults with learning disabilities may have acquired some complex vocabulary in relation to the rest of their communication, owing to experiences such as blood transfusions.
- Complexity of ideas: for example, words connected to time may be difficult to understand because the underlying concept is very abstract, e.g. tomorrow, yesterday, next week. This can lead to the person repeatedly asking the same question, such as 'When's my sister coming?' Ways to make this clearer might revolve around having a diary, simple Filofax or chart, where the keyworker can draw pictures or symbols to indicate when things will be happening. It can be helpful for this to be compiled with the person on a daily basis, or to have see-through pockets or Velcro on the back of the symbols or pictures. In this way it is possible to remove any items or activities which will not be happening on that particular day, and so avoid potential confusion.
- Sentence construction: some features of sentence construction can be especially difficult. For example, negatives can be embedded in sentences in a variety of ways: 'There's no bread'; 'There isn't any bread'; 'There's no more bread'. These can be easily missed so that the person thinks the sentence has the opposite meaning to that intended by the speaker. This can lead to confusion, where, for example, the person repeatedly hears the word bread but still does not receive any. In the case of an instruction the person may appear deliberately to do the opposite, having misunderstood what was said.
- Sentence length: the person may understand the individual components of the sentence but have difficulty assimilating the whole: 'Please

may I borrow your knife to cut my orange?' is a polite, reasonable and explanatory request, but the person may repeatedly proffer an orange, since it is the last-named thing.

Tips to ensure you are understood

- Address people by name and ensure you have their attention, visually if you are using signs or symbols to communicate.
- Aim to be consistent in the vocabulary you use yourself, and also check to see if this is the same vocabulary used by the other carers involved with the person. Note important points in the care plan to assist with this.
- Use short, simple sentences, making sure that these are still age appropriate in style.
- Ensure that you talk to the person frequently – language is learnt through repetition. Even where someone is unable to respond verbally, there may be understanding of what is said or, if not, general responsiveness to tones of voice.
- Do not overwhelm the person with too much at a time. Where an instruction has several parts, break it down into several sentences as necessary: for example, instead of 'Go and bring the eggs, butter and flour and put them in a bowl', the request could be broken down as follows: 'Bring the eggs' 'Now bring the butter; great' 'Bring the flour' 'Please put them in the bowl'.
- Avoid complex sentence structures such as negatives and complex time dimensions.
- Judge pace carefully. Speak slowly and give the person time to respond, as necessary.
- Supplement what you say with gestures and other cues. Be aware that some people find apparently simple gestures difficult to understand: for example, pointing may be ambiguous. Head nods and shakes may be difficult for some people to distinguish, and they do not always have the same meanings across cultures.

Alternative and augmentative communication systems

When someone has no speech, has speech which is difficult to understand and/or finds it difficult to understand other people's speech, it may be helpful to use an alternative or augmentative communication system. 'Alternative' refers to the possibility that it may be used by the person as an alternative to speech; 'augmentative' means it may be used to support (or augment) any existing speech or other means of communication. This is likely to involve either signs or symbols, or a combination of both.

Systems which use signs are sometimes referred to as manual or unaided systems, since they involve using the hands and no other equipment. Systems which use symbols are sometimes referred to as graphic or aided systems, since they involve drawing or writing, which may be displayed on a chart, book or computer VDU. Regardless of the system, the overall aim is to help the person communicate in everyday circumstances, and for those in contact with the person to be able to communicate back.

The Makaton vocabulary

One of the most widely used methods for people with learning disabilities is the Makaton Vocabulary Language Programme, which involves the use of signs, symbols and speech. It was originally designed to meet the needs of people with learning disabilities who also had a hearing loss and were living in a hospital. Designed by Margaret Walker in the early 1970s, it is now used with both adults and children with learning disabilities whose communication difficulties may be related to a variety of factors, not just hearing loss. It has also been used with some people who have communication problems unrelated to learning difficulties, e.g. after a 'stroke' (see Grove & Walker 1990 for a full description).

The Makaton vocabulary was revised and updated in 1996, to take account of community living, multi-cultural issues and technological advances and to include a selection of grammatical items. It now consists of a core vocabulary of 450 words, signs and symbols, with an additional resource vocabulary of approximately 7000. The signs are derived from British Sign Language (BSL) for deaf people, but have been standardised, i.e. the dialectical variations in signs, which are a striking feature of BSL, have been eliminated to avoid possible confusion for people with learning disabilities and their carers. The symbols have been designed by the Makaton Vocabulary Development Project and are similar to Rebus (originally a reading scheme using symbols, now also used as a primary means of communication).

Makaton has been adapted for use in 40 other countries. In these instances, cultural changes are made to the words used in the core vocabulary. Signs from that country's sign language are used. Although the symbols are more universal, occasional changes are also made to the symbols, for cultural reasons.

The Makaton core vocabulary is designed to be used flexibly according to need. It is grouped into eight stages, which serve as a guideline for teaching everyday essential vocabulary in a meaningful sequence, progressing from simple to more abstract concepts. For example, in Stage 1 everyday ideas such as 'bus', 'cup', 'I', 'you', 'where' and 'what' occur, while in Stage 7 more abstract ideas, such as 'late', 'early', 'how much' and 'how many' are included. However, an important feature is personalisation of the vocabulary to suit individual needs, i.e. at each stage vocabulary should be selected which is relevant to the individual in terms of their interests, daily activities and environment. This can be very convenient for learning disability nurses, as well as other nurses who work with people with mental health problems or children with learning disabilities, or for adult nurses who may care for people with learning disabilities during acute or chronic illness. Also other carers will find it convenient because it means that it is possible to learn a variety of useful signs and then adapt the precise selection according to the needs of the individual. It is important that everyone who knows the person is kept updated about the signs they use. There have been recent debates about the processes involved in selecting vocabulary for inclusion in sign and symbol systems and whether these should be nationally or locally based (Graves 2000). However, there are pragmatic issues for practitioners in using a widely known system which can be personalised for individual use and yet will be transferable if the person moves from one area to another (and from children's to adult services).

One of the important features of Makaton is economy of use, i.e. building up from teaching a small selection of important everyday concepts and expanding where necessary. Normal grammatical speech should be used by nurses and other carers, although generally only key words are signed. The additional resource vocabulary, which is grouped into topic areas (e.g. sexuality, emotions and relationships, the early attainment targets of the national curriculum, fire and its hazards), contains concepts which can be introduced as necessary. The national curriculum resource also contains many additional grammatical items which can be introduced if needed.

Another key aspect is that Makaton offers the opportunity for multimodal communication. Symbols can be used in the following ways:

- As a basic means of communication for learning-disabled people who have an additional physical disability. They can be mounted on a chart, in a book or on computer, so that the person can indicate choices.
- To assist with learning language. Since symbols provide a more permanent message than either speech or signs, they may help those with memory difficulties. They can be used to help build up language structure.
- To help with understanding of the written word (by being paired with it) or as a means in itself of 'writing' notes, shopping lists, instructions, postcards etc. The symbols are designed to be simple and quick to draw by hand. Some organisations have started to use Makaton symbols in everyday life, to promote better access for people who cannot read. For example, the Benefits Agency has leaflets translated into Makaton symbols to explain eligibility to receive benefit and how to make an application. The London Transport Museum has notices and worksheets translated into symbols. Frimley Park Hospital in Surrey uses symbols plus written words on outpatient department notices.
- As an additional means of communication, to give flexibility so that people can select their preferred mode or vary the mode according to circumstances (in the same way that we do in our own communication). Autistic people may

prefer symbols because of their concrete nature, which allows repeated examination over time and the likelihood that using symbols involves less intense interaction with others (Mirenda & Schuler 1988).

British Sign Language (BSL)

This is a language in its own right and is used mainly by children and adults who are born deaf. It cannot therefore be accurately described as an alternative or augmentative communication system. It has its own structure and word order, which differ from that of spoken English, and it is not generally used with speech (see Miles 1988 for a description). Some profoundly deaf people with mild learning disabilities may use BSL. If so, it is important that others learn to use it and that the person has contact with other BSL users via the deaf community.

Signed English

This was developed as a means of encouraging reading, writing and spoken English among deaf children, and is based on signs from British Sign Language. For this reason, it is used with speech and follows English word order and structure. Every word in a sentence is signed, and additional signs are devised to convey the grammatical elements of spoken English. Signed English may be used by people with learning disabilities.

Paget–Gorman Sign System

This was devised to represent all the elements of spoken English. As in Signed English, all the words in the sentence are signed. There are precise rules about how to produce the signs, which require very fine coordination. Although in the past the Paget–Gorman Sign System was used with people with learning disabilities, it is now used chiefly with children with specific language disorders.

Blissymbols

These were originally devised in the 1940s by Charles Bliss, with the intention of being an inter-national graphic language. During the 1970s they were adapted for use as a communication system for non-speaking people with cerebral palsy. The symbols are composed of nine abstract geometric shapes of differing sizes and orientation, which represent different meanings when combined. The written word is always used with the symbol. Because of their complexity, both visually and conceptually, they are often thought to be too complicated for people with learning disabilities

Picture Communication System (PCS)

This is a set of symbols devised in the USA by Mayer Johnson. The system comprises 3160 symbols, developed to provide a communication aid using simple drawings with or without words, which can be produced in colour.

Compic

This symbol system originates from Australia and has recently been introduced into the UK. It consists of 1670 black and white pictograms based on international symbol style.

Picture charts

These can be developed on an ad hoc basis, according to the needs of the individual. Pictures or photographs can be used, based on things within the person's experience. Although these have the advantage of being easy to understand, provided the person has sufficient symbolic understanding to comprehend pictures, there is the disadvantage that it is difficult to convey abstract ideas.

Picture Exchange Communication System (PECS)

This is a training method rather than a symbol system, designed to be used with autistic children. It is a systematic way of teaching a child to approach others and give them a picture of a wanted item in exchange for it, so that the child begins to understand the purpose of communication. PECS can be used with pictures or any of the symbol systems described above.

Tangible symbols

These are manipulable symbols with raised, tactile features which bear a close perceptual relationship to the item they represent. They can be very useful for people who are not able to understand abstract symbol systems. They will need to be individually developed for each person who needs them (Clark-Kehoe 1992, Rowland & Schweigert 1989).

Objects of reference

These are similar to tangible symbols and may be very useful to help orientate a person with severe learning disabilities and additional sensory impairments. Objects are used in a systematic way to help the person understand and begin to anticipate what is happening next, for example a swimming costume and towel to indicate swimming, or a spoon to indicate kitchen. Gradually, once the person has understood this link, the object could be made more symbolic, for example a small piece of towel instead of the whole towel. People could also be encouraged to use the items to communicate their own wishes.

Rebus

These simple symbols were originally derived from a reading scheme (the Peabody Rebus Scheme) and adapted for use as a communication tool. The original reading scheme contained many verbal puns (e.g. a picture of a tin can to represent the verb 'can'). Although these are amusing for children learning to read, they may be very confusing to people with learning disabilities. These puns have been deleted from the use of Rebus symbols as a communication system. The symbols are arranged alphabetically in a dictionary, so that they can easily be selected by professionals and carers (Devereux & Van Oosterum 1985).

Facilitated communication

This method was originally used with people with physical and communication disabilities, but has also been used with people with autism. Specially trained facilitators use emotional and physical support to enable the person to use communication boards. Although there have been enthusiastic reports of success (e.g. Scrivener 1993), many of the claims have not been upheld by objective research (see Howlin 1994 for a summary).

Why might signs and symbols facilitate communication?

Possible reasons include:

- The nature of signs and symbols: words are very fleeting, whereas signs can be held still long enough for the individual to process them. Symbols are even more permanent.
- The visual nature of signs and symbols: many people with learning disabilities show a preference for visuospatial information. Therefore, this information may be easier for some people to process than spoken language, which relies on auditory vocal processing.
- The iconic nature of some signs and symbols may assist in learning the sign and, ultimately, the corresponding word. 'Iconicity' means the strength of association between the sign and the idea it represents. For example, the sign for 'cup' gives more links to the corresponding idea than the word, which is arbitrary.
- The motivational nature of a sign may make it easier to learn. Although iconicity is likely to be an important factor, a person with learning disabilities may learn a less iconic sign such as 'biscuit', from the Makaton vocabulary, relatively easily if this represents something they enjoy and want (see Powell 1999 for a fuller discussion).

Important considerations

Choice of system It is important to obtain a thorough assessment of the individual's communication skills and professional advice about the most appropriate method to use. There are various guidelines which include issues to consider in system selection (Allen 1989, Walker & Ferris-Taylor 1991).

Individual preferences Owing to the nature of the communication difficulty it may not be possible to involve the person in choosing the system. This makes it important to take into account any apparent preferences (e.g. like or dislike of using gesture or pictorial materials), both at the outset and once the system is in use.

Training It is important that everyone who uses the system on a regular basis feels confident about using it. Some methods, such as Makaton, offer a range of formal and informal courses tailored to meet different needs.

Real-life use The success of any method of communication depends upon the extent to which it is used by the person concerned and everyone else. Often, practice is sufficient to enable carers to feel comfortable using it, both indoors and outdoors.

Although training is crucial, everyday use may be facilitated by memory joggers and sufficient repetition, so that use becomes automatic rather than consciously thought out. Some establishments have adopted a 'signs of the week' approach, where the emphasis is on gradual practice/relearning of a few signs each week, with one staff member taking responsibility for teaching others a small number of signs as selected and prioritised by the staff group (Spragale & Micucci 1990).

Real-life use can also be encouraged by the extent to which signs and symbols are available in everyday settings. See, for example, the Hull and Holderness NHS Trust *Patient's Charter*. (Fig. 15.2).

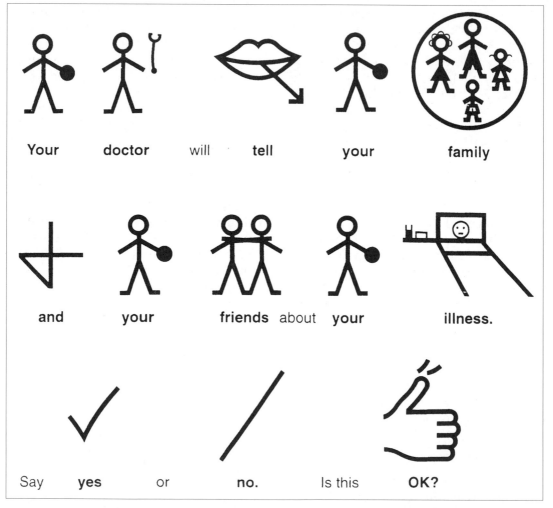

Figure 15.2 Examples of Makaton symbols from the Hull and Holderness NHS Trust Patient's Charter (with permission from the Makaton Vocabulary Development Project).

Given the wide range of carers who may come into contact with those with learning difficulties, it is important to have convenient and effective ways to pass on information about their methods of communication. Personal 'passports' have been used with deaf–blind people and their carers. Caldwell et al (1995) have described these as 'a booklet which described in a human way everything a carer needed to know about the person and, in particular, his or her unique style of communicating with others'.

Individualised use The person's coordination, vision or visual perception may mean that symbols or signs are used in ways which carers need to 'tune in to'. For example, someone using a communication board or chart may access the board in a variety of ways, such as pointing with the finger or fist, or eye pointing. Particularly where eye pointing is concerned, carers will need to take time to adjust and respond.

Many people with learning disabilities will produce Makaton signs which are very unlike the standardised versions taught in workshops and reproduced in booklets. This may be due to factors outlined above. However, it may also be a component of learning signs, analogous to the phonological processes involved in learning speech (Dunn-Klein 1988). It is useful to analyse the person's sign production, looking for patterns or themes rather than just thinking it is 'wrong'.

Makaton can be adapted for one-handed use. It has also been used with people with visual impairments, once again with adaptations to maximise the use of kinaesthetic and tactile features of signs (Mountain 1984). The symbols can be adapted in size or made tangible for students with visual disabilities.

Making best use of a system Using a sign or symbol system will not, in itself, automatically solve all communication difficulties. It is important to bear in mind the principles of positive communication contained throughout this chapter. The following points are particularly important:

- Help the person understand and use the system; they may not automatically understand the meaning of the signs and symbols without clear links being made. They also may not understand the principle that the signs or symbols can convey ideas and help them to express their wishes. This may need to be demonstrated.

- Provide reasons to communicate and opportunities to do so, in the context of pleasurable social activities. If it is difficult to ascertain the person's preferred activities then it is important to spend more time observing and noting preferences and, where necessary, providing the opportunity for a wider range of activities.

- Use the system in everyday life yourself. People will need to see others communicating with signs or symbols in order to recognise that this is an acceptable and valued means of communication. Also, in order to extend skills, they need to see a model of sign or symbol use which is a little beyond their own capacity. Some research has suggested that individuals tend to use signs most in the presence of interactors who use them too (Grove & McDougall 1988, 1989).

- Encourage friends and peers to use the signs and symbols. Effective Makaton peer tutoring courses have been developed, where people with learning disabilities can learn to teach others to use Makaton. There have been exciting developments in the use of peer tutoring, which can involve social and linguistic gains for both tutors and their peers (Hooper & Bowler 1991, Hooper & Newnham 1994) (see Figs. 15.3–15.5). In one inner London Health Trust, peer tutors have been employed as part of a team, teaching signs to peers with communication disabilities as well as to staff and medical students (Ambalu & McClean 1995).

Expression

Speech

Speech is the spoken output of the language system. It involves the movements we make with our lips, tongue, jaws, teeth and hard and soft palates. The energy source comes from air via the lungs activating the vocal folds in the larynx.

Speech involves the fastest movements and the finest coordination of any part of our body. As an example, think of what you are doing when you produce an 's' sound. Your tongue is raised to the

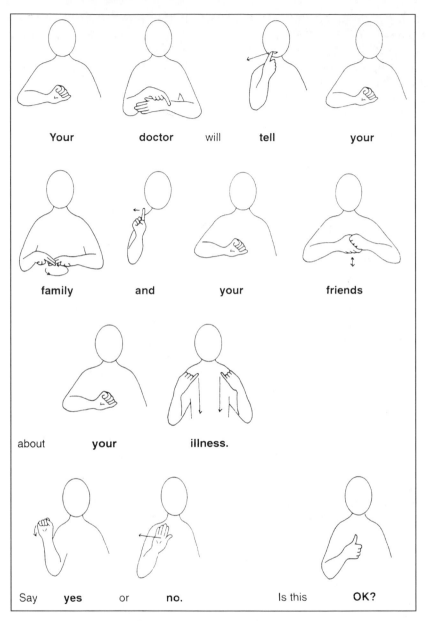

Figure 15.3   Example of Makaton signs from Hull and Holderness NHS Trust Patient's Charter, corresponding to symbols in Figure 15.2 (with permission from the Makaton Vocabulary Development Project).

roof of your mouth, with the tongue tip usually positioned just behind the teeth. The sides of the tongue are raised and touching the sides of the hard palate, and the tongue is grooved all the way along the centre. The vocal folds are close together but not touching, so that air from the lungs passes through the larynx on an outward breath without causing the vocal folds to vibrate. The soft palate is raised so that the uvula touches the back wall of the pharynx. This means that air is channelled

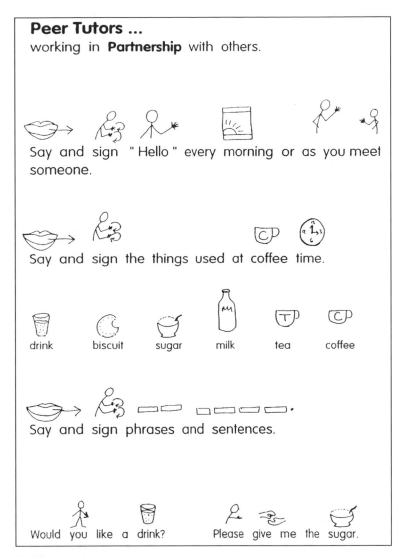

Figure 15.4 Example of Makaton symbol use from a Peer Tutor's Manual (Hooper and Newham 1994) (with permission from Helen Hooper and the Makaton Vocabulary Development Project).

through the mouth, rather than entering the nasal cavity. The air is channelled continuously along the groove along the middle of the tongue, creating friction. And all this for one sound! (See Nolan & Warner 1984 for a fuller description of speech production.)

Owing to this complexity, it follows that there are many factors which can make it difficult for someone to produce clear speech. Some examples are:

- Dysarthria: a difficulty in speaking due to neurological damage affecting coordination of the muscles of the mouth, tongue, throat etc. Severity may vary, so that the person's speech may be so mildly affected that only a few speech sounds are distorted, or it may be so severe that speech is completely unintelligible or absent.
- Dyspraxia: a difficulty in voluntary programming affecting the functional use of a group of muscles. The person has no visible paralysis.

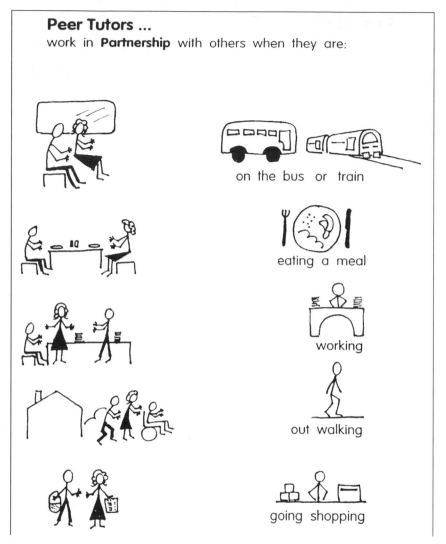

Figure 15.5 Further examples of Makaton symbol use in a Peer Tutor's Manual (Hooper and Newnham 1994) (with permission from Helen Hooper and the Makaton Vocabulary Development Project).

Dyspraxia affects the motor programming of speech, making it difficult for the person to produce and sequence sounds within a word. On some occasions the person may be able to make some sounds/words clearly and effortlessly. This may particularly be the case with emotional words, such as swear words. Dyspraxia may also occur in the limbs, and may therefore give rise to difficulty in producing signs.

- Hearing impairment: we use our hearing to learn language, but also to maintain our communication by tuning in to the sound of our own speech. Therefore, a hearing loss may make it difficult for someone to develop speech and produce all sounds clearly. For example, if someone has a high-frequency hearing loss they will find it difficult to hear high-pitched speech sounds such as 's', 'p', 't' and 'k', and therefore these sounds may be distorted in their own speech. People developing a hearing loss in later life may gradually show signs of deterioration in their speech, depending on the level of the loss.

- Phonological difficulties: phonology is the rules for combining speech sounds together. The person may be able to produce a range of speech sounds in isolation but may have difficulty in organising them into the required sequence within words. For example:

  —clusters of sounds may be simplified, e.g. 'blue' may be produced as 'bu'.

  —unstressed syllables may be deleted, e.g. 'tomato' may be produced as 'mato'.

  —one sound may replace another, e.g. 'car' may be produced as 'ta'.

  —one sound in a word may affect the production of another e.g. 'dog' may be produced as 'gog' or 'dod'.

  It may be that these processes simplify the complexity of speech production or are related to the way the person perceives speech.
- Difficulties with fluency of speech, such as stammering (or stuttering, which is the same). This is a pattern of speech which involves hesitations, repetitions of syllables or words and silent blocks (getting stuck on a sound). Difficulty in speaking may be accompanied by altered breathing patterns and physical gestures. The person may avoid feared sounds, words or situations, so that the actual stammering may appear mild or infrequent to others, but it can come to dominate the person's choice of words and social situations. The causes of stammering are not known.

There is considerable debate about whether 'stammering' in adults with learning disabilities is, in fact, stammering, or is part of a person's overall communication development (analogous to children, who often pass through a period where their speech is non-fluent owing to underdeveloped control over speech musculature and speech patterns), rather than being perceived as a difficulty. Defining factors would involve the degree of awareness and anticipation of difficulty and struggle in the actual production of speech. Although speech modification techniques, such as prolonged speech (which tries to shape speech towards fluency) can be introduced, these can be difficult for anyone to monitor and maintain in everyday life. It can be helpful to analyse when the difficulties occur, e.g. with particular people, or in particular situations. The difficulties of these situations and the emotions involved can then be discussed. Perhaps the most productive approach is to consider your own communication. In particular:

- Maintain an unhurried pace of communication yourself and do not rush the person.
- Allow the person to finish what they were going to say – do not finish it for them (you may get it wrong).
- Keep eye contact with the person.
- Do not put the person 'on the spot' by making them speak in front of others, unless they have indicated that they wish to do so.
- Communicate with the person's family, if applicable, so that they avoid pressuring the person to 'speak normally'.

Helping people to improve the clarity of their speech will probably be a very slow process, if it is appropriate at all within the context of their overall strengths and difficulties in communicating. There are likely to be severe limits to the changes which can be made by adulthood.

It is important that a full assessment is made by a speech and language therapist. This will look at the sounds someone can produce, those which are omitted and distorted, and how this differs in different sequences within words and connected speech. For example, someone may be able to produce the sound 's' in isolation, and in the word 'sun', but omit it in the word 'spider'. Another person may produce fairly intelligible single words but become difficult to understand in connected speech.

The speech and language therapist would also consider the range, speed and accuracy of movements the person can make and, combined with analysing the speech patterns, attempt to make a differential diagnosis. This is important because, depending on the cause, a different approach might be appropriate. For example, if the cause is dyspraxia, a carefully structured approach involving much repetition and building up to practice of sequences of sounds may be adopted. Dyspraxia is now being much more frequently identified in childhood, among children both with and without learning disabilities. Comprehensive programmes, such as the Nuffield Dyspraxia Programme, have been developed.

If the speech difficulty is related to hearing loss, then assistance in using a hearing aid may be beneficial. Some individuals may adjust their speech spontaneously when using their hearing aids, because they can hear themselves more clearly.

From the assessment it may be possible to devise a realistic programme, working from what the person can do and gradually building up, so that confidence is developed and maintained. Motivation is also a crucial factor here: the person needs to have sufficient awareness and the wish to change their speech patterns. Practice will need to be done little and often, so the therapist would devise and supervise the programme but would be unlikely to carry it out in its entirety. The active involvement of nurses, social workers, family members and others concerned with the person on a daily basis is crucial.

It must be borne in mind that the cause of the speech difficulty may be a combination of factors: for example, someone with cerebral palsy may have dysarthria and a hearing loss. In addition, people's level of learning disability will have an overall impact on their speech and language development. If the vocabulary is small it may be easier to differentiate the words being attempted and more important to extend this vocabulary, than to attempt to improve actual speech production.

It may be helpful, in the first instance, to try to 'tune in' to what the person is saying and for the carers to develop a shared 'glossary' of the words/meanings the person is trying to get across. This may be more helpful, and reduce frustration for both parties, than immediately trying to improve the person's speech. It may be that peers, through their familiarity, can understand one another more readily. This was most strikingly exemplified by Joseph Deacon (1974), in his book *Tongue tied*, a testimony to communication between people with learning disabilities.

Other pragmatic approaches include building up a list of target words which the individual needs to use more frequently, or which are particularly important. This may be done by accompanying the person in everyday situations, noting the words used or attempted, and drawing up a priority list. The person can then be helped to practise producing these words more clearly, supplemented by facial expressions and gestures to get the meaning across. Such practice can include role play of the relevant situation, progressing to the actual situation.

If the person's speech is particularly unclear or absent altogether, it can be helpful to use a supplementary means of communication, such as Makaton. This may be used to get meaning across to the listener and so reduce frustration. There are many anecdotal suggestions among speech and language therapists that the use of such systems can reduce the pressure on being understood by using speech, and some suggestions from research that the person's speech may spontaneously improve without specific work on speech production being undertaken (Reid et al 1983).

Earlier in this chapter there was a discussion of the close links between speech and gesture in communication development. From a neurological point of view, speech movements are represented in the brain in the precentral gyrus, adjacent to the area responsible for the control of hand and arm movements. It is possible that encouraging communication through signs may stimulate the adjacent areas of the brain, thereby stimulating speech development. When Makaton is used with children with learning disabilities, the aim is always to develop speech where possible and fade out the use of signs when they are no longer needed. We would not realistically expect this in adults, where it may be a means of communication in itself. Nevertheless, it is important also to encourage any concurrent vocalisation or speech.

Use of language

Many adults with learning disabilities may have difficulty in using the syntax of spoken language and may produce sentences which are telegram-like in form. One of the most helpful approaches can be to ensure that an expanded version of what the person has said is available; for example, if the person says 'Kevin's eating', you could respond with 'Yes, Kevin's eating a cake'.

Games involving modelling the use of the target language structure and encouraging the person to copy, in a variety of contexts, can be used (see Warner & McCartney 1984 for useful ideas). However, it may not always be considered necessary or appropriate to try to do this.

Some individuals can appear to express themselves reasonably clearly, but sometimes closer acquaintance shows that their use of language masks underlying problems of understanding. Two particularly striking features to look out for are echoed speech and preservation.

Echoed speech

This is the repetition of words or sentences spoken by other people. For instance, a person who is asked 'Where are you going?' may echo the last word, 'going', or perhaps the whole sentence. This may indicate that the person has not understood and it may be beneficial to simplify the level of language. However, it can be easy to overlook this in everyday circumstances. For instance, coffee might always be chosen by a person because this is always the last-named thing when the offer of 'tea or coffee' is made.

Some people will use echoed speech in a delayed way, so that the echo is not obvious, and these phrases may be used over and over again. Alternatively, they may be related to particular circumstances. For example, one woman used the phrase 'Give me a twirl' whenever she had her hair done, because this phrase had been used once when she had shown others her new hair-do. She remembered, associated and used it within that situation, but when its origin was not apparent to new people its use was very puzzling. Although she remembered the phrase and had no difficulty in producing it clearly, she did not really understand it, and she could not use the individual words outside this fixed phrase or situation. Nevertheless, it was helpful to her carers to understand its origin.

Many autistic people echo phrases in this way, often remembering and reproducing very elaborate conversation. However, we should not be misled by this into developing very high expectations of the person's expressive language. Aarons &

Gittens (1992) have produced a useful checklist for assessing in detail the subtle and often very confusing aspects of autistic people's communication, with suggestions for development. Bebko (1990) has argued that mitigation in echolalia (i.e. a change in some feature of the utterance being repeated, rather than a verbatim repetition) is a crucial characteristic, because it implies a degree of voluntary control and symbolic functioning. By contrast, exact repetition implies little evidence of the ability to understand or use speech meaningfully. This argument is developed to suggest that those with no speech or unmitigated echolalia may fare best with a sign or symbol system, whereas those with mitigated echolalia may have a more positive prognosis for developing speech. However, this model is derived from studies of existing research and is a theoretical one which so far has been untested.

Perseveration

Perseveration means the continuation of speech or activity which was appropriate in one context but is now no longer appropriate. For example, the person may continue to repeat the same word, phrase or sign even when others have responded. This may also be more evident in more general conversation, where the person may find switches from one topic to another confusing. Factors such as the pace of conversation, or the person's hearing acuity, can make it difficult to keep up with topic changes in a group setting. It may be neurologically based, i.e. a difficulty in initiating and terminating responses, or it can be habitual or, once again, related to a lack of understanding of what others have said. Perseveration may also occur in a broader sense. The person may keep on entering into a dialogue about the same event or theme, and this may go on for weeks, months or even years. Once again, the reasons may be very diverse. For example, such conversation may be the person's sole focus of interest (e.g. the royal family, or a particular TV programme). It may be a way of trying to come to terms with a particularly significant or distressing event (for example, if we are upset by a divorce or bereavement, we may wish to discuss it repeatedly with different friends, or a counsellor. However, because of our language skills we have a wider range of possible things to say about it). It may be related to limited appreciation of time and the words used to express various timescales. In elderly people with learning disabilities it may be that the long-term memory is better than the short-term, so that it is easier to refer to events remembered from the more distant past. Such repetitive and insistent speech can be very irritating, difficult and puzzling for those in daily contact with the person. This should not be underestimated, particularly where it persists, relatively unchanged, for very long periods. The approach will vary, depending on the cause. However, in general it is helpful to be aware of the person's level of understanding of language and tailor your own speech accordingly. It is also important to be aware of changes in either the form or the tone of voice used, in order to cue in to the person's emotions.

Finally, where someone has relatively good understanding of speech but little or no speech themselves, full assessment may be helpful to determine whether they have a specific speech or language disorder.

CONCLUSION

There is a range of factors specific to individuals which may adversely affect their communication. However, in seeking to minimise communication difficulties, it may often be more appropriate and hopeful to focus on environmental factors and the impact of our own communication on the dialogue.

The importance of communication is crucial. As Anne McDonald (Crossley & McDonald 1982) has said, 'Communication falls into the same category as food, drink and shelter: it is essential for life. Without it life becomes worthless.'

ACKNOWLEDGEMENTS

The author is grateful to the Makaton Vocabulary Development Project for kind permission to reproduce examples of signs and symbols from the Makaton Vocabulary, and to Tom Reid, for helpful discussions during preparation of this chapter.

REFERENCES

Aarons M, Gittens T 1992 The autistic continuum: an assessment and intervention schedule. NFER-Nelson, Windsor

Abercrombie K 1968 Paralanguage. British Journal of Disorders of Communication

Allen J 1989 Augmentative communication: more than just words. ACE Centre, Oxford

Ambalu S, McClean B 1995 Makaton peer tutors find jobs. College of Speech and Language Therapist's Bulletin 517: 1–2

Argyle M 1977 The psychology of interpersonal behaviour. Pelican, Harmondsworth

Bartlett C, Bunning K 1997 The importance of communication partnerships: a study to investigate the communicative exchanges between staff and adults with learning disabilities. British Journal of Learning Disabilities 25(4): 148–153

Basil C 1992 Social interaction and learned helplessness in severely disabled children. Augmentative and Alternative Communication Journal 8: 361–368

Baumgart D, Johnson J, Helmstether E 1990 Augmentative and alternative communication systems for persons with moderate and severe disabilities. Paul H Brookes, Baltimore

Baxter C, Poonia K, Ward L, Nadirshaw Z 1990 Double discrimination – issues and services for people with learning disabilities from black and ethnic minority communities. Kings Fund Centre, London

Bebko J M 1990 Echolalia, mitigation and autism: indicators from child characteristics for the use of sign language and other augmentative systems. Sign Language Studies 66: 78–88

Best A B 1987 Steps to independence. BIMH, Kidderminster

Bradley J, Snow B (undated) Making sense of the world sense. National Deaf Blind and Rubella Organisation, London

Bradshaw J 1998 Assessing and intervening in the communication environment. Brtish Journal of Learning Disabilities 26(2): 62-66

Bruce T 1993 Time to play in early childhood education. Hodder and Stoughton, London

Caldwell M, Calder J, Aitken S, Millar S 1995 Use of personal passports with deaf–blind people. Talking Sense 43(3): 9–12

Campbell J, Oliver M 1996 Disability politics. Routledge, London

Campbell P, Wilcox J 1986 Communication effectiveness of movement patterns used by non-verbal children with severe handicaps. Abstracts from the 4th International ISAAC Conference, St David's Hall, Cardiff

Clarke-Kehoe A 1992 Towards effective communication. In: Brown H, Benson S (eds) A practical guide to working with people with learning disabilities. Care Concern/Hawker Publications, London

Crawley B 1988 Learning about self advocacy. Values Into Action, London

Crompton S 2000 How babies can use signs. The Times, Tuesday October 10, p. 13

Crossley A, McDonald R 1982 Annie's coming out. Pelican, Harmondsworth

Crystal D 1984 Listen to your child. Penguin, Harmondsworth

Crystal D 1987 Teaching vocabulary: the case for a semantic curriculum. Child Language Teaching and Therapy 3(1): 40–56

Crystal D 1992 The Cambridge encyclopaedia of language. Cambridge University Press, Cambridge

Daw R 2000 The impact of the Human Rights Act on disabled people. RNID, London

Deacon J 1974 Tongue tied. Mencap, London

Devereux K, VanOosterum J 1985 Learning with rebuses glossary. EARO/LDA, Ely

Dobson S, Stanley S, Maley L 1999 An integrated communication and exercise programme in a day centre for adults with challenging behaviours. British Journal of Learning Disabilities 27(1): 20–24

Dobson S, Dodsworth S, Miller M 2000 Problem solving in small multidisciplinary teams; a means of improving the communication environment for people with profound learning disabilities. British Journal of Learning Disabilities 28(1): March 2000

DOH 2001 Valuing people: a new strategy for learning disability for the 21st century. Cm 5086. The Stationery Office, London

Downes R 1996 Know your rights. Greater London Association of Disabled People, London

Dunn-Klein M 1988 Pre-sign language motor skills. Communication Skill Builders, Texas, Arizona

Ferris-Taylor R 1999 Learn to listen. SITRA Bulletin, February 1999, pp 10-11

Ferris-Taylor R, Pinney S 1994 How to help with hearing loss. Hexagon, New Malden, Surrey

Grant G 1997 Consulting to involve or consulting to empower? In: Ramcharan P, Roberts G, Grant G, Borland J (eds) Empowerment in everyday life. Jessica Kingsley Publishers, London

Graves J 2000 Vocabulary needs in augmentative and alternative communication: a sample of conversational topics between staff providing services to adults with learning difficulties and their service users. British Journal of Learning Disabilities 28(3): 113–119

Grove N, McDougall S 1988, 1989 An exploration of the communication skills of Makaton students: Part I: The children (1988); Part II: Interviews with teachers and speech therapists (1989). Report to the Leverhulme Trust, St George's Hospital Medical School, London

Grove N, Walker M 1990 The Makaton vocabulary: using manual signs and graphic symbols to develop interpersonal communication. Augmentative and Alternative Communication 6(1): 15–28

Halle J W, Baer D M, Spradlin J E 1981 Teachers' generalised use of delay as a stimulus control procedure to increase language use in handicapped children. Journal of Applied Behaviour Analysis 14(4): 389–409

Heider F 1958 The psychology of interpersonal relations. Wiley, New York

Hewitt D, Ephraim G 1994 Access to communication: developing the basics of communication with people with severe learning difficulties through intensive interaction. David Fulton, London

Holland S, Ward C 1990 Assertiveness: a practical approach. Winslow Press, Bicester, Oxon

Hooper H, Bowler D M 1991 Peer tutoring of manual signs by adults with mental handicaps. Mental Handicap Research 4(2): 207–215

Hooper H, Newnham C, MVDP 1994 Peer tutor manual. Makaton Vocabulary Development Project, Camberley, Surrey

Howlin P 1994 Recent research into facilitated communication. Abstracts from Forum on Learning Disability – Communication and Learning Disability: a briefing and update on recent developments. Royal Society of Medicine, London

Hughes A, Coombs P 2001 Easy guide to the Human Rights Act 1998. BILD Publications, Kidderminster

Jones S E 1990 Intercom. NFER, Windsor

Kozleski E B 1991 Expectant delay procedure for teaching requests. Alternative and Augmentative Communication 7(1): 112–131

Lavis D, Cullen P, Roy A 1997 Identification of hearing impairment in people with a learning disability: from questioning to testing. British Journal of Learning Disabilities 25(3): 100-105

Lee M, MacWilliam L 1996 Movement, gesture and sign. RNIB, London

Levy G 2000 Eye operations for adults with learning disabilities. RNIB Update 130, September 2000, p. 10

Mansell J L 1992 Services for people with learning disabilities and challenging behaviour or mental health needs. HMSO, London

Miles D 1988 British Sign Language – a beginner's guide. BBC Publications, London

Millner L, Ash A, Ritchie P 1991 Quality in action – a resource pack for improving services for people with learning difficulties. Norah Fry Research Centre, Bristol

Minkes J, Robinson C, Weston C 1994 Consulting the children: interviews with children using residential respite care services. Disability and Society 9(1): 47–57

Miranda P, Schuler A L 1988 Augmenting communication for persons with autism: issues and strategies. Topics in Language Disorders 9(1)

Morris D 1987 Manwatching – a field guide to human behaviour. Grafton Books, London

Morris J 1991 Pride before prejudice. Women's Press, London

Mountain M 1984 Signing with the visually and mentally handicapped non-communicating child. College of Speech Therapists Bulletin 386: 12

Noland M, Warner J 1984 Hearing and speech: the structure and function of the ear and speech organs. In: McCartney E (ed) Helping ATC students to communicate. BIMH, Kidderminster

O'Brien J 1986 A guide to personal futures planning. In: Bellamy G G, Wilcox B (eds) A comprehensive guide to the activities catalog: an alternative curriculum for youth and adults with severe disabilities. Paul H Brookes, Baltimore, Maryland

Oliver M 1990 The politics of disablement. Macmillan, London

Powell, G 1999 Current research findings to support the use of signs with adults and children who have intellectual and communication difficulties. Paper available from the Makaton Vocabulary Development Project, 31 Firwood Drive, Camberley, Surrey GU15 3QD

Reid B, Jones L, Kiernan C 1983 Signs and symbols: the 1982 survey of use. Special Education, Forward Trends 10: 27–28

Reiser R, Mason M 1992 The medical model and the social model of disability. In: Reiser R, Mason M (eds) Disability equality in the classroom: a human rights issue. Disability Equality in Education, London

Rowland C, Schweigert P 1989 Tangible symbols: symbolic communication for individuals with multisensory impairments. Augmentative and Alternative Communication 5(4): 226–234

Royal National Institute for the Deaf/Coast Project 1990 Hearing matters! A training pack on hearing loss and older people. RNID, London

Sacks O 1990 Seeing voices. Picador, London

Sanderson H, Harrison J 1992 Aromatherapy and massage for people with learning difficulties. Hands On Publishing/John Abbott Ltd, Leicestershire

Scrivener T 1993 Somebody inside with something to say. Community Living 6(4): 10

Shakespeare T, Watson N 1997 Defending the social model. Disability and Society 12(2): 293-300

Spragale D, Micucci D 1990 Signs of the week: a functional approach to manual sign training. Alternative and Augmentative Communication: 96–104

Tizard B, Hughes M 1984 Young children learning. Fontana, London

Tizard B, Cooperman O, Tizard J 1972 Environmental effects on language development: a study of young children in long stay residential nurseries. Child Development 43: 337–358

Trevarthen C 1977 Descriptive analysis of infant communicative behaviour: theory and method sign language studies 21: 317–352

Van der Gaag A 1998 Communication skills and adults with learning disabilities: eliminating professional myopia. British Journal of Learning Disabilities 26(3): 88–93

Van der Gaag A, Dormandy K 1993 Communication and adults with learning difficulties. Whurr Publishers, London

Walker M, Ferris-Taylor R 1991 Guidelines for selection of children and adults with communication difficulties for a Makaton vocabulary programme. Makaton Vocabulary Development Project, Camberley, Surrey

Warner J, McCartney E 1984 Teaching language forms: phonology and syntax. In: McCartney E (ed) Helping ATC students to communicate. BIMH, Kidderminster

Weston C, Went F 1999 Speaking up for yourself: description and evaluation of an assertiveness training group for people with learning disabilities. British Journal of Learning Disabilities 27(3): 110–115

Williams M, Grove N 1989 Getting to grips with aided communication: an overview of the literature. British Journal of Special Education 16(2) Research Supplement: 63–68

Wolfensberger W 1980 The definiton of normalisation: updates, problems, disagreements and misunderstandings. In: Flynn RJ, Nitsch KE (eds) Normalisation, social integration and community services. University Park Press, Baltimore

Yeates S 1995 The incidence and importance of hearing loss in people with severe learning disability: the evaluation of a service. British Journal of Learning Disabilities 23: 79–84

FURTHER READING

Beukelman D R, Mirenda P 1998 Augmentative and alternative communication – management of severe communication disorders in children and adults. Brookes Publishing Company, London

Miller J F, Leddy M, Leavitt L A (eds) 1999 Improving the communication of people with Down syndrome. Brookes Publishing Company, London

Murphy J, Scott J 1998 Talking to people with severe communication problems. Winslow Press, Bicester

USEFUL ADDRESSES

Action for Blind People
14–16 Verney Road
London
SE16 3DZ
Tel: 020 7732 8771
email: info@ afbp.org
www.demon.co.uk/afbp

British Association for the Hard of Hearing
(BAHOH)/Hearing Concern
7 Armstrong Road
London
W3 7JL
Tel: 020 8743 1110
www.hearingconcern.com
email: info@ hearingconcern.com
textphone 0208 742 9151

British Deaf Association (BDA)
1–3 Worship Street
London

EC2A 2AB
Helpdesk: 0845 074 4600
Minicom: 020 7588 3529
www.bda.org.uk

Change (*a national organisation for people with learning disabilities who are blind or deaf*)
First Floor
69–85 Old Street
London
EC1V 9HY
Tel: 020 7490 2668
Fax: 0207 490 3581
Minicom: 0207 490 3483

Learning Development Aids (LDA)
Duke Street
Wisbech
Cambridge
PE13 2AB
Tel: 01945 63441

Makaton Vocabulary Development Project
31 Firwood Drive
Camberley
Surrey
GU15 2QD
Tel/ fax: 01276 61390
Training office: telephone/fax 01276 681368
www.makaton.org
email: mvdp@makaton.org

Paget–Gorman Sign System
3 Gipsey Lane
Headington
Oxford
OX3 7PT

Plain English Campaign
PO Box 3
New Mills
High Peak
SK22 4QP
Tel: 01663 744409
Fax: 01663 747038
Info@plainenglish.co.uk
www.plainenglish.co.uk

Royal Association in Aid of Deaf People
27 Old Oak Road
Acton
London
W3 6HN
Tel: 01206 509509

www.royaldeaf.org.uk
email: info@royaldeaf.org.uk
minicom: 01206 577090

Royal National Institute for the Blind (RNIB)
105 Judd Street
London
WC1H 9NE
Tel: 020 7388 1266
www.rnib.org.uk
email: rnib.org.uk
minicom: 0845 758 5691

Royal National Institute for the Deaf (RNID)
19–23 Featherstone Street
London
EC1Y 8SL
Tel: 0808 808 0123
www.rnid.org.uk
email: helpline@ rnid.org.uk
minicom: 0808 808 9000

The National Deaf Blind and Rubella Association – SENSE
11–13 Clifton Terrace
Finsbury Park
London
N4 3SR
Tel: 0207 272 7774
www.sense.org.uk
minicom: 020 7272 9648

16

Health and health promotion

Sue Hart

CHAPTER CONTENTS

KEY ISSUES

- Most people with learning disabilities do not receive good quality health services. Evidence from research in primary and secondary health service provision often finds people and their carers dissatisfied with the care provided (Hart 1998, Kerr et al 1996, Mencap, 1997).
- People with learning disabilities often struggle to access preventive measures such as screening, and those who would benefit from spectacles, hearing aids and dentures are less likely to have them, than people who do not have a learning disability (Barr et al 1999).
- Of the many obstacles to receiving good health care access, communication with the health provision and actually getting to the service remain significant problems (NHSE 1999). This is alongside the negative attitudes from generic health care providers leading to often chronically low levels of expectation on behalf of people with learning disabilities and their carers and supporters.
- Rigorous evidence indicates that people with learning disabilities have generally higher health needs than the general population (Mencap 1997).
- The role of learning disability nurses in enabling people to access the health care they need is changing. The new role emphasises that nurses need to work in partnerships with people with learning disabilities and with generic health providers to help empower people to receive the service they need.

INTRODUCTION

This chapter outlines the state of contemporary primary and secondary health services for people with learning disabilities. A brief history will trace the shift from institutional based health provision to the expectation, following the re-provision of services into the community, that health care would be provided in local settings. This is followed by a consideration of the health needs of people with learning disabilities and by evidence from service users about the health care they have received.

Health promotion involving people with learning disabilities has evolved in recent years, with interventions to support and enable people to learn important messages about health. Some of these developments will be considered.

Drawing on current literature, policy initiatives and research, as well as examples from practice, the chapter will examine how people with learning disabilities experience health care provision.

Health and health promotion

Maintaining good levels of general health and wellbeing are a concern to most people, irrespective of whether or not they have learning disabilities. Established in the UK in 1948, the National Health Service exists to provide comprehensive health care for all its citizens, accessible to all, free at the point of delivery, financed by income tax and National Insurance (Lock 1996). People with learning disabilities have an absolute equal right to access health services on a par with anyone else.

Reader activity 16.1

Can you recall a time when you felt unwell, telephoned your general practitioner (GP) to make an appointment, and later the next day saw your doctor in the surgery? Think of someone you know who has learning disabilities. Are there any of the stages in the process you went through (self-recognition of possible illness, contacting the surgery and accessing the service of your GP) with which a person with learning disabilities may have difficulties?

However, there is accumulating evidence which suggests that people with learning disabilities are not entirely satisfied with the health care they receive.

Ensuring that people with learning disabilities access the health care to which they have a right is important, not least because it is implied as a principle of community integration and participation (O'Brien 1986). It should be regarded as a fundamental human right. For learning disability nurses, ensuring that the health needs of people in their care is met is an important role dimension (DOH 1996) and if genuine community participation is to be achieved, one which will continue to require considerable adjustment from old style working practices.

With the publication of *Valuing People* (DOH 2001a, p. 59) has come a clear statement from the government that people with learning disabilities should be enabled to access a 'health service designed around their individual needs.' This recognises that good health is a necessary prerequisite if people are to be able to achieve the goal of living independently and being included in society.

Although most people who have learning disabilities now live in community-based settings of one type or another, as Chapter 3 has shown this was not always the case. The closure of the long-stay hospitals has led to significant changes in how health care is provided. Of course some people with learning disabilities have always lived in the community with their families or independently, and have been known to and cared for by generic locally based health services. These numbers were always fairly small, with people being known as individuals with particular needs. At the same time however, all over the country and in various locations, hundreds of people with learning disabilities were living together in large institutions (Wing 1989). Although hospitalised for reasons other than being physically ill, it was inevitably the case that the physical health of some residents would deteriorate as they grew older. Economies of scale together with the culture of care at the time (which sought to keep people with learning disabilities hidden from public view) combined to ensure that most health needs were managed in the institution. Ironically this situation meant that psychiatrists (doctors based in the institutions who were there primarily to attend to the mental health of the residents) were often required to call upon their basic skills as physicians to assess and treat physical ill health.

Most often the physical health of residents would be attended to in a specially designated 'sick' ward, often but not always staffed by nurses who had undertaken some additional training for example as a Registered Nurse (Adult).

Indeed, many units established their own acute medical treatment facilities, and general hospital admission was rarely needed . . . This system was far from perfect. However the care of these individuals has now moved to the community, and there is a danger that specialist knowledge and related skills will be lost (Aspray 1999).

Now that community relocation has occurred, large numbers of people with learning disabilities are eligible to receive generic health services. This change has posed, and continues to pose a challenge to the service, and needs to be addressed (Hayward & Kerr 1998). For instance, the NHS Executive good practice guidelines (NHSE 1999a) has alerted GPs that in a list of 2000 patients 40 are likely to have learning disabilities, and of these, eight will have severe learning disabilities. Further, as increasingly more children with learning disabilities are surviving into adulthood (Burke & Cigno 2000) and more people are living into old age (DOH 2000, Walker & Walker 1998) the demand for health services from this group is likely to rise. Thus in their everyday practice, nurses in general hospital settings, specialists in outpatient departments, GPs and practice nurses are routinely being required to provide for the health needs of people with learning disabilities. The challenge is that invariably few (although occasionally some) of these professionals have had any training or direction in how to manage, or understand the sometimes special needs of people with learning disabilities. Such a challenge is further compounded by evidence that indicates that people with learning disabilities have greater health needs than the general population. Yet, research undertaken by Mencap has shown that 'despite their greater medical needs, people with

learning disabilities make fewer visits to their GPs than do the general population' (Mencap 1997, p. 1).

WHY IS A CONSIDERATION OF HEALTH NEEDS FOR PEOPLE WITH LEARNING DISABILITIES NOW IMPORTANT?

There is a growing body of knowledge that suggests people with learning disabilities do not always receive the standard of health care service expected by people who do not have learning disabilities. This has been found across both primary and secondary services, and is now so well evidenced that it can be seen as a widespread and systematic failure to meet the health needs of this particular group. Research shows that the health needs of people with learning disabilities are too often unreported or undetected (Beange et al 1995, Cumella et al 1992, Howells 1986, Martin et al 1997, Meehan et al 1995, Wells et al 1997, Wilson & Haire 1990).

For example, when Howells (1986) examined 151 members of a day service for people with learning disabilities, he found 279 medical needs of which only 76 were being properly managed. The remainder were either newly detected in his study, or previously known but being inadequately managed. In a further study of day service members' health Wilson & Haire (1990) found 103 medical conditions in 65 people, of which they considered only 13% to be well managed.

Additionally, people with learning disabilities have difficulties receiving all types of NHS screening services, with women often being denied routine breast and cervical screening (Hall et al 1999, NHSE 1999a, Pearson 1998). But simply gaining access to the service is not always the issue; it is what happens during the consultation or hospitalisation that must be considered.

Langan et al (1994) have noted that health services for people with learning disabilities tend to be reactive, i.e. sought by individuals or their carers only when they recognise they have a need. This suggests that important notions such as health education and preventive activities may not be effectively reaching this group. Further evidence

Reader activity 16.2

Consider how the following situations may have been prevented:

- 'She has suffered a lot from the cancer in her bones that spread from her breast. We feel angry because, when she went for a mammogram two years ago, she got upset and they told us not to come back. If they had been more patient things might have been different' (NHSE 1999a, p. 20).
- 'The doctor gave me some tablets, but I had no idea what they were. He explained to me, but I didn't understand. It was Latin. People with learning difficulties find it hard to take tablets. They don't know what they are. They're afraid they will take the wrong kind of tablet and die' (Building Expectations 1996;58).
- 'I, I, I sort of take it all in as I can understand it, but sometimes it is hard to understand, because sometimes the doctors and that use long words which I don't quite understand. Then, if I've got my mum with me she tries to explain it to me, what they mean. But you know its just that the big long words that they use sometimes, I don't understand what they are on about. . . .' (Hart 1997).

has indicated that people with learning disabilities do not contact their GPs any more than the general population, despite the well-documented increased incidence of health and medical needs (DOH 1998, Wells et al 1997, Wilson & Haire 1990). Commonly raised obstacles to health care are also poor staff attitudes, and inadequate or ineffective communication (Hart 1998, Law et al 2000, Lennox & Kerr 1997). Low expectations, fear and anxiety are other frequently occurring themes in the literature (Foreman 1997, Hart 1998, Wells et al 1997).

The failure in health provision for people with learning disabilities is now fairly well-established and questions of quality and value for money in the public sector highlight the deficiency. Numerous strategies have been implemented to address this situation locally, however to date these have been impotent in effecting major change, and this is a concern because as the following will highlight, several indicators predict that people with learning disabilities will require increased health care in the future.

First, as more people with learning disabilities are living longer there is an increased likelihood that more people will develop illnesses of old age

(DOH 1998, Edgerton et al 1994, Jenkins et al 1994) and we are already witnessing an increased incidence of people with Down syndrome developing Alzheimer's disease (Holland & Oliver 1995, Whitehouse et al 2000). Patterns of illness are already altering as a result of longevity and are increasingly reflecting the mortality and morbidity levels in the general population (Barr et al 1999).

Secondly, and as noted earlier, increased numbers of younger multiply disabled children are surviving into adulthood with severe and complex health needs (DOH 1998).

Thirdly, as deinstitutionalisation nears completion the few remaining segregated services, once located in long-stay hospitals, will close, and yet more people with learning disabilities will access health care across generic services. In a truly inclusive health service, there will be no role for 'specialist' dentists, physiotherapists and chiropodists who offer their services to individuals primarily because they have learning disabilities. There may be a future for a small number of specialist services that focus on particular needs, for example sensory disability, epilepsy, mental health (DOH 1998). Significantly these will offer additional specialist input, rather than (as before) being a poor relation in what was essentially a two tier health care system (DOH 2001a). This is not to criticise some of the excellent services provided to people with learning disabilities by hospital-based health care professionals, and the high order skills many people developed to work effectively with the more challenging of their patients. But it nevertheless remained the case that health services delivered outside of the mainstream (in segregated institutional environments) were largely disengaged and isolated geographically from their mainstream counterparts.

Lastly, we now understand and should act where people with learning disabilities are known to have an increased health risk. Conditions such as epilepsy, cerebral palsy and other physical disabilities are found in about one third of all people with learning disabilities. Also, hypertension, chronic bronchitis and gross obesity all occur more frequently than in people without learning disabilities. Physical disability affects many people with learning disability, and is also associated with spinal and postural deformities, hip dislocation, eating and swallowing problems, gastro-oesophageal reflux, constipation and incontinence (NHSE 1999a, Vernon 1997).

Research has demonstrated that people with learning disabilities also have an increased likelihood of experiencing mental health problems (HoNOS-LD 1998) with some suggestions that there is occurrence in up to 50% of the population (NHSE 1999a). *Once a Day* (NHSE 1999a, p. 17) also suggests that depressive illnesses and withdrawal are frequently not diagnosed or treated.

Certain syndromes have come to be associated with specific health needs. People with Down syndrome are known to be prone particularly to cardiac disorders, respiratory problems, frequent chest infections, megaloblastic anaemia, acute lymphoblastic leukaemia, disorders of the thyroid, hearing impairments and orthopaedic problems (Vernon 1997). Tuberous sclerosis is associated with epilepsy, tumours, respiratory disorders and disorders of the central nervous system (Vernon 1997). Klinefelter syndrome is linked with cardiac disease, osteoporosis, kidney problems and gastrointestinal bleeding (DOH 1995, NHSE 1999a, Vernon 1997).

There is also evidence to suggest an underdetection of sensory disabilities, in particular hearing and vision problems. Somewhere in the region of 40% of people with learning disabilities are believed to have some problems with hearing, and as many as one-third may have problems with their eyesight (NHSE 1999a). Of course as people grow older these needs are likely to increase.

Now, midwives, dentists, operating department practitioners, dieticians, radiographers, health visitors, outpatient department personnel, porters, surgeons, GPs, practice nurses and receptionists, as well as doctors and nurses in general hospitals to name but some, will most days be meeting people with learning disabilities in the course of their work. This constitutes an enormous challenge for the National Health Service, as well as for people with learning disabilities and their families and supporters. It also requires learning disability nurses and other learning disability professionals to embrace the guidelines in *Valuing People* (DOH 2001a) and reconsider signifi-

cantly their roles and activities in relation to health care delivery for their clients.

WHERE ARE WE NOW?

Barely a week passes without the NHS featuring in the media, for what are often negative reasons. Recent concerns have been doctors (Rodney Ledwood, Harold Shipman) and the Alder Hey hospital pathologist (Professor Dick van Velzen), whose practices have all given rise to an ongoing debate about the autonomy and often alleged arrogance of senior members of the medical profession. Other headline news stories have included: a case of medical negligence 'Doctors may face charges for injecting the wrong drug' (Guardian 3 February 2001); and the dehydration of elderly patients 'She was dying for a cuppa. Literally' (Observer 1 November 1998).

Any consideration of how people with learning disabilities find the experience of care and treatment in the health care system has to be realistic. Despite anecdotal evidence that the NHS is the envy of much of the world, the UK National Health Service is, in reality, subject both to criticism from its users as well as, at times, to praise from the many grateful patients and their families satisfied with the care they have received. Clearly, it can be argued that many people who do not have learning disabilities have good reason to be dissatisfied with aspects of the health care they receive. Why should this be any different for people with learning disabilities? Of course some people with learning disabilities are satisfied with the service they receive, although research has identified that when asked people with learning disabilities do voice dissatisfaction (Hart 1998).

What is now emerging, is accumulating evidence that people with learning disabilities have particular reasons to be displeased with aspects of the health service they receive, over and above any of the 'mainstream' complaints about which all citizens may have a view. These inequalities are emerging as more and more people are being asked their views about health care. This is coming to light as a result of the welcome recent trend in research in reporting directly the views of people with learning disabilities (Booth & Booth 1994,

Northway 2000, Richardson 1997). Recent research has focused on how people with learning disabilities actually experience the health care they have received (Hart 1998, Fovargue et al 2000). Evidence of what people with learning disabilities themselves say about general hospitals, nurses and GPs is growing. In a climate of consumerism, where service users' views are actively being sought, these findings should be regarded as especially significant. Even if it makes for some uncomfortable reading for professionals, there can be no better judgements about the quality of health care than from those who receive the service.

People with learning disabilities in general hospitals

Research undertaken specifically to harness the views and experiences of people with learning

Reader activity 16.3

Imagine you are the manager responsible overall for a group of small community residences for people with learning disabilities, run by an independent sector provider. Elsie, who is in her mid-50s, moved in to one of the houses from a long-stay hospital 8 years ago, and has adjusted well to life in the community. She has her own room, is entirely self-caring and very independent. Elsie needs to go into the local general hospital for exploratory surgery to investigate anal bleeding. All screening and day surgery investigations so far have been inconclusive. Mainly for moral support, the house manager Lynn accompanies Elsie to the pre-admission clinic; she could have managed alone. The clinic nurse asks to speak privately to Lynn. Lynn says that Elsie should hear anything that is about her. The clinic nurse says that because Elsie has learning disabilities she must have an escort with her all the time during her forthcoming admission. When Lynn insists that Elsie can manage as well as anyone else the nurse retorts: 'It is hospital policy. I don't make the rules. I have been told to tell you, no escort no operation. We just don't have the staff to manage people like her. We don't have the training.' Lynn is very angry and telephones you later in the day. Elsie is in tears because she feels cross and humiliated.

   What action can you take? It may be useful to think about short-term as well as long-term actions. Imagine how Elsie may feel. How can you best support her through this crisis? How do you manage Lynn and your other house managers to address similar situations in the future?

disabilities in general hospital settings (Hart 1998) found a catalogue of dissatisfaction, that weighed unevenly against the one or two positive comments people offered. This small-scale project used grounded theory techniques to analyse a series of tape-recorded interviews with the subjects. All the respondents had been either hospital inpatients, day patients or had attended as outpatients in the past 3 years. Whilst acknowledging the unacceptability of categorising people with learning disabilities, it is important at least to comment that the informants were all fairly able, most were active self advocates, and none could be regarded as having severe learning disabilities. The most frequently occurring themes in the research, 'fear about treatment', 'general nursing care', 'consent to treatment', 'communication about treatment' and 'doctors' will now be explored. All informants' names have been changed.

Fear

This research identified that people with learning disabilities demonstrated varying degrees of fear about general hospitals. Some were able to express this directly, others were not. For some people the fear was rooted in their dislike of nursing or medical interventions, for others it was rooted in their lack of understanding about what was happening to them. In some instances people's fear was responsive to reason and explanation, but for others it was not so, and several respondents reported uncomfortably high levels of anxiety.

   'Ned' had been in hospital for surgery on his back. He needs a lot of help with basic and life care skills, but is able to speak for himself. In response to an emerging theme he was asked further questions by the interviewer (Int).

Int: 'What do you think you were frightened of?'
Ned: 'The people.'
Int: 'How frightened?'
Ned: 'A lot.'
Int: 'You were very frightened?'
Ned: 'Yes.'

Again in response to a developing theme:

Int: 'So when you are having treatment and you don't understand . . .'
Ned: 'Yeah'.
Int: 'What does that feel like?'
Ned: 'Frightening it is, frightening.'

'Jan' had to have an infected wisdom tooth extracted in day surgery. She told the interviewer 'I was a bit er, nervous. Because, um, somebody told me, I can't remember who, somebody said to me I had a tooth growing out of the root, and if I had that out, I wouldn't be able to talk. . . . I told my mum, I am not going into that hospital to have my tooth out . . . I was ever so upset.' Having had several operations on her mouth as a child losing the ability to speak was a very real fear for Jan. But her fear responded to reason and careful explanations about the treatment. 'It was um, getting worse, and it could give me problems later on in life' and she reluctantly agreed to have the tooth removed.

Although somewhat reassured by his surgeon who took the trouble to ask if he felt nervous about his forthcoming operation, Michael had found his own way of managing his particular fear. 'Sometimes when I was in hospital um, they come with a needle and that and I have to look away, I don't like the sight of needles. I have to look away, you know what I mean?'

General nursing care

Biley (1994) has reported that nurses' negative attitudes to people with disabilities admitted to acute settings often result in traumatic experiences in hospital. This research (Hart 1998, p. 473) has reported that only one informant gave an account of a nurse appearing to be quite spontaneous and genuinely caring. Of concern is the finding that;

Not only were nurses seldom praised, but also they were the subject of criticism from several respondents. In these instances, situations are described where nurses lacked initiative and where spontaneous caring was simply not there. Where respondents say positive things about nurses, it is usually linked to their 'hands-on' skills, or dispensing medications when they were called by the patient's own call bell. Evidence is minimal of nurses interacting with their patients, talking with and observing them.

'Jon' had a 6-week admission on an orthopaedic ward and is the one respondent who reported real kindness from one nurse; they are still friends today. 'She used to keep me company, tell me . . . Talk to me and all things. And all the other nurses, they think, all the other nurses, all the other ones were alright, they all guessed who was, who my number one nurse was.' But it was not always so. As the interview proceeded it became clear that for the first 2 weeks of his admission Jon had been largely neglected and left to fend for himself. It was not until his frustration reached critical levels and he demanded his discharge that the problem emerged. Jon cannot read or write.

Jon: '. . . when I was in there I used to have salad for dinner and salad for tea . . . Yeah, because nobody tell me that . . . nobody help me read the menu, and in the end Claire and the other nurses, give me a hand with the menu.'
Int: 'Oh, so you had the salad because you didn't know which other box to tick?'
Jon: 'That's right.'
Int: 'Did you ask them for help or did they notice?'
Jon: 'I asked them for help and they said yeah we will, so that's how come I got chatting with Claire and the other nurses.'
Int: 'How long had you been having the salads before you . . .?'
Jon: '2 weeks, 2 weeks I did.'
Int: 'But once you got the proper help, you could get what you wanted?'
Jon: 'Yeah . . . I wanted to walk out because I was so bored with salad, and Claire said 'No, if you walk out, if you sign out, you are gonna hurt your leg and get worse and worse.' And in the end I stayed in. In the end it was better.'

Jan, finally admitted for her tooth extraction, was asked about the care she received from her nurses.

Well I was a bit cold for a start . . . because I was dozing. I was a bit cold. All I had on was one of those gowns that they put on you when you are in hospital . . . The sheet was here (draws a line across her body at mid chest point) under my arms and, she [pause] um, kept taking my blood pressure, and that was it. And I didn't have nothing to drink.

It emerged that Jan had only a sheet covering her, no blanket. Pulled down for routine observations it was not pulled up again. Jan says she felt too uncomfortable to ask for more covers, and yet pointedly remarks in exasperation: 'The gown was short, I had bare arms.' Later Jan expressed a wish to have had the means to complain formally about the care she received.

Consent to treatment

Although as adults they were legally eligible to consent or not to consent to their own treatment (NHSE 1999a) Hart (1999) found that the people in the study experienced very variable attitudes from the medical staff. All would have had the capacity to understand what they were consenting for in general terms, if the details had been explained using accessible language.

'Ellen' is an able and independent woman. She attended outpatients departments alone and seemed to have a very clear understanding about her operation – a hysterectomy.

Int: 'Do you remember signing the consent form?'
Ellen: 'I didn't. I think, I think, I did, I don't, I think I did and then was it? I don't know. No my mum did. My mum did. When she came to see me the day I had it. My mum signed the consent form.'
Int: 'Why did your mum do it and not you?'
Ellen: 'I don't know Sue, I don't know. Why do they do that?'

Another man had given consent for treatment to his back, but was ignored when he attempted to withdraw consent. 'I said to the doctor I don't want it, I don't like it.' Nevertheless the procedure continued. If a non-learning disabled person, for example a bank manager, had reacted in this way, would the outcome have been different?

Fovargue et al (2000, pp 342–343) have examined the question of who really decides. It was reported that in a series of workshops with people with learning disabilities 'many participants told us that they did not sign consent forms themselves, but that their carers were asked to do so.' This behaviour 'appeared to reinforce the erroneous belief that parents and carers can consent to medical treatment on behalf of a person with a learning disability.'

Valuing People (DOH, 2001a, 6.21) acknowledges that in general hospitals 'staff may be unfamiliar with seeking consent from people who have learning disabilities.' It is therefore important to know what the guidelines and good practice recommend (see Box 16.1).

Communication about treatment

Several studies (Daniels et al 1989, Leino-Kilpin 1993) have concluded that the main cause of dissatisfaction with hospital care per se, has been the poor communication of information. That doctors would be subject to criticism for using jargon or complicated medical words was anticipated, and did feature in the research. The reverse, however, had not been expected. When asked why she had gone into hospital Ellen uses the correct word to describe her forthcoming operation – a hysterectomy. However when reporting what the consultant said: 'She said they were going to take your womb away, when you have your period operation and that.' How frustrating to be spoken to in a manner which so undermines ability!

'David' had many inpatient admissions when he was younger. He said of the doctors. 'They used to, sort of, they used to ask my mum or dad. Then they asked me after, but first of all it used to be my mum or dad, when I went in to hospital.'

Box 16.1 Good practice in obtaining consent from people with learning disabilities

NHS Executive Health Service Circular HSC 1999/031 (NHSE 1999b)
'A patient has the right under common law to give or withhold consent to medical examination or treatment. This is one of the basic principles of health care.'
  'Every person is presumed to have the capacity to consent to or to refuse medical treatment unless and until that presumption is rebutted.'

Reference Guide to Consent for Examination or Treatment (DOH 2001b: 12)
'Consent may be expressed verbally or non-verbally: an example of non-verbal consent would be where a patient, after receiving appropriate information, holds out an arm for their blood pressure to be taken.'
  See also UKCC 1998 and DOH 2001c.

Int: 'So even when you were an adult, they'd ask your mum and dad first?'

David: 'Yes, yes.'

Int: 'What did you feel about that?'

David: 'I felt that I was in there for the operation, in my chest and that. I was the one having the operation.'

Int: 'And that they should ask you?'

David: 'Yes, yes.'

Int: 'When doctors behave as though you don't understand, and they talk to your mum, what does that make you feel like?'

David: 'Feel like I'm not there, just I'm there, but oh well, he can't understand.'

Doctors

Few interpersonal interactions have been as thoroughly investigated as those between doctors and patients. However the notion of the remote consultant still endures today. Some people established a very good rapport with their doctors. Michael clearly liked his doctor very much and when asked why this was so replied: 'Because I felt, I thought, I felt that I could get on with him. First time I went in for a check up he shook my hand and that. "Come in Mr A. Take a seat." He shook me, he shook me hand. "How do you do, morning!" '

This positive encounter stands in contrast to the accounts of other respondents. One spoke about a doctor being 'really nasty' and raising his voice. With relief she said, 'He's retired now.'

Primary care for people with learning disabilities

There are many issues that may affect the smooth access of people with learning disabilities to primary health care services. Some people with learning disabilities have been very critical of their primary care. One person was sensitive to age discrimination: 'If you turn 56, God help you – because they're more for the youngsters than when you get to a certain age. They don't focus on people with learning disabilities who are elderly. You're completely finished' (Building Expectations 1996, p. 63).

Box 16.2 Barriers to receiving good primary health care services

- Some people have low expectations, both for their own health and of the service they may receive. Many individuals and their carers tolerate unnecessarily quite unacceptable standards of health care services
- Some people are not able to read letters, make appointments, tell the time or read instructions on medication
- Some people may be fearful of coming to their doctor's surgery
- Some people may find waiting very difficult, particularly if they have a poor understanding of time or if the area is very noisy or crowded
- Some people may not understand the process of consultation, or what they need to know, including what certain equipment may be used for and how it will feel
- Some people may find the standard appointment times too short to fully understand what they need to know
- Some people struggle with the concept of time. Questions such as when symptoms were first noticed may not be understood
- Some people do not mention all of their symptoms to their doctor or carers

---

A further comment captured the low self-esteem resulting from attitudes: 'some doctors treat me [as] if I am a waste of space' (Building Expectations 1996, p. 59).

In Box 16.2 below are some obstacles identified as potential barriers to people with learning disabilities receiving a good primary health care service.

It is now being recognised that access for people with learning disabilities to primary health care may also be impeded by the GP's and other professionals' lack of skills. In a large study, *Prescription for Change*, Mencap (1997) sent postal questionnaires to 543 GPs, 821 people with learning disabilities and 547 carers. It was found that:

whilst many GPs are trying to provide a high standard of care, there are major shortfalls in services provided for people with learning disabilities. This is directly affecting the health of many of the 1.2 million people with learning disabilities in the UK. In fact 81% of GPs thought that the health care needs of people with learning disabilities were less well met than those of the rest of the population.

Also of great concern was the finding that a small number of GPs were withdrawing their service for people with learning disabilities (Caplan 1997).

Developments to address concerns with health matters for people with learning disabilities

There have been numerous developments in recent years to address the concern that people with learning disabilities have not been receiving a good enough health service. These can be categorised broadly into three areas: Department of Health and National Health Service Executive guidelines; service user focused initiatives; and finally the development of good practice in services for people with learning disabilities. However, despite some excellent ideas and good work in the delivery of health services to people with learning disabilities, a note of caution must be sounded. Russell (1999) has observed that the:

Evidence of what could be achieved was unfortunately matched by equally convincing evidence that it was not being achieved; with large gaps between policy and practice, rhetoric and reality, design and delivery. People were by no means guaranteed ready access to good quality health care . . .

Department of health guidelines

Almost a decade ago, the NHS Executive circulated the guidelines HSG(92) 42 (NHS Executive 1992). Had the health service mobilised in response to some of the excellent recommendations made then, the situation today may have been much better. The guidelines begin:

People with learning disabilities have the same right of access to NHS services as everyone else but they may require assistance to use the service. Special care must be taken to ensure that they are not denied health care because of their disability, and that steps are taken to ensure that any barriers to access are minimised.

Practical suggestions for GPs to help to minimise stress caused by unfamiliar surroundings include offering domiciliary visits instead, or an early or late appointment, when the health centre may be less busy. Unfortunately, there is no evidence to suggest that these guidelines had any impact whatever on the question of health service provision for this group.

The foreword to *Signposts for Success* (NHS Executive 1998) acknowledged that many people with learning disabilities are not getting a fair deal from the health service. The report, aimed at the providers and commissioners of health services for people with a learning disability, is far reaching in its scope. Although it acknowledged the need for some specialist service provision to continue, in the spheres of mental health, epilepsy, physical and sensory disabilities, overwhelmingly the message is that people with learning disabilities must access mainstream generic health services and be enabled to do so. Good practice in all health services is defined and models to work to are suggested. These cover the issues of rights, information, access, attitudes and communication. The good practice guidelines also elucidate how people with learning disabilities in general hospitals, those having routine health checks, and those receiving community health care can all be enabled to have a better service.

Once a day one or more people with learning disabilities are likely to be in contact with your primary health care team. How can you help them?

This statement is on the cover of the NHS good practice guideline *Once a Day* (NHSE 1999a) which targets all members of primary health care teams. The handbook offers practical advice in key areas such as what is a learning disability, supporting families who have discovered their child has learning disabilities and enabling people with learning disabilities to cope with various life events. Difficulties with access to services are clearly outlined and associated health problems that GPs may encounter in their patients are explained. Helping people with learning disabilities to be responsive to health promotion initiatives and strategies to ensure access to screening are also featured in the handbook.

The Health of the Nation: a Strategy for People with Learning Disabilities (DOH 1995) followed publication of an earlier document, *The Health of the Nation: A Strategy for Health in England* (DOH 1992). The same five key areas of coronary heart disease and stroke, cancer, HIV/Aids and sexual health, accidents and mental illness are included in both documents, with the former including particular reference to the needs of people with learning disabilities. The same document also acknowledged that people with learning disabilities have a greater number of health problems than the general population, while the uptake of health care remains low. There is an emphasis on the need for health promotion and health surveillance for this group and also on the value of forming health alliances, where colleagues from the general and specialist spheres can work together to enhance the wellbeing of a person with learning disabilities. An example of a health alliance could be a community learning disability nurse making contact with a local general hospital accident and emergency department, and agreeing to give telephone advice, in the event of staff struggling to meet the needs of a person with a learning disability.

User-based initiatives

Various creative strategies have been developed to help support people with learning disabilities to receive the health service they need.

In 1995 Hull and Holderness Community Health NHS Trust collaborated with the Makaton Vocabulary Development Project to produce *The Patient's Charter and You* (Hull & Holderness Community Health NHS Trust 1995). *The Patient's Charter* was one initiative of the Citizen's Charter scheme, launched during the government of John Major to make the public sector more directly accountable to its customers. The charter made explicit the standard of service that patients in the health care system should expect in certain aspects of their care. Waiting times, right to health checks, and a standard time for an ambulance response to an emergency are some of the expectations included.

In the collaborative project, *The Patient's Charter* was interpreted to be more user friendly. A simple re-wording of more complex statements was accompanied by line drawings of Makaton signs, as well as the statement repeated with symbols and photographs. For example, where the original text reads 'You can expect a thorough eye examination that should include checks for any disease or abnormality as well as checking your sight', the interpretation reads 'An optician will examine your eyes'. This statement appears with symbols,

Makaton signs and is further supported by a photograph of an optician undertaking an eye test on a patient.

This work aimed to ensure that the charter would be more accessible for anyone who may have struggled to understand its text, and to address the problem of poor communication with people with learning disabilities in health care settings. It did this by using more than just one means of communication, for example the spoken word supported by Makaton signs, or by the use of photographs or symbols. Through this it was hoped that people with learning disabilities might be able to understand the charter and, as a consequence, take more responsibility for aspects of their own health care.

The OK Health Check (Mathews 1997) is a system of assessing and planning for the health care needs of people with learning disabilities, which was developed in response to the recognition that the new community services were not attending adequately to the health needs of their clients. *The OK Health Check* aims to enable the carers of people with learning disabilities, both qualified and unqualified practitioners, to recognise the health needs of their clients. The assessment works through a series of questions focused on the body systems (for example circulation and breathing, digestion and elimination) as well as monitoring body measurements. By including reference back to previous health records (or last year's OK check) it is possible to identify changes in a client's wellbeing, which may not have come to light due to the very gradual nature of the deterioration.

This systematic approach invites carers to consider critically all aspects of their clients' health and, importantly, aims to provoke concern that there may be a breakdown in good health in an area not previously identified. *The OK Health Check* may in some cases detect illness that would otherwise have been identified through health screening, an area where we know that people with learning disabilities have less good access than the general population.

Feedback from colleagues who have used the *OK Health Check* is generally positive. However, as the assessment is to be undertaken by carers its use is not indicated as a means of carrying out routine health checks on people with learning disabilities living independently in the community.

Feeling Poorly (Dodd & Brunker 1998) is a resource package that has been designed to enable people with learning disabilities to develop the skills to communicate more effectively any discomfort or symptoms of ill health. The materials include an assessment tool, teaching resources and evaluation strategies.

In a similar vein *Getting Better* (Band 1997) is a video resource pack that aims to teach people with learning disabilities how to get what they need from their GP. Acknowledging that people often avoid going to the doctor even when they are ill, the resource offers people practical suggestions and guidelines about how to proceed, for instance in making and then preparing for an appointment with their GP.

Other teaching and learning packages addressing health concerns are listed in the Further reading section, and are suitable for people with learning disabilities. These include work in the areas of going to the doctor (Hollins et al 1996), going into hospital (Hollins et al 1997) and going to outpatients (Hollins et al 1998). *The Healthy Way* was published by the Department of Health (1998) at the same time as *Signposts for Success* (NHS Executive 1998) and includes an easy to read booklet, poster game and cassette. The *Your Good Health* series was published by the British Institute of Learning Disability (BILD 1997) and comprises a series of leaflets. Topics include 'If you are ill', 'Looking after your teeth', 'Coping with stress' and several others on health related themes.

All of the above initiatives aim to enable people with learning disabilities to access and receive better health care. These aims are laudable, however a note of caution must again be sounded: These days there seems to be a training pack for almost any challenge anyone with a learning disability may present or experience, and for their carers too. No problem, except the aim of many is explicitly to simplify – and they do so (often) with resounding success.

Some of these are costly, particularly the resource packages. Potential buyers would be well advised to view expensive packs before purchase. Further, to state the obvious, the purchase of a training package is in itself not a solution to any challenge. Such packages are tools which, depending on the subject area, require skilled facilitation. The limitations of these tools, as well as their possibilities, must be addressed in a realistic way, and ideally considerations about facilitation should be made before purchase.

Good practice in services

The Continuing the Commitment Project in learning disability nursing (DOH 1996) recognised that the learning disability nurse had a central role to play in the surveillance and promotion of health for people with learning disabilities. At Bournewood Community and Mental Health NHS Trust in Surrey a community learning disability nurse was given a specific health surveillance role. The nurse needed to identify if there were people with learning disabilities resident in the community who were not having their health needs met. Once contact had been made the nurse could support the people in identifying their own health needs, and assist them in obtaining the help they needed. Explanations about health matters and health promotion information are further dimensions of the role. Recent developments have included facilitating a programme designed to enable general hospital staff members to develop an awareness of the needs of people with learning disabilities.

Some positive developments have also been made in the area of consent to treatment for people with learning disabilities. In one of the London boroughs, a joint health and social services learning disability service has established comprehensive guidelines for staff, including a procedure to ensure that an accurate and swift response can be made where any difficulty arises with regard to consent.

THE ROLE OF LEARNING DISABILITY NURSES IN HELPING PEOPLE WITH LEARNING DISABILITIES ACCESS HEALTH SERVICES

The resettlement into the community of individuals who had lived in long-stay hospitals heralded a momentous change in the lives of those people with learning disabilities who were involved. What is less often acknowledged, is both the extent to which learning disability nurses have been required to change their practice in order to work in the new style of service provision, and the challenge that this has posed for the profession. There have been some worrying examples of working practices more typical of a long-stay hospital environment being transferred almost wholesale in to the community (Brown & Walmsley 1989). As Collins (1995) has argued, genuine community presence and participation for people with learning disabilities means something more than just being resident in the community.

Learning disability nurses share responsibility for the future of our profession, through their supervision of student nurses in practice, and the mentorship of newly qualified nurses. It is essential for the future development of the profession that practice is contemporary, building on the positive ideologies of today, and abandoning any routine and segregated practices of the past. How learning disability nurses' new roles have needed to evolve can be illustrated well through the example of health care.

Earlier in this chapter, it was noted how health care was once provided in the isolated setting of the long-stay hospital. Here many nurses were responsible for the physical health of people with learning disabilities. Now learning disability nurses must see their focus mainly as one where they enable people with learning disability to access the health care they require, rather than as in the past, seeing themselves as responsible in the

first instance for providing such care. The role of 'health facilitators' (DOH 2001a) has been developed in order to support people with learning disabilities in overcoming some of the barriers they encounter in accessing health services. The report notes (DOH 2001a, 6.12) 'learning disability nurses will be well placed to fulfil this role.'

This shift in the role of learning disability nurses needs to be reflected in practice, in attitudes and in interactions with others (see Box 16.3).

In the new culture of community care learning disability nurses have a very important and central role. But this is not the same as it was, and we do a disservice to our clients if we do not accept the challenge of our new role in relation to helping people with learning disability obtain the health services they need.

Box 16.4 Illustrates some of the ways in which learning disability nurses may work towards enabling better health for their clients.

Box 16.3 Changing role of learning disability nurses

- In practice – as in a residential service for people with learning disability we make a referral to local district nurses, to perform a general health nursing care activity (e.g. to give an injection)
- In attitudes – as we re-evaluate our role and recognise it is one where we enable and assist people to access generic health care services wherever possible
- In interactions – as we appraise other professionals of the new role of learning disability nurses in contemporary learning disability services (DOH 1996)

Box 16.4 Role of learning disability nurses in health care for people with learning disabilities

- Enabling access, by supporting clients to telephone their GPs
- Enabling choice and decision making in health care matters by counselling a client about healthy eating and weight loss
- Helping people to give informed consent to treatment
- A teaching and advisory role with a mother who has learning disabilities, enabling her to provide nutritious meals for her children
- Health surveillance role, for example raising the health awareness of clients, leading people to recognise their own health needs
- Helping people to make and maintain contacts – for example supporting a person with learning disabilities to attend a well man or well woman clinic
- Working with and supporting families and other professionals to manage health care needs for their family members or clients who have learning disabilities
- Liaison in a general practice setting, where several patients have learning disabilities and effective communication can be problematic
- Using symbolic language or illustrations to explain to clients about the treatment they need
- Using available resources to convey health education messages
- Using resources, for example a breast screening awareness pack, to work with women with learning disabilities

Areas requiring further development to ensure good health services for people with learning disabilities

The current focus on the health care of people with learning disabilities is good, and with the plethora of guidelines, research and resources available some noticeable shift towards improved services should be imminent. But as Oliver Russell has acknowledged (Russell 1999), there is compelling evidence to show that progress is scant. What can be done now to make a difference?

A helpful start would be the *actual implementation* of some of the good practice guidelines. Too often useful work (*Signposts for Success*, NHS Executive 1998, *Once a Day*, NHS Executive 1999a) is published with a flourish, but without any corresponding implementation programme, and is left to gather dust on the bookshelves of senior managers, whose attention inevitably has been drawn to today's priority. A named individual in each general hospital, charged with actually implementing *Signposts for Success*, could have had an impact at a local level, which would have considerably improved the experience of health care for service users with learning disability.

A further development of our understanding of health matters associated with people with learning disabilities would be useful. We now know of many areas where people have an increased likelihood of being affected (see earlier in chapter). There could be routine screening and investigation of these conditions, to diagnose early and minimise the impact of any ill health (Barr et al 1999).

Learning disability nurses also need to develop skills in surveillance of the health of people with learning disabilities, in order to make referrals on to specialist health care professionals (DOH 1996). For community learning disability nurses working with people who live independently, this may be using a health care assessment tool designed to enable people with learning disability to recognise for themselves that they may have a health need. When working with non-speaking people with more severe learning disabilities, nurses need to develop enhanced skills in the interpretation of non-verbal communication, gesture and facial expression as well as behaviours, and consider whether the person may be communicating that they are unwell.

Health care providers would do well to consider some of the structural obstacles to people accessing their services. Special consideration needs to be given to the needs of people with learning disabilities in regard to appointment times, consent and understanding. Ensuring access to screening, health monitoring and health checking is obtained would also be a useful development (DOH 1998).

The particular health needs of people with learning disabilities who are from different cultures and ethnic backgrounds could be further examined. Also the education of health service staff (nurses, doctors and others in multidisciplinary health care teams) in key areas such as communication with people with learning disabilities, attitudes and awareness must also be seen as a priority (Mencap 1997).

Finally, as there is likely to be an increase in learning disability nursing activity in the future in health promotion, health education and health surveillance for people with learning disabilities, it is useful to consider the knowledge and skills in this area.

HEALTH PROMOTION

Learning disability nurses, and other professionals such as health visitors specialising in learning disability, have a very important role to play in enabling people with learning disabilities to stay healthy, and in the event of ill health, to access and receive the best possible health care.

It is suggested above that *some* learning disability nurses may need to reflect on how they relinquish aspects of their earlier roles in actually *providing* health care for people with learning disability. By contrast, many learning disability nurses usefully could reflect now on their important role with regard to health promotion, through strategies such as health gain, health surveillance, health awareness and encouraging healthy lifestyles for their clients.

The Alma Ata Declaration (WHO 1978) has defined health promotion as a process of enabling people to increase control over and improve their health. In the UK a standard definition of health promotion in practice is that developed by Ewles & Simnett (1985). It refers to 'health' in a broad sense, including physical, mental and social health. Health promotion can be seen as having three main goals: primary prevention, with a focus on preventing ill health and disease; secondary prevention, which includes early detection and treatment; and tertiary prevention which aims to stop the needless progression of disease (Nightingale 1992).

Continuing the Commitment, the report of the learning disability nursing project (DOH 1996, p. 20) made explicit that 'health surveillance and health promotion' should be seen as areas where learning disability nurses need to develop their knowledge and skills. This was considered to be necessary if learning disability nurses were to be able to 'have a direct or indirect role in the assessment, provision and evaluation of support that contributes to bringing about the optimum health status of the individual.'

The Health of the Nation: A Strategy for People with Learning Disabilities (DOH 1995) has stressed that people with learning disabilities should be included in all the programmes offered to the rest of the community. Also that all health promotion programmes should be presented in such a way as to make them accessible to all people, including those who may have difficulty in understanding some of the concepts.

Signposts for Success (NHS Executive 1998) recognised that an increasing number of people with learning disabilities needed help in managing aspects of their health and lifestyles. The increasing numbers of people with learning disabilities who have become involved in the misuse of alcohol and/or drugs has heightened the need for specialist health promotion in these areas (Parrish & Kay 1998).

Recent trends in generic health promotion have included an emphasis on the notion of 'positive and healthy lifestyles' (Cowley 1996). Here health is emphasised more from a social than a medical perspective, recognising self-determination and lifestyle choices. Health promotion activities may aim to increase positive health behaviours such as

eating a healthy diet, but they may also focus on strategies to decrease behaviours which may be damaging to health, such as the over-use of alcohol. It is also important that health promotion can be seen as potentially enjoyable as well as good for the individual, such as in the Cardiff Pedal Power fitness programme. Here more than 100 adults with learning disabilities have participated in the scheme that developed from a 'Try a bike day' in summer 1996. Now, following a programme of regular supported cycling sessions:

Every twelve weeks a series of measurements are taken including blood pressure, height, weight and pulse rate before and after exercise. The psychological and social effects of the programme are measured, using pictures to check participants' enjoyment levels. The results have been spectacular all round. After 12 weeks, cardiovascular fitness levels among the first 25 participants were up by 100%, and nearly three quarters of participants had lost weight (Hobden 1999).

This is heartening especially as physical inactivity, with all its associated health risks, is considered to be prevalent in people with learning disabilities, who as a group are regarded as 'amongst the most inactive and sedentary members of the population' (Messent et al 2000).

In generic health promotion services there is a debate about the usefulness of various approaches to convey most effectively to the general public messages about health. Single focus health issues are in some quarters viewed as ineffective as they may be regarded as targeting professionally defined 'problems'.

However, in work with people with learning disabilities there is value in keeping messages clear and simple, and 'single focus health promotion programmes to modify lifestyles' (Cowley 1996, p. 449) are likely to be the most effective. Here for example, topics such as weight loss, smoking cessation, safer sex, improved nutrition, exercise for health and relaxation, are dealt with individually. Goal directed programmes, using techniques grounded in our understanding of how people with learning disabilities may learn most effectively, can be successful. Effective communication of health related information is essential. To ensure maximum effectiveness this needs to be accessible and user-friendly. Complicated health promotion images such as the 'Aids Iceberg' campaign some years ago may be incomprehensible to a person who struggles with concepts, and who may have a tendency to literal interpretations. Health promotion messages which dwell on giving up existing behaviours may unintentionally imply that to be healthy is to adopt a miserable and undesired lifestyle. However, care must be taken to ensure that people with learning disabilities understand health promotion messages in a balanced way; for example ensuring that people understand that three or four times a week short episodes of vigorous aerobic exercise can be beneficial to health, and conversely that over-exercising can, in the long run, be detrimental to health.

Box 16.5 explains some of the health related terms used when working with people with learning disabilities.

Recent 'health' based initiatives have been the development of health clinics for people with learning disabilities, for example where learning

---

Box 16.5 Health related terms used when working with people with learning disabilities

- Health gain – where a person's health is improved as a result of an intervention, such as education or screening
- Health surveillance – describes a role, often undertaken by community learning disability nurses, where the health and wellbeing of clients is a focus. Where necessary, referral on to general health services or health promotion specialists may result from these interventions
- Health facilitator – people with learning disabilities who need support to ensure their health needs are met are to have a named health facilitator from the local community learning disability team by Spring 2003 (DOH 2001a, p. 63, 6.12)
- Health awareness – where people have an understanding of their own health and the relationship between certain activities and behaviours, for example that over-eating can lead to obesity; that neglecting teeth cleaning could lead to dental caries
- Healthy lifestyles – where individuals attempt to live their lives in a 'healthy' way. For instance, to eat five portions of fruit and vegetables per day, engage in 20 minutes of brisk exercise, to refrain from smoking and only to consume alcohol in moderation would be considered some of the foundations of a healthy lifestyle

disability specialist health visitors or nurses have set up drop-in style health clinics in day service settings. In Scotland (Allan 1999) a drop-in health clinic was established in two adult training centres, facilitated by a health visitor. The research shows that people with learning disabilities used the clinic for a variety of reasons such as advice about weight loss and healthy eating. Other consultations concerned bereavement and loss. A similar project in Watford (Milligan 1999) has been reported, where community learning disability nurses run two half day health improvement clinics a month in a day centre for people with learning disabilities.

The obvious advantage of both these schemes is that clients are seen in familiar surroundings, and can be supported by people whom they know. Regular health monitoring can uncover health needs that may otherwise remain undiagnosed. For instance, high blood pressure is reported as one of the main health needs detected in the Watford project. In terms of addressing the inequalities in health care provision for people with learning disabilities these projects appear to be successful. Yet the fact that such health input needs to be provided in these segregated settings reflects the failure of mainstream health services to properly provide for the health needs of people with learning disabilities in the community on equal terms with non-disabled people. The success of such projects in meeting health needs must be weighed against the long-term harm that may come from the perpetuation of separate provisions for our clients. This is not what was intended when community care services were being developed.

In East Yorkshire another development sought to address health needs for people with learning

 Reader activity 16.4

Consider some of the ways in which the health needs of people with learning disabilities could be met, without compromising any of the principles of the right to access health services in the same way as would any other person.

disabilities, with a specific focus on healthy lifestyles and the early self-identification of illness (Graham 2001). Local research was undertaken to try to understand why people did not use primary health services. 'Where people accessed primary health care independently, this was encouraged, but recognition was given to those who needed practical help to do so. This was achieved by developing a tailor-made well person clinic *in the client's own GP practice*' (Graham 2001, p. 41). Here a similar outcome to the earlier two examples is achieved. But the more typical environment of the GP surgery as a location in which to focus on health concerns must be considered a more suitable model for the service provision.

In the project above there has also been encouragement for people with learning disabilities to participate in some of the local health initiatives, alongside other service users who do not have a learning disability. In terms of community participation and presence this is a positive development (Graham 2001).

Other health promotion initiatives have involved actual collaboration between learning disability services and mainstream health service providers. In one project in Dundee a 'Women's health issues group' was created when it was identified through local research that women with learning disabilities were sometimes missing out on some basic health education messages (McRae 1997). Research locally had revealed that a majority of women with learning disabilities had not accessed a well woman or family planning clinic. Also smear tests, vaginal or breast examination or contraceptive advice was not generally being obtained. The research showed a marginally better access to such services from women who lived independently, than those who were still resident in a hospital. Here learning disability nurses collaborated with local well woman and family planning services. It is through such professional liaisons that best practice in health can be developed. Learning disability nurses are in the best possible position both to advocate on behalf of their clients, and to help professional colleagues who are less used to working with people with learning disabilities to become aware of some of the particular needs people may have. For ex-

ample, communication is often difficult with some people with learning disabilities and simple messages about keeping language simple and jargon-free may enable a more satisfactory consultation for both the professional and the person involved.

Earlier in this chapter reference was made to the evidence which demonstrates that people with learning disabilities tend to be excluded from health screening checks, and other preventive measures such as immunisations (Barr et al 1999, Wilson & Haire 1990). It is clear from earlier research that health screening could contribute to the improvement of health for people with learning disabilities, and there have been several attempts to raise an awareness of the need for screening. In South East England collaboration between a volunteer service user, practitioners from three learning disability NHS Trust providers and West Surrey Health Promotion Service has produced a breast screening package. Now any woman with learning disabilities in this locality can be talked through the whole process of breast examination and mammography while looking at pictures of the clinic, and some of the staff based there. Those who are able can read the clear explanations of the process (which include some symbols) and respond to the 'yes' or 'no' consent prompts.

Other health promotion activities directly aim to improve health knowledge, awareness and management. An important topic for people with learning disabilities is sexual health. There are examples of projects that focus on teaching people about sexuality, and other intimate or personal subjects such as hygiene, interpersonal relationships and sociosexual knowledge and skills (Antram & Phillips 1992, McCarthy et al 1998, Rushton 1994).

One project used group work techniques to present information and raise awareness and understanding about sociosexual matters and, importantly, to examine with the group how this information could be used in their everyday lives. This work was undertaken with people described as having moderate to severe learning disabilities, people unlikely to pick up health education messages without direct specialist input. The project leader devised a non-verbal (pictorial) assessment tool to measure the sociosexual knowledge of group members. There was also a series of questions about gender identity, sexual language, body parts and sexual behaviour. She then facilitated a series of workshops for adults with learning disabilities, with the aim of improving the social functioning of the participants, and increasing their sociosexual knowledge and understanding of socially acceptable sociosexual behaviour. Pre- and post-programme testing indicated that workshop participants had increased their understanding of the three key areas. A control group that did not have the training showed almost no change in their understanding of these areas over the same period of time.

It is now recognised that teaching teenagers and adults with learning disabilities about sexuality is important, especially where evidence exists that people may not have a good enough understanding of this area. This may be evidenced in a variety of ways. A collaborative project was instigated by a nurse and a special needs teacher, to develop and run a practical programme to teach social skills, hygiene and basic sex education to teenagers with severe learning difficulties. The programme was devised initially to address the behaviour of a pupil who 'exhibited inappropriate behaviour in public places' (Antram & Phillips 1992). However, rather than just do work with the pupil directly it was decided to involve the entire class of teenagers. The programme needed to address the following behaviours:

- interactions with strangers, ranging from extreme shyness to complete trust
- the distinction between private and public behaviours
- expressing sexual interest in a manner which did not cause offence or embarrassment to others.

Other work in the sphere of health promotion already undertaken with people with learning disabilities includes smoking education (Kelman et al 1997), the 'pleasures and problems of alcohol' (Manthorpe 1997), menstruation (Rodgers 2001) and HIV/AIDS (Senker 1997). Access to studies such as these prior to considering any work of this nature is strongly recommended. Reviewing the existing literature in learning disability journals, establishing what research has already been undertaken to evaluate the methods used, and the use of electronic search methods such as accessing web pages on the internet can often provide very useful information. Health promotion activities grounded in evidence-based practice initiatives are likely to be better received by service managers, and by avoiding the mistakes of others who may have pioneered initiatives, are more likely to be successful for clients.

Finally, the use of alternative and complementary health approaches in learning disability services (for example massage, aromatherapy, reflexology) is discussed elsewhere (Ch. 20). The positive influences on health of these initiatives are important. Learning disability nurses are encouraged to consider accessing such services for clients.

CONCLUSION

This chapter has explored health care for people with learning disabilities. It has highlighted how long-stay hospital-based health care provision and health care expertise were lost forever when services for people with learning disabilities were relocated in the community. Although acknowledged to have been an imperfect system (Aspray 1999), it was nevertheless easily accessed by those who needed medical attention.

It was hoped that genuine community integration for people with learning disabilities would result from the hospital closures, but, arguably, this goal is still distant as the example of health care demonstrates. Research evidence consistently shows that people with learning disabilities are generally not satisfied with the health care they receive. Whether it is, for example, that health needs go unmet, that screening is overlooked, or that consent to treatment is deferred to a relative, when they are asked, people with learning disabilities often express dissatisfaction with aspects of the service they receive.

Now many initiatives and developments are in place or underway to address these concerns. This chapter has highlighted some of the innovative work going on, and by reference to the Department

Box 16.6   Key actions for health (DOH, 2001a, p. 61)

- Action to reduce health inequalities: explore feasibility of establishing a confidential inquiry into mortality among people with learning disabilities
- Action to challenge discrimination against people with learning disabilities from minority ethnic communities
- Health facilitators identified for people with learning disabilities by Spring 2003
- All people with a learning disability to be registered with a GP by June 2004
- All people with a learning disability to have a Health Action Plan by June 2005
- NHS to ensure that all mainstream hospital services are accessible to people with learning disabilities
- Development of local specialist services for people with severe challenging behaviour to be a priority for the capital element of the Learning Disability Fund
- Mental Health NSF (National Service Framework) will bring new benefits to people with learning disabilities
- New role for specialist learning disability services, making most effective use of their expertise

of Health publications (DOH 1998, DOH 2001a,b,c, NHS Executive, 1999a,b) has demonstrated that improved health care for people with learning disabilities is a government priority.

The publication of the first White Paper for learning disabilities for 30 years (DOH 2001a) has served to harness some of the disparate initiatives that have been going on in the sphere of health. It demonstrates unequivocally the Government's commitment to person-centred health services, which people with learning disabilities can access according to their particular needs. The White Paper describes the failure of mainstream health services to consider the needs of people with learning disabilities, highlighting that the NHS has been slow to develop the capacity and skills needed to meet the particular needs of this group (DOH 2001a, p. 59).

If the 'Key Actions' for health (DOH 2001a, p. 61) outlined in the White Paper are effectively implemented (see Box 16.6), and if there is commitment in local health services to ensure the actions are achieved, then there can be room for cautious optimism that health care for people with learning disabilities is set to improve.

REFERENCES

Allan E 1999 Learning disability: promoting health equality in the community. Nursing Standard 13(44): 32–37

Antram M, Phillips S 1992 Straight talk. Special Children (March): 7–19

Aspray T J 1999 Patients with learning disability in the community. British Medical Journal 318: 476–477

Band R 1997 Getting better – how people with learning disabilities can get the best from their GP. Pavilion Publishing, Brighton

Barr O, Gilgunn J, Kane T, Moore G 1999 Health screening for people with learning disabilities by a community learning disability nursing service in Northern Ireland. Journal of Advanced Nursing 29(6): 1482–1491

Beange H, McElduff A, Baker W 1995 Medical disorders of adults with mental retardation: a population study. American Journal of Mental Retardation 99: 595–604

BILD 1997 Your good health series. Bild publications, Plymbridge Distributors, Plymbridge House, Estover Road, Plymouth PL6 7PZ

Biley A 1994 A handicap of negative attitudes and lack of choice: caring for in-patients with disabilities. Professional Nurse 9(12): 786–788

Booth T, Booth W 1994 Parental adequacy, parenting failure and parents with learning difficulties. Health and Social Care in the Community 2: 161–172

Booth T, Booth W 1996 Sounds of silence: narrative research with inarticulate subjects. Disability & Society 11(1): 55–69

Brown H, Walmsley J 1989 In: Brechin A, Walmsley J (eds) Making connections. Reflecting on the lives and experiences of people with learning disabilities. Hodder & Stoughton, London

Building Expectations 1996 Opportunities and services for people with a learning disability. The Mental Health Foundation, London

Burke P, Cigno K 2000 Learning disabilities in children. Blackwell Science, London

Caplan P 1997 Now doctors are having to ration. Viewpoint, Mencap, London

Collins J 1995 Moving forward or back? Institutional trends in services for people with learning disabilities. In: Philpot T, Ward L (eds) Values and visions: changing ideas in services for people with learning disabilities. Butterworth Heinemann, London, ch 8

Cowley S 1996 Promoting positive and healthy lifestyles. In: Twinn S, Roberts B, Andrews S (eds) Community health care nursing: principles for practice. Butterworth Heinemann, London, ch 26

Centre for Research and Information into Mental Disability, University of Birmingham, Birmingham

Cumella S, Corbett J, Clark D et al 1992 Primary health care for people with a learning disability. Mental Handicap 2: 23–125

Daniels L, Rose A, Wall E et al 1989 Road to recovery: the effect of successful patient education. Intensive Care Nursing 5(1): 19–24

Dodd K, Brunker J 1998 Feeling poorly: Pavilion Publishing, Brighton

Department of Health 1992 The health of the nation: a strategy for health in England. HMSO, London

Department of Health 1995 The health of the nation: a strategy for people with learning disabilities. HMSO, London

Department of Health 1996 Continuing the commitment: the report of the learning disability nursing project. HMSO, London

Department of Health 1998 The healthy way. HMSO, London

Department of Health 2000 The NHS plan. HMSO, London

Department of Health 2001a Valuing people: a new strategy for learning disability for the 21st century. Cm 5086. The Stationery Office, London

Department of Health 2001b Reference guide to consent for examination or treatment. The Stationery Office, London

Department of Health 2001c Seeking consent: working with people with learning disabilities. The Stationery Office, London

Edgerton R B, Gasto M A, Kelly H et al 1994 Health care for ageing people with mental retardation. Mental Retardation 32(2): 146–150

Ewles L, Simnett I 1985 Promoting health: a practical guide to health education. Wiley, Chichester

Foreman P 1997 Medicine health and intellectual disability. Journal of Intellectual Disability 22(4): 225–226

Fovargue S, Keywood K, Flynn M 2000 Participation in health care decision-making by adults with learning disabilities. Mental Health & Learning Disabilities Care 3(10): 341–344

Graham K 2001 Better health care and learning disability. Nursing Times 97(8): 39–41

Hall P, Ward E 1999 Cervical screening for women with learning disability. British Medical Journal 7182 (318 Index): 536–537

Hart S L 1997 Learning disabled people in general hospitals – towards a better understanding of their care and treatment. Unpublished MSc dissertation. University of Portsmouth

Hart S L 1998 Learning-disabled people's experience of general hospitals. British Journal of Nursing 7(8): 470–477

Hart S L 1999 Meaningful choices: consent to treatment in general health care settings for people with learning disabilities. Journal of Learning Disabilities for Nursing, Health and Social Care 3(1): 20–26

Hayward B, Kerr M 1998 Accessing primary health care: pathways to care. In: Kerr M (ed) Innovations in health care for people with intellectual disabilites. Lisieux Hall, Chorley, Lancashire, ch 2

Hobden J 1999 Pedal power and collaboration. Frontline (February 3)

Holland A J, Oliver C 1995 Down's syndrome and the links with Alzheimer's disease. Journal of Neurology, Neurosurgery and Psychiatry 59: 111–114

Hollins S, Bernal J, Gregory M et al 1996 Going to the doctor. Books Beyond Word Series (available from the Royal College of Psychiatrists, 17 Belgrave Square, London SW1X 8PG)

Hollins S, Avis A, Chevertan S et al 1998 Going into hospital. Books Beyond Word Series (available from the Royal College of Psychiatrists, 17 Belgrave Square, London SW1X 8PG)

Hollins S, Bernal J, Gregory M et al 1998 Going to outpatients. Books Beyond Word Series (available from the Royal College of Psychiatrists, 17 Belgrave Square, London SW1X 8PG)

HoNOS-LD Version 2 1998 Health of the nation outcome scales for people with learning disabilities. Royal College of Psychiatrists, London

Howells G 1986 Are the health needs of mentally handicapped adults being met? Journal of the Royal College of General Practitioners 36: 449–453.

Hull and Holderness Community Health NHS Trust 1995 The Patient's Charter and you with signs and symbols. Hull and Holderness NHS Trust and Makaton Vocabulary Development Project,

Jenkins R, Brooksbank D, Miller E et al 1994 Ageing in learning difficulties: the development of health care outcome indicators. Journal of Intellectual Disability Research 38(3): 257–264

Kelman L, Lindsay W, McPherson F, Mathewson Z 1997 Smoking education for people with learning disabilities. British Journal of Learning Disabilities 25: 95–99

Kerr M, Fraser D, Felce D 1996 Primary health care for people with a learniing disability; a keynote review. British Journal of Learning Disabilities 24: 2–8

Langan J, Whitfield M, Russell O 1994 Paid and unpaid carers; their role in and satisfaction with primary health care for people with learning disabilities. Health and Social Care 2: 357–365

Law J, Byng S, Bunning A, Seeff B 2000 Communication disability in primary care, NHS Executive, City University, London

Leino-Kilpin H 1993 Client and information: a literature review. Journal of Clinical Nursing 2(6): 331–340

Lennox N, Kerr M 1997 The general practice care of people with intellectual disability; barriers and solutions. Journal of Intellectual Disability Research 41(5): 380–390

Lock K 1996 The changing organisation of health care: setting the scene. In: Twinn S, Roberts B, Andrews S (eds) Community health care nursing principles for practice. Butterworth Heinemann, London, ch 2

McCarthy M, Thompson D 1998 Sex and the 3R's rights, responsibilities and risks. Pavilion Publishing, Brighton

McRae D 1997 Health care for women with learning disabilities. Nursing Times 93(15): 58–59

Manthorpe J 1997 Service challenges: the pleasure and problems of alcohol. Journal of Learning Disabilities for Nursing Health and Social care 1(1): 31–36

Mathews D R 1997 The OK health check: a health assessment checklist for people with learning disabilities. British Journal of Learning Disabilities 25: 139–143

Martin D M et al 1997 Health gain through screening – users' and carers' perspectives in health care. Journal of Intellectual and Developmental Disability 22(4): 241–249

Meehan S, Moore G, Barr O 1995 Specialist services for people with learning disabilities. Nursing Times 91(13): 33–35

Mencap 1997 Prescription for change (summary). Mencap Research,

Messent P, Cooke C, Long J 2000 Secondary barriers to physical activity for adults with mild and moderate learning disabilities. Journal of Learning Disabilities 4(3): 247–263

Milligan C 1999 Targeting unmet needs. Community Nurse (June): 14

Nightingale C 1992 Pointing to the way ahead in health education for people with learning disabilities. Professional Nurse 7(9): 612–615.

NHS Executive 1992 Guidelines HSG (92) 42 Health services for people with learning disabilities (mental health). HMSO, London

NHS Executive 1998 Signposts for success in commissioning and providing health services for people with learning disabilities. HMSO, London

NHS Executive 1999a Once a day. HMSO, London

NHS Executive 1999b Health Service Circular HSC 1999/031 Consent to treatment. HMSO, London

Northway R 2000 Finding out together: lessons in participatory research for the learning disability nurse. Mental Health and Learning Disabilities Care 3(7): 229–232

O'Brien J 1986 A guide to personal futures planning. In: Bellamy G T, Wilcox B (eds) The activities catalogue. Responsive Systems Associates, Georgia, USA

Parrish A, Kay B 1998 Exploring the NHS Executive document Signposts for success. British Journal of Nursing 7(8): 478–480

Pearson V, Davis C, Ruoff C, Dyer J 1998 Only one quarter of women in Exeter have cervical screening. British Medical Journal 316: 1979 (letter)

Richardson M 1997 Participatory research methods: people with learning difficulties. British Journal of Nursing 6(19): 1114–1121

Rodgers J 2001 The experience and management of menstruation for women with learning disabilities. Tizard Learning Disability Review 6(1): 36–44

Rushton J 1994 Learning together. Nursing Times March 90(9): 44–46

Russell O 1999 The way in – guaranteeing access to a healthier future for people with learning disabilities. Note of a breakfast meeting held at the King's Fund on Wednesday 23 June 1999

Senker J 1997 Gender, race and sexual behaviour: issues in service responses to HIV/AIDS. British Journal of Learning Disabilities 25: 58–63

United Kingdom Central Council for Nursing, Midwifery and Health Visiting 1998 Guidelines for mental health and learning disabilities nursing. UKCC, London

Vernon D 1997 Health. In: Gates B (ed) Learning disabilities, 3rd edn. Churchill Livingstone, Edinburgh, ch 6

Walker C, Walker A 1998 Uncertain futures: people with learning difficulties and their ageing family carers. Pavilion Publishing, Brighton

Wells M, Turner S, Martin D, Roy A 1997 Health gain through screening – coronary heart disease and stroke: developing primary health care services for people with intellectual disability. Journal of Intellectual and Developmental Disability 22(4): 251–263

Whitehouse R, Chamberlain P, Tunna K 2000 Dementia in people with learning disability: a preliminary study into care staff knowledge and attributions. British Journal of Learning Disabilities 28(4): 148–153

Wilson D N, Haire A 1990 Health care screening for people with a mental handicap living in the community. British Medical Journal 301: 1379–1381

Wing L 1989 Hospital closure and the resettlement of residents: the case of Darenth Park. Gower, Aldershot

World Health Organisation (WHO) 1978 Alma Ata declaration. Copenhagen, Denmark

FUTHER READING

Band R 1997 The Healthy Living Series – 5 booklets 'Food', 'Keep Clean', 'Safety in the Home', 'Epilepsy' and 'Coming for a Drink?' Available from: The Elfrida Society, The Tom Blythe Centre, 34 Islington Park Street Road, London N1 1PX

BILD Publications 1997 Your Good Health Services – 10 booklets (If you are ill; Looking after your teeth; Coping with stress; Eating and Drinking; Breathe Easy; Alcohol and Smoking; Exercise; Seeing and hearing; Sex; Using medicine safely) Available from BILD publications, Plymbridge Distributors, Plymbridge House, Estover Road, Plymouth PL6 7PZ

Department of Health 1998 The Healthy Way. Published simultaneously with 'Signposts for Success', this resource consists of an illustrated and easy to read booklet, a cassette and a poster/game which may be suitable for some service users and their carers 1998.

Dodd K, Brunker J 1998 Feeling Poorly. Pocketed ring binder providing a training programme and resources for people with learning disabilities and their support workers. Pavilion Publishing, Freepost (BR458) 8 St George's Place Brighton, East Sussex BN1 4ZZ

McCarthy M, Thompson D 1998 Sex and the 3R's Rights, Responsibilities and Risks, 2nd edn. A sex education package for working with people with learning difficulties. Pavilion Publishing, Brighton Available from Pavilion Publishing Ltd 8 St George's Place, Brighton, East Sussex BN1 4GB

USEFUL ADDRESSES

Department of Health website is a useful source of any information about health www.doh.gov.uk

British Medical Association www.bma.org.uk
Health Evidence Bulletins: medical conditions in people with intellectual disability

http://hebw.uwcm.ac.uk./learningdisabilities/chapter7.htm
West Surrey Health Authority, Breast Screening at the Jarvis Centre. Information from Diane McCormack, Health Promotion Service, The Jarvis Centre, 60 Stoughton Road, Guildford, Surrey GU1 1LJ

17

Profound and multiple disability

Eileen Wake

KEY ISSUES

- The prevalence of profound and multiple disability has increased in the last 25 years (Hack et al 1996, Kohlhauser et al 2000, Lorenn et al 1998).
- This increase of prevalence is due to a number of reasons, for example, increased survival

rate in early gestation and very low birth weight neonates, and technological advances assisting in reduction of mortality rates (Newacheck et al 1998).

- Increased survival has not automatically meant reduced morbidity. It has resulted in increased incidence of infants surviving with neurological sequelae, for example cerebral palsy and cognition problems as well as profound and multiple disabilities (Msall et al 1993, Sanderson and Hall 1995, Vohr et al 2000).

INTRODUCTION

This chapter considers, in some depth, the holistic needs of people with profound and/or multiple disabilities, within the context of family-based care. It intends to promote further study by readers by exposing them to a wide range of relevant literature and research.

What does 'profound and multiple disability' mean?

This is a term that is often used yet difficult to define. Kay et al (1995a) have stated that it is important to move away from definitions that are 'static', and move 'towards a more person centred approach'. Using this approach, profound and multiple disability might be construed as referring to an individual requiring maximum assistance in most if not all aspects of everyday life, in terms of 24-hour care and supervision. For example, the person may have difficulty in communication, eating and drinking, continence and mobilisation.

Multiple disability means that the individual has additional needs, for example in terms of physical disabilities and/or sensory impairment, and this often includes a range of additional, complex health needs, as acknowledged by the Department of Health (DoH 2001a). It may also include life limiting/threatening condition in addition to, or as a consequence of the cause of a person's learning disabilities.

It is important that carers working with people who have profound and multiple disabilities stop and reflect upon the meanings that are attached to

such terms. As carers, it is vital that we question such labels from a psychosocial perspective. Words that we invariably use in our schemas, and which create our view of everyday life, include a wide range of attributions about others in terms of our own attitudes, beliefs and values. It is important that all carers involved in the care of people with profound and multiple disabilities examine and re-examine their attitudes, beliefs and values regarding this group of people.

It is essential that carers working with people with profound and multiple disabilities act as advocates for their clients, and focus on their abilities and strengths, rather than concentrating on what they are unable to do. In the past the medical model (Jones 1994) had a tendency to focus upon what a person could not do, and nurses should challenge this, celebrating the uniqueness of every individual and focusing care on their strengths. This does not mean that needs are not acknowledged, simply that the person's strengths should be used in helping to meet these needs. This can involve a high degree of health care input, much of which is aimed at maintaining health and preventing ill health.

The traditional nursing models used within health care are very limiting when working with people with profound disabilities, as acknowledged above. The increased use of critical care pathways within the acute sector has to be viewed with caution in terms of meeting the acute health care needs of people with profound disabilities. This systems approach focuses upon the biological/physiological needs of the individual and would not provide sufficient insight into that person's holistic needs. One way to address these issues would be to use the person-centred planning approach (Kennedy 1995, Rudkin and Rowe 1999, Stalker and Campbell 1998), (also see Ch. 19) in conjunction with the Health Action Plan (HAP), as recommended within the current DOH (2001a) strategy for learning disability. However, all approaches carry a risk of over documentation and loss of focus on the person one is caring for.

Therefore it would seem prudent to adopt a collaborative stance such as that acknowledged in Fruin's (1998) SSI report on services for adults with learning disabilities and such as HemiHelp (1999), with all dimensions of care integrated within the information. This is particularly useful if the person has ongoing health needs that require intervention, as one would be able to map the episodes of ill health/exacerbation of a chronic illness such as epilepsy, and seek to review any long-term issues that arise. This would enable appropriate health promotion strategies to be undertaken with and on behalf of the client to promote wellbeing. An example of this could be when a young woman with profound learning disabilities has increased tonic–clonic seizures prior to the onset of menstruation on a regular basis. This increased incidence of seizures correlated with the menstrual cycle is known as 'catamenial epilepsy' (British Epilepsy Association 2001, p. 1). This would identify a need for medication review as acknowledged by Robertson (1999) and Zahn et al (1998), in terms of anticonvulsant therapy (and possible introduction of clobozam along with the introduction of the contraceptive pill to aid cycle regulation, and continued regular blood serum anticonvulsant therapy monitoring). The introduction of the contraceptive pill to regulate hormonal activity will in itself lead to health promotion and maintenance needs, for example regular blood pressure monitoring. Consideration must also be given to the ethical dimensions of using this approach and to informed consent concerns (DOH 2001b).

The health status of every individual is unique. For example, if someone receives enteral feeding, it will be usual for that person to have a daily nutritional assessment to maintain good hydration and nutrition. However, for another person, who is able to eat and drink normally, either with or without help, such an intervention would be unnecessary. Yet those who have enteral feeding are not ill, they are just not able to have all their nutritional needs met orally. The enteral feeding therefore maintains their health.

This issue will be further explored when nutrition is discussed, especially with regard to whether enteral feeding is therapy or treatment; this is an ongoing ethical issue within learning disabilities nursing and the legal system in the UK.

Holistic care: a multidisciplinary/ multi-agency approach?

It is important that professionals recognise the boundaries of their knowledge and skills. People with profound and/or multiple disabilities will have a wide range of needs, as will their carers. It would be wrong to assume that the adult client will need to be under the care of a consultant psychiatrist and not require the full range of services that the rest of the community uses. This is especially so as many people with profound disabilities live in the community; therefore, their care should be in and by the community (Brown & Smith 1992, DOH 1999a). People with profound disabilities may require help from the primary, secondary and tertiary health sectors, as well as from social services and other statutory and non-statutory agencies, which may cause difficulties. They may also find they have to deal with a multitude of professionals, and there can be a significant lack in consistency of approach by those professionals as well as a poorly resourced service (HemiHelp 1999). Thus the 'key' or 'link' worker or 'named nurse' approach has been used to minimise the difficulties of multi-agency working. This named individual acts as the main link with clients and their carers, and seeks to coordinate services with them, thus avoiding duplication, as recommended by the DOH (2001a). One problem that has been identified with this approach is that each agency will appoint a named person to work with the family; this is not a true key worker approach. Indeed it is of concern that the recommendation for a key worker approach and the inherent difficulties with multi-agency working have yet to be addressed within all aspects of service provision. Parents/carers wish and need the key worker approach to work; the problems of poor inter-agency communication, and service gaps and overlaps continue to limit the ability of services to be truly needs-led.

Agencies involved should acknowledge that one person from the service that is most involved should coordinate services. Central to this arrangement is the need for this person to be someone with whom the client and the carer can identify, and whom they feel will best act as a facilitator, advocate and enabler. This also ensures that the professional workers gain more appropriate opportunities to build upon their interactions with the client and so offer a more needs-led service, as acknowledged by Griffiths & Cowman (1999).

Regular reviews of service input should be arranged, and these meetings must include the service users, i.e. the clients and their carers. Practitioners must be familiar with the recommendations and the implications for practice of legislation such as the Carers (Recognition and Services) Act 1995, the 'Quality protects' management plan for disabled children (DOH 1999b), and the Carers and Disabled Children's Act (2000). Practitioners also need to consider the implications of the forthcoming Children's NHS Plan (DOH 2001c), and the Learning Disability Task Force (adult and children's task forces) as recommended by the DOH (2001a).

Need for holistic and lifelong planning of care

This focuses on how people with profound and/or multiple disabilities can be supported to maximise their quality of life. One of the ways in which this can be achieved is the maintenance of the individual's health. Health gains are also considered where appropriate, but it needs to be appreciated that health gains cannot be met if the individual is not being supported in the maintenance of health and in strategies to avoid ill health. In addition to considering the person with profound and multiple disabilities one must remember that the person does not live in isolation and therefore the needs of the family and carers must also be considered. There is a multitude of published articles which explore the impact on the family of caring roles, for example Cameron et al (1992), Greenberg et al (1993), Barnett & Boyce (1995), Cahill & Glidden (1996), Cunningham (1996), Chisholm (2000), Van Riper (2000), Button et al (2001). It would require an additional chapter to do justice to the complexity and diversity of family needs and experiences. Practitioners are advised to consider this aspect in depth when working with families and to read the material with the purpose of enabling, empower-

ing and listening for families. Readers should refer to Chapter 24 for a more detailed account of family-centred approaches to care.

When exploring a person's health care requirements one needs to consider the impact of meeting these on the family if the person is cared for at home. With an increase in medical technology such as enteral feeding equipment and portable oropharyngeal suction and a range of other care interventions this may result in parents and even siblings perhaps having to provide a wide range of care ranging from oral hygiene to intimate care and 'nursing interventions'.

Practitioners working with families need to be aware of the potential problem of 'obligate parenting' (Darbyshire 1994) and ensure that service provision is in place to reduce the potential burden of care on the family and thus free up family time to enable positive family functioning. In addition to this, practitioners need to be aware of the accountability and responsibility dimensions (UKCC 1992) in teaching a family member or other informal carers to undertake a 'nursing intervention' such as oropharyngeal suction. There are also issues of audit to ensure quality of teaching and review of skills acquired to ensure that the needs of the person are not compromised in any way (as well as the health and safety issues for the carer). An additional facet to this is in relation to formal carers within the local authority when a person is receiving care (day or residential) or education, and the support these carers need to ensure safe and evidence-based provision of appropriate health care for clients. This has significant implications for health care providers in terms of which (if any) nursing care is going to be provided by the local authority staff. The accountability and responsibility of the health care providers in relation to education, training, support and audit of such care provision must be acknowledged in order to ensure that the client's health care needs are indeed met.

ISSUES RELATED TO EATING AND DRINKING

People with disabilities may have problems related to muscle tone around the mouth and face or in the body generally. A person with severe cerebral palsy, for example, may have a problem with all of these that will express itself in terms of general posture, i.e. seating position difficulties, as well as problems with the ability to suck, chew and swallow without aspirating (Rogers et al 1993).

Important reflexes such as coughing and gag may be limited, and the person may still have some of the reflexes that are present in infancy, such as the startle reflex. The implications of the startle reflex are commented on in the next section.

Such problems may be in addition to other problems common in the general population, such as food intolerance and allergies, malabsorption syndromes, and specific oral/dental and skeletal problems. The implications for eating and drinking of conditions such as cerebral palsy (and the resultant increased energy expenditure in addition to actual feeding problems as highlighted by Stallings et al 1996), cleft lip and palate, Pierre Robin syndrome and Goldenhar syndrome, for example, cannot be underestimated. It is also important to consider the impact of underlying health problems, such as congenital heart disease and respiratory difficulties, both of which can greatly affect a person's ability to eat and drink. Gastrointestinal problems such as oesophageal reflux are relatively common in people with severe cerebral palsy, and cause a great deal of discomfort (Halpern et al 1991). Management of gastro-oesophageal reflux is usually via conservative medical treatment, initially using drugs such as cimetidine. Practitioners should be aware that cisapride, which previously was widely recommended, has been suspended from use in the UK as a result of ongoing concerns in relation to its potentially harmful pharmacodynamics upon the heart in neonates, as commented upon by Premjj & Paes (1999) and Ferriman (2000).

Medication should be used in conjunction with advice to carers on techniques that may alleviate the symptoms, such as ensuring that the person is in a comfortable, upright sitting position during the meal, and is not laid down for at least 30 minutes afterwards. Close observation is needed after meals, especially if the person is prone to reflux problems. Any discomfort or vomiting could have serious consequences (for example if the individual is lying down there is an increased risk of gastro-oesophageal reflux and resultant aspiration, which could lead to significant respiratory distress). The avoidance of drugs and food or drink that are linked with gastro-oesophageal irritation should be encouraged, and everyone involved in the person's care should be aware of what foods can cause such problems. Offering smaller meals more often, rather than the traditional 'three square meals a day' will also help, especially if there is an underlying medical condition such as cardiac or respiratory disease.

It may be necessary for a specialist in gastro-oesophageal problems to become involved if the condition continues despite conservative management, as the discomfort and distress of reflux and its potential complications, such as oesophageal erosion, should not be underestimated. It may therefore be necessary for surgery to be performed (the Nissen fundoplication, Heine et al 1995) to lessen the likelihood of reflux. For some people this may be done as a precursor to insertion of a gastrostomy. However, this should be in view of the reflux difficulties and not just routinely part of PEG insertion (Puntis et al 2000), in which case insertion will be part of the overall surgical procedure, rather than via endoscopy as described below. However, the good feeding regimens should continue after surgery and the person will continue to require careful monitoring.

Another aspect of feeding problems to be considered relates to the level of learning disabilities the person may have. Some may have very immature feeding skills, such as sucking food rather than attempting to chew it, or even being unable to take food off a spoon correctly, except by tongue thrusting and licking movements. As a result some clients may be unable to manage food, even in a semisolid form, without distress. Traughton & Hill (2001) commented that this inability to feed without difficulties is understandably strongly linked to malnutrition in such clients. A strong body of published material (Dahl et al 1996, Gisel and Patrick 1998, Ramsey et al 1993, Sines 1992, Sullivan et al 2000, and Zickler and Dodge 1994) supports this, all of whom have highlighted that people with profound and multiple learning disabilities, particularly children, are often mal-nourished and underweight due to a variety of reasons, including feeding problems. It is an area of care that has also raised both professional and public interest in relation to the ethical dimensions of the introduction of enteral feeding for some individuals.

Management of eating and drinking skills

It essential that people with profound and multiple disabilities and their carers have regular access to speech and language therapists with specific training in feeding difficulties and management. It is important to obtain advice and guidance from the therapist on, for example, feeding techniques, food consistency, and the management of problems specific to the individual.

The therapist may advise that non-oral feeding is in the person's best interests (see below). The involvement of the physiotherapist, occupational therapist and orthodontist (Avery-Smith 1998, Haberfuller et al 2000) are also invaluable in the assessment and management of feeding difficulties.

In residential and professionally run units/homes it is important to have specific policies with regard to the management of feeding difficulties of each individual who utilises the service. The reader is strongly advised to use the contacts, addresses and texts that are mentioned at end of the chapter for further information.

Nutrition and feeding

There are many people with profound and multiple disabilities who have difficulty with feeding skills, particularly the ability to suck, chew and swallow, as well as drinking adequate volumes of fluids. The main issue here is the potential risk of aspiration (Gisel et al 1995). This is in addition to the difficulty of feeding oneself, and thus being reliant on carers for food and drink. This relates to the issue raised earlier in the chapter regarding accountability and responsibility of health care practitioners, for example when carers vary in their abilities as regards appropriate and safe oral feeding techniques. This is in addition to the more complex issues when enteral feeding is being used. Practitioners need also to be aware of additional nutritional issues with this client group. One example is that of poor vitamin dietary intake and physiological uptake, particularly vitamin C (Cahill et al 2000). This is further exacerbated by the implications of gaps and misunderstandings in terms of caregivers' nutritional knowledge, beliefs and skills regarding the needs of the person with a multiple disability (Verrall et al 2000).

Before one can consider feeding techniques, it is essential that the physical handling and positioning of the person is correct, otherwise this will exacerbate the above problems as well as being uncomfortable for the individual. For this it is essential to liaise closely with the occupational therapist and physiotherapist. The correct seating position and equipment are essential.

The person with severe muscle spasms due to cerebral palsy will, for example, require a seating system that enables the correct posture to be maintained, thereby minimising the impact of extensor spasms. If this is not achieved and the person experiences extensor spasms while eating or drinking, there is a high risk of choking and aspiration. However, carers also need advice about the whole environment in which the person will be having meals.

It is important to consider the opportunities available to enhance the quality of the individual's mealtime experience. A quiet period beforehand to reduce the impact of the mealtime activity itself can be useful, for example approaching the person gently, talking quietly and massaging their face can help, and mealtimes should be unhurried. The carer should sit face to face with the individual, allowing better eye contact and ensuring that being fed is a sociable occasion, rather than something you have 'done to' you. Certainly with new staff it can be useful to spend time on role play, giving carers the opportunity to find out how it feels to be fed, and how not to feed someone, before they engage in such an activity. It is vital that a new member of staff does not attempt to feed someone with feeding difficulties, owing to the increased risk of causing the person to choke and aspirate. In units or homes that care for people with extensive feeding difficulties it is recommended that there is supervision by a medical practitioner and a speech and language therapist trained in this aspect of care, in addition to the support offered by the community learning disability nurse. It is also advisable that someone trained in the use of emergency suction techniques is always available at mealtimes. This raises concern within current provision for people with complex and profound disabilities in that staff may not have undertaken courses that have exposed them to the nursing care needs of such individuals. One does not wish to medicalise the needs of the person with a profound and multiple disability, however there must be a comprehensive risk assessment (DOH 1998) of the person's health care needs and there should be staff available, where a need is identified, to perform such basic yet life-saving interventions. This has implications for parents/informal carers within the family setting as there may be a need for training and resources to be made available within the home for emergency oropharyngeal suction to be performed.

Within the author's own area of clinical experience families are usually provided with two suction machines (one as back up) and it is preferable that both are portable and able to be operated, for example, from a car battery.

It is not acceptable to expect families to provide complex care for their child, or for other care providers to do so, without adequate and well-maintained resources. Again this raises issues of accountability and responsibility for the health care practitioner, and it is necessary to monitor closely whether the person's needs are being safely met. Given the critical nature of ensuring that care is regularly evaluated and adapted to meet needs, it is essential for all practitioners to ensure that record keeping in relation to the care provision is exemplary and compliant with the guidelines for record keeping of the UKCC (1998) and/or other appropriate regulatory bodies where appropriate. This is applicable to all aspects of health care provision.

When people with such difficulties are cared for at home, the main carers should be taught how to use suction equipment, and have appropriate

Reader activity 17.1

Paul is having his meal in the residential home for ten adults in which he lives. Paul has severe cerebral palsy, and as a result tends to have a lot of problems with extensor spasms and an exaggerated startle reflex. He is therefore easy startled, which results in involuntary movements. The dining room in which he has his meals has a heavy swing door into the kitchen, which is constantly in use. The door bangs shut each time it is used and each time this happens Paul is startled and starts to cough and choke. As Paul's main carer, what would you do to ensure that he is able to eat his meals with the minimum of difficulty?

portable equipment available. Supportive nursing services should also be available 24 hours a day where necessary, so that eating and drinking are not restricted to mealtimes only. This needs to be arranged as part of the person's overall care package as otherwise some health and social care providers will not be able to provide such a level of health care provision within current services.

Severe swallowing difficulties – a management strategy

It is important to seek the advice and support of the speech and language therapist trained in feeding skills (Caudery & Russell 1995). Those people who have significant feeding difficulties may not be receiving their full nutritional and hydration requirements. Added to this is the problem that a person with, for example, severe cerebral palsy may have an increased energy requirement owing to increased metabolism and frequent involuntary movements. Thus it is also important to refer to the dietician for advice and for strategies that can be used to ensure that nutritional needs are being met. Such strategies can include the use of a wide range of nutritional supplements based on the person's age, weight, calorie needs, abilities and tastes. These can include fortified drinks, such as juices and milk shakes, fortified puddings, whole meal supplements in drink form, and high-calorie powders that can be added to the meal and which do not alter its taste.

The use of thickened drinks, meal supplements and puddings has an added benefit in that they are easier to swallow than fluids on their own. Fluid thickeners (with no calorie content) that promote easier swallowing are also available.

If it is felt that individuals are not taking adequate nutrition orally, it may be in their interests for oral feeding to be supplemented with enteral feeding, via a nasogastric tube or gastrostomy, the latter being much more suitable as a long-term approach. The benefits of this are that:

- it ensures that the person has adequate fluid and nutritional intake in a given 24-hour period
- it enables people to take in orally whatever they wish and are able to, without carers having to worry about the amount taken that day.

The disadvantages focus mainly on the fact that enteral feeding may be viewed as an intrusion or 'unnatural', and on the cost involved. However, it is a strategy that is increasingly being used. It could be argued that the benefits of such feeding techniques outweigh the difficulties in terms of reducing the risk of aspiration. Also, if oesophageal reflux is minimised the associated discomfort and potential distress of oesophagitis may be alleviated (Heine et al 1995).

Key professionals should work together with people with feeding difficulties and their main carers to assess particular feeding problems and to ensure that any strategies implemented are regularly evaluated. Additional opportunities to review the extent of feeding problems may arise if the client and family access short-term breaks, which enable a more intensive assessment and review to take place if there are significant problems (Sharpe 2000). As mentioned earlier, an individual with serious swallowing difficulties is at risk of aspiration, hence the importance of lifesaving suction skills. There is a wealth of effective portable suction equipment available, and the community nurse will be able to offer advice, as well as access to an equipment loan scheme. In such cases it is important to question whether oral feeding techniques are really in the person's best interests. Videofluoroscopy is currently regarded as the best technique available for identifying a person's overall swallowing abilities (Gisel et al

Reader activity 17.2

Christopher is 39 years old and has profound and multiple disabilities. He is unable to sit up properly even with the support of a seating system. He has all his meals and drinks orally. However, his father has noticed that Christopher is coughing more and more often when being fed, and is repeatedly suffering severe chest infections. After much discussion and consultation Christopher had a videofluoroscopy performed, which showed he was aspirating a considerable amount.

It was decided by his father and the professionals involved that it would be best if Christopher had a gastrostomy, and no longer took food or fluids orally, because of the significant risk of aspiration. A month after the operation Christopher's father said he was finding the new regimen difficult, because he felt that Christopher did not understand why he could not have any more drinks or food. He was now wondering whether the gastrostomy was the best approach.

There are a number of issues within the above scenario that are important to consider.

- If the gastrostomy had not been performed there was a significant risk of aspiration-induced respiratory problems. Given that this is known, does it justify the approach taken?
- Although it can clearly be argued that the action taken was in Christopher's best interests, perhaps there is an alternative argument when making such a decision, given that Christopher has had oral feeds for 39 years. Does this make the decision more difficult, and why?
- In view of the current debate regarding enteral feeding as 'ordinary' treatment, what if Christopher's father later wished for feeding to be stopped?

1995, Mirret et al 1994, Morton et al 1993). However, there is a need to standardise clinical recommendations, which vary greatly depending on whether procedures are to be performed on an adult or a child (O'Donoghue & Bagnall 1999).

It may be considered that the risk of aspiration is too high: indeed, the person may have experienced episodes of aspiration resulting in respiratory difficulties, or even aspiration pneumonia. In this instance non-oral feeding may be the best option, with no oral feeding taking place.

The benefits of enteral feeding, especially gastrostomy feeding, cannot be ignored, especially as it is argued that up to 80% of children with profound learning disabilities are considered to be at risk of aspiration (Morton et al 1993, Mirret et al 1994). Techniques for gastrostomy insertion have become simpler and the equipment has become more user friendly.

Gastrostomies can now be inserted through endoscopy, hence the term percutaneous endoscopic gastrostomy (PEG); this means that usually only a short general anaesthetic is needed for the procedure. Overall this has tremendous benefits for individuals with underlying respiratory problems. However, whilst there are health gains from this approach the practitioner needs to work very closely with the client and the family and be mindful of the long-term implications of enteral feeding for the client and carers. Adams et al (1999) and O'Brien (1999) have highlighted that it is likely that the enteral feeding and care will be undertaken by family members or other non-nursing colleagues. Studies such as that by Bannerman et al (2000) have demonstrated a positive view of the value of gastrostomy feeding.

Thorne et al (1997) and Townsley and Robinson (1999) highlighted the need for national guidance in relation to enteral feeding provision and the varying levels of support/interventions needed for carers who are not health care professionals. This is a particular issue that needs to be taken on board by health care providers as carers do appear to be taking on more and more extended caring roles without the prerequisite levels of support and training in place.

Once a gastrostomy tube has been in place for approximately 6 months (the time element is very much based on individual needs) it may be changed for what is termed a 'button gastrostomy', such as the MIC-Key device, which is almost flush with the skin. The button gastrostomy is easy to use and the design ensures that there are no free moving parts that could be accidentally pulled or damaged (see Fig. 17.1). Each button will have its own attachments for feeding use. Several manufacturers provide a wide range of gastrostomy devices, and they are usually very helpful with basic troubleshooting information as well as aids and adaptations to make the system easier to use. Many manufacturers also supply portable electrical pump systems, which are small and lightweight and would enable a person to have a continuous feed over time if necessary, without having to be dependent on a mains supply to operate the pump.

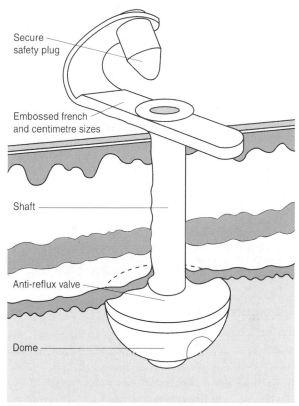

Figure 17.1 Button gastrostomy. (With permission from Merck Biomaterial, after illustration of button in information Sheet on Corpak® Button.)

Access to the full range of equipment for gastrostomy feeding is usually via the dietician and community nurse. The feeds to be used and the dietary regimen must be under the strict supervision of a dietician, and the feeds are available on prescription. The equipment may also be available on prescription, but it is most often ordered via the dietician, who liaises with the medical practitioner and community nurse. Many manufacturers provide a 'door-to-door' service to the individual's place of residence.

Care of a gastrostomy

Oral hygiene

Individuals having all or some of their nutritional intake through a gastrostomy still need a regular oral hygiene routine. It is a common misunderstanding that if someone does not take fluids or food orally they will not suffer from dental decay; on the contrary, plaque continues to form on the teeth whether one eats or not. Moreover, if people are unable to ask for a drink, they are likely to be given drinks whenever their carers feel they need them, rather than when they want them, so it is likely that their mouths will be more dry and that the need for mouth care will be increased. This will be discussed more fully later in the chapter.

 Reader activity 17.3

Consider how you would feel if you had no oral intake and were reliant on carers to provide your oral hygiene needs. How often would you like to have this? How would you like to have it performed for you?

The gastrostomy itself

Gastrostomy care is reasonably straightforward and involves certain basic principles regardless of the type of tube used. There are additional guidelines that refer specifically to each gastrostomy design, which must be adhered to and would be explained by a health care practitioner such as the community nurse. Again, manufacturers provide specific information about their products, including management advice. There may be additional guidelines to be considered depending on the age and the ongoing health needs of the individual; these can be explored with, for example, the community nurse.

Basic care principles include good hand hygiene and skin care around the gastrostomy site. The following should also be observed:

- Keep the site clean and dry.
- Gently wash around the site with cool boiled water or Normasol at least once daily. Pat gently dry, ensuring that the area is thoroughly dried.
- Watch for any leakage, excoriation or redness around the site. The advice of the community nurse or medical practitioner should be sought if any of these occur.
- The gastrostomy itself should not be covered by a dressing or taped down, unless this has been specifically advised by the medical practitioner.

Feeding techniques

- Always use the equipment specific to the type of gastrostomy being used.
- Only use the type of feeds and amounts of feeds that are prescribed for that person.
- The tube should be gently flushed with cool boiled water before and after feeds – the amount is dependent on the needs of the person and on the dietitcian's advice.
- When bolus feeding with a large syringe the feed should *never* be forced in using the syringe plunger – it must always be allowed to go in via gravity. The community nurse will advise on management if it appears that feeds are blocking the tube.
- A large syringe should be used for bolus feeding – ideally 50 or 60 mL syringes and no smaller than 30 mL.
- When continuous feeding is used the correct electrical pump for that type of commercial feed should be used, with its own giving set designed for single use.

Carers are advised to consult the relevant health professionals and appropriate texts for further information. There are also videos and leaflets that can be helpful.

It is important that, even if individuals have some or all of their meals via the gastrostomy, they do not miss the social experience of mealtimes, and are able to have the same care offered to others. Mouth care during the gastrostomy feed is essential, and for many people a range of small amounts of food in the mouth, if appropriate, can be very important in terms of oral stimulation. Mealtimes are part of the collective culture of the UK, and often a time of relaxed socialising. It is important that the person who is having gastrostomy feeds should not miss out on such occasions.

ISSUES OF MOBILISATION

The importance of correct seating positions and being comfortable is something that is often overlooked. Many people with profound learning and multiple disabilities are unable to move around independently, and are completely dependent on their carers for their every move. Because of this carers need to stop and reflect on the full impact of what it means to be fully dependent on others. This requires a degree of empathy in considering ways in which such people can be empowered to make their needs and wishes known, using the abilities they have. This may be through facial expression, eye pointing or verbal methods, for example. Communication is essential and must be valued, whatever method is used.

For the person with mobility difficulties the input of physiotherapist and occupational therapist is essential. These team members should be included in the planning of everyday care provision for all individuals with such problems.

The key areas considered in this section are:

- The promotion of an individual's potential in terms of everyday functional skills and the role of the therapists in this
- The minimisation of additional physical disabilities
- The prevention of pressure sores
- Strategies to enhance mobilisation and ensure optimum comfort and positioning for the individual.

In relation to people with Down syndrome, the Department of Health (DOH 1995a) issued guidelines which reaffirmed the need to avoid subluxation in an individual with Down syndrome. This is a problem that is considered rare, yet difficult to exclude due to ligament problems and potentially poorly developed bones. The Department of Health (1995a), supported by Dennis (2001a) for the Down Syndrome Association, has acknowledged that previous advice, which supported the use of neck X-rays to identify individuals at risk, could not be relied upon. This supported a 5-year study by Morton et al (1995), which considered this problem in particular. The condition should always alert health care professionals to act with caution, although Dennis (2001a) has advised that it should not be a reason to exclude clients with Down syndrome from sporting activities unless there is a known problem.

Promoting the individual's potential

Perhaps the most important issue here is the inherent right of individuals to have access to

therapists and resources to enable them to gain the most from their own motor and sensory skills. Therapists are then able to complete regular functional assessments of the client as suggested in Pope's (1992) description of a continual programme. This not only means that clients have the opportunity to develop their own potential, and enhance their quality of life, it also ensures that therapists can identify potential mobility problems. Active measures can then be taken to minimise the impact of potential complications. However, this relies on good inter-agency communication (O'Connor 1995) and the practitioner having a sound understanding of the roles of therapists. Knowledge of the assessment tools for orthofunction, for example the Edinburgh Rehabilitation Scale (Mattison et al 1992), the Chailey levels of ability (Poutney et al 1999) and the Gross Motor Function Measure (Russell et al, 1998) are also beneficial in order to identify appropriate therapeutic interventions that may benefit a client. Hopefully this would ensure prompter referrals and earlier highlighting of problems to therapists. Because of the variety and complexity of the issues, for example in relation to importance of early intervention for hand functioning (Eliasson et al 1998) and management of windswept hip deformity (Young et al, 1998), readers are advised to explore the wide range of articles and texts on this topic. Multi-level surgery for hip and tendon problems for this client group (Ross et al 2001, Wong et al 2000) requires the practitioner's attention, as it is increasingly being used for clients with cerebral palsy, although there have been concerns raised in relation to its clinical effectiveness and the potential post-surgical implications (HemiHelp1999). Practitioners should consult this latter document when working with clients requiring planned orthopaedic interventions.

Role of the therapist

As mentioned earlier, a good seating system is important. The physiotherapist and occupational therapist should therefore work with clients and their main carers to identify seating systems that are comfortable as well as providing the correct body posture in terms of hip alignment and limb and trunk positioning, in order to minimise any potential further disabilities.

It has been argued that poor seating systems are linked to and exacerbate hip problems (Smith & Emans 1992). Neck support is also important. Some people with profound physical disabilities may need a seating system that includes a body mould, i.e. an insert moulded to the shape of their body to encourage a more upright position. The introduction of such an insert must be very gradual, especially if the person has always previously been in a supine or prone position. Children in particular, as acknowledged by Reid (1995) require regular reassessment of their seating systems due to growth and maturation, and all clients using such systems will require regular reviews in order to ensure that any exacerbation of musculoskeletal problems is addressed.

Safety in the use of seating and mobility systems is essential. The positioning straps and supports are there not only to encourage the best position, but also to provide safety for individuals who cannot support themselves. Therapists spend a great deal of time with individuals and their carers considering possible options, such as the ability of the system to help minimise the effects of involuntary movements, and providing reliable and comfortable safety devices which are also easy to keep clean. From the author's own clinical experience, for individuals who may be at risk of aspiration, or who have severe seizures on a regular basis, quick-release safety and positioning devices are essential within seating systems.

The design of the seat must also be age appropriate, so as not to reinforce the negative view of individuals with profound learning and multiple disabilities as 'eternal children'. Families may express concern that the seating system should not be cumbersome or significantly different from furniture in their homes. There is a wide range of systems available that seek to overcome these concerns, and most manufacturers endeavour to provide equipment that is not only therapeutic but also aesthetic, catering for the needs and wishes of different individuals and their families. Most equipment is relatively portable, thereby overcoming transport difficulties, and it is important that services such as short-term breaks have

access to the equipment used by an individual. Usually one system is provided for the individual to use in the usual care setting and one in the educational or day care setting, but there is perhaps a need for a system to be available in every care setting used by the client, because of the problem of limited transport facilities and the inconvenience for carers of having to transport equipment around.

Therapists' roles are diverse, and can be seen to have a demonstrable and positive effect on a person's quality of life in terms of posture, balance, coordination, and strengthening of function in the limbs. One intervention is the use of tilting tables, which encourage a more upright posture in a secure, supported standing position. This has many benefits and these include:

- improvement of circulation
- promoting bone strength and limiting the impact of spontaneous fractures
- improving breathing, and also neck control
- the opportunity to see everyday life from a different perspective.

Communication skills may also be enhanced, as the individual has an opportunity to communicate at a different physical level; this can help limit the negative impact of being 'talked down to' which can occur when someone is in a wheelchair.

It is important that equipment is used with guidance from the physiotherapist, who will advise on how to ensure that the individual is comfortable, and in a safe as well as a beneficial position. Clients should not be left unattended while using the equipment, especially if they have a tendency for powerful involuntary movements that could affect their safety.

Physiotherapy can be provided in both formal and informal settings. Formal methods can include strategies such as conductive education, patterning and concentrating on specific movements. These methods can be very helpful, and are practised in conjunction with an occupational therapist, focusing on movement as well as on the prevention of problems such as contractures. It is important that children in particular are referred to therapists at an early stage and the value of intensive therapist involvement cannot be underestimated (Hodgson 2000, Bower et al 2001). Informal methods can include activities such as horse riding, which is valuable in encouraging good posture and balance, as well as being an important social occasion (Lehrman & Ross 2001). Swimming, formal hydrotherapy sessions and aquatic therapy using 'water shiatsu' (Vogtle et al 1998, p. 250) also help to promote good breathing techniques and to relax stiff and contracted muscles, as well as providing the obvious benefits of buoyancy and freedom of movement.

Minimising additional physical disabilities

A great deal of the time spent caring for a person with profound learning and multiple disabilities is aimed at maintaining health, which is very important for quality of life. This is particularly so given the increased long-term survival rates of individuals in this client group. There is controversy in the debate surrounding the assessment of anticipated orthofunction, i.e. limb flexibility. Despite the benefits of, for example, vibrotactile work by occupational therapists (Boakes 1990) to promote optimum functioning, orthofunction is often described as being particularly poor in this client group; yet many of these same individuals are later seen as having better orthofunction than initially predicted (O'Grady et al 1995).

Physical disabilities can be exacerbated in many ways, and a range of strategies must be used to ensure that this is prevented, or at least minimised. Potential problems include:

* muscle atrophy
* contractures
* loss of limb flexibility (orthofunction)
* increased difficulty in using seating, hoists and wheelchairs, necessitating more and more adaptations
* podiatry-related problems.

The above problems can also mean that an individual is more at risk of respiratory problems, pressure sores and perhaps even fractures. People with profound learning disabilities who are immobile are estimated to be most at risk of developing deformities (Bottos et al 1995). Indeed

development of the musculoskeletal system per se can differ for the person with a profound disability, particularly in relation to cerebral palsy as there are potentially significant hip and spinal problems than must be prevented or minimised.

Practitioners need to be aware of the risk factors that can lead to additional hip and/or spinal problems, which must be addressed by therapists. Gudjonsdottir & Mercer (1997) have described the risk factors as being due to primary causes such as muscle imbalance, poor seating and delayed or insufficient weight bearing. They also identified that these can then exacerbate or even cause contracture development and increase the risk of fractures due to problems related to decreased bone density. This links directly to the nutritional issues explored earlier in the chapter.

Immobility-related problems are an issue for people with profound and multiple disabilities, because of muscle atrophy and reductions in muscle size, caused by lack of oxygen. As muscle contraction increases this further limits joint movement, and this can be difficult to prevent, even with high levels of physiotherapy intervention. For people with cerebral palsy, as well as those with Down syndrome in particular, the risk of hip dislocation cannot be ignored.

Physiotherapy and occupational therapy devices such as splints and body braces can be invaluable in enabling the person to maintain optimal posture and limb positioning. However, surgery may become the main option to alleviate the discomfort of hip subluxation or dislocation as the person enters adulthood. This problem is exacerbated in individuals with muscle contraction, in that at present the only reliable intervention for excessive muscle tone, particularly in the lower limbs, is surgery in the form of a tenotomy. Intensive physiotherapy built into the individual's everyday activities is essential. Passive physiotherapy techniques can be particularly beneficial when used in conjunction with hydrotherapy, either formal or informal. Surgery may also be considered for the client with severe cerebral palsy and resultant scoliosis. Spinal fusion may be an option for adult (in terms of skeletal maturity) clients and their carers to consider, to reduce the effects of the scoliosis

(Comstock et al 1998) and so enhance seating ability whilst promoting comfort. However, there needs to be considerable discussion regarding the complexity of the surgery, potential significant complications and the long-term postoperative care and rehabilitation that may be required (see earlier in the chapter in relation to the guidelines from HemiHelp (1999).

Medication can also be beneficial in helping to reduce potential muscle spasms, which can exacerbate contractures, and the associated discomfort. Medication such as baclofen (Lioresal), the current drug of choice, and dantrolene (Dantrium), aim to reduce muscle tone and can be very beneficial. Diazepam (Valium), a benzodiazepine, is also used, but is associated with increased sedation and even occasionally extensor hypotonus. All drugs used for muscle relaxation, particularly those such as baclofen and dantrolene, must be introduced very gradually and the dose slowly titred to ensure the optimum effect with the minimal dose. These drugs must always be reduced gradually if they are being withdrawn. Dantrolene should *not* be used with children (BMA & RPS 2001).

There has been some discussion, particularly in North American journals (see Wiens 1998 and Ward 2001), in relation to the value of intrathecal baclofen, using a surgically implanted pump for adults, for improving orthofunction and reducing discomfort. However, regardless of the approach used, medication should be an adjunct to other supportive methods rather than a single treatment option. Practitioners need to constantly evaluate their understanding of current research in order to ensure the best practice options are available for clients. One therapeutic approach that has relatively recently gained momentum is the use of botulinum toxin with clients with cerebral palsy, and enhanced orthofunction has been achieved with the therapy, particularly with children. There is a wealth of material published on this particular therapeutic intervention and practitioners are advised to review the current studies in the medical and nursing journals. However, the work to date has focused on relatively mobile clients with no or mild learning disability, where there have been positive results (Ubhi et al, 2000), rather than on clients with profound and multiple disabilities.

As stated earlier, physiotherapy is essential, and one should consider the range of massage techniques that can be used to help reduce muscular spasms, as well as the use of complementary therapies such as aromatherapy and homoeopathy (see Ch. 20). The use of TENS – transcutaneous electrical nerve stimulation – should also be considered as a non-invasive yet very effective way in which the discomfort and pain of muscle spasm can be reduced.

Good seating and positioning are also essential to minimise muscle spasms, and can even inhibit the full extent of extensor spasms, for example, by enabling the person to be more in the midline, or perhaps even in a position of mild flexion. This would have to be maintained in any moving and handling techniques used.

There is a wide range of mobilisation aids that the physiotherapist and occupational therapist may use to promote orthofunction and thus enhance daily living. Arm gaiters, for example, can be very useful for support when sitting balance is being attempted. They can also help minimise involuntary muscle actions and thus perhaps enable the person to use an adapted motorised wheelchair. The lycra-based dynamic splinting suit (Blair et al 1995) has also been publicised as promoting orthofunction. The 'Upsuit', as it is termed, is tailor-made to meet the needs of the individual and is considered to be very effective. It is argued that an adaptation of this, in the form of dynamic splinting on the limbs only, may be easier to use and is certainly better for the individual for whom lung function is a concern, or where carer compliance is an issue (Blair et al 1995).

Flotron therapy is also used to assist mobilisation as it can alleviate muscle spasm and help prevent contractures. It is often used following the removal of plaster or delta casts, which may have been applied after a tenotomy has been performed. Another example of how flotron therapy can be used is for a specified period of time before the person is helped to get up after a night's sleep.

Prevention of podiatry problems

This is an area of care that is often forgotten, possibly because it is overshadowed by the other mobilisation difficulties that are predominant. However, this does not mean that regular podiatry assessment and preventive care is not important. The simplest issue is the need to ensure that any footwear, whether specialist or not, fits well and does not rub or irritate the skin (Prasher et al 1995). The use of ankle–foot orthoses (AFOs) can be very effective in promoting and maintaining transfer ability, balance and orthofunction (Chang & Cardenas 2000, p. 435). However, if an individual wears AFOs as well as specialist footwear, there is the chance that the orthosis may be put on incorrectly by carers, causing sore areas on the feet.

Carers should not attempt to apply AFOs without demonstration and supervision by the physiotherapist, and the effectiveness of the AFO must be reviewed on a regular basis through, for example, gait assessment (Abel et al 1998). This is particularly important in childhood when there is rapid growth in foot size, especially in young children.

Regular podiatry assessment is an essential component of everyday care for the individual, and is readily available without financial cost for people with learning disabilities through local Primary Care Groups and/or Trusts.

Management of pressure areas and the prevention of pressure sores

People who are immobile are at high risk of potential skin breakdown as a direct result of their immobility. If they are left in the same position for long periods, with no attempt to change that position either by themselves or by others, then skin integrity will be compromised and skin may break down. This can be so severe as to cause extensive tissue and muscle damage, as well as being a potential site for localised or systemic infection. A multidisciplinary/multi-agency approach is needed to ensure pressure sore prevention is a priority (Cave 1998).

Prevention involves a range of strategies:

- Ensuring that individuals have the correct nutritional and fluid intake to meet their daily needs.

- Ensuring that these nutritional needs are re-evaluated when individuals are unwell or having elective surgery, so as not to compromise their overall health status and hence to promote their wellbeing.

- Regular evaluation of the range of equipment used daily for the individual's comfort; checking for any areas where skin may come into contact with straps, fastenings and the general framework of the equipment is essential.

- Ensuring that the person's position is changed regularly to maintain skin integrity, including during sleep. However, the practice of changing a sleeping person's position hourly or 2-hourly should be questioned, and the time period altered according to the individual's sleep pattern and in light of evidence-based practice (DOH 1993a,b).

- Specialist equipment such as sleep systems and alternating pressure mattresses can be of use, especially if the person has significant physical disabilities and limited movement. (Some individuals with severe muscle contractures are only able to lie or sit in a limited number of positions, and are therefore more at risk of pressure sores). This requires easy access to a range of such specialist equipment for clients and may be an issue in terms of identifying resources in the community (Clark & Cullum 1992, Collier 1996 and Hallett 1996).

- Daily calculation and recording of the potential risk of skin deterioration; if the individual is being cared for in a residential facility or by multiple formal carers, difficulties could arise in identifying potential skin integrity problems and taking action as soon as possible. Using an appropriate risk calculator, such as that of Waterlow (1992, 1997), can assist in identifying the level of risk as well as acting as a means by which to monitor the effectiveness of any related intervention.

- Prompt action is important if there are any concerns regarding skin integrity, in order to minimise skin breakdown.

Strategies to enhance mobilisation

Caring for someone who is immobile involves difficult and time-consuming activities, such as dressing, undressing, moving and bathing the person, which leaves less time for carers to spend considering the individual's leisure and recreational needs. Families should be encouraged to seek the best equipment available that will enable them to care for their relative, and occupational therapists can suggest a range of ways in which routine activities can be made easier.

Dressing and undressing someone with severe contractures and muscle spasms can be extremely difficult, and can be responsible for back and neck injuries in carers (Aldridge & Becker 1993, DOH 1999c); this should be considered in the carers' assessments within the Carers (Recognition and Services) Act (1995). The occupational therapist may suggest loose-fitting clothing for the client, so as to ease the difficulties of dressing and undressing. Changing the way in which a garment is fastened can also help, for example front fastening bras can be useful for women with profound and multiple disabilities. There is a range of aids for assisted bathing, such as bath hoists, cradles, alternating-height baths, shower trolleys, overhead tracking and other individualised adaptations. The cost of such equipment can be considerable, but the cost of providing extra carers to support the family is much greater, and thus helping families in any way possible is of benefit to all concerned. In addition to the need to ensure adequate assessment, training and equipment there are health and safety issues in relation to safe moving and handling techniques (Health and Safety Executive (HSE) 1998). This places resultant obligations on statutory care providers to ensure that the needs of carers are fully taken into consideration and to reduce the risk of injury to carers, family members and clients.

In summary, direct carers need to consider the following:

- Be aware of the impact of nutrition and fluids on maintaining health.
- Ensure that therapists such as physiotherapists and occupational therapists are involved in caring for the individual: their input is essential.
- Consider moving and handling strategies that maximise comfort and safety for the individual and carers at all times.

- Carers should never lift a person on their own if at all possible. Formal carers working in residential facilities, for example, will be in breach of the HSE (1998) regulations if they attempt to lift someone on their own.
- Do use the range of pressure-relieving equipment available to meet the individual's needs.

ISSUES OF VISUAL IMPAIRMENT

There are many factors to which visual impairment may be attributed in clients with learning disabilities. However, due to the wide variations in types and severity of problems and in consensus on prevalence it is difficult to ascertain the significance of visual impairment amongst this client group (Mamer 1999, RNIB 1995 and Warburg 1994). This is further compounded by difficulties in evaluating visual function, highlighted by Dundon & Mann (1995) and Ciner et al (1996). However, there are some particular issues that practitioners need to be aware of and these are briefly explored below.

Retinopathy of prematurity is stated to be a common cause of visual impairment, where retinal blood vessels spasm and complete retinal detachment can occur (Dodds 1993, Msall et al 2000); this has multifactorial causes. It has a significant impact on the individual, and can affect general development in that the young child has to maximise the use of the other senses to explore the environment; it also affects the child's spatial awareness (Dodds et al 1991).

Other causes of visual impairment include conditions that are generally associated with the elderly, although it should be remembered that this is not always necessarily the case. Macular degeneration, in which central vision deteriorates, is a common cause of significant visual impairment. Peripheral vision is often still present, and carers need to be aware of the need to maximise any residual peripheral vision that the person may have.

Glaucoma can also affect the individual's vision. This involves the build-up of aqueous fluid in the ducts of the eye, resulting in pressure on the optic nerve as well as on the retina. (For further explanation of the physiology in relation to ophthalmic problems, the practitioner could consult texts such as Hinchcliff et al (1996)). Glaucoma can occur gradually, and thus not be identified until individuals express concern regarding their sight, or it can occur over a short period of time and is associated with pain and discomfort. Given that either form may develop, it is important that visual screening is regularly performed, especially if there is a known familial tendency to the condition. Carers might otherwise not notice the chronic form, especially if the individual has limited communication skills. A key worker is important if the person is being cared for in a formal setting, so that any difference in the individual's behaviour can be identified and the cause linked to deterioration in vision. A potential tendency to develop glaucoma can be identified in children; indeed, there is a form of glaucoma known as buphthalmos that occurs in young children (Beck 1997, Gardell and McGuinn 1999).

Damage to the optic nerve and the areas of the brain associated with vision in utero or postnatally owing to, for example, meningitis or trauma, is also an associated reason for visual impairment in people with profound and multiple disabilities. Conditions linked with learning disabilities such as Sturge–Weber syndrome (Sullivan et al 1993) and CHARGE Association also require close screening for visual impairment by practitioners.

Visual impairment in people who are immobile is of particular concern, as their only means of independent 'mobility' within their environment is through sight. If an individual is dependent on visual cues as a means of communication, when verbal communication is not possible, this could be seen as a fundamental need. Thus the promotion of optimal visual health is not an extra but a necessity. Regular visits to the optician and attendance at an ophthalmology clinic should be maintained, if appropriate. It is important that common conditions such as myopia (short-sightedness), hypermetropia (long-sightedness) and presbyopia (far-sightedness, which is more prevalent in older people) are screened for in people with profound and multiple disabilities. Correction of these conditions via the use of spectacles can be invaluable in ensuring that they have

the best possible quality of life. However, there is a range of other visual health issues that are more prominent in people with profound and multiple disabilities. These include, for example, tear production problems and resultant blepharitis, cataracts and hemianopia.

Tear production problems are common in people with Down syndrome, in that the tears contain excessively high amounts of protein. This causes a chronic eye infection known as blepharitis, owing to the eyelash follicles becoming irritated and inflamed. If the individual is susceptible it is important that carers perform eye care as part of their daily routine and ensure that any resultant infection is promptly reviewed by the GP.

Cataracts can seriously impair an individual's vision and clients should be screened for this at all ages (Crofts 1997). Cataracts can be congenital, but may not be detected until young adulthood, or can develop later in life. Given the significance of visual skills for people with profound and multiple disabilities, it would appear to be prudent to check their visual status at least annually and more often in childhood.

Hemianopia usually presents as part of the person's overall physical disabilities, in that it is often associated with hemiparesis. This can be particularly difficult for immobile people as it means that their visual field is often significantly impaired on the affected side of their body. As with all visual impairments, it is important that the extent of such a condition is known by carers, so that they can seek support and advice from therapists as to how the person's residual vision can be optimised. Advice from the local service for the visually impaired is invaluable, as is the range of equipment and advice available from support groups such as the Royal National Institute for the Blind (RNIB) – The website address can be found at the end of the chapter.

Visual impairment can also include nystagmus and squint as well as those problems already considered in this section.

Caring strategies

It is important that those involved in the day-to-day care of an individual with profound and multiple disabilities are aware of the significance of visual impairment. It is acknowledged that inappropriate self-stimulatory behaviour can be a result of significant visual impairment (Moller 1993); hence the need to ensure that any residual sight is maximised, and the emphasis on using the person's other skills must be paramount, in order to discourage the development of any such behaviour.

A range of strategies can be used to meet the needs such individuals. Multisensory techniques can be invaluable, but they must be used with care and understanding to prevent a distressing sensory overload. Techniques such as Snoezelen (Ashby et al 1995, Doble et al 1992, Laurent 1992, Thompson & Martin 1994) can be beneficial to both individual and carers when used properly, although, as Thurtle & Wyatt (1999) have acknowledged, there is not yet a firm evidence base in support of its use and there is a need for clinical guidance on this matter.

The use of relaxation techniques and the gradual introduction of auditory and olfactory stimulation while maximising the person's residual vision, can also be extremely satisfying. Other strategies can also be used, such as tactile and auditory equipment that is age appropriate in design and use. Altering the lighting in an individual's home can help promote the use of residual sight, for example by using bright light and primary colours in eating utensils and crockery. The development of a 'multisensory garden' or window box can be very worthwhile: this involves maximising the use of the fragrances given off from flowers and herbs.

ISSUES CONCERNING HEARING IMPAIRMENTS

Hearing impairment and visual impairment are among a range of health needs that have been acknowledged by the Department of Health (Kay et al 1995a, Lindsay 1998). However, it is most disappointing not to see this acknowledged in the Department's latest strategy documentation (DOH 2001a).

Carers, both informal and formal, need support in developing their understanding of the impact of hearing impairment. This is particularly pertinent given that studies by such as Marcell & Cohen (1992), Ashman & Suttie (1996) and Evenhuis et al (1997) have identified a significant incidence of hearing impairment amongst people with learning disabilities, particular in older clients. Clients with Down syndrome are more at risk and the problem is further exacerbated as the client grows older in terms of the risk of vision and hearing loss (Janicki & Dalton 1998).

Definitive statistics are difficult to obtain, possibly because the screening of such individuals is still inadequate (RNIB 1996, Janicki & Dalton 1998). However, as more infants and young children are screened for hearing impairment, realistic statistical information should emerge. The interpretation of the statistics could be argued to be more important, in that it may enable more people with profound and multiple disabilities to access the range of hearing impairment services they require, which could help improve their quality of life.

It is argued that currently approximately 0.16% of the general population of the UK have severe learning disabilities, and approximately 33% of these have sensory impairments (Harries 1991). There is growing evidence, for example Janicki & Dalton (1998), that sensory impairment is a significant problem for older clients with learning disabilities, particular for those with Down syndrome. The extent of the problem is difficult to define, as there is still a lack of consensus on what would be considered a significant sensory impairment (Hatton & Emerson 1995). Also, understandably, there is less self-reporting of such problems amongst clients with learning disabilities (Warburg 1994). Therefore there is a need for regular screening of clients for sensory problems and guidelines are available for practitioners from, for example, the RNIB.

Hatton & Emerson (1995) have highlighted problems in providing services for people with profound and multiple disabilities who have a hearing impairment, owing to the difficulty of identifying such people. They argued that even though health care Trusts expressed a willingness to offer services, provision remained patchy due to lack of availability of appropriate screening facilities and lack of understanding of the complex needs of this client group. This problem is evident in all areas of health care provision for people with profound and multiple disabilities and is not limited to hearing impairment.

There are a number of options that one could use to support the individual and the family which should assist service purchasers in reflecting on the need to develop service provision further. The advent of the multi-agency Children with Disabilities registers as a result of the Children Act (1989) may be regarded as a means to highlight service provision needs within localities. Although registers are seen by some as further labelling and segregating individuals with learning disabilities, the need to overcome the problems highlighted by Hatton & Emerson (1995) perhaps tips the balance in their favour, if it means that service provision will ultimately improve.

As with vision, it is important that residual hearing is maximised. A programme of positive approaches that professionals can use with the individual and the family includes:

- screening of individuals who are seen as being at risk of hearing impairment
- early identification of any hearing difficulties
- prompt and systematic management strategies to minimise the impact of hearing impairment (including exploration of the value of therapeutic interventions such as auditory integration training. However Zollweg et al (1997) have argued that this has mixed success with clients with profound and multiple disabilities)
- information for families regarding the diagnosis and management of hearing impairment, and the support networks and services available.

Risk factors would include prematurity, prenatal infection, maternal illness during pregnancy (for example rubella and herpes zoster), neurological impairment such as severe cerebral palsy (particularly athetoid linked), meningitis and other central nervous system infections, and trauma. Possible iatrogenic causes of sensorineural (perceptive) hearing impairment should also be con-

sidered, for example intravenous antibiotic therapy used to treat meningitis.

Serum otitis media, generally known as 'glue ear', is a form of conductive hearing impairment that should be suspected, particularly in people with Down syndrome, as the problem tends to persist. Indeed Dennis (1995) has advised on behalf of the Down Syndrome Association that clients with Down syndrome have additional problems with the effectiveness of the medical and surgical interventions available and so require ongoing monitoring for potentially significant hearing loss; clients may also need hearing aids. Practitioners need to ensure those clients with Down syndrome, particularly infants and children, have their hearing reviewed by an audiologist rather than through routine child health surveillance methods.

Familial incidence of hearing impairment should also be regarded as a significant indicator to consider screening the child with profound and multiple disabilities. Engelman et al (1998) highlighted that an increased risk of significant sensory impairments is also linked to a wide range of both genetic and acquired antenatal and postnatal causes for this client group.

Care issues

Treatment of any underlying medical cause of the hearing impairment is essential. With any other type of hearing impairment it is important that, as stated above, residual hearing is maximised. This may involve the use of appropriate hearing aids and adaptations to the person's environment, for example an audio loop to enhance hearing aid performance within the home. It is important that the effectiveness of any aids is regularly evaluated, particularly as compliance with their use may be a problem (Yeates 1995).

For an individual with profound hearing loss, as well as profound and multiple disabilities, verbal communication can be severely affected, and so the development of non-verbal communication skills is essential. If an individual has motor and mobilisation difficulties, the use of non-verbal signing systems, such as Makaton, may be more difficult to achieve. However, a personalised version of Makaton and/or the use of electronic touch-sensitive talkers can be of considerable benefit. It may be argued that personalised signing systems limit communication with others in the fullest sense, but the ability to use them with carers should not be disregarded, as it represents an opportunity for individuals to express their needs. In formal care settings care plans should reflect a person's own communication needs and abilities.

CARDIOVASCULAR ISSUES

Cardiovascular problems were cited as an important health care issue in the DOH (1995) publication *The Health of the Nation: a Strategy for People with Learning Disabilities*. It is not possible here to explore the range of cardiovascular disorders that may affect the person with profound and multiple disabilities: none the less, it is important to acknowledge the need for a better understanding of any underlying cardiovascular condition an individual has. There are a number of support groups for carers, which can be found through a GP. The community learning disabilities nurse should also be able to provide further details. The initial *Health of the Nation* document (DOH 1991) and the later strategy document *Saving Lives: Our Healthier Nation* (DOH 1999d) also highlighted cardiovascular problems as an area that should be targeted for action to reduce the incidence of cardiac disease. A range of strategies can be used by carers, for example offering a varied, nutritional choice of foods. Even for those who have to be fed by a carer and have their food chosen for them, it is important to encourage a varied and nutritional diet. Professionals working with carers are advised to use the guidance provided, for example by the Department of Health Committee on Medical Aspects of Food (COMA) (DOH 1996) and NACNE (National Advisory Committee on Nutritional Education). Carers can also seek the advice of a dietician regarding the nutritional and fluid needs of an individual. It is a common misperception that someone who is immobile needs fewer calories; often an individual who has frequent involuntary movements and muscle spasms will require more calories to replace the energy expended.

Lack of physical mobility can predispose the individual to the risk of circulatory problems, such as peripheral vascular disease. There is therefore a need for a daily range of passive and/or active physiotherapy routines that will help maintain the cardiovascular system's effective functioning. Excess weight gain may be a difficulty for some individuals with profound and multiple disabilities, and if this is the case it is important to seek advice.

The individual's GP should be contacted prior to considering any weight loss programme, to ensure that any underlying cause such as thyroid problems are eliminated. The dietician and physiotherapist can help in identifying strategies to promote weight control.

Given that up to 50% of clients with Down syndrome will have a congenital cardiac condition (Cohen 1999) it is clear that screening for such problems in infants and children with Down syndrome is essential as part of the long-term follow-up health care. Understanding the skills, knowledge and experience practitioners need in supporting a client with Down syndrome who has a cardiac condition requires more in-depth material than can be expressed within this chapter. Practitioners are therefore recommended to consider the reading list at the end of the chapter and utilise the excellent Down Syndrome Association (DSA) website (see end of chapter).

ORAL HYGIENE ISSUES

This area of care has already been discussed in reference to individuals who are unable to manage food and/or fluids orally. However, there are some additional general guidelines that should be explored, as well as some specific issues of importance for carers of individuals with profound and multiple disabilities. Oral hygiene is something we tend to take for granted until we are unable to perform it ourselves. Much criticism has been aimed at the low level of priority given to such a basic need when caring for people with profound disabilities (Griffiths & Boyle 1993). Access to dental services should be equitable, and most (if not all) health authority trusts offer a domiciliary dental health service to meet the needs of this client group. Dental hygiene routines may be difficult for carers to perform, perhaps because the individual has an exaggerated bite reflex, or simply does not enjoy the experience of having his or her teeth cleaned. A range of techniques can be employed to make teeth cleaning much easier, such as using desensitisation techniques for the individual's face and mouth prior to attempting to brush the teeth, or the use of an electric tooth brush if tolerated. Plaque disclosing tablets may give the carer some reassurance regarding the effectiveness of the teeth cleaning, particularly as there is a higher incidence of tooth abrasion in clients with cerebral palsy, especially, as Shaw et al (1998) highlighted, where there are gastroesophageal reflux problems. Also, where possible, the avoidance of high sugar-content food and drinks may also be worth considering. Some specific issues that should be considered by carers are:

- the impact of medication, particularly some anticonvulsants, on oral health
- the particular problems that the individual with Down syndrome may have
- general feeding difficulties.

An important issue that needs to be remembered in relation to people with learning disabilities within routine primary health care is the need for oral antibiotic cover before and after dental surgery, including routine procedures such as descaling. The rationale for this is to prevent endocarditis caused by bacteria present in the mouth entering the blood stream.

The impact of medication on oral hygiene

High sugar-content versions of medications, especially if they have to be taken on a regular basis, should be avoided where possible, and sugar-free alternatives considered. For example, if an individual has paracetamol in an elixir form, there is a sugar-free option available.

Another issue regarding medication relates to a frequently used group of drugs, the anticonvulsants (drugs taken orally for various forms of epilepsy). The most common problems here concern phenytoin, which is linked to a condition known as gingival hyperplasia, in which the gums become tender and sensitive and may bleed. Gingival hypertrophy is also a problem. The important care issue here is not to stop the phenytoin but to implement good oral hygiene strategies and to make sure that the dentist is aware of any medication being taken.

Feeding difficulties and oral hygiene

An individual with severe cerebral palsy may have a range of feeding problems, including exaggerated bite reflex, malocclusion and swallowing difficulties. The exaggerated reflex can pose problems for carers trying to clean the individual's teeth; also, if the individual has particular difficulty in chewing and swallowing, there could be a build-up of food in the mouth. This can be a particular problem if the person has to be fed by a carer who is not experienced in assisting someone with such needs. Again, it is important to reiterate the need for good regular oral hygiene care for the individual.

Given that attitudes toward people with profound and multiple disabilities still focus upon the 'tragedy model', and that although attitudes may be professed to be positive, unconscious attitudes of 'I'm glad it's not me' still prevail, one needs to give some attention to the image that the general public has of such individuals. What has this to do with oral health? Dribbling and mouth breathing, and hence halitosis, can be a major problem for the individual and should not be marginalised. Carers and practitioners need to spend time with the individual to seek to identify whether the cause is sensory based or due to muscle dysfunction (Palmer & Heyman 1998).

Consideration needs to be given to ways in which to minimise the impact of the dribbling, for example oral motor stimulation (Domaracki & Sisson 1990), using age-appropriate scarves rather than bibs, and consideration of appropriate medication. Surgical approaches to the management of drooling are an option to consider (Cheng 2001), however this may give limited benefits and practitioners should liaise with regional specialists to ascertain the value of this technique for clients. The problem of halitosis can be increased if the individual is unable to tolerate oral food and fluids, and so oral hygiene is very important. In such cases carers should seek advice from the individual's GP, as there may be a need to use artificial saliva products such as Glandosane to minimise the discomfort of a dry mouth.

RESPIRATORY ISSUES

People with multiple disabilities often have respiratory problems. There are many reasons for this: for example poor swallowing and/or gag reflex, poor cough reflex, immobility, inability to be in the upright position, as well as common problems such as asthma and colds. The reason for including respiratory problems in this chapter is that because of their existing problems individuals with profound and multiple disabilities may have more difficulties with ailments such as colds. Some conditions associated with varying degrees of learning disability are also linked with various respiratory disorders (Down syndrome, Goldenhar syndrome, chromosome 4 problems and CHARGE association problems, for example), as are some conditions that are life limiting and associated with learning disabilities, such as Batten's disease and other metabolic conditions. There are also links between extreme prematurity of neonates with learning disabilities and additional respiratory problems. For example, bronchopulmonary dysplasia is linked with immature lung function as a result of prematurity, and with the treatment such neonates require (Habel & Scott 1998).

The main aims of caring for this client group in relation to respiratory function are:

- to maintain the individual's health
- to promote ways in which respiratory function can be enhanced
- promotion of awareness in carers, both formal and informal, of the risks associated with feeding, in terms of aspiration and potential aspiration pneumonia
- to ensure that any respiratory infections or difficulties are promptly identified
- to ensure that the range of treatment options for respiratory conditions meets the needs of the individual.

Prevention/minimisation

It is important that carers work closely with the physiotherapist in considering ways in which an individual's respiratory health can be promoted. This can include daily chest physiotherapy, including postural drainage to prevent the build-up of excess secretions, especially if the individual is relatively immobile. Oral and nasal suction techniques may be necessary to assist in clearing excess secretions, so that the individual can breathe without discomfort. Also, the removal of excess secretions helps reduce the incidence of respiratory infection.

Changing the individual's position at regular intervals is useful in maximising respiratory function, as well as in maintaining comfort and helping prevent pressure sores.

Promoting good respiratory function need not be expensive or time consuming for carers; simple things that may help include the way in which pillows are positioned while the person is in bed, and making use of times when an individual is perhaps lying over a wedge to encourage head control, to facilitate drainage of excess secretions.

CONTINENCE ISSUES

Continence care can be a major issue for people with profound and multiple disabilities. In childhood particularly, it is important to ensure that there are no underlying factors that could be exacerbating the continence difficulties, rather than presuming, as Stanley (1997) warns, that the only approach needed is a behavioural one. The primary cause of incontinence is likely to be related to the degree of learning and physical disability (Roijen et al 2001), and continence, where achievable, is often delayed later into childhood. Practitioners should be aware that urinary tract infections and renal abnormalities could exacerbate the problem, as for all individuals, and should be treated.

Once all the above are excluded then a behavioural approach may be effective (Bradley et al 1995, Roe & Williams 1994, Williams et al 1995) for those clients who have a degree of understanding of the biological signals in relation to urination and defecation.

Incontinence can be urinary and/or fecal, and there are a number of strategies that carers should be aware of, particularly concerning the individual who is relatively immobile.

Continence aids will be required to meet the individual's needs. These are available through local health authority trusts, many of which have a nurse practitioner who is a designated continence advisor, and who works closely with the professionals involved in supporting clients and carers. It is important to consider the impact of incontinence on the individual in terms of body image, comfort (some continence aids can be very bulky to wear), and skin care; prompt skin care regimens and the use of appropriate barrier creams are important.

Care issues

The most common form of incontinence is urinary, and a range of continence aids is available. Intermittent or long-term catheterisation may be an option and can be very successful for people with neurological conditions such as spina bifida, or paraplegia-related difficulties. There are a number of points that carers should be aware of in catheter care management, to ensure the individual's comfort and prevent problems. For example, if long-term catheters are being used then the choice of type is important: silicone catheters are more comfortable and less likely to be associated with problems of urinary crystallisation. Monitoring the pH of the urine may seem 'over the top', but can be useful to assist in the early identification of a urinary tract infection if this is a significant problem for the individual, and thus ensure prompt treatment. The consumption of up to 400 mL of cranberry juice daily is currently suggested as being beneficial in minimising the incidence of urinary tract infections (Nazarko 1995). A good fluid intake generally is very beneficial, especially in this client group, because urinary stasis and the potential problem of urinary tract infection are exacerbated by immobility.

Fecal incontinence is particularly distressing, and carers need to consider ways in which, for example, the odour can be minimised. The most effective strategy is simply prompt skin care after defecation, and the effective use of the appropriate continence aids. However, fecal incontinence does not mean that an individual should have to endure diarrhoea or constipation. Constipation is a problem considered to be associated with immobility, and it is therefore important for the individual to have a well balanced diet that is high in fibre (unless medically contraindicated) and an adequate fluid intake, as well as opportunities for mobilisation, both passive and active. Medication is often prescribed to aid defecation, e.g. stool softeners and aperients, but the use of medication for constipation should be minimal and only under the guidance of a person's GP.

EPILEPSY

Epilepsy is a condition often associated with profound and multiple disabilities (Kay et al 1995a). Before all the aspects of this subject are explored in relation to the client group being considered in this chapter, the reader is advised to turn to Reader activity 17.4.

What is meant by the term epilepsy? McMenamin & Bird (1993, p. 4) define epilepsy as: 'recurrent, episodic, uncontrolled electrical discharge from the brain. Epilepsy is the term for recurrent, unprovoked seizures or convulsions.'

Epilepsy is a condition that produces a range of images for both professionals and the general public, and it is important that readers examine their attitudes, beliefs and values regarding this condition.

It is essential that professionals have a significant understanding of epilepsy, given the incidence of epilepsy in this client group. Indeed the

 Reader activity 17.4

- What do you understand by the term epilepsy?
- How do you envisage that epilepsy can affect the life of the individual with profound and multiple disabilities?
- What information do you think carers may want as regards caring for someone with profound and multiple disabilities who also has epilepsy?
- How would you access that information?

British Epilepsy Association (BEA), in partnership with the British Institute of Learning Disabilities (BILD) (BEA/BILD 2001b) cited the incidence of 200 000 clients with learning disabilities severely affected by epilepsy. However, it is important to stress that having epilepsy does not equate with learning disability, and this must not be assumed. A number of studies have attempted to identify the factors that would signify a link between learning disability and epilepsy. Certainly epilepsy within the first year of life is seen as a significant (although not definite) related factor with learning disability (BEA/BILD 2001b, Curatolo et al 1995). However, it should be emphasised that there are a number of reasons why this may be so, such as prenatal malformations within the brain, and all the other linked pre- and postnatal conditions that are associated with learning disabilities. A case control study by Curatolo et al (1995) has highlighted the multitude of factors that can influence the development of learning disabilities alongside epilepsy, and also cerebral palsy.

If carers suspect that the individual has epilepsy, how is it diagnosed? Epilepsy is not usually diagnosed as a result of a single seizure, but rather if and when a second seizure occurs. The reason for this is that we all have the potential for a single isolated seizure. However, this does not mean that medical advice should not be sought when a seizure occurs, as it may be a sign of an underlying medical condition that requires investigation and treatment. However, it may be more difficult to diagnose epilepsy in the client with a learning disability due to communication issues and the complexity and diversity of types of epilepsy. It is important that carers maintain a diary of an individual's seizures before and after formal diagnosis, as this will help ensure that the treatment prescribed is appropriate and meets the individual's needs.

Diagnosis is made primarily on the clinical history and using diagnostic tools such as EEG (electroencephalogram) and CT (computed tomography); both are non-invasive procedures. The medical practitioner will wish to exclude any underlying medical condition, and blood samples may be taken for analysis.

Types of epilepsy and medications used

Epilepsy can manifest itself in many forms, although most people tend to be aware of the more common types: tonic–clonic seizures (often referred to as *grand mal* seizures, a term now disregarded owing to the limitations of its meaning) and absence seizures (again often inappropriately referred to by the traditional term *petit mal*). All areas of the brain can be affected, although the frontal, parietal and temporal lobes of the cortex are most often linked with epilepsy.

Simple partial seizures

This is when symptoms affect only one side of the body. Consciousness is not affected and the person often experiences unusual feelings. Simple partial seizures often occur while the person is asleep.

Complex partial seizures

This form of seizure is often difficult to describe, and maintaining a thorough diary will help in assessing whether seizures are of this type. The temporal lobe of the brain is associated with this type of seizure, and those suffering these seizures are often said to be unaware of their surroundings, as consciousness is affected to a degree. The person may experience what is termed as an aura beforehand, for example an unusual smell. Automatisms – the term used to describe repetitive behavioural responses such as 'finger flapping' – can be evident. Partial seizures are often treated with carbamazepine (Tegretol), phenytoin (Epanutin), lamotrigine (Lamictal) or vigabatrin (Sabril).

Absence seizures

These may be described as 'a brief loss of awareness, without any obvious jerking or falling down' (McMenamin & Bird 1993, p. 3). These can occur frequently throughout the day, and again the carer's diary may indicate that a review of medication to limit the frequency of such episodes is required. It is sometimes possible to take steps to minimise recurrent episodes by ensuring that the individual is not over-tired or under undue stress, and that blood sugar levels are not low. As with all forms of epilepsy, medication prescribed to control the seizures must never be stopped except on medical advice. Absence seizures are usually treated with sodium valproate (Epilim) or ethosuximide (Zarontin) (specifically for absence seizures).

Generalised tonic–clonic seizures

As stated earlier, this type of seizure is the best-known form of epilepsy, and carers often refer to it as causing the greatest anxiety, because of its manifestations. It can be the primary form of epilepsy, but it can also occur as a secondary form following other types of seizures, such as complex partial seizures. The seizure involves two stages, tonic and clonic, although it may be difficult for onlookers to differentiate between them. The tonic stage involves loss of consciousness, with an appearance of becoming rigid as the muscles go into extension. This is followed by a clonic period, which is typically seen as the muscles alternately rapidly contracting and relaxing. There may be urinary incontinence during the seizure and also biting of the tongue. After the convulsing has ceased a period known as the postictal phase follows, in which the person often is very drowsy yet rousable. The person may wish to sleep for a time after the tonic–clonic phase has ended. It is important that carers are aware of the usual pattern of the individual's seizures so that any digression from that pattern can be investigated. Tonic–clonic seizures are usually treated with sodium valproate (Epilim) or phenytoin (Epanutin). The relatively new generation of anticonvulsants, vigabatrin (Sabril) (Dichter & Brodie, 1996), or lamotrigine (Lamictal) have been used particularly to manage partial seizures, whether with tonic–clonic seizures or in isolation (Stephen & Brodie 1998).

Lamotrigine has now been recognised for use as a monotherapy in the UK (Feely 1999). Newer medications such as gabapentin (Neurontin) and topiramate (Topamax) are also now available, with gabapentin useful in newly diagnosed clients with epilepsy (UK Gabapentin Study Group 1990) as it has less side effects, but it is potentially less effective. Topiramate is more powerful but fraught currently with side effects, even with gradual introduction (Faught et al 1996). Practitioners need to ensure that they remain up-to-date with current and future therapies to ensure that they can advocate appropriately on behalf of clients with epilepsy who would benefit from medication review.

As a practitioner one finds it unacceptable that even now, according to a BEA (1996) study, people who have epilepsy are still not receiving the most appropriate therapeutic management. This raises the profile even more of the need for practitioners to act as informed advocates on behalf of clients with learning disabilities (particularly those with profound and multiple disabilities) to ensure the best care is provided.

There are other types of epilepsy that carers may need to be aware of, and professionals should always be aware of the number of ways in which epilepsy can manifest. These include myoclonic seizures, atonic seizures and seizures as a result of Lennox Gestaut syndrome. Carers and other professionals also need to be aware of the potential problem of what is termed status epilepticus, where a tonic–clonic seizure is prolonged (that is, longer than usual for that individual) or the seizure is followed by another within a short time without the person regaining consciousness. This is classed as a medical emergency and requires prompt treatment in terms of immediate first aid and advanced management, and will almost certainly require medical treatment unless the problem is rectified by the administration (if prescribed) of diazepam in a specially prepared format for rectal administration (Stesolid).

There is ongoing discussion by such as Scott et al (1999) and Wiebe (2000) in relation to the value of buccal midazolam as an alternative/addition to management of such situations. Readers are advised to review further updates as they emerge within the medical press and the BEA website in terms of the potential value of this drug as a less invasive therapeutic intervention.

Given the potential range of physical effects of epilepsy on the daily life of an individual with profound and multiple disabilities, it is a condition that cannot be ignored because of its psychosocial impact on individuals and their families. When the seizures are frequent and severe, the impact on everyday life may be phenomenal and the level of care required may seem inordinate. Readers are advised to contact the British Epilepsy Association for more detailed information (website in Useful addresses section).

OTHER ISSUES IN THE CARE OF PEOPLE WITH PROFOUND AND MULTIPLE DISABILITIES

This section, by no means exhaustive, covers only few of the many aspects of care that could be explored. Each person with profound and multiple disabilities has unique needs, and it is hoped that this chapter will act as a catalyst for the reader to develop a wider and more empathetic understanding of these needs. Thus this final section will consider:

- aspects of pain management
- health surveillance regarding thyroid problems and diabetes mellitus
- the need for health screening in relation to thyroid problems and diabetes mellitus
- the impact of the life expectancy debate
- age and ageing
- leisure
- support for carers.

Readers are advised to consult other chapters for more in-depth consideration of leisure needs (Ch. 9) sexual identity and sexual health (Ch. 16 and 23). Ch. 12 explores the relevant mental health issues for this client group.

Pain management

There are many misconceptions regarding pain, its existence, manifestations and treatment. The purpose of this section is to direct readers to challenge their beliefs, values and knowledge concerning pain. It is of concern that studies such as that by Twycross (2000) have highlighted the

limited input on pain assessment and management within learning disabilities branch courses (pre-registration). As a result there is a need for further work at both pre- and post-registration levels in nursing to address this important issue.

Aside from the above educational issue, practitioners and carers in general need to be aware of the wide variety of ways in which profound and multiple disability in itself can generate specific pain experiences, as well as those experienced by all in ill health.

One particular issue is that of involuntary muscle spasms, post-seizure aches and, as highlighted in Schwartz et al's (1999) study, limb and lower back pain in clients with cerebral palsy. This is exacerbated by the inability to communicate verbally, and the limited ability of some individuals with profound and multiple disabilities to communicate non-verbally could mean that they are marginalised in terms of pain management, as the assessment of pain is subjective. If the carer is not familiar with the means by which clients communicate, the ways in which they express pain may be misinterpreted. The measure of someone's pain should not rely solely on verbal expression of its existence, and professionals should work with clients and their carers to ensure that pain relief is given where appropriate and its effectiveness monitored. There has been some success with work with clients to build upon their understanding and ability to communicate how they feel when they are ill (Dodd & Brunker 1999), and there is a need to explore the effectiveness of such an approach with this client group. It should not be assumed that pain will be relieved just by prescribing analgesia.

Pain management tools should be adapted to enable the person's behaviour to be measured objectively, especially when the client has limited or no verbal communication. Behavioural pain assessment tools such as that of Tarbell et al (1992), may be extremely effective if modified and adapted to be age appropriate. However, as with all behaviour-based assessments, they are dependent on observable behaviour. Thus carers who use them must be aware of how clients behave when well, in addition to when they are ill, or in pain. There must be agreement regarding the subjective interpretation of an individual's behaviour to ensure a consistent and effective approach to pain management. Carers need to be aware that behavioural tools can only suggest, rather than represent an absolute indicator of pain (Carter 1994). Also, carers must be aware that the generally construed signs of pain, such as crying, will not necessarily be present, and pain may be felt even if the individual does not cry (Grunau et al 1990, Krechel & Bildner 1995).

This is an important factor, as some people have negative perceptions regarding individuals with profound and multiple disabilities and may assume that 'they can't feel anything anyway'; hence one of the benefits of pain assessment tools is to objectively demonstrate pain and pain control responses. They also have the added benefit of ensuring a consistent approach and enabling pain control strategies to be evaluated. Readers are directed to the Royal College of Nursing (2001) clinical practice guidelines on the recognition and assessment of pain in children.

There is a range of pain management strategies that may be particularly useful with this client group, in addition to the more traditional pharmacological methods. These include distraction (including the use of the Snoezelen, as explored in a research project on chronic pain by Schofield et al (1998)), relaxation through touch and massage, aromatherapy, acupuncture and all the other complementary therapies. The use of TENS (transcutaneous electrical nerve stimulation) has already been described and could be given further consideration as it is effective, safe and non-invasive. Whatever is used, it is important that the strategy is tailored to the individual's needs. Inadequate and ineffective pain management is unacceptable.

Health surveillance in relation to thyroid problems and diabetes mellitus

Hyper and hypothyroid problems.

There is a higher incidence of thyroid function problems both congenital and in adolescence and older age, in clients with Down syndrome (Dennis 1995b, Prasher 1994). There is also evidence that older clients may have more problems with thyroid function in later life (Pueschel et al 1991). The implication for practice is that a client with Down syndrome should have annual screening of thyroid function as part of a well person's check. Also practitioners working with children need to be aware that children with Down syndrome may have transiently high levels of the thyroid stimulating hormone (TSH), however this may reduce to normal in some children. Regardless of this all children with Down syndrome with high levels of TSH require frequent monitoring, as acknowledged by Selikowitz (1993).

Diabetes mellitus (type 1)

In people with Down syndrome, particularly children, and often alongside hypothyroidism, may be found diabetes mellitus (type 1) (Selby 1997). Clients with Down syndrome who develop diabetes require the same support and therapeutic care as clients in the general population. Practitioners should be aware of this increased incidence and include screening for this within other routine medical care/health reviews. The British Diabetic Association (now DiabetesUK) has an excellent website for further study, which is given at the end of the chapter.

Life expectancy

It is important to acknowledge that there are a number of health issues for this client group, but the expectation of morbidity should not be encouraged. The focus of work with this client group needs to be on the maintenance and promotion of health in terms of emotional and physical wellbeing as well as self-esteem (Evans et al 1990, King et al 2000, Woodhill et al 1994). A study by Murphy et al (1995) highlighted that the care of adults with cerebral palsy with acute health care needs was satisfactory, but there were significant gaps in preventive health care. Cerebral palsy does not necessarily equate with profound and multiple disabilities, but the need to provide adequate preventive health care is a global one.

Diagnosis and management of profound and multiple disability have improved in the last 25 years. This has to be considered in relation to the life expectancy of children with severe learning disabilities, which has increased considerably (Evans et al 1990, Eyman et al 1993, Hutton et al 1994, Katz 2001, Strauss et al 1998). A study by Crichton et al (1995) highlighted some factors that are still considered as concerns, these being epilepsy, the degree of the learning disability, respiratory conditions and impaired mobility. These studies are particularly pertinent given the current medicolegal and ethical debates regarding infants and children and quality of life, and even the right to life itself. Hence the requests to discontinue medical care, in relation to enteral feeding being debated as an extraordinary treatment for a young child with profound and multiple disabilities, and for C (wardship: a minor) [1996], who was a ventilated premature infant with a prognosis of profound and multiple disabilities, are particularly poignant. Similar cases are Re B (wardship: a minor) [1981 All ER 927], in relation to an infant with Down syndrome, and Re J (wardship: a minor) [1990 All ER 930], in relation to a ventilated 27-week gestation infant (Campbell & McHaffie 1995).

Practitioners need to review the current Royal College of Paediatrics and Child Health (1997) guidance/framework on withholding or withdrawing life saving treatment in children. There are specific practice situations and recommendations in relation to children with severe neurological impairment that practitioners need to explore in light of their current practice and in view of The Human Rights Act (1998) and primary legislation in the UK such as the Children Act (1989). Readers are strongly advised to consult recent medical/legal/ethical journals regarding these most important issues. It is likely that these debates will become more pertinent and frequent, given the current climate within medicine. Readers should also be aware that there are a number of conditions associated with profound and multiple disabilities that are considered to be life-limiting. Examples of these are Batten's disease and other metabolic conditions, degenerative conditions such as Tay–Sachs syndrome, and other inherited conditions, as well as the range of neurodegenerative conditions such as leukodystrophy and spinal muscular atrophy. Readers are advised to consult specific texts regarding the care of an individual with a life-limiting condition, as there is too much material to cover here. Some texts are included in the reference list, including the good practice guidelines in relation to caring for children with life-limiting conditions (NHSE 1998). It is important that both professionals and informal carers should seek to network with colleagues in the locality, as clients and their carers have a right to the full range of information and options regarding support. Support may include hospices, home care, short-term breaks and family-to-family support, as well as practical support and symptom control (such as pain management clinics).

Age and ageing

Readers may be aware of the negative stereotypes associated with people who have learning disabilities. These include the 'Peter Pan syndrome' and the 'everlasting child', and this is particularly the case as regards individuals with profound and multiple disabilities. Consider the scenario described in Reader activity 17.5 and spend some time reflecting on these questions.

Adolescence is a time when identity synthesis is evolving. It is a time when people explore what 'I' and 'self' mean to them and to their peers and family. In the UK and other western societies, adolescence is seen as a time that leads to self- definition (Kroger 1996). However, this process of self- definition is often not fulfilled by adolescents with profound and multiple disabilities, because of the identity they have been 'given' since infancy, of being profoundly disabled, and because of a perception of them as 'eternal children'. Subsequently it is important that carers (and professionals) are supported in re-evaluating their beliefs regarding adolescence in this client group (Baker 1991), enabling the developmental aspects of adolescence and young adulthood to be acknowledged (King et al 2000, Marn & Koch 1999). Indeed this is particularly important when planning transition to adult services appropriately in partnership with the parents/carers and the client (American Academy of Pediatrics 1996, Betz 1998).

The period of transition can be a time of great turmoil within the family, with questions such as:

- When does my son/daughter have to move from children's to adult services?
- Do I have a choice, does my son/daughter have a choice about when that should happen?
- I have known these professionals throughout my son/daughter's life; will the 'new' staff ever know him/her?
- What happens after school finishes?
- What services are there, and will they provide sufficient care and stimulation on a daily basis?

It is a time that could poignantly remind the family of 'what might have been', as friends' children prepare for further education or work. At this time, parents often express concern about what will happen if they themselves become ill and are unable to carry on caring; it is a time when the individual can no longer truly be seen as a child. This reminds the parents of their own age, adding to their concerns for their son or daughter's future.

Adulthood is a vast subject area, and so only one other major lifetime continuum event or state will be discussed, i.e. the older person with profound and multiple disabilities. This may appear a contentious subject, but readers are referred to the section earlier in this chapter regarding health care needs, life expectancy and this client group, and asked to reflect upon recent papers which have completed longitudinal studies on this issue.

 Reader activity 17.5

Imagine you are a newly qualified nurse and for the past 6 months since qualifying you have been assigned to the local community team for children with learning disabilities. You are visiting one of the special schools that you have been asked to liaise with. One of the teachers, while in general conversation with you, asks if you could 'go and talk to one of her mums'. She expresses concern that Zoë, one of the teenagers in the special care group, always seems to be dressed in clothes that are more suitable for a 5-year-old rather than a 15-year-old. The teacher then shrugs her shoulders and says that she feels that Zoë's mother 'might listen to you more as you are a nurse'. What should you do?

Before one can consider specific issues surrounding the care of the older person with profound and multiple disabilities, readers are asked to look at Reader activity 17.6.

It has been argued that individuals in this client group should be considered 'older' from the ages of 40–50 years, because of premature ageing and reduced life expectancy (Dalton & Wisviewski 1993). However, the reader is asked to consider all the information available before accepting this as a definitive view, and to consider clients on an individual basis. Indeed it should be remembered that people with learning disabilities are living much longer (Barr 2001), including those clients with profound and multiple disabilities, therefore health and social care provisions must be adequate to meet the additional health care needs of this growing client group (Harris et al 1997, Livingstone & Tindale 2000). This includes consideration of strategies to maintain mobility. Most studies, such as Rantanen et al (1999) and Eldar and Marincek (2000), focus on exercise in older people per se or those with physical disability, without consideration of learning disability as an additional factor. However, given the benefits of appropriate exercise in promotion of wellbeing in older people (Dustman et al 1990, King et al 1997) This is clearly an area that requires further attention for clients with learning disabilities.

It is acknowledged that people with Down syndrome have specific needs, as they are known to be more at risk of developing Alzheimer's disease in middle age (Holland et al 2000, Soliman & Hawkins 1998). However, the papers that explore the links with learning disability and premature ageing tend not to include people with profound and multiple disabilities. Indeed they tend to focus on people with mild learning disabilities as a client group with mental health needs and ageing concerns (Cooper & Collacott 1994, Van Minnen et al 1994). It is important to consider the issue of ageing in our client group further, particularly regarding leisure and health needs, considering osteoporosis and reduced joint flexibility as well as sensory impairment (Matteson et al 1993), for example, along with the right to access services designed to meet the needs of people in their 'third age'. Therapies such as validation and

Reader activity 17.6

- What do we mean by the terms 'older person' and 'ageing'?
- Are these terms different when one is discussing the individual with profound and multiple disabilities? If so why, and if not why not?

resolution therapy, reality orientation and multisensory approaches are useful in the management of dementia (Hope 1998, Morrissey & Biela 1997, Woodrow, 1998), however it could be argued that there is a need to consider the appropriateness of these therapies for older people with profound learning disabilities. The most realistic and successful approach would therefore be the multisensory approach (highlighted by Hutchinson & Haggar (1994) and Ashby et al (1995)) in conjunction with reality orientation, but this is reliant on the practitioners involved having the relevant skills, knowledge and experience to utilise these approaches. Savage (1996) has highlighted this in a paper raising concerns regarding Snoezelen use for confused older people.

Leisure

Providing for the leisure and occupational needs of this client group may appear to be a challenge for carers. It is important that leisure needs are not disregarded, and facilities and activities should be age-appropriate and wide ranging, so as to provide stimulation and pleasure as well as exercise.

There are a number of activities which can incorporate care needs while creating a leisure focus. Massage and multisensory activities can also incorporate some of the individual's physiotherapy needs, although it is important that there are times in the day that are purely for relaxation and leisure. Another important aspect in terms of leisure/stimulation is the need to experience different environments, as well as having some time outdoors. For individuals cared for in a formal unit, it is likely that all their care will be provided in one building, and so there will be no specific

need to go outdoors. This can also be the case even when individuals are cared for at home, as they may be taken to designated day centres or other services via specialised transport, only experiencing being outdoors on transferring to and from the transport. This can inhibit the opportunity to experience wind, the sun or even rain.

Leisure needs, as well as education/occupational needs, must therefore be carefully integrated into lifelong planning. There is a wide variety of leisure experiences that the individual may enjoy, depending on personal preference. It is access in terms of transport, moving and handling and carer support for these leisure activities that can and does make the difference. Readers are advised to build upon their knowledge network regarding leisure facilities and the level of access available for this client group.

Support for carers

It is important that carers are seen as equal partners with professionals. Consider the comment made by Madden (1995) regarding the parents of children with learning disabilities. It could be seen as a poignant statement on behalf of all carers:

Parents are at the start of a lifelong journey they did not bargain for. They need to know that professionals are going to be with them. Professionals need to learn to think and act collaboratively so that parents have fewer experiences of duplication, confusion or professional rivalries (Madden 1995, p. 90).

Supporting the carers thus requires commitment from professionals, who can act as enablers and facilitators. It involves implicit recognition that it is the carers who are actually doing the caring, and this is a 24-hour, 7-days-a-week responsibility. Support involves recognising the unique needs and coping strategies of each family. Some may wish for regular contact from professionals, and others would rather just have access to a 24-hour professional helpline. Professionals also need to realise that the level of support required will vary over time.

Requests for information, advice, just listening for rather than to the carer, or even formal counselling may be services that the carer may require at some time or another. There are key times when it is recognised that perhaps additional support will be needed. These include:

- the diagnosis (or identification) of disability (and the time preceding diagnosis)
- the care of the preschool child
- formal education assessment and statementing
- educational statementing reviews
- before transition to adult services
- times when the individual is unwell
- ill health of the main carer
- general increasing care needs of the individual.

This list is endless and should never be seen as prescriptive. Professionals need to adopt the 'key worker' approach, as stated earlier in the chapter, and need to be able to offer a comprehensive range of services to carers.

Short-term breaks

Many families regard access to such services as an essential part of service provision. Professionals need to be aware of the range of short-term breaks available for this client group. It can be difficult to access family-based care for individuals with profound and multiple disabilities, owing to the level of care that may be required. This is especially so if the individual has additional complex health needs. Robinson & Stalker (1990) identified, in a UK study, that short-term break services for this client group are generally under-resourced, despite being in demand and highly valued by parents/carers. Short-term breaks are not a 'panacea for all ills', but should be regarded as an integral part of service provision and practitioners are advised to explore all potential options in relation to short-term breaks, both family- and building-based, to ensure that service provision is proactively needs-led. The need to involve parents/main carers in service planning and review cannot be underestimated.

CONCLUSION

The health care needs of children and adults with profound and/or multiple disabilities presents practitioners with numerous challenges, however this should not mean that these needs are overlooked. Practitioners need to work proactively with clients and their families to promote and maintain health and to ensure that additional acute and/or chronic health care needs are met accordingly and always to the highest standards. Clinical excellence should be the hallmark of health care provision for this client group as for all other service users. The essence of all professional involvement has to be to meet the needs of those individuals and their families as people first and foremost.

REFERENCES

Abel M F, Juhl G A, Vaughan C L, Damiano D L 1998 Gait assessment of fixed ankle-foot orthoses in children with spastic diplegia. Archives of Physical Medicine and Rehabilitation 79: 126–133

Adams R A, Gordon C, Spangler A A 1999 Perspectives in practice: maternal stress in caring for children with feeding disabilities: implications for health care providers. Journal of the American Dietetic Association 99(8): 962–966

Aldridge J, Becker S 1993 Children who care – inside the world of young carers. Loughborough University, Loughborough

American Academy of Pediatrics Council for Disabilities and Committee on Adolescence 1996 Transition of care provided for adolescents with special health care needs. Pediatrics 98(6): 1203–1206

Ashby M, Lindsay W, Pitcaithly Broxholme S, Greelen N 1995 Snoezelen: its effects on concentration and responsiveness in people with profound multiple handicaps. British Journal of Occupational Therapy 58(7): 303–307

Ashman A F, Suttie J 1996 Vision in aging and dementia. Optometry and Vision Science 70: 800–813

Avery-Smith W 1998 An occupational therapist co-ordinated dysphagia programme. OT Practice 3(10): 20–23

Baker P A 1991 The denial of adolescence for people with mental handicaps: an unwitting conspiracy? Mental Handicap 19(2): 61–65

Bannerman E, Pendlebury J, Phillips F, Ghosh S 2000 A cross sectional and longitudinal study of health related quality of life after percutaneous gastrostomy. European Journal of Gastroenterology and Hepatology 12(10): 1101–1109

Barnett W S, Boyce G 1995 Effects of children with Down Syndrome on parents' activities. American Journal of Mental Retardation 100: 115–127

Barr O 2001 Towards successful ageing: meeting the health and social care needs of older people with learning disabilities. Mental Health Care and Learning Disabilities 4(6): 194–198

Beck A D 1997 Advances in pediatric glaucoma. Seminars in Ophthalmology 12(4): 176–189

Betz C L 1998 Facilitating the transition of adolescents with chronic conditions from pediatric to adult health care and community settings. Issues in Comprehensive Pediatric Nursing 21(2): 97–115

Blair E, Ballentyne J, Horsman S, Chauvel P 1995 A study of dynamic, proximal stability splint in the management of children with cerebral palsy. Developmental Medicine and Child Neurology 37(6): 544–554

Boakes M 1990 Vibrotactile stimulation. British Journal of Occupational Therapy 53(6): 220–224

Bottos M, Paato M L, Vianello A, Facchin P 1995 Locomotion patterns in cerebral palsy syndromes. Developmental Medicine and Child Neurology 37(1): 883–899

Bower E, Michell D, Burnett M, Campbell M J, McLellan D L 2001 Randomised controlled trial of physiotherapy in 56 children with cerebral palsy followed for eighteen months. Developmental Medicine and Child Neurology 43(1): 4–15

Bradley M, Ferris W, Barr O 1995 Continence promotion in adults with learning disabilities. Nursing Times 91(39): 38–39

British Epilepsy Association 1996 The treatment of epilepsy – a patient's viewpoint (survey results). BEA, Leeds

British Epilepsy Association 2001a Epilepsy and women. www.epilepsy.org.uk/info/

British Epilepsy Association 2001b Epilepsy and learning difficulties. www.epilepsy.org.uk/info/

British Medical Association and the Royal Pharmaceutical Society of Great Britain 2001

British National Formulary No. 31, March 2001. British Medical Association and the Royal Pharmaceutical Society of Great Britain, London

Brown H, Smith H 1992 Normalisation. A reader for the nineties. Routledge, London

Button S, Pianta R C, Marvin R S 2001 Partner support and maternal stress in families raising young children with cerebral palsy. Journal of Developmental and Physical Disabilities 13(1): 61–81

Cahill B M, Glidden R M 1996 Influence of diagnosis on family and parental functioning: Down's Syndrome vs. other disabilities. American Journal of Mental Retardation 101: 149–160

Cahill K M, Burri B J, Sucher K 2000 Dietary intakes and plasma concentrations of vitamin C are lowered in healthy people with chronic, non-progressive physical disabilities. Journal of the American Dietetic Association 100(9): 1065–1067

Cameron S J, Snowtown A, Orr R R 1992 Emotions experienced by mothers of children with developmental disabilities. Children's Health Care 21(2): 96–102

Campbell A G M, McHaffie H E 1995 Prolonging life and allowing death: infants. Journal of Medical Ethics 21: 339–344

Carter B 1994 Child and infant pain. Principles of nursing care and management. Chapman & Hall, London

Caudery A, Russell O 1995 Vitamin C status and dietary intake in a long stay unit for clients with learning disabilities: implications for community care. British Journal of Learning Disabilities 23: 70–73

Cave J 1998 Tissue viability: pressure area care in the community setting. British Journal of Community Nursing 3(10): 477–478, 480–482

Chang M W, Cardenas D D 2000 Ankle-foot orthoses: clinical implications. Physical and Medicine Rehabilitation State of the Art Review 14(3): 435–454

Cheng J C 2001 Intraductal laser photocoagulation of the bilateral parotid ducts for the reduction of drooling in patients with cerebral palsy. Plastic and Reconstructive Surgery 107(4): 907–913

Chisholm J 2000 The context, content and consequences of mothering a child with disabilities. AXON 22(2): 22–28

Ciner E B, Appel S, Graboyes M, Zambone A M 1996 Grand rounds. Assessment and rehabilitation of children with special needs. Optometry Clinics 5(2): 187–226

Clark M, Cullum N 1992 Matching patient need for pressure sore prevention with the supply of pressure redistributing mattresses. Journal of Advanced Nursing 17: 310–316

Cohen W I 1999 Health care guidelines for individuals with Down's Syndrome: 1999 revision. Down Syndrome Quarterly 4(3): 1–31. Available also: www.denison.edu/dsq

Collier ME 1996 Pressure reducing mattresses. Journal of Wound Care 5(5): 207–211

Comstock C P, Leach J, Wenger D R 1998 Scoliosis in total-body-involvement in cerebral palsy: analysis of surgical treatment and patient and caregiver satisfaction, including commentary by Lubicky J B. Spine 23(12): 1412–1415

Cooper S A, Collacott R A 1994 Relapse of depression in people with Down's syndrome. British Journal of Developmental Disabilities XL 1(78): 32–37

Crofts B 1997 Eye problems in children with Down's Syndrome. Notes for parents and carers. DSA, London

Crichton J U, Mackinnon M, White C P 1995 The life expectancy of persons with cerebral palsy. Developmental Medicine and Child Neurology 37: 567–576

Cunningham C 1996 Families of children with Down's Syndrome. Down's Syndrome Research and Practice 4: 87–95

Curatolo P, Arpino C, Stazi M A, Medda E 1995 Risk factors for the co-occurrence of partial epilepsy, cerebral palsy and mental retardation. Developmental Medicine and Child Neurology 37: 776–782

Dahl M, Thommessen M, Ramussen M 1996 Feeding and nutritional characteristics in children with moderate or severe cerebral palsy. Acta Paediatrica 85: 697–701

Dalton A J, Wisviewski H M 1993 In: Roberto K A (ed) 1993 The elderly care giver. Caring for adults with developmental disabilities. Sage Publications, London

Darbyshire P 1994 Living with a sick child in hospital. The experiences of parents and nurses. Chapman Hall, London

Dennis J 1995 Hearing problems in people with Down's Syndrome. Notes for parents and carers. DSA, London

Dennis J 2001a Atlanto-axial instability among people with Down's Syndrome. Notes for parents and carers. DSA, London

Dennis J 2001b Thyroid disorder among people with Down's Syndrome. Notes for doctors. DSA, London

Department of Health 1991 Health of the nation. HMSO, London

Department of Health 1993a Pressure sores: a key quality indicator. HMSO, London

Department of Health 1993b PSI foam mattresses: a comparative evaluation. HMSO, London

Department of Health 1995a Standing Medical Committee (CMO (86) 9). Cervical spine instability in people with Downs Syndrome. Department of Health, London

Department of Health 1995b Carers (recognition and services) Act 1995: policy guidance and practice guide. HMSO, London

Department of Health 1995c The health of the nation: a strategy for people with learning disabilities. HMSO, London

Department of Health 1996 COMA. Report on nutritional aspects of cardiovascular disease. HMSO, London

Department of Health 1999a Facing the facts: services for people with learning disabilities: policy impact study of social care and health services. Department of Health, London

Department of Health 1999b Quality protects: first analysis of management action plans with reference to disabled children and families. Department of Health, London.

Department of Health 1999c Caring about carers: a national strategy for carers. Department of Health, London

Department of Health 1999d Saving lives: our healthier nation. Executive summary. www.doh.gov.uk/ohn/execsum

Department of Health 2001a Valuing people: a new strategy for learning disability for the 21st Century. Department of Health, London

Department of Health 2001b Reference guide to consent for examination or treatment. Department of Health, London

Department of Health 2001c Children's NHS plan. www.DoH.org.uk

Dichter M A, Brodie M A 1996 New antiepileptic drugs. New England Journal of Medicine. 334: 1583–1590

Doble D, Goldie C, Kewell C 1992 The White approach. Nursing Times 88(40): 36–37

Dodd K, Brunker J 1999 'Feeling poorly': report of a pilot study aimed to increase the ability of people with learning disabilities to understand and communicate about physical illness. British Journal of Learning Disabilities 27(1): 10–15

Dodds A 1993 Rehabilitating blind and visually impaired people. Chapman & Hall, London

Dodds A G, Helawell D J, Lee M D 1991 Congenitally blind children with and without retrolental fibroplasia: do they perform differently? Journal of Visual Impairment and Blindness 85(7): 306–310

Domaracki L S, Sisson L A 1990 Decreasing drooling with oral motor stimulation in children with multiple disabilities. American Journal of Occupational Therapy 44(8): 680–684

Dundon M, Mann R 1995 Using visual assessment to identify a client's needs. Nursing Times 91(22): 40–41

Dustman R E, Emerson R Y, Shearer D E 1990 Aerobic fitness may contribute to CNS health: electro-physiological, visual and neuro-cognitive evidence. Journal of Neurological Rehabilitation 4: 241–254

Eldar R, Marincek C 2000 Physical activity for elderly persons with neurological impairment: a review. Scandinavian Journal of Rehabilitation Medicine 32(3): 99–103

Eliasson A, Ekholm C, Carlstedt T 1998 Hand function in children with cerebral palsy after upper limb tendon transfer and muscle release. Developmental Medicine and Child Neurology 40(9): 612–621

Engleman M D, Griffin H C, Wheeler L 1998 Deaf-blindness and communication: practical knowledge and strategies. Journal of Visual Impairment and Blindness 92(11): 783–798

Evans P M, Evans S J W, Alberman E 1990 Cerebral palsy: why we must plan for survival. Archives of Disease in Childhood 65: 1329–1333

Evenhuis H M, Mul M, Lemaire E K G, de Wijs J P M 1997 Diagnosis of sensory impairment in people with intellectual disability in general practice. Journal of Intellectual Disability Research 41: 422–429

Eyman R K, Grossman H J, Chaney R 1993 Survival of profoundly disabled people with severe mental retardation. American Journal of Disability in Childhood 147: 329–336

Faught E, Wilder B J, Ramsay R E et al 1996 Topiramate placebo controlled dose ranging trial in refractory partial epilepsy using 200, 400 and 600 mgm daily dosages. Neurology 46: 1684–1690

Feely M 1999 Drug treatment of epilepsy. British Medical Journal 318(7176): 106–110

Ferriman A 2000 A UK licence for cisapride is suspended. British Medical Journal. 321(7256): 259

Fruin D 1998 Social Services Inspectorate. Moving into the mainstream: the report of a national inspection of services for adults with learning disabilities. Department of Health, London

Gardell C, McGuinn J 1999 Childhood glaucoma. Insight 24(3): 81–85

Gisel E G, Applegate-Ferrante T, Benson J E, Bosma J F 1995 Effect of oral sensori-motor treatment on measures of growth, eating efficiency and aspiration in the dysphagic child with cerebral palsy. Developmental Medicine and Child Neurology 37(6): 528–543

Gisel E G, Patrick J 1998 Identification of children with cerebral palsy unable to maintain a normal nutritional state. Lancet 1(8580): 283–286

Greenberg J S, Seltzer M M, Greenley J R 1993 Aging parents of adults with disabilities: the gratifications and frustrations of later-life caregiving. The Gerontologist 33: 542–550

Griffiths J, Boyle S 1993 Colour guide to holistic oral care. A practical approach. Mosby Year Book, London

Griffiths C, Cowman S 1999 Towards understanding the interactions with people with a profound learning disability: a pilot study. Nursing Review (Ireland) 17(1/2): 35–39

Grunau R V E, Johnston C C, Craig K D 1990 Neonatal facial and cry responses to invasive and non-invasive procedures. Pain 42: 293–305

Gudjonsdottir B, Mercer V S 1997 Hip and spine in children with cerebral palsy: musculoskeletal development and clinical implications. Pediatric Physical Therapy 9(4): 179–185

Habel A, Scott R 1998 Notes on paediatrics: neonatology. Butterworth Heinemann, Oxford

Haberfuller H, Schwartz M S D, Gisel E G 2001 Feeding skills and growth after one year of intraoral appliance therapy in moderately dysphagic children with cerebral palsy. Dysphagia 16(2): 83–96

Hack M, Friedman H, Farnhoff A A 1996 Outcomes of extremely low birth weight infants. Pediatrics 98: 931–937

Hallett A 1996 Managing pressure sores in the community. Journal of Wound Care. 5(3): 105–107

Halpern L M, Jolley S G, Johnson D G 1991 Gastrooesophageal reflux: a significant association with central nervous disease. Journal of Paediatric Surgery 26: 171–173

Harries D 1991 A sense of worth: a report on services for people with learning disabilities and sensory impairment. Committee on the Multi-handicapped Blind, London

Harris J, Bennett L, Hogg J, Moss S 1997 Ageing matters: pathways for older people with a learning disability. British Institute of Learning Disabilities, Kidderminster

Hatton C, Emerson E 1995 Services for adults with learning disabilities and sensory impairments. British Journal of Learning Disabilities 23: 11–17

Health and Safety Executive (HSE) 1998 Manual handling: operational regulations 1992, 2nd edn. HSE, Suderbury

Heine R G, Reddihough D S, Catho-Smith A G 1995 Gastrooesophageal reflux and feeding problems after gastrostomy in children with severe neurological impairment. Developmental Medicine and Child Neurology 37: 320–329

HemiHelp 1999 Recommendations for minimum standards of health care for children with cerebral palsy. HemiHelp, London

Hinchcliff S M, Montague S E, Watson R 1996 Physiology for nursing practice. Baillière Tindall, London

Hodgson K 2000 Horseback riding as therapy for children. Physiotherapy Frontline 6(23): 18

Hope K W 1998 The effects of multi sensory environments on older people with dementia. Journal of Psychiatric Mental Health Nursing 5(5): 377–385

Holland A J, Hon J, Huppert F A, Stevens F 2000 Incidence and course of dementia in people with Down's Syndrome: findings from a population based study. Journal of Intellectual Disability Research 44(2): 138–146

Hutchinson R, Haggar L 1994 The development and evaluation of a Snoezelen leisure resource for people with severe multiple disability. In: Hutchinson R (ed) 1994 Sensations and disability: sensory environments for leisure, Snoezelen, education and therapy. ROMPA, Chesterfield, p. 48

Hutton J L, Cooke T, Pharoah M 1994 Life expectancy in children with cerebral palsy. British Medical Journal 309: 431–435

Janicki M P, Dalton A J 1997 Pending impact of dementia related care on intellectual disability providers. Paper presented at the International Congress on the Dually Diagnosed Mental Health Aspects of Mental Retardation, Montreal. Cited in: Janicki M P, Dalton A J 1998 Sensory impairments among older adults with intellectual disability. Journal of Intellectual and Developmental Disability 23(1): 3–11

Human Rights Act 1998 www.hmso.gov.uk/acts/acts1998

Janicki M P, Dalton A J 1998 Sensory impairments among older adults with intellectual disability. Journal of Intellectual and developmental disability 23(1): 3–11

Jones L J 1994 The social context of health and health work. Macmillan, London

Katz R T 2001 Life care planning for the child with cerebral palsy. Journal of Legal Nurse Consultants 12(2): 3–9

Kay B, Rose S, Turnbull J 1995a Continuing the commitment. The report of the Learning Disability Nursing Project. Department of Health, London

Kay B, Rose S, Turnbull J 1995b Learning Disability Nursing Project Resource Package. Department of Health, London

Kennedy J 1995 Person centred planning. Information Sheet. Scottish Human Services, Edinburgh

King A C, Omar R F, Brassington G S, Bliwise D L, Haskell W L 1997 Moderate intensity exercise and self rated quality of sleep in older adults. A randomised controlled trial. Journal of American Geriatric Society 277: 32–37

King G A, Cathers T, Polgar J M, Mackinnon E, Havens L 2000 Success in life for older adolescents with cerebral palsy. Qualitative Health Research 10(6): 734–749

Kohlhauser C, Fuiko R, Panagl A et al 2000 Outcome of very low birth weight infants at one and two years of age. Clinical Pediatrics 39(8): 441

Krechel S, Bildner J 1995 CRIES: a new neonatal postoperative pain measurement score. Initial testing of reliability and validity. Paediatric Anesthesia 5: 53–61

Kroger J 1996 Identity in adolescence. The balance between self and other, 2nd edn. Routledge, London

Laurent S 1992 Atmospherics. Bulletin 90/9. British Institute for Learning Disabilities, Bristol

Lehrman J, Ross D B 2001 Therapeutic riding for a student with multiple disabilities and visual impairment. A case study. Journal of Visual Impairment and Blindness 95(2): 108–110

Lindsay M 1998 Signposts for success in commissioning and providing health services for people with learning disabilities. NHSE/Department of Health, London

Livingstone S R, Tindale J A 2000 Community focus: growing old with a developmental disability. Canadian Nurse 96(9): 28–31

Lorenz J M, Wooliever D E, Jetton J R, Paneth N 1998 A quantitative review of mortality and developmental disability in extremely premature infants. Archives of Pediatric Adolescent Medicine 152: 425–435

McMenamin J, Bird M 1993 Epilepsy. A parents guide. Brainwave (The Irish Epilepsy Association), Dublin, pp 3, 4

Madden P 1995 Why parents: how parents. A keynote review. British Journal of Learning Disabilities 23: 90–93

Mann L M, Koch L C 1999 The major tasks of adolescence: implications for planning with youths with cerebral palsy. Work: a journal of prevention, assessment and rehabilitation 13(1): 51–58

Mamer L 1999 Visual development in students with visual and additional impairments. Journal of Visual Impairment and Blindness 93(6): 360–370

Marcell M M, Cohen S 1992 Hearing and visual impairments. Clinics in Geriatric Medicine 8: 173–182

Matteson M A, Linton A, Byers V 1993 Vision and hearing in cognitively impaired older adults. Geriatric Nursing 14(6): 294–297

Mattison P G, Aitken R C B, Prescott R J 1992 Rehabilitation status in multiple handicap. Archives of Physical and Medical Rehabilitation 73(10): 926–929

Mirrett P L, Riski J E, Glascott J, Johnson V 1994 Videofluoroscapic assessment of dysphagia in children with severe spastic cerebral palsy. Dysphagia 9(3): 174–179

Moller M A 1993 Working with visually impaired children and their families. Pediatric ophthalmology. Pediatric Clinics of North America 40(4): 881–890

Morrissey M, Biela C 1997 Care of older people. Snoezelen: benefits for nursing older clients. Nursing Standard 12(3): 38–40

Morton R E, Bonas R, Foune B, Minford J 1993 Videofluoroscopy in the assessment of feeding disorders of children with neurological problems. Developmental Medicine and Child Neurology 35(5): 388–395

Morton R E, Khan M A, Murray-Leslie C, Elliott S 1995 Atlantoaxial instability in Down's syndrome: a five year follow up study. Archives of Diseases in Childhood 72(2): 115–118

Msall M E, Buck G M, Rogers B T 1993 Prediction of mortality, morbidity and disability in a cohort of infants 28 weeks gestation. Clinical Pediatrics 32: 512–527

Msall M E, Phelps D l, DiGaudio K M et al 2000 Severity of neonatal retinopathy of prematurity is predictive of neurodevelopmental functional outcome at age 5.5yrs. Pediatrics 106(5pt1): 998–1005

Murphy K P, Molnar G E, Lankasky K 1995 Medical and functional status of adults with cerebral palsy. Developmental Medicine and Child Neurology 37: 1075–1084

Nazarko L 1995 The therapeutic uses of cranberry juice. Nursing Standard 9(34): 33–35

Newacheck P W, Strickland B, Shonkoff J P 1998 An epidemiological profile of children with special health care needs. Pediatrics 102: 117–123

NHSE 1998 Evaluation of the pilot project programme for children with life threatening illnesses. Department of Health, London

O'Brien M E 1999 Special section: care technologies. Commentary on Spalding K, McKeever P 1998 Mothers' experiences caring for children with disabilities who require a gastrostomy tube. Journal of Pediatric Nursing 13(4): 234–243

O'Connor B 1995 Challenges of inter agency collaboration: serving a young child with severe disabilities. Physical and Occupational Therapy in Pediatrics 15(2): 89–109

O'Donoghue S, Bagnall A 1999 Videofluoroscopic evaluation in the assessment of eating disorders in paediatric and adult populations. Folia Phoniatricia and Logopaedica 51(4–5): 158–171

O'Grady R S, Grain L S, Kohn J 1995 The prediction of long term functional outcomes of children with cerebral palsy. Developmental Medicine and Child Neurology 37: 997–1005

Palmer M M, Heyman M B 1998 The effects of sensory based treatment of drooling in children: a preliminary study. Physical and Occupational Therapy Pediatrics 18(3/4): 85–95

Pope P M 1992 Management of the physical condition in patients with chronic and severe neurological pathologies. Physiotherapy 78(12): 897–903

Poutney T E, Cheek L, Green E, Mulcahy C, Nelham R 1999 Content and criterion validation of the Chailey levels of ability. Physiotherapy 85(8): 410–416

Prasher V P 1994 Thyroid function in adults with Down's Syndrome. Conference proceedings: medical issues in Down's Syndrome – consensus and controversy. DSA, London

Prasher V P, Robinson L, Krishnan V H R, Chung M C 1995 Podiatric disorders among children with Downs syndrome and learning disability. Developmental Medicine and Child Neurology 37: 131–134

Premjj S S, Paes B 1999 Cisapride: the heart of the problem. Neonatal Network 18(7): 21–25, 29–31

Pueschel S M, Jackson I M D, Giesswein P 1991 Thyroid function in Down's Syndrome. Developmental Disabilities Resumé 12: 287–296

Puntis J W L, Thwaites R, Abel G, Stringer M D 2000 Children with neurological disorders do not always need fundoplication concomitant with percutaneous endoscopic gastrostomy. Developmental Medicine and Child Neurology 42(2): 97–99

Ramsey M, Gisel E, Boutry M 1993 Non-organic failure to thrive: growth failure secondary to feeding skills disorders. Developmental Medicine and Child Neurology 35: 285–297

Rantanen T, Guralnik J M, Sakari-Rantala R et al 1999 Disability, physical activity and muscle strength in older women, the 'Women's Health and Ageing Study'. Archives Physical Medicine 80: 130–136

Reid D T 1995 Development and preliminary validation of an instrument to assess quality of sitting of children with neuromotor dysfunction. Sitting Assessment for Children with Neuromotor Dysfunction (SANCD). Physical and Occupational Therapy in Pediatrics 15(1): 53–81

RNIB 1995 Looking for eye problems in people with learning difficulties. RNIB, London

RNIB 1996 Looking for hearing problems in people with learning difficulties. RNIB, London

Robinson C, Stalker K 1990 Respite care – the consumer's view. Norah Fry Research Centre, University of Bristol

Robertson M 1999 Management of epilepsy throughout the reproductive cycle – an overview of treatment issues. AXON 21(1): 18–20

Roe B, Williams K 1994 Clinical handbook for continence care. Scutari, London

Rogers B T, Arvendson J, Msall M, Demerath R R 1993 Hypoxaemia during oral feeding of children with severe cerebral palsy. Developmental Medicine and Child Neurology 35: 3–10

Roijen L E G, Postema K, Limbeek V J, Kuppevelt J M 2001 Development of bladder control in children and adolescents with cerebral palsy. Developmental Medicine and Child Neurology 43(2): 103–107

Ross S A, Engsberg J R, Olree K S, Park T S 2001 Quadriceps and hamstring strength changes as a function of selective dorsal rhizotomy surgery and rehabilitation. Pediatric Physical Therapy 13(10): 2–9

Royal College of Paediatrics and Child Health 1997 Withholding or withdrawing life saving treatment in children. Framework for practice. RCPCH, London

Royal College of Nursing 2001 Clinical practice guidelines. The recognition and assessment of acute pain in children. Implementation guide. RCN, London

Rudkin A, Rowe D 1999 A systematic review of the evidence base for lifestyle planning in adults with learning disabilities: implications for other disabled populations. Clinical Rehabilitation 13(5): 363–372

Russell D, Palisano R, Walter S et al 1998 Evaluating motor function in children with Down's Syndrome: validity of the GMFM. Developmental Medicine and Child Neurology 40(10): 693–701

Sanderson C, Hall D M B 1995 The outcomes of neonatal intensive care. British Medical Journal 310 (6981): 681–682

Savage P 1996 Snoezelen for confused older people: some concerns. Elder Care 8(6): 20–21

Schofield P, Davies B, Hutchinson R 1998 Evaluating the use of Snoezelen and chronic pain: the findings of an investigation into its use (part II). Complementary Therapy Nursing and Midwifery 4(5): 137–143

Schwartz L, Engel J M, Jensen M P 1999 Pain in persons with cerebral palsy. Archives of Physical Medical Rehabilitation 80(10): 1243–1246

Scott R C, Besag F M, Neville B G 1999 Buccal midazolam and rectal diazepam for treatment of prolonged seizures in childhood and adolescence: a randomised trial. Lancet 20(353): 623–626

Selby P 1997 Diabetes and Down's Syndrome. Notes for parents and carers. DSA, London

Selikowitz M 1993 A five year longitudinal study of thyroid function in children with Down's Syndrome. Developmental Medicine and Child Neurology 35: 396–401

Shaw L, Weatherill S, Smith A 1998 Tooth wear in children: an investigation of etiological factors in children with cerebral palsy and gastroesophageal reflux. ASDC Journal of Dental Needs of Children 65(6): 484–486

Sines D 1992 Meeting the nutritional needs of people with multiple handicaps. Journal of Clinical Nursing 1(2): 57–58

Smith R M, Emans J B 1992 Sitting balance in spinal deformity. Spine 17: 1103–1109

Soliman A, Hawkins D 1998 The link between Down's Syndrome and Alzheimer's' Disease. British Journal of Nursing 7(13): 779–784, 847–850

Stalker K, Campbell V 1998 Person centred planning: an evaluation of a training programme. Health and Social Care in the Community 6(2): 130–134

Stallings V A, Stemel B S, Davies J C, Cronk C E, Charney F B 1996 Energy expenditure of children and adolescents with severe disabilities: a cerebral palsy model. American Journal of Clinical Nutrition 64(4): 627–634

Stanley R 1997 Treatment of continence in people with learning disabilities: 3. British Journal of Nursing 6(1): 12,14,16

Stephen L J, Brodie M J 1998 New drug treatments for epilepsy. Prescribers Journal 38: 98–106

Strauss D, Shavelle R M, Anderson T W 1998 Life expectancy of children with cerebral palsy. Pediatric Neurology 18: 143–149

Sullivan P B, Lambert B, Rose M, Ford-Adams M, Johnson A, Griffiths P 2000 Prevalence and severity of feeding and nutritional problems in children with neurological impairment. Oxford Feeding Study. Developmental Medicine and Child Neurology 42(10): 674–680

Sullivan T J, Clarke M P, Morin J D 1993 Ocular manifestations of Sturge-Weber Syndrome. Journal of Ophthalmic Nursing and Technology 12(6): 271–279

Tarbell S, Cohen T, Marsh J 1992 The toddler-preschool postoperative pain scale: an observational scale for measuring post operative pain in children aged 1–5yrs. Pain 50: 273–280

Thompson S B N, Martin S 1994 Making sense of multisensory rooms for people with learning disabilities. British Journal of Occupational Therapy 57(9): 341–344

Thorne S E, Radford M J, McCormick J 1997 The multiple meanings of long-term gastrostomy in children with severe disability. Journal of Pediatric Nursing 12(2): 89–99

Thurtle V, Wyatt L 1999 Evidence based practice. Multi sensory environments and evidence based practice. British Journal of Community Nursing 4(9): 442–445

Townsley R, Robinson C 1999 More than a health issue: a review of the current issues in the care of enterally fed children living in the community. Health and Social Care in the Community 7(3): 216–224

Traughton E V, Hill A E 2001 Relation between objectively measured feeding competence and nutrition in children with cerebral palsy. Developmental Medicine and Child Neurology 43(3): 187–190

Twycross A 2000 Education about pain: a neglected area? Nurse Education Today 20(3): 244–253

UKCC 1992 The Code of Professional Conduct for nurses, midwives and health visitors. UKCC, London

UKCC 1998 Guidelines for records and record keeping. UKCC, London

UK Gabapentin Study Group 1990 Gabapentin in partial epilepsy. Lancet 335: 114–117

Van Minnen A, Hoelsgens I, Hoogduin K 1994 Specialised treatment of mildly mentally retarded adults with psychiatric and/or behavioural disorders: inpatient or outreach service? British Journal of Developmental Disabilities XL(1)(78): 24–31

Van Riper M 2000 Family variables associated with well being of siblings of children with Down Syndrome. Journal of Family Nursing 6(3): 267–286

Verrall T C, Berenbaum S, Chad K E, Nanson J L, Zello G A 2000 Children with cerebral palsy: caregivers' nutrition knowledge, attitudes and beliefs. Canadian Journal of Dietetic Practice and Research 61(3): 128–134

Vogtle L K, Morris D M, Denton B G 1998 An aquatic program for adults with cerebral palsy living in group homes. Physical Therapy Case Reports 1(5): 250–259

Vohr B R, Wright L L, Dusick A M et al 2000 Neurodevelopmental and functional outcomes of extremely low birth weight infants in the National Institute of Child Health and Human Development. Neonatal Research Network. Pediatrics 105(6): 1216–1226

Warburg M 1994 Visual impairment among people with developmental delay. Journal of Intellectual Disability Research 38: 423–432

Ward C L A 2001 An intrathecal option. Registered Nurse 64(1): 39–41

Waterlow J 1992 The Waterlow scale. Newlands, Curland, Taunton

Waterlow J 1997 Practical use of the Waterlow tool in the community. British Journal of Community Health Nursing 2(2): 83–86

Wiebe S 2000 Buccal midazolam may be a useful alternative to rectal diazepam for treating acute seizures in refractory epilepsy. ACP Journal Club 132(1): 22

Wiens H D 1998 Spasticity in children with cerebral palsy: a retrospective review of intrathecal baclofen. Issues in Comprehensive Pediatric Nursing 21(9): 49

Williams K, Roe B, Sindhu F 1995 An evaluation of nursing developments in continence care. National Institute of Nursing, Oxford

Wong A M, Chen C, Hong W et al 2000 Motor control assessment for rhizotomy in cerebral palsy. American Journal of Physical Medicine 79(5): 441–454

Woodhill G, Renwick R, Brown I, Raphael D 1994 Being, belonging, becoming: an approach to the quality of life of persons with developmental disabilities. Brookline Books, MA

Woodrow P 1998 Interventions for confusion and dementia 4: alternative approaches. British Journal of Nursing 7(20): 1247–1250

Yeates S 1995 The incidence and importance of hearing loss in people with severe learning disability: the evaluation of a service. British Journal of Learning Disabilities 23: 79–84

Young N L, Wright J G, Lam T P, Rajaratnam K, Stephens D, Wedge J H 1998 Windswept hip deformity in spastic quadriplegic cerebral palsy. Pediatric Physical Therapy 10(3): 94–100

Zahn C A, Morrell M J, Collins S D 1998 Management issues for women with epilepsy – a review of the literature. Neurology 51: 949–956

Zickler C F, Dodge N N 1994 Office management of the young child with cerebral palsy and difficulty in growing. Journal of Pediatric Health Care 8(3): 111–120

Zollweg W, Palm D, Vance V 1997 The efficacy of auditory integration training: a double blind study. American Journal of Audiology 6(3): 39–47

USEFUL ADDRESSES

A number of useful web sites are identified that will assist the reader to further explore aspects of profound and multiple disabilities.

For information on Asthma: www.asthma.org.uk
For information on syndromes and support groups for families: Contact a Family: www.cafamily.org.uk
For information from the Department of Health (England, UK) www.doh.org.uk
For information on Down syndrome: www.dsa.org.uk, www.ndss.org, www.nads.org.
For information on diabetes: www.Diabetesuk.org.uk
For information on enuresis and encopresis: www.eric.org.uk

For information on epilepsy: www.BEA.org.uk
For information on hearing impairments: www.RNID.org.uk, www.ndcs.org.uk (for children)
For information on mental health: www.youngminds.org.uk, www.mhf.org.uk
For information on cerebral palsy contact Scope: www.scope.org.uk
For information on sensory impairments – Sense: National Deaf – Blind and Rubella Assocation: www.sense.org.uk
For information on Spina-bifida and hydrocephalus: www.asbah.org.uk
For information on visual impairments: www.RNIB.org.uk

18 Specialist learning disability services in the UK

Robert Jenkins, Ian Mansell, Ruth Northway

KEY ISSUES

- People with learning disabilities and their families/carers may require access to a range of specialist services.
- These services may assist the person with learning disabilities in gaining access to generic services or may provide an additional, separate service to meet specific needs.
- A range of agencies and professionals are involved in the provision of such services.
- Careful coordination and close collaboration are, therefore, required.
- In the coming years a range of demographic, professional, service user and policy challenges are likely to influence the demand for and provision of specialist services.

INTRODUCTION

The aim of this chapter is to provide an overview of specialist services for people with learning disabilities within the UK. It will first introduce some of the debates concerning the provision of specialist services before giving an overview of the agencies and professionals who are involved in the delivery of such services. The importance of collaboration and coordination will then be explored before examining the role of community-based teams. The role of specialist services in supporting two key groups of clients (those whose behaviour challenges and older people with learning disabilities) will then be examined. Finally, the chapter will conclude by reflecting upon some of the key influences which are likely to shape the provision of specialist services for people with learning disabilities in coming years.

Three case illustrations are provided to assist the reader in applying some of the principles discussed to the lives of people with learning disabilities. In addition other activities will be suggested, which will help the reader to reflect critically on historical, present and future patterns of specialist services.

First, however, it is important to clarify what the term 'specialist services' means, how such services relate to other forms of service provision, and the role that they play in helping people with learning disabilities to achieve independence and wellbeing.

THE CONTEXT OF SPECIALIST SERVICES

Within the UK we have an established system of public services designed to meet the needs of our citizens. However, what is considered to be a need, and what is deemed to be an appropriate public response to such need, changes over time. Resulting patterns of service provision are thus the product of a complex interaction between policy, practice and social values. This is very evident when the history of learning disabilities services is considered, as was discussed in Chapter 3.

As a group, people with learning disabilities have been misunderstood in different ways at different points in history, and patterns of service provision have reflected such views. At the end of the nineteenth century they were viewed as being in need of education and thus educational institutions developed with a view to educating, training and then returning people to their own communities. By the beginning of the twentieth century they were seen as a threat to society and segregation became a prime function of institutional provision. From the early 1970s there was recognition that people with learning disabilities should be supported to live in their local communities using many of the services provided for other local citizens (Jones 1972). However, a recent English policy document recognises that some 30 years later they remain one of the most excluded groups within society (DOH 2001).

Baldwin (1991) has distinguished between three different types of service provision – specialist, generic and special needs. This framework is useful when considering what we mean by 'specialist services' for people with learning disabilities, and how they relate to other forms of service provision.

According to Baldwin (1991) *specialist services* are those which are provided for a specific client group (for example people with learning disabilities). These services often meet needs which members of that client group share with other members of society (for example educational, residential, health and recreational needs). However, they are provided in a separate and parallel manner. The large institutions, which were once the major form of service provision for people with learning disabilities, were examples of such a service. Residential, educational, recreational and health care needs were all met within one facility provided specifically for people with a learning disability. Segregation was promoted as a way of ensuring that their 'special needs' could be met (Clarke 1986), but such separation from mainstream society reinforced negative notions of difference. Examples of such service provision are not, however, confined to history. Today we still have a system of special schools, specialist day centres and specialist residential accommodation.

Generic services, according to Baldwin (1991), are those designed to meet needs shared by all members of society. Examples of such services might include public transport, education, health care facilities and local leisure facilities. The impetus to support people with learning disabilities in accessing such services originates primarily from the various philosophies of normalisation and social role valorisation (Wolfensberger 1972, 1992). However, some concerns have been expressed about the current capacity of generic services to meet adequately the needs of people with learning disabilities (DOH 2001). Additional support to access such services may, therefore, be required.

Special needs services are those required by some people who have specific, less common needs (Baldwin 1991). Some people with learning disabilities have additional physical disabilities, challenging behaviour, mental health problems and sensory impairments (Fruin 1998). In some areas services have been developed to meet the special needs of such groups of people. However, they have not been exempt from criticism. For example Rapley & Clements (1994) have suggested that the provision of such services for people who have challenging behaviour can deskill staff working within mainstream services, and further reinforce notions of difference.

It can be seen from the above discussion that the term 'specialist services' currently refers to a range of things in relation to people with learning disabilities. There may be special services, special needs services and specialist support to access generic services. Each form of service provision has possible strengths and weaknesses. It is also important to remember that people with learning disabilities are not a homogeneous group. Needs vary from person to person and individual needs may vary over time. Some people will not require specialist services whereas others will require ongoing and intensive support, if independence and wellbeing are to be promoted. Flexible forms of service provision are thus required. The following sections provide examples of how services are currently seeking to respond to such challenges.

A range of specialist services is available to support people with learning disabilities and their families. The exact pattern of service provision will vary from one area to another but certain key elements are common. This section will, therefore, provide an overview of agencies, and the types of services they might provide before considering the contribution which individual professional groups might make.

AN OVERVIEW OF AGENCIES

Specialist services for people with learning disabilities may include educational, day, employment, residential and domiciliary services. These are provided by both the statutory agencies, and the independent sector.

Statutory

A number of statutory agencies may be involved in the provision of specialist services to people

Reader activity 18.1

Think about the services available to people with learning disabilities living in your area. What specialist, generic and special needs services are there? Has the balance between the different types of service provision changed over recent years?

who have learning disabilities. This can include (for example) housing, leisure and the Benefits Agency. The focus in this section will be on three key agencies – health, social services and education. However, it should be noted that in Northern Ireland combined Health and Social Services Trusts exist.

Health

Historically professionals within health have provided much of the care for people with learning disabilities. Within long stay institutions the main providers tended to be doctors and nurses. The institution provided total care for the person with learning disabilities and departments such as physiotherapy and occupational therapy were frequently found within the hospital site. Following the development of community care ideologies, and the acceptance of the need to close the long-stay hospitals, the role of the health service in delivering care to people with learning disabilities has undergone progressive change.

The White Paper *Better services for the mentally handicapped* (DHSS 1971) and subsequent reports such as the Jay report (DHSS 1979) called for changes in the way services were structured, highlighting the need to develop the role taken by local authorities. Jay highlighted three major principles, which have had a significant impact on the development of services to date. These were that people with learning disability have a right to valued life experiences in community settings; that they have the right to be treated as individuals; and the right to help from both professionals and their communities to develop their potential (DHSS 1979).

These sentiments were reinforced within the 'Ordinary life principles' adopted by the King's Fund (Towell 1980) and the *All Wales Strategy* (Welsh Office 1983). The challenge for health, then, was to modernise service provision within changing social structures. This has resulted in health provision refocusing its energies in meeting the health needs of people with learning disabilities.

Health service provision for people with learning disabilities thus now includes both residential and community services. Hospital provision still remains in some parts of the UK but this is much reduced. For example, the recent English White Paper (DOH 2001) states that in 2000 there were nearly 10 000 places in NHS facilities, of which 1570 are classified as long-stay places, 1550 as specialist places, 1520 as campus places and 5100 places in other residential accommodation provided by the NHS. The stated aim is to enable those still living in long-stay hospital provision to move to more appropriate accommodation by 2004 (DOH 2001). Within Scotland the aim is to close the largest institutions by 2002 (Scottish Executive 2000).

Where the NHS continues to provide residential accommodation this is usually to support those with continuing health care needs (for example those with complex physical needs, or those whose behaviour challenges). In a community setting health personnel are often key members of community-based teams.

Social services

The role and function of local authorities in the provision of learning disability services has also changed significantly, and continues to evolve.

As well as the involvement of social workers within community-based teams (discussed below), social services have long been responsible for a range of other services for people with learning disabilities. These historically included day services and a wide range of residential provision such as hostels, group homes and more recently a range of ordinary life accommodation.

Since their inception in the 1970s, legislative and philosophical changes have influenced how services have been delivered. The *All Wales Strategy* (Welsh Office 1983) made local authorities in Wales the lead agency in the provision of services to people with learning disabilities. This was reinforced within the NHS and Community Care Act reforms (DOH 1990), which identified local authorities as being responsible for social care needs whilst health services remained responsible for meeting health care needs. There was thus an attempt to clarify responsibilities for the provision of community based services.

Lloyd (1998) has pointed to the changing role of social service departments. He has highlighted the potential change from being providers of services, and the perceived 'helping' role of the social worker, through to a social service department becoming resource managers and inspectors through systems such as Care Management, with the emphasis on arranging and monitoring services, rather than delivering them. However, it needs to be recognised that not all care managers are social workers, and not all social workers are care managers.

Education

Schools for children with severe learning disabilities are relatively new. Prior to the 1970 Education Act children in this client group were considered to be uneducable. However, over the past 30 years significant strides have been made in the delivery of education to children with special needs (see Ch. 7). One of the problems of contrasting educational services with broader learning disability services is the differing terminology used. For example, the definition of special educational need used by education services includes children who may present with difficult behaviour or language difficulties (such as dyslexia) and even gifted children.

A key area of debate in relation to educational services for children who have learning disabilities is whether they should be educated within special schools, or whether they should be integrated into, or included within, mainstream educational provision. The Warnock report (DHSS 1978) highlighted a range of possible options, which included the development of specialised units within the grounds of mainstream schools

Case illustration 18.1   Alison

Alison is 15 years old and lives with her parents and younger brother at home. She very much enjoys the company of other people, going out with her family and has a good sense of humour. As with many other girls of her age she likes pop music and fashionable clothes.

Alison has cerebral palsy and this affects her in a number of ways. She needs to use a wheelchair as she cannot stand unaided and she needs assistance with most activities of daily living. She does not communicate verbally but makes her needs and views known by facial expressions, vocalisations and body posture. Eating and drinking are difficult for her and so a few years ago it was decided that she would have a Percutaneous Endoscopic Gastrostomy (PEG) fitted (see Chapter 17). She is also said to have severe learning disabilities and has regular epileptic seizures.

Reader activity 18.2

Look at Case Illustration 1. What would you consider to be the most appropriate form of educational provision for Alison? What are your reasons for your choice? What arguments could be put against your choice?

through to children being educated in mainstream classes with additional support. Whilst the drive for inclusion continues to grow, there is some concern that the bid to raise educational standards, and the introduction of educational league tables, may limit progress. It is then important to balance the benefits of inclusive education against the possible advantages that smaller, more focused special needs education can provide. A fuller discussion of the issues surrounding this can be found in Chapters 7 and 8.

The independent sector

The term 'the independent sector' developed during the late 1980s and early 1990s as an umbrella term to cover those services not provided by the statutory sector (Churchill 1998). It includes those residential, day and domiciliary services provided by voluntary, private and charitable organisations.

The Community Care White Paper (DOH 1989) proposed that there should be an increased range of service providers involved in the delivery of community care. Thus, whilst voluntary and private agencies have always been involved in the provision of community-based services, this role has expanded over recent years. This situation has not only affected services for people with learning disabilities but all care services. Society in general has moved away from services being delivered by the state through the increased use of the independent sector, where it is believed that services can be delivered in a more efficient and cost effective way. A diverse range of service providers has thus emerged and patterns of service delivery differ from one area of the UK to another.

Reader activity 18.3

Look back on the list of local services you identified in Reader activity 18.1. Which agencies provide the services? Could one agency provide all of the services, or are there benefits from having a range of service providers?

AN OVERVIEW OF PROFESSIONS

A wide range of professionals can be involved in the provision of specialist services to people who have learning disabilities. It is not possible here to discuss in depth the role of all professionals but Box 18.1 below provides an overview of some of the professions who might be involved in supporting people who have learning disabilities. It should be noted that this list is not definitive, and that only key areas of expertise are highlighted.

It can be seen from Box 18.1 that, even though individual professions have their own areas of expertise, there are also areas of overlap. In addition individual professionals may also have developed their own personal areas of interest and expertise.

This section has provided an overview of some of the agencies and professionals involved in the provision of specialist services, but it is important to recognise that whilst differing agencies and

---

Box 18.1   Some professionals who might be involved in supporting people who have learning disabilities

Dietician
Assessment of nutritional needs, advice regarding healthy eating, health promotion, advice regarding special diets, provision of dietary supplements.

Learning disability nurse
Assessment of health needs, health promotion, behavioural assessment and intervention, advice regarding medication, provision of residential services/support. Development and coordination of care packages.

Occupational therapist
Assessment of occupational, functional and interpersonal skills, assessment of the environment, provision of aids and adaptations, advice regarding housing design, occupational and leisure opportunities.

Psychiatrist
Assessment of mental health, diagnosis of mental health problems, prescription of medication and other therapies, forensic and legal matters.

Psychologist
Assessment of behaviour, development and social interaction, focused interventions (for example behavioural, cognitive, counselling), group-work.

Physiotherapist
Assessment and analysis of movement, prevention of deformities and contractures, provision of aids and adaptations, advice regarding orthopaedic, respiratory and cardiac problems, advice regarding exercise.

Speech and language therapist
Assessment of communication and feeding difficulties, enhancement of communication skills, developing communication systems, advice regarding feeding difficulties.

Social worker
Assessment of social care needs, developing, managing and evaluating packages of care, family therapy, provision of residential services/support, child protection issues. Welfare benefits. Approved social worker role.

---

professional groups bring skills and expertise to help meet the needs of people with learning disabilities, no one single group can provide all the services required. It is also important to recognise that services are constantly responding to legislative changes, broader changes within society and client need. This means that careful coordination and collaboration are required if services are to effectively meet the sometimes complex needs of some people with learning disabilities.

THE IMPORTANCE OF COORDINATION AND COLLABORATION

Services for people with learning disabilities have changed significantly over the past 20 years (Barr 1998). Two major elements within the changing nature of services have been the introduction of multi-professional team working and the introduction of care management as a means of assessing needs, and developing packages of support. If people have complex support needs then they are more likely to require complex packages of support which require careful coordination and collabora-

Reader activity 18.4

Take another look at Case illustration 18.1. As Alison moves into adulthood what services and professionals do you feel might be involved in providing support to her and her family? How could these services best be coordinated?

tive working between professionals and agencies. Team working and care management have been viewed as strategies which facilitate this.

Team working

The concept of teams of professionals combining to provide services is not new. The National Development Group (1976) has highlighted the need for collaboration between the various providers of services, both at strategic and service delivery levels. They proposed a model of teamwork within which members from differing professional backgrounds come together to provide coordinated services to service users. They suggested that such teams might include social workers, nurses, psychologists, educationalists and therapists.

Ovretveit (1993) has described a multidisciplinary team as 'A group of practitioners with different professional training (multidisciplinary) employed by more than one agency (multiagency) who meet regularly to co-ordinate their work providing services to one or more clients in a defined area' (p. 9). Further, Ovretveit (1997) has indicated that teams can be located on a continuum between a loose knit networked team of professionals, who have limited contact and ownership of the team, to a closely integrated team operating to a team manager responsible for the delivery of services within the team's catchment area (see Fig. 18.1).

A range of authors have noted that there are strengths to multi-professional working (for example Brown 1994, McGrath 1991, 1993). The strengths of community teams have been highlighted as being: improved inter-professional working and a focus on the clients' needs (Moss 1994); improved team dynamics and better working environment (McGrath 1993).

However, not all commentators have shared an enthusiasm for community-based teams. Iles & Auluck (1990) have argued that personal contact between professionals may not be enough to facilitate good working relationships. They point out that for teams to be effective there needs to be a feeling of equal status between members. Team aims, objectives and priorities to guide action also need to be agreed (Barr 1997).

There remains a danger that if professionals within teams are not clear of their role within the team, then there is the risk of role blurring which leads to the potential loss of the skill which initially brought the professionals together (Mansell & Harris 1998). In an article critical of community teams in mental health services, Galvin & McCarthy (1994) concluded that teams deliver poorly focused, low quality services and indicate that team members are frequently de-skilled and demoralised.

The team model has, until recently, become the accepted ideal for delivering services to people with learning disabilities. However, the recent White Paper on learning disability (DOH 2001) has suggested that whereas community learning disability teams were the 'forerunner' in joint working between professionals, they have failed to consolidate their position, and changes to the way these teams function are needed. To place this statement in context it is important to understand how community teams have been developed, and the service they have provided.

The development of community-based teams

Cowen (1999) has highlighted that 'community mental handicap teams' were a major plank of the All Wales strategy (Welsh Office 1983), and the continued need for multidisciplinary working

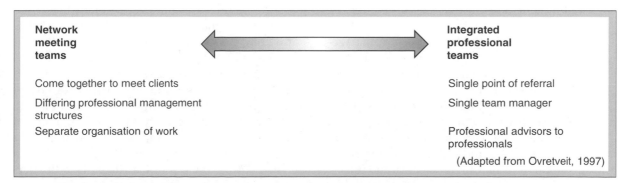

Figure 18.1 Community team structures (teams may develop across this continuum)

has been reinforced within subsequent policy frameworks, such as the NHS and Community Care Act (DOH 1990). Wales was very much seen as the forerunner in community learning disability teams, as these were a major element within the All Wales mental handicap strategy (Welsh Office 1983). As previously discussed the strategy made the local authority the lead agency in the provision of services to people with a learning disability and introduced learning disability teams as the means of coordinating and delivering the community services envisaged. Prior to the All Wales strategy (AWS), the Welsh Office acknowledge that services tended to be piecemeal and poorly coordinated; the development of community teams was seen as a means of overcoming these difficulties (Felce et al 1998).

Although community teams have been developed throughout the UK the extent of their growth and the nature of their provision has varied from area to area. For example, within Northern Ireland the need for community-based teams was identified back in 1978, but a recent review of services found that whilst most areas claimed to have such teams the available evidence suggested that the team concept was still developing and that such services varied from area to area (DHSS 1995). The future of community-based teams is thus a focus for current discussion, some of which is detailed below.

Care management

Care management was a cornerstone of the NHS and Community Care Act (1990). The principle behind the care management process, was that each care manager would be responsible for the process of securing a package of care on behalf of the service user. Griffiths (1988) saw care management as 'The assessment, planning, co-ordination and monitoring, offering the targeting of resources to those clients most in need, full involvement of service users, speed of co-ordination of services and accountability for planned resources' (p. 225).

Underpinning the care management process was the assessment of individual need, including a written plan, whilst noting the views and preferences of the service user (Northway 1996).

Beardshaw & Towell (1990) have suggested that there are three models of care management: social entrepreneurship, a service brokerage model and thirdly the care manager as the person responsible for both identifying need and also providing services through practice.

Where next for community teams and care management?

The English White Paper on the development of learning disability services (DOH 2001) has indicated that community learning disability teams have not consolidated their initial progress, and more needs to be done. Care management arrangements are to be maintained in learning disability services in England.

However, in relation to the health care of people with learning disabilities there is recognition that their needs are not currently being met appropriately within teams. Two key elements are to be developed within England to rectify this situation. Health facilitators are to be introduced to help clients access the appropriate health care, whether this is from primary or secondary health care. The White Paper suggests that any member of the community learning disability team could take this role, but that the learning disability nurse is 'well placed to fulfil the role' (DOH 2001, p. 63). The second element to be introduced is health action plans. Each person with learning disabilities will be offered the opportunity of having his or her own health action plan. This plan will include information about the person's broad health needs, dental records, medication and information regarding screening tests. In discussing the role of health professionals the White Paper stresses that a key role for this group is facilitating and supporting people with learning disabilities in using generic or 'mainstream services'. The aim is to include and support people with learning disabilities within the health care system available to all citizens, rather than marginalising them within separate services. The ideology of social inclusion is thus to apply within the context of health care provision.

The Scottish review of learning disability services (Scottish Executive 2000) has also questioned the current effectiveness of community teams. This review suggests that assessment, planning and support services do not always work well, and highlights that professionals do not always work well either with families or each other.

This review indicates that very often people are multiply assessed by a variety of professionals and agencies and yet no clear plan of action is available for the individual. The Scottish review, like the White Paper in England, highlights that despite the introduction of community teams and care management, the health needs of people with learning disabilities are frequently unmet.

It could be argued that the Scottish Executive (2000) has gone further in reforming how services will be delivered to people with learning disabilities by indicating that local area coordinators will replace care managers in arranging and supporting care. The review suggests that 'care management' will no longer be used in Scotland, since it has not performed well in meeting need. In a similar move to the English White Paper's health action plans, Scotland is to introduce 'personal life plans'. Personal life plans will include the record of health care need suggested for England.

PROVIDING SPECIALIST SERVICES FOR PEOPLE WITH COMPLEX NEEDS

The above section has set out some of the debates concerning the coordination of specialist services for people who have learning disabilities. To illustrate what this might mean in the relation to clients with specific needs this next section will explore the complex support needs of two groups of people – people whose behaviour challenges and older people who have learning disabilities.

Providing a coordinated service for those whose behaviour challenges

The continued move toward community care has resulted in a renewed focus on the provision of services for people who exhibit challenging behaviour. Historically this client group has almost exclusively received services provided by the health service, in the form of secure accommodation within institutions which primarily con-

tained, or attempted to suppress, such behaviours. Sines (1988) saw the development of needs-based services based on the principles of normalisation as effectively removing this franchise so that other agencies could become involved. Turnbull (1993) however, still believed that there was a role to be played by the health service and professionals such as nurses, but only if they were prepared to learn from their experiences and develop their skills. Blunden & Allen (1987) advocated that a change of emphasis was required. Instead of viewing the individual as the problem, the focus should be on the service. The problem would be for services to rise to the challenge of developing appropriate responses and effective solutions to an individual's particular challenging behaviour. A multi-agency approach was viewed as one of the ways to improve the service to the client.

Newman & Emerson (1991) have promoted a view that there would be benefits to be gained from the development of specialisation, as opposed to specialised services. This view is supported by the Royal College of Psychiatrists (1997) who recommend specialisation as a way of ensuring high standards in services. However, the Mansell report (DOH 1993) advocated the development of locally based specialist services to support good mainstream practice. It also highlighted the need for suitably skilled staff to provide services for people with learning disabilities who exhibited challenging behaviour. Unfortunately, the report failed to identify which group of staff, or what skills they should possess.

In the past, professionals may have been guilty of viewing challenging behaviour as a purely clinical problem rather than what Emerson (2001) described as a complex social phenomenon. The term has been used to encompass a wide range of behaviours from deliberate soiling to physical violence (Harris et al 1994). Qureshi & Alborz (1992) felt that some challenging behaviours, such as aggression and self-injury, could be classed as severe if their impact caused major problems for services. Some definitions include psychiatric disorders whereas other definitions encompass psychiatric disorders within a broad definition of challenging behaviour. Interestingly, a study by

Allen & Kerr (1994) found little difference in the clients who were referred to separate dual diagnosis and specialist challenging behaviour services.

There is also a disparity over the usage of differing definitions by both social and health care agencies in determining whether individuals are exhibiting challenging behaviour. This issue is also explored in depth by Slevin (1995) and Gates (1996). Such divisions lead to differing approaches to service provision being adopted and, as such, highlight the need for greater cooperation to ensure that efficient use is made of scarce resources and that individuals receive a client-focused package of care. Naylor & Clifton (1993) have suggested that definitions ultimately serve the needs of service planners in putting people into categories, and that confusion still reigns between planners and front line workers over the use and meaning of the term 'challenging behaviour'.

Whatever the difficulties and confusion that surround the term, the reality is that behavioural problems will often prevent individuals from reaching their full potential and adapting to the 'ordinary life' experience. There is also a danger of the individual being excluded from society. The key points for planners to consider when developing services (in addition to being aware of environments, relationships and the skills and attitudes of professionals) are outlined in Box 18.2.

Signposts for Success (Lindsay 1998) has provided some useful guidance on the development of services. This document encompasses the term challenging behaviour under the broad heading of mental health services. It states that the services required should aim to promote the emotional wellbeing of clients by working with other agencies and with carers. There should be help with dealing with issues such as loss, abuse, stress and relationship problems. Counselling and psychotherapy services should be made available for people with learning disabilities and their carers. There should also be appropriate treatment for distressing physical health problems. In addition services should provide screening, assessment and treatment for the detection of mental health problems. Support packages need to be individually tailored after comprehensive multidisciplinary clinical assessments. This document highlighted that the 'care of people with challenging behaviour or other mental health problems in social care settings requires sufficient resources, skills, organisation and motivation' (p. 60).

However, the problem facing planners is whether services for people with learning disabilities and mental health problems should be provided by generic services, learning disability services or specialist dual diagnosis services. Jacobson (1999) felt that whichever strategy is adopted it should incorporate a number of facets, such as having suitable numbers of skilled staff, using least–restrictive environments, maintaining high professional standards, providing individually tailored services and utilising standardised diagnostic and assessment methods. In terms of chal-

Case illustration 18.2   Roger

Roger is a 33-year-old man with learning disabilities and severe challenging behaviour. He has recently been admitted to the treatment and assessment unit of a local health service Trust from his parents' home. The reason for admission to the unit was due to an outburst of aggression toward his elderly parents and a neighbour, which resulted in the neighbour being injured and receiving hospital treatment. His parents want his antipsychotic medication changed again as they think it is not keeping him quiet.

Roger's communication skills are very poor, and he tends to grunt if he wants to gain attention. He spends much of the day rocking in his favourite chair, or out on the garden swing in fine weather. He becomes very agitated when demands are made of him, and appears to find the company of others, especially strangers, threatening. He has spent about 15 years of his life in various institutions due to his challenging behaviour.

Box 18.2   Factors which should influence service planning

- Ethically sound approaches
- Value for money
- Quality of life issues
- Clinical effectiveness
- Ordinary life principles
- Decrease in challenging behaviour

Reader activity 18.5

Look at Case illustration 18.2. What would you consider to be Roger's short-term needs for specialist services? What role might specialist services play in supporting Roger on his discharge from the Assessment and Treatment Unit?

lenging behaviour specialist support services, Allen & Felce (1999) have stated that there are two types of approaches, in the shape of peripatetic support teams and residential treatment units. They highlight that the two approaches have benefits and shortcomings and what is needed is more research into the clinical effectiveness of both.

Placing people with learning disabilities and challenging behaviour within ordinary housing remains a contentious issue (Felce et al 1999). However, Felce et al (1999) have pointed out that there have been schemes which have been successful in moving individuals with challenging behaviour from long-stay hospital provision into ordinary housing. They also acknowledged that there will be a very small number of individuals with severe challenging behaviours who will be difficult to place within ordinary housing. Such clients might be considered to have continuing health needs. Services need to ensure that environments offer individuals routine support to engage in the ordinary life experience, have an emphasis on a structured approach and individualised planning, and that staff are skilled in behavioural analysis (Felce et al 1999). Allen (1999), in a study of the key variables of success and failure of community placements, found community placements would be less successful if service settings did not have optimal resource utilisation and internal organisation and staff were not trained in emergency behavioural techniques. The challenge therefore still remains with services to provide the appropriate package of measures to meet the needs of individuals with learning disabilities who have challenging behaviour. Chapters 10, 11, 12 and 13 provide considerably more detail on

issues of challenging behaviour, autistic spectrum disorder, mental health problems and self-injurious behaviour in people with learning disabilities.

Providing a coordinated service for older people with learning disabilities

Generally, people are living longer, due to improvements in social conditions, improved access to health care and advances in medical care (Holland 2000), and the numbers of older people with learning disabilities are predicted to increase over the coming decades (Welsh Health Planning Forum 1992).

Older people with learning disabilities may experience the same physical deterioration as they age, as do the general population. However, there is a suggestion that ageing in people with learning disabilities starts earlier, and that they are at more risk of physical disorders and diseases such as sensory defects, cancer, diabetes and fractures (Jenkins et al 1994) and musculoskeletal, respiratory, cardiovascular and neoplastic illnesses (Day & Jancar 1994). Some genetic disorders, for example Down syndrome, bring with them additional problems such as increased prevalence of vascular disease and hypothyroidism (Cooper 1998; see also Ch. 2). Psychiatric disorders are common due to additional risk factors stemming from old age and a learning disability (Cooper 1999). However, it is reported by Hubert & Hollins (2000) that the higher rates of psychiatric disorders include dementia, anxiety, depression, affective and delusional disorders.

A contributing factor to the development of physical illness is the individual's lifestyle. Barr et al (1999) state that people with learning disabilities often lead unhealthy lifestyles, which contribute to the development of physical ailments in later life. In the past, health promotion activities, which would have been of great benefit to this client group, were never specifically geared to the needs of people with learning disabilities. It is only recently (DOH 1995, 1998) that there has been a move to include people with learning disabilities in strategies to improve health status. It can thus be seen that, as a result of increasing health problems, older people with learning disabilities may require the intervention and support of nurses. These may be nurses who specialise in working with people with learning disabilities or other nurses working in primary care. However, Jenkins (2000) has stated that little attention has been paid in the nursing literature to older people with learning disabilities. The Department of Health (1995) has issued a guide to learning disability nursing illustrating how the health care needs of people with learning disability could be met through targeting skills. In addition, a lack of collaboration between specialist and primary care services has been noted (Rodgers 1994) and the need for nurses to work in collaboration with nurses from other specialisms has not always been viewed as a priority (Northway & Walker 1999).

The majority of people with learning disabilities live in the community with their families and in later life usually with one parent (Hubert & Hollins 2000). The level of professional support tends to diminish with ageing according to McGrath & Grant (1993) who further suggested that there is also a reduction in family support networks leading to increased household isolation. Maggs & Laugharne (1996) believed that life changes and choices by older carers will put a strain on their relationship as the individual with learning disability ages. They also advise that health and social services should work together to support and manage the process of ageing of both client and carers. This is supported by Walker & Walker (1998) and is in keeping with policy developments (DOH 1990, 1992a, 1992b) which have advocated closer working between agencies.

Health and social services are viewed as having a critical role in promoting the health and wellbeing of carers, in the provision of responsive services and in promoting awareness regarding carers' needs (National Assembly for Wales 2000). This requires that agencies work in close collaboration and that both the contribution made by carers and their needs are carefully identified (National Assembly for Wales 2000). The importance of health and social services working closely with people with learning disabilities and their carers to support and manage the process of ageing has thus been stressed (Harris 1997)

A major problem with greater cooperation between services is the adoption of differing models and values. Walker & Walker (1998) have highlighted that services for older people and people with learning disabilities have traditionally followed different paths. They have argued that services for older people tend to view individuals as moving from an independent to a dependent position by stating that 'The idea of a service continuum, based on increased dependency and the inevitability of decline in the abilities of the older person, has dominated policy thinking and service provision' and 'Policy makers and service providers still regard residential care as a legitimate form of provision for older people and older people are almost the last group for whom residential care is regarded as an acceptable and appropriate model of care' (Walker & Walker 1998, p. 128).

This is in stark contrast to the development of services for people with learning disabilities. The wide adoption of the various principles of normalisation, or social role valorisation (SRV) has resulted in a large-scale move away from residential care, with the closure of large hospitals. Service philosophies have encouraged people with learning disabilities to cast off their dependent state by developing a variety of skills and adopting valued social roles. However, if services for older people with learning disabilities were to fully embrace the principles of normalisation then one would expect this client group to use ordinary generic services. This would at the very least cause tensions for professionals who have traditionally worked with learning disability services who would not view large residential settings as a viable option for people to live. The question professionals need to be posing would be which service model would best meet the needs of older people with learning disabilities?

Grant (2001, p. 157) has stated that currently, in terms of designing and planning services, there appears to be three competing models:

- The 'age-integrated' model in which a cradle-to-grave commitment is given in the form of a learning disability dedicated service.
- A 'specialist' model in which older people with learning disabilities are provided with services dedicated to their needs.

- A 'generic' model in which services are shared with elderly people and the wider population at large.

Whereas professionals may be concerned with which service model to follow, service users and carers would probably be more concerned with the values, beliefs and principles guiding such models. Whichever model is adopted then services need to adopt some guiding principles such as those advocated by Jenkins (2000) (see Box 18.3). Barr (2001) has called for health and social services to proactively identify and make available appropriate services to address the problems of age-related ill health that this client group poses. This will inevitably mean that there also needs to be greater cooperation between primary health care teams and learning disability community teams if the needs of older people with learning disabilities are going to be met.

Case illustration 18.3 Ian

Ian is a 67-year-old man with learning disabilities who lives in a small community house with three other gentlemen. He retired from working in the local supermarket some years ago and spends much of the day mooching around the house. He previously led a very active life and was popular in the local neighbourhood because of his connection with the supermarket.

Recently, he has posed difficulties in the household, as he has become very forgetful and confused, often wandering in and out of bedrooms trying to find his room. Support staff have also noticed a steady decline in his motivation to perform everyday tasks and he has become very moody. His fellow tenants are complaining about his behaviour and want him to leave.

Reader activity 18.6

What are some of the strengths and weaknesses of each of the models identified by Grant (2001)? Look at Case illustration 18.3. What do you feel would be the most appropriate form(s) of service provision for Ian? Would you see these changing as Ian gets older?

Box 18.3 Guiding principles of services (Adapted from Jenkins 2000)

Promotion of:

- a client led service
- independence
- empowerment
- self and independent advocacy
- innovation in service delivery
- multidisciplinary approach
- flexibility of service provision
- general proactive response

FUTURE CHALLENGES FOR SPECIALIST SERVICES IN THE UK

In the preceding sections reference has been made a number of times to the changing nature of service provision. This section will, therefore, reflect upon factors that are likely to shape the pattern of specialist service provision over coming years. Three key challenges will be considered – demographic, professional, and service user. It should be noted, however, that whilst they are considered separately here, they are inextricably linked and interdependent. Finally, current policy proposals for the development of specialist services are discussed.

Demographic challenges

There are two key demographic challenges that are likely to influence the need for, and nature of, specialist service provision over the next few years. These are the increased numbers of children with profound and multiple disabilities who are (due to improved medical interventions) living longer, and the generally increased life expectancy within the population of the UK which likewise applies to people with a learning disability (Department of Health and Social Services 1995). The latter has already been discussed.

Increased numbers of children with profound and multiple disabilities present a challenge for health, social services and education authorities both as individual service providers, and (because of the complex needs of the children) as partners in service provision. It also raises questions about the most appropriate form of service provision.

For example, should children with profound and multiple disabilities be supported primarily by specialist learning disability services, or by children's services? What are the strengths and weaknesses of each model? Should this group of children attend a special school, or should they be supported to attend a mainstream school? If it is the latter, how can specialist support best be made available to them in this setting?

This client group also presents major challenges to adult services who (historically) may have had limited experience of meeting this level of need. For example, how can community-based respite services best be provided for people who may have a high level of health needs?

 Reader activity 18.7

Think about service provision in your local area. What provision is there for people with complex needs? What provision is there for older people with learning disabilities? Do you feel that the types of provision and levels of provision may need to change over coming years?

Professional challenges

As patterns of client need and service provision change, so professional preparation to work within these services also needs to be reviewed.

In their draft consultation document, produced as part of the London Learning Disabilities Strategic Framework, the Department of Health, Social Services Inspectorate and the NHS Executive (2001) stated that specialist services will be based on needs and functions, rather than on professions. This suggests that staff working within such services will need to possess the skills of inter-agency and inter-professional working; they will need to be flexible and may share common skills.

The recent English White Paper (DOH 2001) has stated that, within the existing framework of vocational qualifications, a new Learning Disability Awards framework will be developed. This will enable staff to acquire a Level 2 Certificate and a Level 3 Advanced Certificate in

working with people with learning disabilities. The route to specific professional qualifications may, therefore, be through general learning disability preparation. Indeed the Department of Health (1999) have stated that there should be closer links between vocational training and pre-registration nurse training.

Nurse education within the United Kingdom is currently undergoing change with the introduction of the *Fitness for Practice* curriculum (UKCC 1999). This will mean that student learning disability nurses will undertake a one-year common foundation programme shared with other student nurses followed by a two-year specialist branch programme in learning disabilities. However, other possible futures are also being discussed as *Fitness for Practice* (UKCC 1999) has also suggested that the current system of four branches within nursing should be reviewed. This could mean a move towards (in common with other European countries) generic nurse training at a pre-registration level with specialisation in learning disabilities at a post-registration level. In addition, the possibility of shared elements of education with other health care professionals is also being discussed (UKCC 1999).

It would appear, therefore, that there are two key dimensions which need to be considered in relation to the future preparation of professionals to work in specialist services for people who have a learning disability:

- The balance between preparing people who work in generic services to work with people who have learning disabilities and preparing those who work in specialist services for people with learning disabilities.
- The balance between profession-specific and shared educational preparation for those working in specialist services for people with learning disabilities.

Readers may like to refer to Chapters 29 and 30 for further discussion of these issues.

Service user challenges

One of the principles stated in the Scottish learning disability strategy document (Scottish

Executive 2000) is that people with learning disabilities should be consulted about the service they receive, and be involved in making changes where they feel they are necessary. This principle of user involvement in the planning and development of services is one which has been integral to the development of many of the recent policy documents. People with a learning disability, their families and carers have been consulted about what they want and their views used to inform service planning. Future patterns of specialist services will thus be influenced, not just by the views of professionals and policy makers but also by those who use the services. It is likely, however, that a range of views will be evident. For example, some families feel that their children should attend a mainstream school whilst others feel strongly that special schools are the best way to meet the needs of their child. The challenge will be, therefore, to ensure that views are sought, and listened to, and that patterns of service provision are sufficiently flexible to ensure that diverse views and needs are accommodated.

Policy challenges and responses

As has been seen in earlier sections of this chapter, policy has played a major role in shaping service provision. At the end of the chapter it would therefore seem appropriate to consider how recent policy developments seek to respond to the challenges outlined above and hence to shape the future provision of specialist services for people who have learning disabilities.

At the time of writing this chapter three key policy documents have recently been published, each of which have something to say about future service provision. These documents relate specifically to the development of services in London (DOH et al 2001), more broadly to service development in England (DOH 2001) and also within Scotland (Scottish Executive 2000). A new strategy for learning disability services in Wales is currently awaited from the National Assembly for Wales. What should immediately be apparent from this list of developments is the impact that devolution is exerting on the provision of services for people who have learning disabilities.

On a positive note devolution does offer the possibility of developing services that are responsive to local needs. However, it also allows for variation in levels of provision. To some extent this has always been the case and hence the new strategy documents are starting from differing existing patterns of service provision. Nonetheless, it will be important to monitor in future years whether the variations are extended as a consequence of regional policy developments.

It has not been possible, within the confines of this chapter, to provide a detailed review of each of these policy documents, although some key proposals have already been highlighted. However, there are some common themes which are important to note since they are likely to influence service development.

The first recurring theme is inclusion. The 1995 review of policy for people with a learning disability in Northern Ireland (Department of Health and Social Services 1995) stated that the time had come to move beyond the principles of normalisation and instead to focus on the inclusion of people with learning disabilities within society. Inclusion is also identified as a key principle underlying the English White Paper (DOH 2001) and as an area requiring action within the Scottish strategy (Scottish Executive 2000). But what is inclusion and how does it differ from other approaches such as integration?

Inclusion stresses the importance of recognising that people with learning disabilities are citizens and hence should be included within society (Department of Health and Social Services 1995). However, whereas an integrative approach seeks to integrate people into structures and society as they already exist, inclusion recognises that it is these systems and structures which exclude people and which, therefore, need to be changed (Northway 1997). This means that, wherever possible, people with learning disabilities should be enabled to use the same services which are available to other citizens. However, for this to become a reality then some of these services may need to change in order to accommodate specific needs. There may also be a need for additional support to be provided in order to facilitate access. Specialist services should thus be an addition to generic services rather than a replacement (Scottish Executive 2000), their purpose being to promote inclusivity (DOH et al 2001).

This leads to a second recurring theme, namely the need for specialist services to focus on meeting specific areas of client need. The London learning disabilities strategic framework (DOH et al 2001), for example, stresses that specialist services should only be developed where:

- there are needs specific to people with learning disabilities which are not found in the general population
- there is a need for a specialist service to promote access to generic services
- the volume of work generated by a specific need amongst people with learning disabilities is sufficient to justify the development of a specialist service.

Elsewhere it is stressed that there is a need to make best use of the expertise within specialist services (DOH 2001). These points suggest that, in future, specialist services may become more focused on specific areas of need. A possible list of areas for development is identified within the London strategy (DOH et al 2001) and these are set out in Box 18.4.

CONCLUSION

This chapter has explored some of the debates surrounding the provision of specialist services

> **Box 18.4** Possible areas for the development and provision of specialist services (Department of Health, Social Services Inspectorate and NHS Executive 2001)
>
> - Communication
> - Mental health
> - Independence and skills
> - Care management
> - Access to generic health care
> - Eating and drinking
> - Family support
> - Sexuality and relationships
> - Challenging needs
> - Mobility
> - Sensory services
> - Health promotion
> - Adult protection
> - Forensic

to people with learning disabilities in the UK. It has also explored the importance of coordination and collaboration within such services. It has been seen that the nature of such services has changed over time and that currently further changes are being proposed. The challenge in coming years is to develop specialist services that enhance independence and wellbeing whilst promoting the inclusion of people with learning disabilities in both generic services and wider society. This demands that professionals working within specialist services work collaboratively and that they use their skills and expertise in a flexible manner.

REFERENCES

Allen D 1999 Success and failure in community placements for people with learning disabilities and challenging behaviour: an analysis of key variables. Journal of Mental Health 8(3): 307–320

Allen D, Felce D 1999 Service responses to challenging behaviour. In: Bouras N (ed) Psychiatric and behavioural disorders in developmental disabilities and mental retardation. Cambridge University Press, Cambridge, pp 279–294

Allen D, Kerr M 1994 A survey of referrals to specialist services for people with learning disabilities who have dual diagnosis or challenging behaviour. British Journal of Learning Disabilities 22(4): 144–147

Baldwin S 1991 From community to neighbourhood. In: Baldwin S, Hattersley J (eds) Mental handicap. Social science perspectives. Routledge, London, pp 145–166

Barr O 1997 Clinical management. Inter-disciplinary teamwork: consideration of the challenges. British Journal of Nursing 6(17): 1005–1010

Barr O 1998 Community support teams. In: Fraser W, Sines D, Kerr M (eds) Hallas' The care of people with intellectual disabilities, 9th edn. Butterworth-Heinemann, Oxford, pp 99–114

Barr O 2001 Towards successful ageing: meeting the health and social care needs of older people with learning disabilities. Mental Health Care 4(6): 194–198

Barr O, Gilgunn J, Kane T, Moore G 1999 Health screening for people with learning disabilities by a community learning disability service in Northern Ireland. Journal of Advanced Nursing 29(6): 1482–1491

Beardshaw V, Towell D 1990 Assessment and care management: implications for the implementation of Caring for People. Briefing paper 10, King's Fund, London

Blunden R, Allen D 1987 Facing the challenge: an ordinary life for people with learning difficulties and challenging behaviours. Project paper 74. King's Fund Centre, London

Brown J 1994 Analysis of reponses to the consensus statement on the future of the specialist nurse practitioner in learning disabilities. University of York, York

Churchill J 1998 The independent sector. In: Thompson T, Mathias P (eds) Standards and learning disability, 2nd edn. Baillière Tindall, London, pp 46–67

Clarke D 1986 Mentally handicapped people. Living and learning. Baillière Tindall, London

Cooper S A 1998 Clinical study of the effects of age on the physical health of adults with mental retardation. American Journal on Mental Retardation 102(6): 582–589

Cooper S A 1999 Psychiatric disorders in elderly people with developmental disabilities. In: Bouras N (ed) Psychiatric and behavioural disorders in developmental disabilities and mental retardation. Cambridge University Press, Cambridge, pp 212–225

Cowen H 1999 Community care, ideology and social policy. Prentice Hall, Hemel Hempstead

Day K, Jancar J 1994 Mental and physical health in mental handicap: a review. Journal of Intellectual Disability Research 38(3): 257–264

Department of Health 1989 Caring for people. Community care in the next decade and beyond. HMSO, London

Department of Health 1990 The National Health Service and community care act. HMSO, London

Department of Health 1992a Social care for adults with learning disabilities. Department of Health, London

Department of Health 1992b Health services for people with learning disabilities. Department of Health, London

Department of Health 1993 Services for people with learning disabilities and challenging behaviour or mental health needs. HMSO, London

Department of Health 1995 Learning disability: meeting needs through targeting skills. HMSO, London

Department of Health 1998 Our health service. HMSO, London

Department of Health 1999 Making a difference. Strengthening the nursing, midwifery and health visiting contribution to health and health care. Department of Health, London

Department of Health 2001 Valuing people: a new strategy for learning disability for the 21st century. Cmnd 5086, The Stationery Office, London

Department of Health and Social Security 1971 Better services for the mentally handicapped. Cmnd 4683, HMSO, London

Department of Health and Social Services 1978 Report of the committee of enquiry into the education of handicapped children and young people. Special educational needs (Warnock report). Cmnd 7212, HMSO, London

Department of Health and Social Security 1979 Report of the committee of enquiry into mental handicap nursing and care (Jay Report). Cmnd 7468, HMSO, London

Department of Health and Social Services 1995 Review of policy for people with a learning disability. HMSO, Northern Ireland

Department of Health, Social Services Inspectorate and the NHS Executive 2001 London learning disabilities strategic framework. Services to improve people's quality of life (Booklet 2–Consultation Draft). Online. Available: http://www.doh.gov.uk/london/learningdisabilities/services.htm 22 February 2001

Emerson E 2001 Challenging behaviour. Analysis and intervention in people with severe intellectual disabilities, 2nd edn. Cambridge University Press, Cambridge

Felce D, Grant G, Todd S et al 1998 Towards a full life researching policy innovation for people with learning disabilities. Butterworth Heinemann, Oxford

Felce D, Lowe K, De Paiva S 1999 Ordinary housing for people with learning disabilities and challenging behaviours. In: Emerson E, McGill P, Mansell J (eds) Severe learning disabilities and challenging behaviours. Stanley Thornes Publishers, Cheltenham, pp 97–118

Fruin D 1998 Moving into the mainstream: the report of a national inspection of services for adults with learning disabilities. Department of Health, London

Galvin S W, McCarthy S 1994 Multi-disciplinary teams: clinging to the wreckage. Journal of Mental Health 3 (June) 157–166

Gates B 1996 Issues of reliability and validity in the measurement of challenging behaviour (behavioural difficulties) in learning disability: a discussion of implications for nursing research and practice. Journal of Clinical Nursing 5(1): 7–12

Grant G 2001 Older people with learning disabilities: health, community inclusion and family care giving. In: Nolan M, Davies S, Grant G (eds) Working with older people and their families. Open University Press, Buckingham, pp 139–159

Griffiths R 1988 Community care. An agenda for action. HMSO, London

Harris J 1997 Services for older people with learning disabilities. Social Services Inspectorate, Department of Health, London

Harris P, Humphreys J, Thompson G 1994 A checklist of challenging behaviour: the development of a survey instrument. Mental Handicap Research 7(2): 118–133

Holland A J 2000 Ageing and learning disability. British Journal of Psychiatry 176(1): 26–31

Hubert J, Hollins S 2000 Working with elderly carers of people with learning disabilities and planning for the future. Advances in Psychiatric Treatment 6(1): 41–48

Iles P A, Auluck R 1990 From the organisational to inter-organisational development in nursing practice: improving the effectiveness of interdisciplinary working. Journal of Advanced Nursing 15(1): 50–58

Jacobson J W 1999 Dual diagnosis services: history, progress and perspectives. In: Bouras N (ed) Psychiatric and behavioural disorders in developmental disabilities and mental retardation. Cambridge University Press, Cambridge, pp 329–358

Jenkins R 2000 The needs of older people with learning disabilities. British Journal of Nursing 9(19): 2080–2089

Jenkins R, Brooksbank D, Miller E 1994 Ageing in learning difficulties: the development of health care outcome indicators. Journal of Intellectual Disability Research 38(3): 257–264

Jones K 1972 Better services for the mentally handicapped. In: Jones K (ed) The year book of social policy in Britain. 1971. Routledge and Kegan Paul, London, pp 187–203

Lindsay M 1998 Signposts for success in commissioning and providing health services for people with learning disabilities. Department of Health, London

Lloyd M 1998 Local authorities. In: Thompson T, Mathias P (eds) Standards and learning disability, 2nd edn. Baillière Tindall, London, pp 68–80

McGrath M 1991 Multidisciplinary teamwork. Community mental handicap teams. Avebury, Aldershot

McGrath M 1993 Whatever happened to teamwork? Reflections on CMHTs. British Journal of Social Work 23 (Feb): 15–29

McGrath M, Grant G 1993 The life cycle and support networks of families with a person with learning difficulty. Disability, Handicap and Society 8(1): 25–41

Maggs C, Laugharne C 1996 Relationships between elderly carers and the older adult with learning disabilities: an overview of the literature. Journal of Advanced Nursing 23(2): 243–251

Mansell I, Harris P 1998 The role of the registered nurse learning disability within community support teams for people with learning disabilities. Journal of Learning Disabilities for Nursing, Health and Social Care 2(4): 190–194

Moss R S C 1994 Community mental health teams: a developing culture. Journal of Mental Health 3 (June): 167–174

National Assembly for Wales 2000 Caring about carers. A strategy for carers in Wales. National Assembly for Wales, Cardiff

National Development Group for the Mentally Handicapped 1976 Mental handicap: planning together. HMSO, London

Naylor V, Clifton M 1993 People with learning disabilities – meeting complex needs. Health and Social Care in the Community 1(6): 343–353

Newman I, Emerson E 1991 Specialised treatment units for people with challenging behaviours. Mental Handicap 19(3): 113–119

Northway R 1996 The health and social care divide: bridging the gap. Nursing Standard 10(21): 43–47

Northway R 1997 Integration and inclusion: illusion or progress in services for disabled people? Social Policy and Administration 31(2): 157–172

Northway R, Walker G 1999 Promoting collaboration within community health care nursing. Journal of Community Nursing 13(4): 4–8

Ovretveit J 1993 Co-ordinating community care: multi-disciplinary teams and care management. Open University Press, Buckingham

Ovretveit J 1997 How to describe inter-professional working. In: Ovretveit J, Mathias P, Thompson T (eds) Inter-professional working for health and social care. Macmillan, Basingstoke, pp 9–33

Qureshi H, Alborz A 1992 Epidemiology of challenging behaviour. Mental Handicap Research 5(2): 130–145

Rapley M, Clements J 1994 New song: reflections upon the inadequacy of community services for people with learning disabilities. Care in Place 1(3): 248–255

Rodgers J 1994 Primary health care provision for people with learning difficulties. Health and Social Care in the Community 2(1): 11–17

Royal College of Psychiatrists 1997 Meeting the mental health needs of people with learning disabilities. Part 1. Adults with mild learning disability. Part 2. Elderly people with learning disabilities. Council Report CR56. RCPsych London

Scottish Executive 2000 The same as you? A review of services for people with learning disabilities. Scottish Executive, Edinburgh

Sines D 1988 Towards a comprehensive service: its nature and design. In: Sines D (ed) Towards integration: comprehensive services for people with mental handicaps. Harper and Row; London, pp 165–198

Slevin E 1995 A concept analysis of, and proposed new term for, challenging behaviour. Journal of Advanced Nursing 21(5): 928–934

Towell D 1980 An ordinary life. Comprehensive locally based residential services for mentally handicapped people. King's Fund, London

Turnbull J 1993 Learning disabilities: facing up to the challenge. Nursing Times 89(9): 65–66

United Kingdom Central Council for Nursing, Midwifery and Health Visiting (UKCC) 1999 Fitness for practice. The UKCC commission for nursing and midwifery education. UKCC, London

Walker A, Walker C 1998 Normalisation and 'normal' ageing: the social construction of dependency among older people with learning difficulties. Disability and Society 13(1): 125–142

Welsh Health Planning Forum 1992 Protocol for the investment in health gain – mental handicap (learning disabilities). Welsh Office, Cardiff

Welsh Office 1983 The All Wales Strategy for the development of services for mentally handicapped people. Welsh Office, Cardiff

Wolfensberger W 1972 The principle of normalization in human services. The National Institute on Mental Retardation, Toronto

Wolfensberger W 1992 A brief introduction to social role valorization as a high-order concept for structuring human services. Training Institute for Human Service Planning, Leadership and Change Agentry (Syracuse University), Syracuse, NY

FURTHER READING

Felce D, Grant G, Todd S et al 1998 Towards a full life. Researching policy innovation for people with learning disabilities. Butterworth-Heinemann, Oxford

Ovretveit J, Mathias P, Thompson T (eds) 1997 Inter-professional working for health and social care. Macmillan, London

Thompson J, Pickering S (eds) 2001 Meeting the health needs of people who have a learning disability. Baillière Tindall, Edinburgh

Thompson T, Mathias P (eds) 1998 Standards and learning disability, 2nd edn. Baillière Tindall, London

USEFUL ADDRESSES

www.open.gov.uk/ *The Government website containing useful information concerning policy development.*
www.bild.org.uk/ *The website of the British Institute of Learning Disabilities*

www.arcuk.org.uk/ *The website of the Association of Residential Care*
www.ndt.org.uk/ *The website of the National Development Team (N.B. Each of the above also has useful links)*

19 Person centred planning

Helen Sanderson

KEY ISSUES

- Person centred planning is rapidly becoming a focus of interest and activity within human services.
- Person centred planning is a cornerstone of the Department of Health policy for the health and social care of people with learning disabilities (DOH 2001). One of the eleven main objectives of *Valuing People* focuses upon person centred planning.
- Person centred planning places the person with leaning disabilities at the heart of planning support.
- Person centred planning requires listening to people with learning disabilities and using different planning styles than have been used historically.

INTRODUCTION

This chapter first defines person centred planning and then identifies five key features that will be recognised in all approaches to person centred planning. It then introduces different ways of listening and planning, and suggests where different approaches may be useful. Person centred planning, however, is not 'next generation' individual programme planning. Instead, it is based on a completely different way of seeing and working with people with learning disabilities, which is fundamentally about sharing power and developing community inclusion. This presents many challenges for professionals and services, if the promise of person centred planning, as a way to help people get better, valued lives, is to be realised.

WHAT IS PERSON CENTRED PLANNING?

Person centred planning is a process of continual listening and learning, focused on what is important to someone with learning disabilities now, and for the future, and acting upon this in alliance with the person's family and friends. There is a family of approaches to person centred planning. These approaches share common values and principles, and are used to answer two fundamental questions:

- Who are you, and who are we in your life?
- What can we do together to achieve a better life for you now, and in the future?

Person centred planning is a process of learning about a person: who they are; what has happened to them; what is important to them; what they like and dislike; and what they want from life. This takes place over a period of time. It usually begins with an initial planning meeting, which is just the first step (Sanderson et al 1997). Neil's story illustrates what person centred planning is and how it works in practice (Case illustration 19.1).

Reader activity 19.1

We all plan our lives in different ways. You may have very clear ideas about what you want and how to achieve it; or you may simply take opportunities as they arise; or you may have clear dreams, and be working to turn these into reality. Take a few minutes to think about:
- how you have planned for a major change in your life (for example, moving or getting a new job)
- what plans you have for the future
- how the way you plan your life differs from someone you know who has a learning disability.

WHO USES PERSON CENTRED PLANNING?

Person centred planning is used by self-advocates, families, friends and paid support staff.

Case illustration 19.1

Neil's story
Neil is a 27-year-old man who is supported in his own home by a small group of staff. He has learning disabilities, doesn't speak and moves only his right hand very slightly and his eyes. Neil attends a day centre every day and usually sleeps whilst there. People supporting Neil at home describe him as enthusiastic, lively and up for trying anything new. People supporting him during the day describe him as tentative, unadventurous, and unlikely to understand what people suggest to him.

Together with Neil and his mum we decided to get everyone together to plan for the future and to air these different views of who Neil is. Neil and I spent a while together making sure that I understood how Neil communicated. I learned that he would use his eyes to say no and his right hand to say yes. We decide to use the PATH planning process to plan the future. Neil invited staff he liked from both the day service, and his staff from home and his mum. The day centre staff were unsure about whether or not it was worthwhile to come, but in the end did attend. We met together in an evening in Neil's living room. The plan took about four hours.

During the planning Neil worked on a dream for the future which included getting a job, making a video for television, moving to a bigger house, improving his social life, getting married, having children, the usual sorts of ambitions for someone in their late twenties. For Neil, these ambitions had not been considered usual, no one even knew that Neil had these ambitions. So one of the most important things that happened during the planning was that everyone treated Neil as an ordinary person and his dreams as valid. No one said this was unrealistic, Neil was confirmed as a young, ambitious and adventurous man. Day centre staff realised that the reason Neil was different at the centre was probably because he was bored and had nothing meaningful to do. They realised this without having to be told. The people who attended the plan have worked together to change things over the last year. So far they have assisted Neil to apply for a mainstream college course on a part time basis. It has been agreed that he will have a one-to-one worker (who previously worked at the centre). This worker will assist Neil at college and for the rest of the time to do ordinary things in the community instead of going to the day centre. Neil is involved with everything that is happening and is directing the changes. The pace of change is slow but steady; Neil is getting a life.

Neil's story told by Pat Black (reproduced with kind permission).

When people want to think about their lives using person centred planning, they may have the energy and drive to ensure that their plan happens themselves. There are booklets that self-advocates can use themselves, or with some help. One is *Listen to Me* (Allen & Smull 2001), which is a way for individuals to record what is important to them in their everyday lives, and what support they want to be able to do that. *Capacity Works* (Mount 1995) is another approach, which includes recording what someone aspires to for the future.

If people do not want to, or for whatever reason are not able to orchestrate this planning, they may entrust this to a family member or a friend. This is what most of us do when planning changes in our own lives. There are training courses for families to learn to plan with their son or daughter. There is a manual written specially for families learning to lead person centred planning called *Families Planning Together* (Allen & Smull 2000). If people do not have the stamina to organise the process, and have no one in their personal network that can take this on, they will have to rely on a member of staff.

In the UK, over the last few years most training courses have been for support staff. This is now slowly changing, as self-advocates, parents, and friends are being supported to learn how to use person centred planning.

WHERE HAS PERSON CENTRED PLANNING COME FROM?

The dominant model or paradigm in the field of learning disabilities is slowly shifting. There has been a move from the medical model to the developmental model, and now a new paradigm is emerging which focuses on community membership and functional supports to enhance quality of life (Bradley 1994, Kinsella 1993). In the 1970s and into the 1980s, many people working in services for people with learning disabilities developed individual planning systems. To begin with, these were essentially plans for rehabilitation and training of the individual. Traditional planning processes have typically focused on what people could not do, and set goals to develop competencies in these areas with the ultimate goal of increasing independence. Goals were defined by professionals and recorded in terms of what the person needed to do, for example 'Gill will com-

plete a six piece inset puzzle correctly without any prompting' (Peck & Hong 1988). As systems of planning developed there was a shift of language, with more attention being paid to people's 'strengths' as well as their 'needs', and a much greater concern that the person should be present, and should be helped to participate. Individual planning also tended to focus on the process of multidisciplinary meetings rather than on making things happen for a person. The development of shared action planning (Brechin & Swain 1987) is one example of a direct response to disillusionment with individual planning in the UK. These approaches place increased emphasis on self-advocacy, with a greater role being played by the person and their family. Assessment is seen as an ongoing process of discussion and observation rather than measuring people against set criteria. Early practitioners of shared action planning and other styles of person centred planning all had experience of well-developed individual planning systems, which were supposed to be helping people, but these 'service-centred' planning systems all were focused on changing people and keeping them within services.

Person centred planning is a different approach rooted in the values of the new paradigm. Instead of trying to 'fix' people, the aim of person centred planning is to discover what an individual's chosen lifestyle is and how this can be achieved.

Person centred planning developed partly in response to dissatisfaction with individual programme planning, and from societal changes in the ways that people with learning disabilities were seen. Therefore, person centred planning is rooted in the values based on the five service accomplishments (O'Brien 1987), the social model of disability and the inclusion movement. It is a family of styles that challenges services to work actively towards building inclusive communities, as well as seeking valued experiences for people with disabilities and achieving service accomplishments. Table 19.1 illustrates some of the values that underpin services for people with learning disabilities, while Table 19.2 compares the focus of individual programme planning with that of person centred planning.

Table 19.1 Values underpinning services for people with learning disabilities (O'Brien & Lyle O'Brien 1991)

Valued Experiences (for people with learning difficulties)	Community Challenge (the aims we are working to achieve)	Service Accomplishments (what the service should aim to achieve)
Sharing ordinary places	Include all people and activities	Community presence
Making choices	Protect integrity by creatively resolving conflicts	Protecting rights and promoting choice
Developing abilities and sharing personal gifts	Develop all available resources wisely	Recognising interests and gifts; improving competence
Being respected and having a valued social role	Offer valued roles to everyone by confronting limiting beliefs and their historical consequences	Promoting valued roles

WHAT ARE THE KEY FEATURES OF PERSON CENTRED PLANNING AND HOW DOES IT DIFFER FROM TRADITIONAL PLANNING?

There are five key features of person centred planning. For many self-advocates, families and friends leading person centred planning, they will happen naturally. For example, if an individual is organising his own planning, it will be difficult for him not to be at the centre, which is the first key feature of person centred planning! However, many people are dependent upon service systems, and staff and professionals need to struggle with the problems and dilemmas of sharing power in person centred planning. The following assumes that a member of staff is supporting someone to plan his life, and illustrates how for many people person centred planning reflects a different way of thinking about people with disabilities, rather than a new technique.

The person is at the centre

'Person centred planning begins when people decide to listen carefully and in ways that can

Table 19.2 Key questions and answers from individual programme planning and person centred planning (adapted from Bradley 1994)

Key questions	Traditional individual programme planning	Person centred planning
Who is the person of concern?	The client	The citizen
What is the typical setting?	A group home, adult training centre, special school	A person's home, workplace or local schools
How are services organised?	In a continuum of options	Through a unique array of supports tailored to the individual
What is the model?	Developmental/behavioural	Individual support
What are the services?	Programmes/interventions	Supports
How are services planned?	Individual programme plan based on professional assessments	Through a person centred plan
Who controls the planning decision?	An interdisciplinary team	The individual or those family or friends closest to the person
What is the planning context?	Team consensus	A circle of support or person centred team
What is given the highest priority?	Independence/skill development/ behaviour management	Self-determination and relationships
What is the objective?	To develop independence and change undesirable behaviours	To support the person to have the lifestyle that they choose in their local community

strengthen the voice of people who have been or are at risk of being silenced' (John O'Brien in O'Brien & Lyle O'Brien 1998).

Person centred planning is rooted in the principles of shared power and self-determination. Power is an issue because many people are limited in their power in comparison to others; others control their lives. They direct how people spend their time, what they eat, how they behave, even what they say. In this context, planning can become just a further indignity. Person centred planning can be used to redress this balance as far as possible. People using person centred planning make a conscious commitment to share power. Built into the process of person centred planning are a number of specific features designed to shift the locus of power and control towards the person with learning disabilities. In traditional individual programme planning the person was often present at the planning meetings, but not fully included.

Box 19.1 describes the experiences of some people with individual programme planning.

Where person centred planning is used within services, the issues in Box 19.2 should be thoughtfully considered as ways of keeping the person at the centre, whilst remembering that having meetings, involving the person and making the plan is not the outcome. Rather, the outcome is to help the people to be supported to have a better life on their own terms.

Box 19.1 Some of People First's experiences of traditional service planning

People First in Liverpool describe their experiences of individual programme planning:

'Everyone got together, staff, family and did your meeting and got my future sorted out without me.'

'You could say what you wanted but it wouldn't happen – it was the ideas staff had themselves that they did.'

'Plans are not worth bothering about if the same old stuff keeps coming up – it should be good ideas instead.'

'Staff put it in the cupboard and forgot about it – nobody explained it.'

'No point having lots of plans if things don't happen . . . there were things that staff had put down years ago that still haven't happened.'

Box 19.2 Keeping the person at the centre of planning meetings

- **The person is consulted throughout the planning process**
  If people with learning disabilities have been involved in planning before then it makes sense to talk to them about how they want to plan, if they want a meeting, and if so, what kind of meeting, and how they want to be involved. If the people with learning disabilities are new to planning, it is important to spend time with them explaining the purpose of planning and looking at different options.
  One way to help people think about planning is to work through the book *Our Plan for Planning* by Liverpool and Manchester People First (1997). This booklet describes what people want before, during and after planning meetings. Where staff are involved in supporting planning, the booklet specifically describes what support people want from staff, and what they do not want staff to do.

- **The person chooses who to involve in the process**
  Unlike traditional planning, it is for the people with learning disabilities to decide who they want to include in the planning process, and how. This is easy to say, but within existing services this is highly counter-cultural to the way meetings are typically organised. If the people around these with learning disabilities cannot find a way to help them make and communicate that decision for themselves, then they have to decide in good faith who they think those people would want to involve. A good starting-point is 'people who know and care about the person'. This may well yield a different list from 'people who provide a service to this person'.

- **The person chooses the setting and timing of meetings**
  If a meeting does take place it should be at a time convenient to the people with learning disabilities and the people they wish to invite, and be in a place where they feel at home. The planning should be carried out in a way that is accessible to the person with learning disabilities. Graphics, tapes, video or photos are often used.

Using person centred planning involves finding creative ways to involve people with learning disabilities whilst recognising that some people will have limited experience on which to base a choice and others will have limited ability to follow and contribute to the process.

Family members and friends are partners in planning

'Person-centred planning celebrates, relies on, and finds its sober hope in people's interdependence.

At its core, it is a vehicle for people to make worthwhile, and sometimes life changing, promises to one another' (John O'Brien in O'Brien & Lyle O'Brien 1998).

Person centred planning places people in the context of their family and their community. It is therefore not just the people themselves that we seek to share power with, but family, friends and other people from the community who they have invited to become involved. These represent two of the most important challenges for services using person centred planning:

- How can we share power with people and support them to participate as much as possible?
- How can we encourage and include family, friends and non-service people?

Often it is family members who know the person best. They care about the person in a way that is different from everyone else, and they will probably be involved in supporting the individual for the rest of their lives. They often bring huge commitment, energy and knowledge to the planning process. Family members see the person and the situation from their own perspective. They may well have been let down time and again by services. They have probably had many experiences of not being heard unless they shout. They will probably have had professionals smile knowingly when they talk about their son or daughter and will have seen those professionals discount or ignore what they have to say. They will have had experience of being told nothing, or of being passed from pillar to post. They will also have legitimate concerns about safety and security that have to be acknowledged, respected and addressed.

Person centred planning commences from an assumption that families want to make a positive contribution and have the best interests of the person at heart, even if they understand those best interests differently from other people. In person centred planning, families are not caricatured as one dimensional, either 'over-protective' or 'not interested'; instead they are invited to tell their side of the person's story with the richness of detail that can provide clues for change. It is a crucial priority for services to sustain, value and strengthen people's family connections. Sharing power with families means seeking their active involvement and building a partnership. This has to be based on families and professionals getting to know and trust each other.

The plan reflects what is important to the person, her capacities, and what support she requires

Person centred planning seeks to develop a better, shared understanding of the person with learning disabilities and her situation. A person centred plan will describe the balance between what is important to the person, her aspirations and the supports that she requires.

Focus on capacities

The focus of professional effort in the lives of disabled people has traditionally been on a person's impairment. People are channelled into different services depending on the category of their impairment, for example learning disability, sensory impairment or loss of mobility. This leads to a process of assessment, which analyses and quantifies the impairment and its impact on a person's ability to undertake a range of tasks. This assessment results in a description of the person in terms of what they cannot do: their deficits. Professionals then set goals for people to try and overcome these deficits.

The most serious consequence of this is that people's participation in ordinary community life is then seen as dependent on their success in achieving these goals. People are only given opportunities when staff feel they are 'ready'. They have to earn the right to be part of their own community. People who expected services to help them to manage their own lives have instead become trapped in a world where others make judgements about their future. Traditional individual programme planning focused on deficits. Person centred planning focuses on capacities and capabilities, on what people can do, who they are and what their gifts are. Person centred planning challenges us to ask whether the skills professionals seek to teach have any functional meaning for the person in the real world, or whether they are skill acquisition for its own sake. Rather than requiring a person to change and adapt, person centred planning requires that services, supports and environments change instead, and focus on supporting people to develop relationships within the local community and to direct their own lives.

Where services are embracing person centred planning, learning and education are refocused. Instead of asking 'what skills do we need to teach next, and how can we do this?' the question is 'what would it take to support this person to be part of the local community?'

Discovering what is important to the person

Person centred planning therefore focuses on people's capacities and not their deficits, and looks at what supports they need rather than assuming that people need to change. This shared understanding will reflect what is important to the people in their day to day lives, and in the future they desire.

Identifying supports

Professionals have been training people toward 'independence' for years. In discussion John O'Brien has offered two definitions of independence. The first is the familiar rehabilitation model where people are trained to be able to meet their own basic needs with minimum assistance. The second is a 'support model' that portrays independence as choosing and living one's own lifestyle – regardless of the amount and type of assistance necessary. Independence would therefore not be measured by the number of tasks that people can do without assistance, but the quality of life a person can have with whatever support is needed. Person centred planning assumes that people with learning disabilities are ready to do whatever they want as long as they are adequately supported. The 'readiness model' (where people are only given opportunities when they have attained certain skills) is replaced with the 'support model' which acknowledges that everyone needs support and some people need more support than others. A person centred plan clearly records what support someone requires, on that person's own terms.

A shared understanding – rethinking the role of the professional

There are two common points of view about what people with learning disabilities want and need. The first is that professionals know or can find out everything there is to know about learning disabled people's needs. The other is that people with learning disabilities know everything there is to know about what they want. Neither of these is true. People using person centred planning assume that people are the first authority on their own lives and that a dialogue with other people – family, friends, service workers or professionals – can build on this.

Therefore professionals are no longer in charge of collecting and holding information and making decisions about a person's life. Instead, individuals and the people who care about them take the lead in deciding what is important, which community opportunities should be taken or created and what the future could look like. In this style professionals move from being 'experts on the person' to being 'experts in the process of problem solving with others'. People with learning disabilities need good expert advice, information and specific help from skilled professionals – not just nurses, doctors, therapists and social workers, but also lawyers, housing specialists and financial advisors. What they don't need is for those people's opinions to come first, to be the only basis for decision-making. In person centred planning clinical, and/or professional staff move from being the owners of the process, centre-stage, to being backstage technicians, the people who know what is technically possible and how to make it happen.

Information gained from technical assessments of the person can be helpful, but only in the context of a knowledgeable account of a person's history and desired future. Subordinating professional-technical information to personal-knowledge turns the typical agency decision making process on its head (O'Brien & Lovett 1992).

The plan results in actions that are about life, not just services, and reflects what is possible, not just what is available

The focus of person centred planning is getting a shared commitment to action, and that these actions have a bias towards inclusion. By articulating the tension between what is important to the person and what is happening now, person centred planning creates a sense of urgency and a commitment to work for change. It opens up a space in which people can change what they think and do, from the small things they do to assist the person with everyday tasks to the big things they do to help the person have a better life.

Person centred planning is not about standard service packages. Traditional planning has sought to fit people into existing service models and solutions, an available 'bed' or a place in the day centre. Person centred planning describes the support needed from the perspective of the person, and then designs a unique arrangement for getting that support. People who practise person centred planning believe that communities also benefit from including people with learning disabilities. Communities that are more diverse, and which create more opportunities for people to help each other directly, are better places for everyone to live. Person centred planning challenges us to work actively to build more inclusive communities, not just to provide better services.

For most people relationships form the basis of our lives. We all fear rejection and isolation more than anything. We need to belong, to be a part of other people's lives and have them be a part of ours. Many people with learning disabilities end up spending time only with people who are paid to be with them. They have been segregated for so long that they have not had the chance to meet people with whom they have other things in common. Person centred planning seeks to help people create and maintain meaningful connections with people who are not paid to help them. Support staff who want to help people make these connections need to look outside the confines of services. Person centred planning asks 'how could we find someone who knows about this?' and recognises that the service world cannot meet,

and should not seek to meet, a person's every need. It looks for respectful ways to strengthen people's connections with family, friends and community members.

People who practise person centred planning have a bias towards inclusion. They will assume that a person wants to have friends, prefers freedom to captivity, wants somewhere decent to live, would like the chance to contribute, would rather be included in a community than excluded from it – unless the person clearly tells or shows them differently.

The plan results in ongoing listening, learning, and further action

Person centred planning offers people who want to make change a forum for discovering shared images of a desirable future, negotiating conflicts, doing creative problem-solving, making and checking arrangements on action, refining direction while adapting action to changing situations, and offering one another mutual support (John O'Brien in O'Brien & Lyle O'Brien 1998).

Person centred planning should not be a one-off event. It assumes that people have futures, that their aspirations will change and grow with their experiences, and therefore the pattern of supports and services that are agreed now will not work forever. Michael Smull (Smull et al 2001) has described planning as a promise to people. To fulfil this promise we need to reflect on successes and failures, try new things and learn from them and negotiate and resolve conflict together. Acknowledging and resolving conflict is important if people are really to work together to make change.

Person centred planning is based on learning through shared action, and is about finding creative solutions rather than fitting people into boxes and about problem solving and working together over time to create change in the person's life, in the community and in organisations. Table 19.3 illustrates some of the changes required in person centred planning.

DIFFERENT WAYS OF LISTENING

All styles of person centred planning embrace a different way of listening to people with learning disabilities instead of traditional assessments. To

Table 19.3 Moving towards person centred planning (adapted and reproduced with kind permission from Sanderson et al 1997)

Moving from	Moving towards
• planning which focuses on what people can and cannot do	• planning and problem solving which seeks to discover the person's desired lifestyle and preferences for the future
• trying to 'fix' people or wait until they are 'ready'	
• professionals being in charge	• sharing power with individuals, their friends and family. Working to keep the person at the centre of the planning process and participating as much as possible
• people being surrounded only by professionals and paid staff	• people having friends and strengthening community connections
• fitting people into existing service options	• creating individual and unique support arrangements

Reader activity 19.2

How do you record your own life? What are other ways that people might record their lives, and in what circumstances? (For example a parent keeping newspaper cuttings from the day their child was born.)

What information is held about someone you know who has a learning disability?

understand people we need to know who are the people they associate with, the places that they go and the activities that they do. Learning from people about what their lives are like and what they want from them involves spending time with the people and listening to them – to their behaviour as well as their words. John O'Brien (O'Brien & Lyle O'Brien 1998) describes this as 'listening with your heart'. If people do not use words to communicate, then discovering the different ways in which they express themselves would be the first step. Learning about individuals may also involve talking to other significant people in their lives and possibly looking for relevant information from the records and case notes.

Personal profiles and portfolios are ways of people describing their lives themselves. Many people develop collections of videos, photos, certificates, a family tree and other ways of recording their lives and these are sometimes known as personal portfolios. People First in Manchester have made a video called *Our Lives* which describes how to do this and shares the experiences of people who made their own personal portfolios

(People First 1996). A good place to begin to consider recording lives is to think about your own.

Learning about people with learning disabilities in this way often challenges our perceptions and uncovers new insights and stories. This is what happened when Karen supported Stan to plan. Stan was 28 and lived in North Manchester with another man called Pete, supported by staff. When Karen first met Stan one of the staff had said that Steve only had a photo of his sister's wedding but not much else. It was Stan's foster brother's wedding, and Stan brought out three albums, his most precious possessions, that the staff had not been aware of. Stan had not had any photographs taken of him in the last 7 years and had very few from leaving his foster parents at 13 until his 21st birthday in the long-stay hospital. Stan showed Karen some photos that no one else in the house knew about; he had decided that they were too important to show staff in case they got damaged.

Listening in a different frequency requires different sorts of questions that we can ask whilst spending time with people with learning disabilities and supporting them to tell their own stories. These are some of the questions based around the five service accomplishments (see Chapter 3) that you may already be familiar with:

- What choices does the person make now?
- How can the number and significance of these choices increase?
- Who does the person know and spend time with now?
- How can the person meet and get to know more people?
- How can the person's existing relationships be supported?

- Who could help the person make changes in his life?
- What does the person enjoy doing? Where do these activities take place? Who does the person do them with?
- What are the opportunities in the community for the person to pursue his interests, make friends and contribute?
- Where does the person spend his time?
- How can the number of community places that the person shares with other ordinary people be increased?
- What contribution can the person make to the local community?
- Are there any capabilities that would help the person to increase his relationships and contribution in the community?
- What would it take to achieve that?
- Are there aspects of the person's culture or religion that they may like to explore more?

These are general questions that help us to learn about someone. Each style of person centred planning provides other ways of learning about someone's life.

DIFFERENT STYLES OF PLANNING

There are several different approaches or styles of person centred planning. Each style is based on the same principles of person centred planning: all start with who the person is and end with specific actions to be taken. They differ in the way in which information is gathered and whether emphasis is on the detail of day-to-day life, or on dreaming and longer term plans for the future. It is not possible to provide detailed descriptions and examples of the different planning styles here; please refer to the reading and resources at the end. The common planning styles include essential lifestyle planning, PATH and MAPs, and personal futures planning.

Each planning style combines a number of elements: a series of questions for getting to understand people and their situations; a particular process for engaging people, bringing their contributions together and making decisions; and a distinctive role for the facilitator(s).

PATH and MAPs focus strongly on a desirable future or dream and what it would take to move closer to that. Essential lifestyle planning and personal futures planning gather information under more specific headings. Particular sections – such as the section in essential lifestyle planning on how the person communicates and the section in personal futures planning on local community resources – ensure that someone gathers together what is known and records this information so that everyone can use it.

A skilled and experienced facilitator can adapt any style to cover all the areas in a person's life. People may need to focus on different areas of their lives at different times, and therefore use one planning style at one time and another at another time. We need to learn what is important to people on a day-to-day basis and about the future they desire. Sometimes it is important to learn about the day-to-day issues first, and then move on to learning about a desirable future. In other situations we need to hear about people's dreams, and later learn about what is important on a day-to-day basis.

In considering what style to use facilitators need to consider the context and resources available to the person with learning disabilities. The decision about which planning style to use will be influenced by whether the person with learning disabilities has a team to support her, or lots of friends and neighbours who want to get involved, or a circle of support. If the person with learning disabilities has a team who do not know her very well, then starting with a planning style which invests a lot of time in really getting to know the person, for example essential lifestyle planning or personal futures planning, could be a useful place to begin. If the person has family and friends or a circle who know and love her, then starting with dreams through PATH or MAPs is useful. In all person centred planning, the quality of the planning depends more on the skill of the facilitator than on choosing the 'right' style.

When is PATH useful?

Jack Pearpoint, Marsha Forest and John O'Brien (1993) developed PATH. It can be used as a planning style with individuals and with organisations. PATH is a very strongly focused planning style. It helps a group of people with a basic commitment to the person to sharpen that person's sense of a desirable future and to plan how to make progress. It assumes that the people present know and care about the person with learning disabilities, and that they are committed enough to support the person towards her desirable future over the next year. PATH is not a way of gathering information about a person, but a way of planning direct and immediate action.

PATH focuses first on the dream and works back from a positive and possible future, mapping out the actions required along the way. It is very good for refocusing an existing team who are encountering problems or feeling stuck, and mapping out a change in direction. It requires either that the person can clearly describe her dream or, if she does not use words to speak, that the others present know her well enough to describe it for her. PATH needs a skilled facilitator to ensure that the dreams are those of the individual rather than those of the team. It depends on the momentum generated by a group of committed people. With a skilled facilitator, the meetings are powerful and often emotional, and people may make some profound changes in the way they see and understand the person. This then clears the way for specific actions to help the person make significant changes in her life.

When is MAPs useful?

MAPs is a planning style developed by Judith Snow, Jack Pearpoint and Marsha Forest with support from John O'Brien and others. It was used first as a tool for helping disabled children integrate into mainstream schools, but is now used more widely in person centred planning with children and adults. MAPs is more of a picture building style than PATH. It can be used in a meeting or it is possible to use the individual components separately.

For some people there are more important lessons to be learnt from looking at their past. MAPs has a specific section at the beginning of the process for going over the history of an individ-

ual. It goes on to ask the question 'who is the person?' and 'what are the person's gifts?'. Focusing on the gifts often provides the key to unlocking the community so MAPs is a useful process when looking for ways of helping an individual to make connections.

The MAPs process allows people to express both their hopes for the future, in the dreaming section, and their fears about the future, in the nightmares section. The action plan is about working towards the dream and away from the nightmare.

It treads a middle way between PATH and essential lifestyle planning, allowing people to dream and including some 'getting to know you' in the process. It is neither as focused as PATH nor as detailed as essential lifestyle planning. It can be used as a starting point with individuals who feel comfortable with dreaming and who already have a few people around them to support them to work towards their dreams.

When is personal futures planning useful?

Personal futures planning was developed by Beth Mount and John O'Brien (Mount 1990). Personal futures planning provides a way of helping to describe the person's life now and look at what they would like in the future. It helps people to build on areas of their lives that are working well now and to move towards their desirable futures. It is therefore useful when people need to learn more about the person's life (unlike PATH, which assumes this knowledge) and to create a vision for the future (unlike essential lifestyle planning, which focuses on getting a lifestyle which works for the person now). It will not provide the detail about what the person requires on a day-to-day basis in the way that essential lifestyle planning does, but provides an excellent overview from which areas of concern can be considered.

When is essential lifestyle planning useful?

Essential lifestyle planning began in the late 1980s, at the University of Maryland, when Michael Smull and Susan Burke-Harrison (1992) were asked to help people return to their home communities from institutions and residential schools. All of the people that they were asked to help return to their communities had been labelled as 'not ready' for life in the community and their records supported this impression. Escalating interventions had not been effective. For many there was a cycle of placement and failure, and current referrals for community services had resulted in a 'thanks but no thanks' response.

The written description of what they learned with each individual was called an essential lifestyle plan. What they found was that developing an essential lifestyle plan is useful for anyone where it is helpful to:

- Discover what is important to the person in everyday life; and what is important in order for that person to stay healthy and safe
- Describe what they have learned in a way that is easily accessible to those who will help people get what is important to them.

Throughout the 1990s the use of essential lifestyle planning was extended to other people – to individuals living at home, to those using community services, to children and to older adults.

Essential lifestyle planning is a very detailed planning style that focuses on the individual's life now and how that can be improved. It can help people find out who and what is important to the person and what support the person needs to have a good quality of life. It can help the person to get a life that makes more sense to her, now and tomorrow, and will certainly identify what is not working for her at present. It does not address the individual's desirable future or dream, although this can be built in as an extra section.

Essential lifestyle planning specifies the ways that support is to be provided on a day-to-day basis, and this is helpful when different members of staff need to work consistently, or when the person herself or the family is not able to give such detailed direction.

Very little is known about some people who use services, particularly those who are moving out of an institution, or who do not use words to communicate. Essential lifestyle planning is an excellent style to use as a start to getting to know someone and beginning to build a team around them. The appendix at the end of this chapter gives an example of an essential lifestyle plan.

Reader activity 19.3

What can you do now to make your work more person centred? Here are some possibilities to consider
- Start with yourself, by thinking about what planning means in your own life – what are your dreams and aspirations, what is most important to you, what support do you need, what impact has your history had on your life? You may want to use some of the 'maps' from Personal futures planning to do this.
- Share 'Our Plan for Planning' with someone you know to help her think through what she wants from planning in her life.
- Seek training in a particular planning style and begin to learn about what this means in practice.
- Find out how other people are exploring person centred planning locally and start to make networks and allies.
- Find mentors and support from people who have more experience putting person centred planning into practice, through informal meetings or more organised events.
- Compare what you know about person centred planning with the existing practices of assessment used in the service. Could they be changed to become more person centred? Could they be used in a different way that reflects 'power with' rather than 'power over'?
- Think about how training in the service could be changed to focus on person centred values and practices. What would it take to achieve this?
- Think about what it would take to get person centred values and planning on the agenda of the managers and purchasers.
- Begin to focus on community building rather than skill building.
- Explore sharing more of your own life and relationships with people you support.
- Find ways to work more in partnership with the people you support, sharing problems and solving them together.
- Explore with a team what it would mean to become more person centred.
- Learn more, with the people you support, about the local community and what opportunities there are to develop relationships there.

Whatever your role and experience, there are many different ways that you can become more person centred. Reader activity 19.3 provides some suggestions to get started.

CONCLUSION

Person centred planning has been defined in this chapter as a process of continual listening and learning; focused on what is important to someone now, and for the future; and acting upon this in alliance with their family and friends. There are different approaches, however good person centred planning is always recognisable because the person will be at the centre; working in partnership with family and friends, the plan will clearly identify what the person's capacities are, what is important to her and what support she requires; there will be actions that have a bias towards inclusion; and the learning and reflecting are ongoing. Person centred planning creates opportunities for us to change our lives and our relationships, to share power and listen in a deeper way, and discover to what inclusive communities are really about.

REFERENCES

Allen B, Smull M 1999 Listen to me. Online. Available: www.allenshea.com

Allen B, Smull M 1999 Families planning together. Online. Available: www.allenshea.com

Bradley V 1994 Evolution of a new service paradigm. In: Bradley V, Ashbaugh J, Blaney B (eds) Creating individual supports for people with developmental disabilities – a mandate for change at many levels. Paul Brookes, Baltimore

Brechin A, Swain J 1987 Changing relationships – shared action planning with people with a mental handicap. Harper & Rowe, London

Department of Health 2001 Valuing people: a new strategy for learning disability in the 21st century. Cm 5086. HMSO, London

Kinsella 1993 Supported living – a new paradigm? National Development Team, Manchester

Mount B 1990 Making futures happen: a manual for facilitators of personal futures planning. Governor's Council on Developmental Disabilities, Minnesota

Mount B 1995 Capacity works: finding windows for change using personal futures planning. Graphic Futures Inc, New York

O'Brien J 1987 A guide to personal futures planning. In: Bellamy G, Willcox B (eds) A comprehensive guide to the activities catalogue: an alternative curriculum for youth and adults with severe disabilities. Paul H Brookes, Baltimore

O'Brien J, Lovett H 1992 Finding a way toward everyday lives. The contribution of person centred planning. Centre on Human Policy, Syracuse University, New York

O'Brien J, Lyle O'Brien C 1991 Framework for accomplishment: manual for a workshop for people developing better services. Responsive System Associates, Georgia

O'Brien J, Lyle O'Brien C (eds) 1998 A little book about person centred planning. Inclusion Press, Toronto

Pearpoint J, O'Brien J, Forest M 1993 PATH: a workbook for planning positive possible futures. Inclusion Press, Toronto (available from Inclusion Press UK Distribution)

Peck C, Hong C S 1988 Living skills for mentally handicapped people. Croom Helm, London

People First Liverpool and Manchester 1996 Our plan for planning. People First, Manchester

People First 1996 Our lives. People First, Manchester

Sanderson H, Kennedy J, Ritchie P, Goodwin G 1997 People, plans and possibilities – exploring person centred planning. Scottish Human Services Publications, Edinburgh

Smull M, Burke-Harrison S 1992 Supporting people with severe reputations in the community. National Association of State Directors of Developmental Disabilities Services Inc., Virginia

Smull M, Sanderson H, Allen B 2001 Essential lifestyle planning – a handbook for facilitators. North West Training and Development Team, Manchester

FUTHER READING

Forest M, Pearpoint J, Rosenberg R L 1997 All my life's a circle. Using the tools: circles, MAPs and PATHs, 2nd edn. Inclusion Press, Toronto

Manchester People First 1998 My life – my story. Making personal portfolios. Manchester People First, Manchester

O'Brien J, O'Brien C L (eds) 1998 A little book about person centred planning. Inclusion Press, Toronto

People First Manchester and Liverpool 1997 Our plan for planning. People First, Manchester

Sanderson H, Kennedy J, Ritchie P, Goodwin G 1997 People, plans and possibilities – exploring person centred planning. SHS, Edinburgh

Smull M, Sanderson H, with Allen B 2001 Essential lifestyle planning: a handbook for facilitators. North West Training and Development Team

Person Centred Planning website: www.nwtdt.com

APPENDIX: KATH'S ESSENTIAL LIFESTYLE PLAN

The following information is from Kath's plan, but it has been edited to illustrate the components of an essential lifestyle plan and is not her complete plan. It is written in the third person as Kath has significant support needs and does not use words to speak. What is recorded here represents our 'best guesses' and ongoing learning.

Note that the statement below refers to who contributed to the development of Kath's plan, not who attended her meeting. It is helpful to list not only the names of the people who contributed but also their relationship.

Kath's plan was developed by:

Kath
Karen – the team leader
Dean – team member
Andy – team member
Lucy – team member
Joan – team member
Sue – day centre officer
Lynne – aromatherapist
Judy – who used to be a team member
Kate – Kath's Aunty
Father Rivers – priest from St. Joseph's

Facilitated by Helen Sanderson

What People Like and Admire about Kath

Kath is:

Warm	Loving
Gentle	Calming
Caring	Peaceful
Assertive	Sensitive
Feminine	Sociable

Most important to Kath

The next sections of the plan describe what is important to the person. It is critical that they reflect only what is important to the person whose plan this is and not what others think should be important or what is important to the service. It is also helpful to organise the information into themes, with different headings (whilst remembering that not all information will fit neatly into themes).

About her relationships

- To visit her Aunt every 2 months
- To be supported by people who know her well, and know how she communicates.

About places to go

- At least once a month to go to a noisy, bustling place with music and a lot going on, for example live music, discos.
- To go to mass on Sunday. Kath goes to St. Joseph's at 11 a.m.

About things to do

- To have a long bath with bubbles in the morning for about 20 minutes, about an hour after she has woken up. She enjoys bursting the bubbles with her tongue.
- To be tickled by people she knows well – she will grab your hand to let you know that she wants to be tickled.

About food and drink

- To have chocolate (usually a bar of Galaxy) every day.

And

- To wear her glasses all the time.

Kath must not

- Be around loud, sudden noises as these frighten her.
- Have long periods (more than 45 minutes) where there is nothing happening. She must have a structured day and go out and about.
- Have strangers supporting her.
- Go for very long walks (more than 20 minutes is a long walk to Kath). She will sit down when she has had enough.
- Be cold.
- Be rushed.

Second in importance to Kath

*What is important to a person is usually divided up into three categories so that we can know **how** important something is, as well as **what** is important.*

About food and drink

- Kath's tipples are: Martini and lemonade, advocaat and fruit juice (orange or pineapple juice), snowballs and Baileys, although she does like to try different drinks as well. If she is not going out on a Friday or Saturday night then she has a drink at home.
- She likes a full English breakfast once at the weekend (scrambled egg, bacon and fried bread with tomatoes).

About 'pampering'

- Aromatherapy and Massage: Kath goes to Lynne for aromatherapy every 2 weeks on a Wednesday. It is important that staff massage her hands and feet at least once a week.
- Manicure, pedicures and facials: Kath likes to have a manicure, pedicure and facial with skin care masks every month. When she has enough money she goes to the Fabfit leisure centre, if not, one of the team does it. Kath particularly enjoys the 'fruity' masks.
- Footspa: Kath uses the footspa once a week with relaxing essential oils (Lynne makes these up for her).
- Listening to music at home in the morning (usually the radio on Galaxy 102).
- A lie-in in the morning at weekends (until 10 a.m.).

Third in importance to Kath

Things to do

- Sunbathing in the garden whenever the weather is warm enough.
- A 2-week holiday each year, preferably somewhere hot.
- Eating out once a month and trying different foods. Her favourites are the Saleem curry house (for a Korma strength curry) and Est Est Est Italian restaurant (for any pasta dish) and Pizza Land (Kath likes all pizza except those with anchovies).
- Spa baths and swimming about every month.
- Being involved in cooking and baking – smelling and touching the ingredients, and eating the finished product when it is still warm.
- Having relaxing essential oils burning in the evening and invigorating ones in her bubble bath in the morning (made up by Lynne).
- Playing her keyboard, when she feels like it, for about a minute at a time, usually with Anne.

About relationships

- See Judy about once every couple of months.

To be successful in supporting Kath

This section describes the general rules for support so that Kath gets what is important to her and stays healthy and safe. This is the section where something that is important to those who support the person (but not to the person) would be described. For example, we know that Kath needs to have medication to prevent her from having seizures; however, taking medication is not something that is important to Kath and therefore does not appear on the first three sections, but we know that it is important for Kath to keep her healthy and safe and therefore it goes in this section.

As Kath has significant support needs, her routines are described in detail. This section of Kath's plan is long, and the following are extracts from it.

Kath's morning routine

During the week Kath gets up about 8.30 a.m. unless she wakes earlier.

1. Kath takes her tablets (see medication section of this plan) with water whilst still in bed. Staff turn Kath's radio on (Galaxy 102) and run her bath whilst Kath wakes up properly. (Staff must ensure that the blue bath mat is securely placed in the bath.)

2. Staff support Kath to sit on the edge of the bed. Holding both hands staff assist Kath to stand

up. If unsuccessful, leave Kath for a couple of minutes and then try again.

3. Kath is then prompted (by gently touching her elbow, and guiding her towards the bathroom) to walk into the bathroom.

4. Staff enable Kath to undress, for example asking her to hold her arms up to remove her nightwear.

5. Kath is then prompted into the bath. Kath holds on to the bar grab rail with her right hand and with her left hand she holds the left rail on the bath or bath side. Kath then lifts her right leg into the bath and then her left with staff ensuring that she does not slip.

6. Kath enjoys a soak in the bath for about 20 minutes. Kath can be left in the bath, however staff must stay upstairs, because of the danger if Kath had a seizure in their absence.

7. Kath is then supported to wash and has her hair washed using both shampoo and conditioner. Kath then has
   a. pineapple facial wash
   b. cucumber cleanser and toner and moisturiser applied.

8. Kath needs to be physically helped out of the bath. Staff offer both hands to Kath to encourage Kath to stand up and step out of the bath.

9. Kath is then supported while getting dressed. Kath, when asked, will move her arms or legs whilst you put her clothes on for her. Kath wears a pad in the morning.

10. Kath is then prompted to come downstairs. Kath's right hand is placed on the banister. Her left hand is held by staff until she gets round the first corner. She then holds both banisters and is prompted to walk downstairs herself. If Kath stops on the stairs, put her hand back on the banister and she will begin walking down again.

11. Once downstairs, Kath goes into the dining room and is supported whilst eating breakfast. Usually a high fibre cereal and a cup of tea, and one glass of fruit juice.

12. Kath then has her hair dried, comes into the living room, and has her glasses put on.

In a taxi

If Kath is getting into a black cab, she will need help getting in and out. Staff get in taxi first, hold both of Kath's hands and Kath will lift her right foot into the taxi. Kath is then physically supported to get into taxi. If getting in a private hire, Kath prefers to sit in the front seat.

Mealtimes

1. Kath uses a raised plate for her main meals. Her food needs to be cut up (not chopped, pureed etc.).

2. Staff sit on Kath's right side to enable Kath to eat her meals.

3. Kath uses a fork in her right hand.

4. Towards the end of the meal, Kath will need some help to pick up food.

5. When using a spoon, Kath does not need any help.

People who are paid or volunteer to work with Kath should

- Be close to her age
- Be prepared to do everything at Kath's pace and be willing to learn how she communicates, and how to communicate with her
- Like sharing personal space, to support Kath in her 'pampering' activities.

This completes the first three sections of the plan: the administrative section, the person's section and the support section. What follows are the unresolved issues and what is working and not working in Kath's life, which are then developed into the action plan.

Other sections of the plan are done as required; for example, where the plan is being implemented within a service, an implementation plan is included. The implementation plan from Kath's team is included later in this plan.

Unresolved issues/questions to ask

One of the traps in planning is thinking that we need to answer all of the questions and resolve all of the challenges. This section provides a place to list those questions and issues that are left at the end of the information collection. They then become part of the action plan.

Table 19.4 Kath's communication chart How Kath communicates with us

At this time	When Kath does this	We think it means	And we should
In the morning	Kath sits up in bed, blowing	Kath wants to get up	Enable Kath to have a bath (see support section for details)
In the morning	Despite noise around her Kath lies in bed	Kath does not want to get up	Depending on time: ● If Kath does not need to get up – attempt to decrease noise and enable Kath to lie in ● If Kath needs to get up – gently encourage Kath to wake up, give her time to stretch and come round, then give Kath a drink with her medication and then usual bathroom routine (see support section for details)
Anytime of day/ night	Kath appears quite agitated, lots of blowing, flapping things in front of her eyes and shaking her head from side to side	Kath may have had or is going to have a seizure	● Ensure Kath is comfortable and safe, especially if in bed during the night ● Reassure her and talk calmly to her
Any time of day	Kath looks to the left or right with a fixed expression for anything up to a couple of minutes.	Kath is having an absence	Reassure her and talk calmly to her. Stay with Kath till she has recovered
Any time of day	Kath makes loud 'shouting' noises	Kath is unhappy with demands being made on her	If you can stop the activity, do so. If it is something that Kath needs to continue with, e.g. crossing the road, continue, but explain why in a calm, reassuring voice
In the jacuzzi	Kath reaches out towards staff	Kath is feeling unsafe	Make Kath more safe, if she is sitting on the edge of the seat, help Kath to sit back and if Kath wishes carry on holding her hand
Any time of day	Kath holds hand of staff	Kath wants physical contact	Tickle and/or stroke Kath's hand

Table 19.5   Kath's communication chart How We communicate with Kath

At this time	When we want to let Kath know . . .	We do/say this	And encourage Kath to
At mealtimes	It is time for lunch/dinner/supper	Say 'Kath, it is lunchtime' and give her her fork	Come into the kitchen for lunch/dinner or supper
When you are about to go swimming	It is time to go swimming	Say 'Kath, let's go swimming' and hand her her swimming costume	Walk with you towards the door

- Kath has not seen her parents for 3 years. Is there anything we can do to enable them to be part of Kath's life again?
- Kath does not get any exercise other than swimming once a month. How could we enable Kath to get fitter?
- When was the last time that Kath had her eyes tested?
- Could Kath get more involved in the Church?
- Could Kath benefit from 'Intensive Interaction'?

The two sections labelled 'what makes sense . . . ' and 'what does not make sense' are ways to take people from planning to implementation.

Action Plan

The action plan is developed from:
- *unresolved issues/questions to ask*
- *anything that is working that requires actions to maintain it*
- *and the what is not working sections.*

Implementation plan for Kath's ELP

1. How can we ensure that the plan happens?
   a. All the activities from Kath's essential lifestyle plan, and other domestic activities (e.g. collecting benefits) are put into a monthly plan. This plan tells everyone what needs to happen on each shift, or within that week, or within that month.
   b. After each activity there is a space to initial that you supported Kath in that activity.

Box 19.3   Planning to implementation: Kath's perspective (our best guess)

What makes sense?
What works? What needs to be maintained from Kath's perspective?

About relationships
- Her relationship with her Aunt
- The team working at her pace

About places to go, things to do
- Being pampered
- Having regular aromatherapy

What does not make sense?
What is not working? What needs to change from Kath's perspective?

About relationships
- She sometimes has agency staff supporting her who do not know her

About places to go, things to do
- Sometimes Kath seems bored
- Sometimes Kath cannot have 20 minutes in the bath because Derek needs to get ready
- Kath did not go out for a meal last month because money was tight
- Kath did not have a holiday last year

Box 19.4 Planning to implementation: others' perspective

What makes sense?
What works? What needs to be maintained from others' perspective?

About relationships
- Kath is seeing her Aunty regularly
- The team are working at her pace

About places to go, things to do
- Kath really seems to be enjoying cooking
- The aromatherapy is going well

Generally
- The team are all consistently using the communication sections of the plan

What does not make sense?
What is not working? What needs to change from others' perspective?

About relationships
- Most of the people in Kath's life are paid to be with her
- She sometimes has agency staff supporting her who do not know her
- Different people support Kath to go to Mass which might make it difficult to get to know people there

About places to go, things to do
- The keyboard has broken
- Sometimes Kath seems bored
- Kath is attending the day service three days a week, and not doing much there

Generally
- Kath does not always wear her glasses
- Kath having to go to bed before the second member of staff leaves at 10 p.m.

2. How will we know how well we are doing?
   a. At the end of each month Kath's key-worker, Lucy, goes through the monthly plan and compares this with Kath's essential lifestyle plan to see how we are doing.
   b. We devote one of our monthly team meetings to looking at how well we are doing. Firstly, we hear from Lucy about the monthly plan, then we hear from each team member about what they think is working well or not working. We set actions from this.
   c. We also have Kath's essential lifestyle plan as the first item on the agenda for our supervision sessions.

3. How will we share and record what we are learning about the person?
   a. We have the essential lifestyle plan in landscape with space for everyone to write what we are learning, and amend the plan and what we do from this (either in a team meeting or at the 6-montly review).
   b. We use the 'learning log' to record activities and amend the plan and what we do from this.
   c. We have a review every 6 months that involves everyone involved in developing the first plan. At this we ask: What have we learned? What have we tried? What else might we try? What do we need to do next?

Table 19.6   The action plan

What?	Who?	By When?
Actions addressing the 'questions to ask'		
1. To send Kath's parents: 　a. photographs of Kath involved in different activities 　b. cards for birthdays and Christmas 　c. a copy of the plan for information (so that we can invite them to contribute at the review)	Karen	Within 6 weeks (by January 24th)
2. To increase the amount that Kath goes swimming to once a week, to help her get fitter	Andy	From next week
3. To enable Kath to have her eyes tested and talk to the optician about enabling Kath to keep her glasses on.	Dean	Within 2 weeks (by Xmas)
4. To talk to Father Waters to see if Kath can become more involved in the Church	Karen	Within 2 weeks (by Xmas)
5. To investigate 'Intensive Interation'	Karen	Within 2 weeks (by Xmas)
Actions addressing 'what makes sense' that need to be maintained		
1. Book appointments with Lynne, the aromatherapist, for the next three months so that Kath can keep this appointment time	Joan	Within 2 weeks (by Xmas)
Actions addressing 'what does not make sense' that needs to change		
1. To see whether Judy (who used to be part of Kath's team) could cover the extra shifts that we have been using agency staff for	Karen	Next week (by 17th December)
2. To 'blue sky' different activities that Kath may like to try, and develop a plan to enable her to try them	Karen	At the team day on January 24th
3. To 'blue sky' how we could enable Kath to develop more relationships	Karen	At the team day on January 24th
4. To see whether Derek would be happy to have his breakfast before her bath to enable Kath to have her 20 minutes in the bath (on her day centre days)	Lucy	Next week (by 17th December)
5. To explore whether we are maximising Kath's benefits	Karen	Within 6 weeks (by January 24th)
6. To try to alter the rota to enable Kath to go to Church supported by either Andy or Joan	Karen	Within 2 weeks (by Xmas)
7. To talk through Kath's ELP with the day centre manager, to do an action plan within the day service in the short term	Karen	Within 6 weeks (by January 24th)
8. For Kath not to attend a day centre, and explore what is possible – work? community connections? To develop an action plan to explore possibilities and then see what can be done locally	Karen	At the team day on January 24th

4. How can we share the successes and barriers of implementation of essential lifestyle plans with others in the service?
   a. Karen takes the successes and the issues that are blocking us to Helen for the implementation group.
   b. Andy and Lucy give feedback to the rest of the network at the network meetings during the feedback session.

5. What can we do to keep learning/supporting the person to have new opportunities?
   a. Every 3 months we devote a team meeting to looking at new opportunities we could be enabling Kath to have.
   b. At one of our annual team days we will start to look at some of the maps from personal futures planning to increase what we know about Kath and her community.

5

Therapeutic interventions for people with learning disabilities

In this section, three chapters are presented that explore different types of therapeutic interventions that can be used when working with some people with learning disabilities. Firstly, in Chapter 20, Jane Wray and Karen Paton describe a range of complementary therapies that might be used with people with learning disabilities. Next, the use of art, drama and music in the field of learning disabilities is described by Richard Manners, Gillian Stevens and Elaine Chaplin. They point to the therapeutic properties of these often-neglected areas that can enrich people's lives. Finally, in Chapter 22, David Wilberforce outlines a range of psychological approaches that are being increasingly used to work in therapeutic relationships with people with learning disabilities. For too long such approaches have been thought inappropriate for this group of people because of cognitive incapacity; it is now known that such approaches are extremely useful for some people with learning disabilities.

20

Complementary therapies

Jane Wray, Karen Paton

CHAPTER CONTENTS

KEY ISSUES

- In this chapter a rationale for the increased use of, and access to, complementary and alternative therapies within health care settings and by the general public is provided.
- Terminology, definitions, and the identification of key factors that promote and facilitate the use of such therapies with people with learning disabilities are discussed. These include the principle of holism, the importance of touch and communication, the client–therapist interaction, and opportunities for client choice and empowerment.
- Common complementary therapies that can be used with people with learning disabilities are outlined, providing a special focus on the most commonly used therapy, aromatherapy (Graham et al 1998).
- A number of implications for health and social care professionals who work with people with learning disabilities are discussed.
- Finally, resources for further reading and investigation are provided.

INTRODUCTION

Complementary and alternative therapies are now widely available throughout the UK, and a recent survey by Ernst & White (2000) has suggested that as many as one-fifth of the UK population have used some form of complementary or alternative therapy in the last year. Complementary therapies have become a multi-million pound industry with spending estimated at £500 million per year (Welcome News 2000), and this is a significant increase compared to previous estimates in 1996 of £60 million per year (Which 1996). In the US, these figures are even higher with as many as 40% of the population using complementary therapies, and spending estimated at £15–20 billion each year.

So why are people turning to alternative and complementary therapies? Within the UK there are a number of possible reasons that can account for this, and these broadly fall into two categories: those instigated by clients or consumers, and those influenced by health care services and/or practitioners. First, clients and consumers of orthodox health care provision have identified a number of factors that include:

- the unpleasant side effects of some conventional drug treatments
- a wish to have more choice about treatment
- a perceived failure of orthodox medicine to provide satisfactory health care (Guardian Educational Supplement 1996).

This appears to be particularly the case for those patients with chronic and intractable diseases who are seeking an alternative treatment as orthodox medicine fails to find a cure, or even relief from their conditions. Research that has explored access to complementary therapies found that almost half of clients had been symptomatic for over a year, and 66% of people were experiencing musculoskeletal problems (Paterson 1997). In addition, there is a high level of satisfaction with the treatment received from complementary practitioners (Pincus et al 2000), particularly in relation to care, communication and competence. Stone (1999) has argued that people want to be treated with respect as educated consumers, and consequently are increasingly 'shopping' for health care. Frequently when choosing a complementary therapy, people's decisions are based not on statistical data regarding treatment outcomes but on lifestyle preferences as well as beliefs about health and illness (Truant & McKenzie 1999). Increased consumer sophistication, and the promotion of rights have led to clients 'choosing' their health care treatment; this has also been facilitated to some extent by the explosion in multimedia access to information, particularly through the world wide web.

Secondly, reform of the National Health Service has provided opportunity for purchasers and providers to reconsider alternative options for the provision of health care, and different types of working relationships (Emanual 1999). Graham et al (1998) undertook a survey of hospitals (NHS Trusts, acute, community and other) and found that 61% of Trusts, and 79% of private hospitals permitted the use of complementary and alternative therapies. Perry & Dowrick (2000) have found that 18% of GPs regularly used complementary therapies, and this indicates an increase from the 10% estimated in previous surveys (Thomas et al 1995). In addition, complementary therapies are offered as special modules in undergraduate medical curricula (Greenfield et al 2000). However, Luff & Thomas (2000) have noted that the ability to sustain complementary therapy provision in primary care is mediated by funding, the need for research and appropriate service delivery mechanisms.

Within the nursing profession, a similar escalation of interest appears to be the case with Trevelyan (1996) indicating that at least 50% of nurses are using at least one form of therapy in practice. Practitioners working within health care settings appear to be influenced by the desire to promote holistic practice, and also to develop their own role. Embracing complementary therapies enables nurses to offer a range of treatments that offer patients choice and reflect the philosophy of individualised patient health care that is at the heart of nursing theory and practice. The additional training required in order to safely offer therapies to patients as an integral part of health care provision, has obvious implications for the extension of the nurse's role and the scope of nurses' professional practice including increased autonomy (Cole & Shanley 1998).

The significant number of articles currently available in the health care press also demonstrates this growing interest in complementary therapies. In addition, professional bodies such as the United Kingdom Central Council for Nursing, Midwifery and Health Visiting (UKCC) and the

Royal College of Nursing (RCN) have been compelled to provide guidelines for nurses, health visitors and midwives. These guidelines are discussed in more detail later in the chapter.

TERMINOLOGY AND DEFINITION

In relation to terminology, the most commonly found term is 'CAM' – Complementary and Alternative Medicine. Whilst this term is generally acceptable, there are a number of semantic issues relating to its use (Furnham 2000). First, the term covers a very broad range of approaches and is used to refer to both specific therapeutic interventions used alongside orthodox health care, such as using lavender oil to promote sleep, and complete systems of medicine, for example homeopathy. Secondly, a number of commonly used terms including unorthodox, unconventional, natural, fringe, and alternative are also used. These are used interchangeably, assuming them to be synonymous, and whilst these concepts are similar, they encompass a range of therapies as diverse as massage and iridology.

Turner (1998) has classified complementary therapies using a taxonomy of six discrete primary care systems (chiropractic, homeopathy, medical herbalism, naturopathy, osteopathy, and acupuncture) that possess professional infrastructures. This system also allowed for 36 derivative modalities or approaches, from yoga to crystal healing. However, any approach to classification will need to be flexible, as many therapies are becoming more acceptable and available to the general public and to health care professionals, and consequently the descriptive term used is less often 'alternative' or 'fringe', and more often 'complementary'. For example, therapies such as chiropractic and osteopathy are increasingly considered to be part of orthodox medicine (Ernst & White 2000).

The distinction between 'complementary' and 'alternative' becomes important when we consider the types of complementary therapies that are being predominantly used by nurses and other care staff within the context of health care and learning disabilities. Rankin-Box (1997) has suggested that the most commonly practised complementary therapies used by nurses are massage, aromatherapy, reflexology, relaxation, visualisation and acupuncture (in rank order). Those therapies usually identified as common in other professional groups, such as doctors, and by the general public include homeopathy, acupuncture, herbalism, chiropractic and osteopathy (Graham et al 1998). These latter approaches tend to be favoured by the medical profession as it appears that doctors are more comfortable with those complementary treatments that approximate their own biomedical training and have a reliable and explainable foundation (Perry & Dowrick 2000).

The most common therapeutic interventions used with people with learning disabilities are those using a 'hands-on' approach, such as massage, aromatherapy and reflexology (Harrison and Ruddle 1995, Sanderson et al 1992, Sanderson and Carter 1994, Wray 1998). These therapies are on the whole not used to replace the selection of treatments available to clients but to complement orthodox health care and treatment (Vickers 1997). These particular therapies are often used by nurses as techniques, rather than whole systems of treatment, and in the sense of an 'add-on' procedure. For the purposes of clarity, the definition used throughout this chapter is provided in Box 20.1.

It is difficult to estimate prevalence rates of complementary therapy usage for a number of reasons. First, the methods used in surveys vary greatly, making comparisons difficult. For example, use is explored in different target populations ranging from health care professionals through to the general public, and it is often not clear whether 'over the counter' medications are included as a

---

Box 20.1 Definition of complementary therapies

The term *complementary therapy* used here will be taken to mean 'The adoption and use of unorthodox treatments that are used to complement (not replace) orthodox treatments in health care' (Gates 1994). An orthodox treatment is one that conforms to the established and widely accepted treatment standards used by health care professionals. 'Complementary' defined in this way describes a therapy which aims to work in conjunction with orthodox methods of treatment, rather than offer an alternative or substitute treatment option.

Reader activity 20.1

Before moving on to the next section, discuss with a colleague or friend your experience and/or knowledge of one particular alternative or complementary therapy. Next, write a list of the potential benefits you think that therapy might offer a person with learning disabilities.

'complementary therapy' or not, when the sample is asked (Ernst & White 2000). Also, there is no standardisation in relation to classification of therapies or the method used in different surveys. Consequently, all findings have to be interpreted with caution and there is a generally acknowledged paucity of reliable research evidence in this field (Graham et al 1998). This is discussed further later in the chapter.

COMPLEMENTARY THERAPIES AND LEARNING DISABILITIES

The literature exploring the use of complementary therapies refers predominantly to use in general hospital settings and clinical practice, in particular palliative care and oncology (Graham et al 1998). With the exception of a few notable texts (see Further reading), information on the use of complementary therapies in learning disability settings is relatively limited in comparison. However, the potential therapeutic benefit of such therapies for people with learning disabilities has been increasingly acknowledged (Vickers 1994), and their introduction into practice is likely to gain momentum. A number of reasons will facilitate the introduction of such therapies into learning disability practice and these are summarised in Box 20.2.

Box 20.2 Summary of key factors promoting the introduction of complementary therapies in learning disability settings

- The principle of holism
- Touch and communication
- The client–therapist interaction
- Opportunities for client choice and empowerment

The principle of holism

The notion of holism is central to the philosophy and practice of complementary therapies (Long et al 2000) and advocates the care of people on a physical, psychosocial and spiritual level, acknowledging the interplay of the mind, body and spirit. Nursing theory and practice have in the past been dominated by the 'biomedical model', which attempted to explain care provision predominantly in terms of disease and illness. Holism within nursing incorporates a belief in the importance of individualised nursing care, emphasising the treatment of the patient as a whole being. *'Increasingly in the West, account is being taken of the fact that in both health and illness, people have to be assessed in their individual physical, psychological, socio-cultural, environmental and politicoeconomic context'* (Roper et al 1990, p. 87).

Within nursing science, Rogers' theory of unitary human beings (Rogers 1970) provided an explanatory framework in which all persons were seen as highly complex fields of various forms of life energy. This energy was coextensive with the universe and in constant interaction with surrounding energy fields. Rogers' theory provided a functional basis for understanding therapies such as therapeutic touch, in which the direction of life energy moves through the hands of the therapist to the recipient. Holism evolved (or re-evolved, as it was never dead) because it represented a desirable option over the biomedical model in caring for the needs of the whole individual. In addition, the 'whole person' approach to the delivery of community care is more consistent with the philosophy underpinning the recent government strategy *Valuing People* (DOH 2001).

Touch and communication

The basis of many of the complementary therapies is touch, and the importance of using appropriate touch in the provision of care of people with learning disabilities is well documented in the literature (Gale & Hegarty 2000, Harrison & Ruddle 1995, Hegarty 1996). Touch can be used to communicate feelings of encouragement, concern and emotional support and warmth. However, in relation to nurses Jackson (1995) has suggested that they perform four types of touch:

- instrumental touch (bathing, giving of injections)
- expressive touch (empathetic promotion of compassion and understanding, e.g. hand-holding)
- systematic touch (deliberate manipulation of soft tissues, e.g. massage)
- therapeutic touch.

Clients with learning disabilities often have little or no choice about how often, and in what ways, they are touched by those who care for them. Much of the touching behaviour carried out by the nurse or carer can be instrumental and functional in character, and massage can offer a different kind of experience (Hegarty 1996, Sanderson et al 1992). This is of particular importance to people with severe or profound learning disabilities who may have a limited range of communicative abilities, and touch can act as a first or primary sense. Touch can provide carers with a form of communication that facilitates and encourages the therapeutic process, in addition to helping the person to have contact with the social world, to receive information and to convey it.

People with learning disabilities may be isolated through sensory or physical impairments and/or challenging behaviour, and touch can provide a point of contact for them. People with profound learning disabilities seldom have high levels of social contact (McGill & Toogood 1994) and this is particularly the case for people exhibiting challenging behaviour. Relaxation is often difficult for clients to achieve, and it has been shown that teaching clients with learning disabilities an individual relaxing posture can reduce noise and disruption levels in a residential setting (Deakin 1995). In addition, Hegarty (1996) has demonstrated in his case study that the structured use of therapeutic touch can reduce a client's severe long-displayed challenging behaviour. The management of behavioural difficulties is just one area of possible use for complementary therapies and already relaxation training is commonly used as a component of any treatment plan aimed at resolving behavioural difficulties.

Proponents of complementary therapies have described touch as providing *'windows through which the healing potential, the unconscious and the intention of the nurse can be expressed'* (Sayre-Adams & Wright 1995, p. 44). The experience of aromatherapy and/or massage can create and provide a stimulating atmosphere that makes use of both touch and smell. Snoezelen rooms provided in many care facilities attempt to stimulate the client in much the same way, i.e. to provide a multisensory experience (Ayer 1998). In the case of complementary therapies, this is coupled with a high level of one-to-one contact.

However, it should be noted that the use of touch, and touching is a very personal issue and individual experiences and expectations vary both for client and carer, and not everyone's experience of touch is pleasurable. Goffman (1961), in his classic study of institutions, noted that some individuals were unused to touch and consequently found it unpleasant and difficult. A client may need to experience the therapy through sensitive introduction, for example it may be inappropriate to have a full body massage, a hand or foot massage may be less invasive. Gale & Hegarty (2000) have suggested that *'the primary goal of the nurse should therefore be to evaluate the client's response towards the touch interaction and be aware of what touch could convey . . . Understanding the use of touch could provide the nurse with a potent therapeutic tool with unexplored potential'* (Gale & Hegarty 2000, p. 105).

Reader activity 20.2

Using Jackson's (1995) classification of touch (instrumental, expressive, systematic, and therapeutic), monitor and record how often you use touch when caring for your clients in one working day. Observe and categorise each of your touching experiences for that day and reflect on your particular use of touch within your practice. Are you satisfied with the way you use touch? Are your clients satisfied? How do they respond to you? What changes in your touch behaviour might be beneficial to your clients? To assist you in this, please read Gale & Hegarty (2000) *The Use of Touch in Caring for People with Learning Disability*.

The client–therapist interaction

Fundamental to the practice of complementary therapies is the concept of client-centred work, allowing the provision of one-to-one attention and close interpersonal contact between client and therapist. In addition, the principle of holism *'further presumes a participatory relationship between practitioner and client which generates a renewed context of hope and empowerment'* (Long et al 2000, p. 27). One of the important psychological effects of, for example, massage, is the establishment of a relationship between the therapist and the client, where touch is used both as a social and a therapeutic medium through which positive regard can be communicated (Hegarty 1996). Holistic health practitioners use touch to enable clients to become more aware of themselves by fostering a 'helping–healing' relationship (Sanderson & Carter 1994).

People choose to visit a complementary practitioner because of the increased amount of time and attention given to the client during a consultation (Sharma 1992), and satisfaction with their relationship with a practitioner (Truant & McKenzie 1999). This is particularly important when we consider the NHS where the time doctors can devote to their clients is increasingly eroded and the average consultation is 4.6 minutes (Welcome News 2000); an average consultation with a complementary practitioner is between 1 and 2 hours.

Traditionally within the professional carer–client relationship, an element of professional distance has been maintained, and has prevented a nurse or therapist from becoming too involved with the client. However, one may argue that maintaining this distinction serves to reinforce the power imbalance inherent within the relationship. The formation of a warm relationship between client and carer is a fundamental goal of complementary therapies, and of other approaches such as gentle teaching (O'Rourke & Wray 2000). The intimacy of interaction that takes place during a massage both permits and provides time, opportunity and confidence to share problems with an assurance that they will be considered sympathetically, without the rush and hurry that too often characterises medical interviews.

Client Choice and Empowerment

Complementary therapies can offer clients opportunities for choice and empowerment and this is especially important for those individuals who have severe or profound learning disabilities, and are frequently excluded from making choices in relation to the services and care they receive. People with profound learning disabilities can make informed and valued choices and judgements, through non-verbal communication, such as facial expressions and body language that act as 'a mediator for communication' (Sanderson et al 1992). Following assessment of the verbal and non-verbal behaviour of an individual, it is possible to gain an understanding of how these interactions communicate a 'language' (Caldwell 1997). With appropriate support, clients can be involved in choosing the essential oils and determine the nature and extent of a massage; this process is described in Box 20.3.

Increasingly sophisticated tools for assessing the communication of individuals with profound and complex needs are being developed, for example the Affective Communication Assessment (Coupe O'Kane & Goldbart 1998) and the Interaction Sequence (McInnes & Teffrey 1982). These

---

Box 20.3   The interaction sequence and client choice

The interaction sequence (Table 20.1) was developed by McInnes & Treffry (1982) whilst working with children who had visual and auditory impairments. The sequence comprises eight stages, resists, tolerates, cooperates passively, enjoys, responds cooperatively, leads, imitates, and imitates independently. The sequence aims to develop trust, communication and choice and also stresses the development of a trusting relationship between an 'intervenor' and child. The sequence has been adapted and used with people with learning disabilities to assess and monitor interaction during massage and aromatherapy (Sanderson et al 1992). The first four stages are referred to as the passive massage stage and, in practice, this stage can take up to a year to achieve. Stages 5–8 are referred to as the interactive stages of the massage sequence.

Table 20.1 The interaction sequence (Sanderson et al 1992)

Stage	Client and therapist interaction
1. Resists	In this stage, the essential oils are introduced gradually, allowing the person time to experience the smell, touch and texture of the base oils, creams, lotions. The therapist strokes the person's hand for as long as he or she is able to tolerate it, allowing the person to leave or move away at any time. People who are touch defensive may find this process difficult to begin with and if they continue to resist or become distressed, then the therapist withdraws. It is important for the therapist to be aware of clients' use of eye contact and body language. Clients may tolerate the strokes for a few seconds only and contact is built gradually on the clients' own terms. Duration of first stage may be 3–4 weeks or up to 6 months.
2. Tolerates	Next, the therapist offers the person essential oils to smell. It is important that the therapist observes clients' reactions and facial expressions. For example, do they follow the bottle if they like a smell, or do they turn their heads away if they dislike it; do they smile? The therapist also looks for signs of the person enjoying the experience, for example allowing longer periods of stroking. If appropriate, symbols are used to augment this process (see Figs 20.1a, b, c). Massage strokes are introduced slowly and the client may remain in contact for periods of up to 5 minutes.
3. Cooperates passively	In this stage the person is more relaxed and will tolerate massage for longer periods of time. The therapist can continue to increase the choice of oils offered and introduce massage to the feet, head and shoulders. The therapist should observe for a relaxed body position and facial expressions.
4. Enjoys	The person may begin to show signs of enjoying the massage, for example smiling, increasing eye contact and letting the body relax. The person will also allow other areas of the body to be massaged, and remains in contact with the therapist. In this stage, the person is not easily distracted, and will indicate when ready to end the session.
5. Responds cooperatively	This is as stage 4, but the client becomes noticeably more relaxed. For example, when the oils are shown clients may offer their hands in anticipation and require less encouragement to become involved.
6. Leads	The client will begin to show choice in relation to the oils used and the massage strokes (Fig. 20.1d). They also may use objects of reference to initiate the session, such as pointing to the oil bottle or the sign for massage (Fig. 20.1e). As the clients' enjoyment increases and they become fully engaged, they may close their eyes. Clients may also begin to anticipate the sequence of the massage, for example offering their other hand when the first is completed.
7. Imitates	With encouragement, the person begins to reciprocate the massage to the giver or therapist and becomes fully engaged in the session.
8. Imitates independently	In the final stage, the client initiates, and controls the massage experience independently. Communication, trust and the relationship have been established and the person is fully engaged in the sessions.

tools provide a starting point in supporting individuals to give consent. Makaton signs and symbols can also be used to complement this process. A person with physical limitations and/or additional sensory impairments can be helped to explore a range of different sensory encounters, and provided with a rewarding therapeutic experience.

COMMON COMPLEMENTARY THERAPIES

This next section briefly explores some of the therapies used with people with learning disabilities.

This is not intended to be an exhaustive list, but introduces the reader to the most common therapies available, and focuses on the research evidence currently available to practitioners. The following therapies are discussed briefly:

- Massage
- Reflexology
- Therapeutic touch
- Aromatherapy.

The most popular complementary therapy used with people with learning disabilities is aromatherapy (Harrison & Ruddle 1995, Sanderson et al 1992, Sanderson & Carter 1994, Wray 1998).

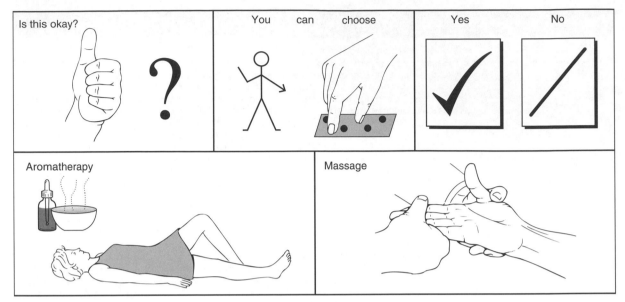

Figure 20.1

Therefore, this section provides a focus upon that approach and three case illustrations are provided later in the section.

Massage

Massage is the therapeutic manipulation of soft tissue involving the touching, kneading and stroking of muscles, tendons, and ligaments of the body with varying degrees of pressure. The basis of massage is touch and this has a number of physiological and psychological effects including the release of stress, tension and pain (Ferrel-Torry & Glick 1993). The movements involved in massage can improve blood and lymph flow, loosen knotted tendons, and relax muscles. It is believed that massage encourages the production of endorphins and these can reduce pain and create a feeling of wellbeing (Oldfield 1992). Field et al's (1992) randomised control trial found that massage, when compared with relaxation, significantly decreased levels of stress and anxiety.

The majority of research into the potential benefits of massage focuses upon it as a form of relaxation, and this can have a positive effect on behavioural difficulties or distressed behaviour (verbal, aggressive and movement) of adults with learning disabilities (Deakin 1995, McPhail & Chamore 1989). Children with anxiety, depression, or behavioural disorders have also been found to benefit from the combined use of yoga exercises, massage, and progressive muscle relaxation (Plantania-Solazzo et al 1992). Other studies evaluating the effect of massage have found that a 10-minute back rub, from a nurse, alleviated anxiety and helped the healing process by stimulating the production of antibodies (Groer et al 1994).

One advantage offered by massage is that its principles and applications are known and understood by a variety of different medical cultures. It can be explained to Western orthodox medicine in terms of anatomy, biology, and psychology and therein lies its perceived legitimacy to the medical profession (Perry & Dowrick 2000).

Reflexology

Also known as 'reflex zone therapy', this is a method of treatment where reflex points in one part of the body are massaged in a particular way so as to produce beneficial effects in other parts of the body. Usually the feet are used but it is also possible to use the hands and face. It is based on the idea that the body is divided into 10 longitudinal zones, from the toes to the head and down the arm to the fingers, through which energy pathways pass (see Fig. 20.2). This is similar, although not identical, to the concepts underlying Chinese Medicine. Exactly how reflexology works is open to conjecture, but it has been suggested that malfunctioning in an organ or one part of the body causes crystalline deposits of uric acid and calcium on the nerve endings of the feet (Thompson 1994). Massaging the reflex zone on the foot corresponding to the malfunctioning part of the body, assists in the breakdown of the crystals, and creates an optimum environment for the body's inherent healing capacity. However, after treatment 'a healing crisis' often occurs due to detoxification (Griffiths 2001).

Reflex zone therapy can be used to treat a number of conditions including back pain, digestive disorders and stress-related problems. People with progressive disorders such as multiple sclerosis may find control of muscle function is improved by reflexology (Booth 1994). However, White et al's study (2000) investigated whether the representation of reflex zones used by therapists could be used as a reliable method of diagnosis. They found that as a diagnostic method, reflex zones were very poor at distinguishing between the presence and/or absence of conditions. Some positive treatment effects for this therapy have been established, but overall the results are ambiguous making it difficult to make a sound clinical judgement regarding its appropriateness for use in the care of people who have learning disabilities.

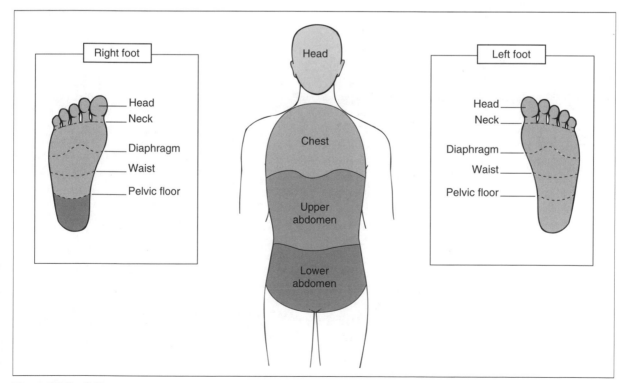

Figure 20.2   Reflex zones

Therapeutic touch

The practice of therapeutic touch (TT) was originally explored by Dolores Krieger (1975) and is the modern day derivative of the ancient practice of the laying on of hands. It differs from this practice in that it is not done within a religious context, requires no professed faith or belief and no direct physical contact between the practitioner and the patient (Sayre-Adams 1994). As an intervention, the practitioner's hands are used to direct energy to the patient with the intent of helping and it involves 'centering', or assuming a meditative state or intention to help the patient. The hands are then used as sensors or scanners to move over the patient's body assessing the energy flow and energy needs of each individual. Using the hands, areas of accumulated tension and energy are identified and re-directed to the patient to restore energy balance. TT represents a 'practical demonstration of the nurses desire to care for and heal the individual, while recognising the interrelatedness of mind, body and spirit' (Rankin-Box 1988, p. 161).

Krieger's (1975) original exploratory studies revealed some degree of effect, however these studies, whilst experimental, were poor in design. Later studies have shown TT to be a fulfilling therapeutic experience for patients (Samarel 1992) and that it can reduce pain (Randolph 1984) and the time needed to calm children after stressful experiences (Kramer 1990). These results were not substantiated by Meehan's (1993) study, in which little statistical significance was obtained when comparing the effects of TT to acknowledged and accepted pain relief treatments. He did conclude the existence of a mild treatment effect but suggested the effect was placebo in nature (see Box 20.4).

In the US, healing touch (HT) was used by nurses to ease pain and anxiety, promote relaxation and accelerate wound healing (Umbreit 2000). TT is non-invasive and has minimal side effects and this natural potential can be used by anyone. Advocates of TT see it as an appropriate modality that can be used by nurses and carers and does not require a doctor's order or supervision.

Aromatherapy

Aromatherapy is the therapeutic use of essential oils extracted from various botanical sources i.e. petals, plants and trees. The essential oils are volatile, highly concentrated and complex substances containing chemical properties, and each essential oil has its own individual properties, specific uses, and actions. Aromatherapy is used to treat illness through the systematic application of the oils, often in conjunction with massage but also in baths, inhalations, compresses, and in restricted cases taken orally (diluted) under the supervision of a qualified aromatologist. The essential oils are potent and should always be diluted in carrier oil when applied to the skin.

Box 20.4 The placebo effect

In double blind clinical testing of new drugs, it is common practice for a control group to be given a 'placebo' instead of the drug itself. The placebo appears to be identical to the drug but does not contain any pharmacological or therapeutic properties. Any effect produced by the placebo (or 'dummy pill') cannot be explained on the basis of the actual drug or treatment, and the effects produced are generally considered to be psychological in nature. This 'placebo effect' is mediated by a number of factors that include: the perception of the therapist, the effect of the therapeutic setting, the credibility of the medication, patient expectations of the medication and patient beliefs (Kleijnen et al 1994).

Within the field of complementary therapies, there is considerable debate as to whether the treatment effect produced by such approaches can be ascribed to the 'placebo effect'. Campbell (2000) has suggested that this debate is unhelpful and that it is necessary to undertake research within a holistic paradigm to establish the subjective mechanisms underlying people's responses to complementary therapies without using terms such as placebo. Others have argued that what is important is whether or not the person with learning disabilities experiences it as beneficial or life enhancing, and not whether the therapeutic change can be attributable to the oils, the massage or the placebo effect. Hanse stated: *'I've worked with people who are deaf and blind with severe mental and physical handicaps who would not understand the concept "placebo" and who are very different after a combination of oils and touch'* (Hanse 1990, p. 43).

Essential oils have their most rapid effect through the olfactory and limbic system so inhalation is commonly the method of choice (for example using an aromatherapy burner).

Aromatherapy massage is the most popular method of administering essential oils to the skin, and appears to interact with the body in different ways. It can act chemically causing changes to occur when the oils react in the bloodstream with hormones and enzymes. It can also act physiologically, affecting stimulation or sedation depending on the oil used. On a psychological level, it can have an emotional or affective consequence, the individual reacting to the smell of the oil and its associations producing an uplifting or relaxing response. Some essential oils may be contraindicated in certain conditions, for example in pregnancy (basil, clary sage and juniper) and hypertension (rosemary and ginger), and it is advisable to consult a qualified aromatherapist before using any oils.

Research evaluating the effectiveness of aromatherapy suggests that beneficial effects for the patient can be derived in certain contexts. However, many of the studies conducted by nurses are individual observations based on the authors' own clinical practice. Research has demonstrated a reduction in behavioural and emotional stress levels with lavender essential oil (Buckle 1993) and neroli essential oil (Stevenson 1992). In addition, aromatherapy has been shown to be more effective than massage, or a 20-minute rest period in reducing patients' heart rate, blood pressure, respiratory rate, pain level and wakefulness (Hewitt 1992), although these results have not, as yet, been replicated. It appears that the psychological effect and influence on the patient may herald the greatest effect. This is supported by Dunn et al's study (1995) in which intensive care patients showed an improvement in mood and perceived anxiety when compared to a control in a study evaluating aromatherapy, massage and periods of rest, although the effect was not sustained nor cumulative. Also, in Wilkinson et al's (1999) study of aromatherapy massage in palliative care, clients showed a statistically significant reduction in anxiety. The largest study to date (Burns et al 2000) indicated a significant reduction in pain for the use of aromatherapy in intrapartum midwifery practice.

Very few studies have focused on the impact of aromatherapy on people with learning disabilities. However, those that have (Armstrong & Heidingsfeld 2000, Harrison & Ruddle 1995, Sanderson & Carter 1994) are predominantly based on anecdotal evidence and case studies. Lindsay et al (1997) compared the effects of four therapy procedures, snoezelen, hand massage/aromatherapy, relaxation but active therapy (a bouncy castle) on concentration and responsiveness in people with profound learning disabilities. The results suggested that both snoezelen and relaxation had a positive effect on concentration and responsiveness but hand massage/aromatherapy had little or no effect. Due to the small number of published research studies into aromatherapy and learning disabilities so far, the evidence base surrounding the effectiveness of such interventions is too small to indicate any real impact (Cawthorn 1995, Stone 1999).

The final part of this section provides three Case illustrations (20.1, 20.2, 20.3) that portray examples of aromatherapy and massage used with people with learning disabilities who presented with a number of different challenges.

These three case illustrations demonstrate how aromatherapy and massage can be used with

Reader activity 20.3

Before reading the next part of the section, consider the following comment made by Sanderson et al (1994): 'We find that the beneficial effects of aromatherapy and massage are the same for everyone, it therefore follows that we have no special 'remedies' specific to people who have learning difficulties, and the basic principles described here are applicable to everyone.' Are people with learning disabilities special cases when we want to use complementary therapies? Do we need to introduce specific guidelines and training? What 'special considerations', if any, would you undertake if you were using a complementary therapy with a person with learning disabilities?

people with learning disabilities in a number of different ways.

The Aromatherapy Organisations Council (AOC) suggests that aromatherapy should only be used on patients by practitioners who have an accepted qualification. Many practitioners are becoming concerned at the ill-informed ways in which some professional groups such as nurses are introducing aromatherapy into their practice. It is considered to be both a danger to patients and disruptive to the aromatherapy profession for non-qualified practitioners to 'dabble' if appropriate advice and consultation has not taken place.

IMPLICATIONS FOR THOSE SUPPORTING PEOPLE WITH LEARNING DISABILITIES

Prior to the introduction of any complementary therapy with people with learning disabilities, there are a number of factors to consider. These include:

- an examination of the research evidence
- the availability of guidelines and protocols
- the education and training of the practitioner
- regulation of therapy

Case illustration 20.1 Client with mild learning disabilities

Background

Helen is 25, has mild learning disabilities and Down syndrome, and lives at home with her mother, a single parent who is her sole carer. Helen works in supported employment at a supermarket and attends a resource centre. The community nurse referred Helen to an aromatherapist and she had a number of presenting symptoms. Helen recognises her symptoms, and was able to communicate them to the therapist. Prior to the commencement of treatment, consent was sought from Helen and her mother. The intervention was fully explained and any queries answered. Helen was given a choice of oils at each session, and these oils were selected to help alleviate her presenting symptoms (see Table 20.2).

Helen had not previously experienced massage and she was anxious, but also eager to begin. A hand massage was initially given to allow Helen to experience this. Helen enjoyed having her hands massaged so in subsequent sessions, massage was introduced to her arms and legs and eventually to her back, neck, shoulders, and feet. Her mother was present at each session and observed the massages. In between sessions with the therapist, Helen and her mother were able to massage each other.

Client outcomes

- Helen's eczema cleared after three sessions (with use of oils between sessions). There has been no recurrence on the most effected areas, the arms, legs and face.
- The eczema on Helen's hands took much longer to clear up and treatment is ongoing.
- Helen and her mother felt that aromatherapy had helped their relationship, by improving communication between them. They would regularly swap massage of hands and feet at home.

- Helen's periods became more regulated, and a stomach massage helped to relieve her discomfort.
- Helen's thyroid is now regulated with GP intervention, and drug treatment.
- Helen feels she is less tense, and finds it easier to relax and looks forward to the aromatherapy sessions.

Table 20.2 Aromatherapy treatment plan for Helen

Presenting picture	Essential oils selected and treatment
Hyperthyroid – tiredness, lethargy, and weight loss	Conventional treatment from GP Geranium (*Pelargonium graveolens*) Frankincense (*Boswellia carteri*)
Eczema – affecting hands, arms and legs	Roman Chamomile (*Anthemis nobilis*) Geranium (*Pelargonium graveolens*)
Pre-menstrual tension – nervous agitation and constipation	Mandarin (*Citrus reticulata*) Neroli (*Citrus aurantium*) Roman Chamomile (*Anthemis nobilis*)
Psychological symptoms – moodswings, tension, tearfulness, aggression and agitation	Clary sage (*Salvia sclerea*) Mandarin (*Citrus reticulata*) Neroli (*Citrus aurantium*) Geranium (*Pelargonium graveolens*)

ARE COMPLEMENTARY THERAPIES EFFECTIVE? EXAMINING RESEARCH AND EVIDENCE

Less than 10% of lay people who use a complementary therapy have based their decision to use that particular therapy on scientific evidence (Jackson 1995). When working with clients with learning disabilities, it is essential that practitioners access, and make use of research evidence upon which to base decisions. Within the relevant literature, the overall paucity of sound research evidence is repeatedly acknowledged (Richardson 2000), and this is particularly the case in the field of learning disability. Systematic evaluation of these therapies to date has been insufficient, the studies conducted often being poor in design and representing mainly case studies and anecdotal evidence. A range of different therapies are being

Case illustration 20.2 Client with learning disabilities and challenging behaviour

Background
Barry is 43 years old and lives in a supported home with four other people. He moved to this house 2 years ago from a long-stay institution. Barry has profound learning disabilities, epilepsy, and asthma and has had considerable professional input from the behavioural team, consultant psychiatrist, asthma clinic, occupational therapist, and speech and language therapist. Barry was referred to an aromatherapist by the multidisciplinary care team as he had difficulties sleeping at night and the team responsible for his care were interested in introducing relaxation therapies as part of his night time plan. Barry also had a number of other difficulties that included: self-induced vomiting, proneness to choking, unsteadiness on his feet, tendency to self-injure, and recurrent chest infections. Barry liked having his head stroked and was tolerant of touch although his attention span was limited. As Barry was unable to give verbal consent, the proposed treatment plan was discussed with his main carer and it was agreed to use the interactive massage sequence (see Box 20.3). The oils were selected to treat specific conditions (such as bronchitis and difficulty sleeping) and to promote relaxation and reduce anxiety (see Table 20.3).

Over the 6 months of Barry's treatment, his response level moved from stage one (resists) to stage two (tolerates). Barry initially accepted no more than a few minutes touch before moving away to another part of the room or leaving the room and returning. As Barry became more tolerant of the touch, he would remain in the same place for longer periods. The massage sequence comprised mostly rhythmic stroking to hands, feet, and head. Barry was most relaxed whilst having his head stroked. Barry is also able to make a basic choice of essential oils for his massage although the therapist selected essential oils that were relaxing and that would help relieve his symptoms. Barry also enjoys water and relaxes in the bath; a blend of essential oils in dispersible bath oil was prescribed and used in his evening bath.

Barry has recently moved into stage three of the interactive sequence, passively cooperative, and is enjoying and relaxing for longer amounts of time. Barry's levels of interaction and engagement, such as eye contact and remaining in contact with the therapist, have increased. Barry's bedroom is being transformed with sensory equipment; he now has coloured lights and music and an electric essential oil diffuser, which enhance his living space.

Client outcomes

- Barry's breathing improves whilst he is receiving aromatherapy as he is more relaxed.
- The sessions have enabled the team to find time to support Barry to relax at bedtime, but they have not resolved his sleep difficulty.

Table 20.3 Aromatherapy treatment plan for Barry

Presenting picture	Essential oils selected and treatment
Asthma and chronic respiratory infections – catarrh, bronchitis	Marjoram (*Origanum marjorana*) Frankincense (*Boswellia carteri*) *Eucalyptus radiata* Cedarwood (*Cedarus atlantica*)
Digestive difficulties – self-induced vomiting and prone to choking	Marjoram (*Origanum marjorana*)
Tendency to self-injure	Cedarwood (*Cedarus atlantica*) Sandalwood (*Santalum album*)
Long term difficulties sleeping at night	Cedarwood (*Cedarus atlantica*) Marjoram (*Origanum marjorana*), lavender (*Lavandula augustifolia*).

Case illustration 20.3 Client with profound learning disabilities

Background

Roger moved into a community house two years ago from a long-stay hospital and lives with two other people in a supported house (the third person had died suddenly prior to treatment commencing). Roger uses a wheelchair but can walk with support and currently receives input from occupational therapy, the district nurse, and day services. Roger has nocturnal epilepsy (controlled) and is prone to constipation and chest infections. He has no verbal communication, but uses eye contact and body language to communicate and has experienced aromatherapy in the past and has enjoyed it. Consent to proceed was sought from Roger's main carer and the interactive massage sequence (see Box 20.3) was commenced using a hand massage. At each session Roger was offered a choice of oils from the aromatherapist's selection (see Table 20.4). Roger was able to indicate choice of where he would like to be massaged.

For the first few sessions Roger was withdrawn and appeared depressed and would not establish eye contact with the therapist. However, Roger was keen to initiate touch and would choose oils by moving his head away if he did not like the oil, or come towards the bottle giving eye contact and smiling when he liked the oil. Roger has a great sense of humour and expresses this within the sessions. The regular sessions and one-to-one gave Roger support with bereavement and continuity through a traumatic few months.

Client outcomes

- Roger now enjoys the contact and interaction and gives eye contact throughout the sessions.
- Roger is less anxious and more relaxed and he wrings his hands less frequently.

Table 20.4 Aromatherapy treatment plan for Roger

Presenting picture	Essential oils selected and treatment
'Stress' since move from long-stay hospital. Emotional agitation, irritability, anxiety and depression	Sandalwood (*Santalum album*) and Neroli (*Citrus aurantium*)
Bereavement and emotional agitation, including irritability, anxiety and depression exacerbated by continual staff changes in the last year	Frankincense (*Boswellia carteri*), Sandalwood (*Santalum album*)
Nervous tension, frustration, irritability and worry. Roger required constant one-to-one attention, was withdrawn, shy, anxious and constantly wringing his hands	Orange sweet (*Citrus sinensis*) Mandarin (*Citrus reticulata*)
Constipation	Managed by regular enemas
Colds and chest infections	*Eucalyptus radiata*
Bronchitis, head colds, asthma	Frankincense (*Boswellia carteri*)

explored primarily by nurses, and aromatherapy has received particular attention. However, as Stevenson (1997) has stated *'the amount of research readily available does not reflect the enthusiasm with which aromatherapy is being introduced into nursing practice'* (p. 46).

Caution must be exercised before the implementation of such therapies into learning disability practice: 'For therapies to become part of professional nursing practice we must also be prepared to undertake research in order to justify that our actions are based upon knowledge rather than belief' (Rankin-Box 1992, p. 103). It has been argued that when evaluating complementary medicine, it is difficult to devise a research protocol that is sufficiently sensitive to measure treatment effects using the current (orthodox) rules for research practice (Long et al 2000). This is not nec-

essarily the case: there is an abundance of different research methods at our disposal. However, it is increasingly important that the method chosen is appropriate to the study, and that the measurement tools are reliable and sensitive enough to detect treatment effects. Consequently, it may be necessary for practitioners to explore the range of research methods available, and there are solid arguments for the devising of more creative methods (Osborne 1994) in which the individual response of a client will be reflected in the research protocol. It might be argued that those quantitative methods with their focus on individuality, holism, humanism, participation and interaction are more suitable to investigate the nature of complementary therapies (Biley & Freshwater 1999).

There is an acute need for the development of a substantive research base in order to critically evaluate and rationalise the use of complementary therapies for specific disorders. In order to achieve this, the following directives are essential (Welcome News 2000):

- a critical review of all currently available evidence undertaken by credible and independent researchers
- the development of a research and development strategy
- the publication and dissemination of all research information in order that informed decisions can be made by practitioners
- an assessment of the potential demand for such therapies including the opinions of local populations and health professionals to inform joint policies in funding.

It is to be hoped that research money will be identified to investigate the efficacy of complementary therapies for people with learning disabilities.

GUIDELINES AND PROTOCOLS

Before implementing aromatherapy, or any other complementary therapy, in a care setting, it is necessary to establish a protocol for practice. 'Any proposal for the integration of complementary medicines must be based on a systematic assessment of health care needs and evidence based practice' (Ernst 2000, p. 42). In Graham et al's (1998) study of NHS Trusts, and private hospitals using complementary therapies, only one-third had a specific protocol in place. In addition, Rankin-Box (1997) has noted that many hospitals had a 'policy' or 'standard' in place, rather than protocols. However, it was evident that protocols were often being established following the introduction of therapy rather than before.

A protocol should consider issues of quality, safety, consent, competence, practice, accountability and risk management. The UKCC (2000) has suggested that employers are responsible for establishing policies to provide a framework for the use of complementary therapies by practitioners in their employment. It is also the practitioner's responsibility to provide insurance to practice.

EDUCATION AND QUALIFICATIONS

It is evident that health care practitioners, and in particular nurses, are practising complementary therapies with a range of expertise, training, and qualifications. Some are gaining formal qualifications, while others are practising after a much shorter course of training, and in some cases this is as little as 10 weeks. Trevelyan (1995) describes these different types of practitioners as 'experts', 'dabblers' and 'facilitators'. The 'experts' are those who hold a recognised qualification in the therapy they practice; 'dabblers' are those who may have a personal and professional interest in a therapy and have usually attended workshops or a short course and then introduce some aspect of that therapy into practice (e.g. using an essential oil). The 'facilitators' are those who are informed about complementary therapies and are able to give information to the client regarding the most appropriate therapy or practitioner for them to consult; they do not practise themselves but ensure informed decision making by the requesting client.

In January 1994, the UKCC produced a position statement on complementary therapies recognising the growing popularity of these therapies within the nursing profession. This position statement refers to various other documents produced by the council that govern the use of complementary therapies by nurses, midwives, and health visitors. This includes the standards set in the *Code of Professional Conduct* (UKCC 1992a) and in particular the application of principles set out in paragraphs 8–11 of the UKCC's document *The Scope of Professional Practice* (UKCC 1992b) which is concerned with developing practice. Specific mention of complementary therapies is made in *Standards for the Administration of Medicines* (UKCC 1992c) (Article 38 and Article 39). The UKCC position is illustrated by the recurrent theme, which states that the nurse is responsible for her or his actions. Therefore, it is vital that those people wishing to use a complementary therapy within their nursing practice should undertake training that has a valid and recognised qualification.

In addition, the RCN have also considered the implications for its nurses, midwives and health visitors with the imminent introduction of complementary therapies into the practice arena. They have formed a special interest group from which has evolved the RCN Complementary Therapies Forum; the forum's six priorities are: '*UKCC recognition of courses, standardisation of education in general, development of and distribution of principles and guidelines for practice, networking, research, increased funds (for courses/research)*' (RCN 1994, p. 5).

The RCN has also constructed guidelines on choosing an appropriate course in a complementary therapy and a 'consumer checklist' (RCN 1993) to allow nurses to give patients advice on how to choose a therapy or therapist. As Frost states: 'one of the great dangers of complementary therapies is that people become interested in one field and rather than take an accepted training course, simply become knowledgeable "dabblers"' (Frost 1992, p. 27).

In relation to other health care workers, most professional groups have been slow to respond to the need for standardisation of education. The College of Occupational Therapists produced a position statement in 1996 stating that complementary therapies were not part of the occupational therapist's core skills, although it acknowledged that there are therapists competent in this field. In addition it noted that in the case of occupational therapists, provision of such therapies ought to be supported by employers through insurance or contract of employment as the College can only advise on standards of practice in occupational therapy.

There is a pressing need for standardised training courses in complementary therapies and courses should aim to receive accreditation by a recognised professional body. However, 'It is the responsibility of the individual practitioner to judge whether a qualification obtained in a complementary therapy has brought the practitioner to an appropriate level of competence to use that skill in patient or client care' (UKCC 2000, p. 5). This UKCC directive states that individuals supplying a service, including medicine, nursing and complementary therapies, will have to justify their actions should a malpractice suit be brought against them. This being the case, adequate pro-

fessional training must be undertaken prior to the inclusion of a complementary therapy into nursing practice to safeguard both the practitioner and the client.

Where a practitioner is working independently, self-evaluation of competence and accountability becomes particularly vital. Membership of a registered professional body, insurance to practice and regular updating of clinical knowledge in the chosen therapy should be a requirement to practise much the same as UKCC requirements for professional development. However, this has yet to be applied to all therapies and not all health care settings have taken the initiative and applied these guidelines to nurses and other professionals. The Aromatherapy Organisations Council (AOC) was established in 1991 as the governing body for aromatherapy and to unify the profession and to develop training standards. The AOC represents 13 professional associations and accredited schools and has set standards for aromatherapy education; a common core curriculum was implemented in 1994 to ensure a standard of recognised training.

The need for information regarding minimum training guidelines is progressively becoming more urgent and these appropriate training levels need to be decided by the professional bodies governing nursing practice. Competence to practise can only be established if standards are set that determine both training and educational levels. When choosing a course in a complementary therapy it should be a professionally validated course, but also the therapy itself should be regulated by one of the two central complementary organisations: the British Complementary Medicine Association (the AOC is a member of the BCMA), and the Institute for Complementary Medicine.

THE REGULATION OF COMPLEMENTARY THERAPIES

As complementary therapies find an increasingly substantial role within health care, it will become vital to ensure that the introduction of these therapies is supported by sound regulatory bodies. Regulation will remove the confusion as to who is, or who is not, qualified and will protect the public from inadequately trained complementary practitioners. Regulation ensures standard setting, organisational codes of conduct and disciplinary procedures for therapy. The recent House of Lords Select Committee on Science and Technology inquiry into complementary and alternative medicine (House of Lords 2000) recommended that complementary therapies move toward statutory or self-regulation. Osteopaths and chiropractors have already achieved this and other approaches are moving in that direction.

The UKCC seeks to regulate nursing practice in relation to complementary therapies, by emphasising the boundaries set by other regulatory documents. This places responsibility firmly with the individual practitioner. It seems likely that the UKCC will be compelled to make a decision regarding those therapies that are acceptable in nursing practice, and those that are not. Nursing autonomy, accountability, health, safety and legal liability all need to be addressed more stringently if therapies are to be integrated into orthodox nursing practice.

All therapeutic interventions, whether they are designated as Western, orthodox, complementary or alternative, carry their own set of contraindications, side effects, warnings and special applications. As with the provision of any treatment and care, a range of precautions should be taken when practising a complementary therapy.

CONCLUSION

Complementary therapies potentially offer people with learning disabilities a range of therapeutic benefits. Evidence supporting the efficacy of some approaches is currently insufficient, however the essential ingredients of the therapies such as support, a positive therapeutic relationship with the practitioner, empathy in treatment and choice are likely to be of considerable value. There are a number of concerns regarding research evidence, guidelines and protocols; education and regulation still need to be addressed. However, if practitioners can 'safely' say they are able to enhance the quality of care provided for people with learning disabilities, then there is every reason to consider incorporating such approaches.

The introduction of *Valuing People: A new strategy for learning disability in the 21st century* (DOH 2001) will necessitate discussions regarding the future role of health care provision for people with learning disabilities (DOH 2001). Whether access to complementary therapies is part of that agenda is yet to be seen. However, the general public and practitioners will continue to demand access to alternative and complementary health care, and it is hoped that people with learning disabilities will be given the opportunity to experience 'rights, independence, choice and inclusion' (DOH 2001) regarding this matter.

REFERENCES

Armstrong F, Heidingsfeld V 2000 Aromatherapy for deaf and deafblind people living in residential accommodation. Complementary Therapies in Nursing and Midwifery 6(4): 180–188

Ayer S 1998 The use of multi-sensory rooms for children with profound and multiple learning disabilities. Journal of Learning Disabilities for Nursing, Health, and Social Care 2(2): 89–97

Biley F, Freshwater D 1999 Trends in nursing and midwifery research and the need for change in complementary therapy research. Complementary Therapies in Nursing and Midwifery 5(4): 99–102

Booth B 1994 Reflexology. Nursing Times 90(1): 38–40

Buckle J 1993 Aromatherapy: does it matter which essential oil is used? Nursing Times 89(20): 32–35

Burns E, Blamey C, Ersser S J, Lloyd A J, Barnetson L 2000 The use of aromatherapy in intrapartum midwifery practice an observational study. Complementary Therapies in Nursing and Midwifery 6(1): 33–34

Caldwell P 1997 'Getting in touch' with people with severe learning disabilities. British Journal of Nursing 6(13): 751–756

Campbell A 2000 Acupuncture, touch and the placebo response. Complementary Therapies in Medicine 8(1): 43–46

Cawthorn A 1995 A review of the literature surrounding the research into complementary therapies. Complementary Therapies in Nursing and Midwifery 1(4): 118–120

Cole A, Shanley E 1998 Complementary therapies as a means of developing the scope of professional nursing practice. Journal of Advanced Nursing 27(6): 1171–1176

College of Occupational Therapists (COT) 1996 Position statement on complementary therapies. Complementary therapies, position statements, standards for practice and clinical guidelines. COT, London

Coupe O'Kane J, Goldbart J 1998 The affective communication assessment. In: Coupe O'Kane J, Goldbart J 1998 Communication before speech: development and assessment, 2nd edn. David Fulton Publishers, London, ch 2

Deakin M 1995 Using relaxation techniques to manage disruptive behaviour. Nursing Times 91(17): 40–41

Department of Health 2001 Valuing people: a new strategy for learning disability in the 21st century. Cm 5086. HMSO, London

Dunn C, Sleep J, Collett D 1995 Sensing an improvement: an experimental study to evaluate the use of aromatherapy, massage and periods of rest in an intensive care unit. Journal of Advanced Nursing 21(1): 34–40

Emanual J 1999 Will the GP commissioner role make a difference? Exploratory findings from a pilot project offering complementary therapy to people with musculo-skeletal problems. Complementary Therapies in Medicine 7(3): 170–174

Ernst E 2000 The complementary/alternative debate: a perpetuation of myths? Complementary Therapies in Medicine 8(3): 214–215

Ernst E, White A 2000 The BBC survey of complementary medicine use in the UK. Complementary Therapies in Medicine 8(1): 32–36

Ferrel-Torry A, Glick O 1993 The use of therapeutic massage as a nursing intervention to modify anxiety and the perception of cancer pain. Cancer Nursing 16(2): 93–101

Field T, Morrow C, Valdeon C 1992 Massage reduces anxiety in child and adolescent psychiatric patients. Journal of the American Academy: Child and Adolescent Psychiatry 31(1): 125–131

Frost J 1992 Herbalism: an overview of ancient art. Professional Nurse (Jan): 47

Furnham A 2000 How the public classify complementary medicine: a factor analytic study. Complementary Therapies in Medicine 8(2): 82–87

Gale E, Hegarty J R 2000 The use of touch in caring for people with learning disability. The British Journal of Developmental Disabilities 46 Part 2 (91): 97–108

Gates B 1994 The use of complementary and alternative therapies in health care: a selective review of the literature and discussion of the implications for nurse practitioners and health care managers. Journal of Clinical Nursing 3(1): 43–47

Goffman E 1961 Asylums; essays on the social situation of mental patients and other inmates. Anchor Books, London (Reprinted in 1987 by Peregrine Books, London)

Graham L, Goldstone L, Ejindu A, Baker J, Asiedu-Addo E 1998 Penetration of complementary therapies into NHS trust and private hospital practice. Complementary Therapies in Nursing and Midwifery 4(6):160–165

Greenfield S M, Wearn A M, Hunton M, Innes M A 2000 Considering the alternatives: a special study module in complementary therapies. Complementary Therapies in Medicine 8(1): 15–20

Griffiths P 2001 Reflexology. Chapter 20 In: Rankin-Box D (ed) 2001 The Nurse's Handbook of Complementary Therapies, 2nd edn. Baillière Tindall and The Royal College of Nursing, London

Groer M, Mozingo J, Droppleman P 1994 Measures of salivary secretory immunoglobulin A and state anxiety after a nursing back rub. Applied Nursing Research 7(1): 2–6

Guardian Educational Supplement 1996 Back to our roots. January 10, The Guardian

Hanse M 1990 Points of view. Nursing Standard 4(48): 43

Harrison J, Ruddle J 1995 An introduction to aromatherapy for people with learning disabilities. British Journal of Learning Disabilities 23(1): 37–40

Hegarty J R 1996 Touch as a therapeutic medium for people with challenging behaviours. British Journal of Learning Disabilities 24(1):26–32

Hewitt D 1992 Massage with lavender essential oil lowered tension. Nursing Times 80(25): 8

House of Lords 2000 House of Lords Science and Technology Committee on Complementary and Alternative Medicine from the 6th report. Session 1999–2000 (HR paper 123). The Stationery Office, Norwich

Jackson A 1995 Alternative update. Nursing Times 91(8): 61

Kleijnen J, de Craen J M, Van Everdingen J, Krol L 1994 Placebo effect in double-blind clinical trials: a review of interactions with medications. Lancet 344: 1347–1349

Kramer N A 1990 Comparison of therapeutic touch and casual touch in stress reduction of hospitalised children. Paediatric Nursing 16(5): 483–485

Krieger D 1975 Therapeutic touch: the imprimatur of nursing. American Journal of Nursing 75: 784–787

Lindsay W R, Pitcaithly D, Geelan N, Buntin L, Broxholme S, Ashby M 1997 A comparison of the effects of four different therapy procedures on concentration and responsiveness in people with profound learning disabilities. Journal of Intellectual Disability Research 41(3): 201–207

Long A F, Mercer G, Hughes K 2000 Developing a tool to measure holistic practice: a missing dimension in outcomes measurement within complementary therapies. Complementary Therapies in Medicine 8(1): 26–31

Luff D, Thomas K J 2000 Sustaining complementary therapy provision in primary care: lessons from existing services. Complementary Therapies in Medicine 8(3): 173–179

McGill P, Toogood S 1994 Organising community placements. In: Emerson E, McGill P, Mansell J (eds) Severe learning disabilities and challenging behaviour: designing high quality services. Chapman and Hall, London, ch 10

McInnes J, Treffry J 1982 Deaf-blind infants and children – a developmental guide. Open University Press, Milton Keynes

McPhail C, Chamore A 1989 Relaxation reduces disruption in mentally handicapped adults. Journal of Mental Deficiency Research 33: 399–406

Meehan T C 1993 Therapeutic touch and post-operative pain: a Rogerian research study. Nursing Science Quarterly 6(2): 69–78

Oldfield V 1992 A healing touch. Nursing Standard 6(44): 21

O'Rourke S, Wray J 2000 Gentle teaching. In: Gates B, Gear J, Wray J 2000 Behavioural distress: concepts and strategies. WB Saunders, London, ch 7

Osborne S E 1994 The future of homeopathy and other complementary therapies as part of the British National Health Service (guest editorial). Journal of Advanced Nursing 20(4): 583–584

Paterson C 1997 Complementary practitioners as part of the primary health care team: consulting pattern, patient characteristics and patient outcomes. Family Practice 14(5): 347–354

Perry R, Dowrick C F 2000 Complementary therapies and general practice: an urban perspective. Complementary Therapies in Medicine 81(2): 71–75

Pincus T, Vogel S, Savage R, Newman S 2000 Patients' satisfaction with osteopathic and GP management of low back pain in the same surgery. Complementary Therapies in Medicine 8(3): 180–186

Plantania-Solazzo A, Field T M, Blank J K 1992 Relaxation therapy reduces anxiety in child and adolescent psychiatric patients. Acta Paedopsychiatrica 55(2): 115–120

Randolph G L 1984 Therapeutic and physical touch: physiological response to stressful stimuli. Nursing Research 33: 33–36

Rankin-Box D F 1988 Complementary health therapies: a guide for nurses and the caring professions. Croom Helm, London

Rankin-Box D 1992 European developments in complementary medicine. British Journal of Nursing 1(2): 103–105

Rankin-Box D 1997 Therapies in practice: a survey assessing nurses' use of complementary therapies. Complementary Therapies in Nursing and Midwifery 3(4): 92–99

Richardson J 2000 The use of randomised control trials in complementary therapies: exploring the evidence. Journal of Advanced Nursing 32(2): 398–406

Rogers M 1970 Introduction to the theoretical basis of nursing. F A Davis, Philadelphia

Roper N, Logan W W, Tierney A J 1990 The elements of nursing: a model for nursing based on a model for living, 3rd edn. Churchill Livingstone, Edinburgh

Royal College of Nursing 1993 Complementary therapies: a consumer checklist. RCN, London

Royal College of Nursing January 1994 Complementary therapies a position statement. RCN, London

Samarel N 1992 The experience of receiving therapeutic touch. Journal of Advanced Nursing 17(6): 651–657

Sanderson H, Carter A 1994 Healing hands. Nursing Times 90(11): 46–48

Sanderson H, Harrison J, Price S 1992 Aromatherapy and massage for people with learning disabilities. Hands On Publishing, London

Sayre-Adams J 1994 Therapeutic touch: a nursing function. Nursing Standard 8(17): 25–28

Sayre-Adams J, Wright S 1995 Change in consciousness. Nursing Times 91(41): 44–45

Sharma U 1992 Complementary medicine today: patients and practitioners. Tavistock/Routledge, London

Stevenson C 1992 Measuring the effect of aromatherapy. Nursing Times 88(41): 62–63

Stevenson C 1997 Complementary therapies and their role in nursing care. Nursing Standard 11: 49–53

Stone J 1999 Using complementary therapies in nursing: some ethical and legal considerations. Complementary Therapies in Nursing and Midwifery 5(2): 46–50

Thomas K, Fall M, Parry G, Nicholl J 1995 National survey of access to complementary health care via general practice: report to the Department of Health. Medical Care Research Unit, Sheffield

Thompson J 1994 Complementary therapy: increasing patient's options. Community Outlook (September) 19–23

Trevelyan J 1995 Incorporating complementary therapy into contemporary nursing practice. Conference paper. Complementary Partnerships Conference, 1.11.95, York

Trevelyan J 1996 A true complement. Nursing Times 92:5

Trevelyan J, Booth B 1994 Aromatherapy. Nursing Times 90(38): 3–15

Truant T, McKenzie M 1999 Discussing complementary therapies: there's more than efficacy to consider. Canadian Medical Association Journal (editorial) 160(3): 351

Turner R 1998 A proposal for classifying complementary therapies. Complementary Therapies in Medicine 6(3): 141–144

Umbreit A W 2000 Healing touch: applications in the acute care setting. AACN Clinical Issues: Advanced Practice in Acute and Critical Care 11(1): 105–119

United Kingdom Central Council for Nursing, Midwifery and Health Visiting 1992a Code of professional conduct, 3rd edn. UKCC, London

United Kingdom Central Council for Nursing, Midwifery and Health Visiting 1992b The Scope of Professional Practice. UKCC, London

United Kingdom Central Council for Nursing, Midwifery and Health Visiting 1992c Standards for the administration of medicines. UKCC, London

United Kingdom Central Council for Nursing, Midwifery and Health Visiting 1994 Complementary therapies position statement. UKCC, London

United Kingdom Central Council for Nursing, Midwifery and Health Visiting 2000 Position statement on complementary therapies. UKCC, London

Vickers A 1994 Health options: complementary therapies for cerebral palsy and related conditions. Element Books Ltd, London

Vickers A 1997 Massage and aromatherapy a guide for health professionals. Stanley Thornes Ltd, Cheltenham, UK

Welcome News 2000 Questioning the alternative Q2: 10–11

Which 1996 Healthy choice. November: 8–13

White A R, Williamson J, Hart A, Ernst E 2000 A blinded investigation into the accuracy of reflexology charts. Complementary Therapies in Medicine 8(3): 166–172

Wilkinson S, Alderidge J, Salmon I, Cain E, Wilson B 1999 An evaluation of aromatherapy massage in palliative care. Palliative Medicine 13(5): 409–417

Wray J 1998 Complementary therapies in learning disabilities: examining the evidence. Journal of Learning Disabilities for Nursing, Health and Social Care 2(1): 10–15

FURTHER READING

Caldwell P 1997 'Getting in touch' with people with severe learning disabilities. British Journal of Nursing 6(13): 751–756
This article describes innovative ways of establishing engagement and interaction with people who are difficult to reach.

Gale E, Hegarty J R 2000 The use of touch in caring for people with learning disability. The British Journal of Developmental Disabilities 46(2)91: 97–108
These research papers consider how we use touch with people who have a learning disability.

Hegarty J R 1996 Touch as a therapeutic medium for people with challenging behaviour. British Journal of Learning Disabilities 24: 26–32

Lindsey W R, Pitcaithly D, Geelan N, Buntin L, Broxholme S, Ashby M 1997 A comparison of four therapy procedures on concentration and responsiveness in people with profound learning disabilities. Journal of Intellectual Disability Research 41(3): 201–207
This paper compared the effects of four therapy procedures, snoezelen, hand massage/aromatherapy, relaxation and active therapy (a bouncy castle) on concentration and responsiveness in people with profound learning disabilities.

Price S, Price L 1999 Aromatherapy for health professionals, 2nd edn. Churchill Livingstone, Edinburgh

Rankin-Box D 2001 The nurse's handbook of complementary therapies, 2nd edn. Baillière Tindall and The Royal College of Nursing, London

Sanderson H, Harrison J, Price S 1992 Aromatherapy and massage for people with learning disabilities. Hands On Publishing, London

Stone J 1999 Using complementary therapies in nursing: some ethical and legal considerations. Complementary Therapies in Nursing and Midwifery 5(2): 46–50

This article considers the ethical and legal considerations raised by nurses using complementary therapies within the NHS and highlights concerns about consent and a lack of evidence base.

Journals
The following journals all provide useful information and resources on a range of complementary therapies and are all published by Churchill Livingstone.

- Complementary therapies in nursing and midwifery
- Complementary Therapies in Medicine
- The International Journal of Aromatherapy

Guidelines for practice
UKCC position statement on complementary medicines from: UKCC, 23 Portland Place, London W1B 1PZ. Fax: 020 7436 2924.
Alternatively, email: publications@ukcc.org.uk, or access the website at: www.ukcc.org
RCN complementary therapies position statement (1994) from:
RCN Complementary Therapies Forum, The Royal College of Nursing, 20 Cavendish Square, London W1M 0AB. Tel: 020 7409 3333.

USEFUL ADDRESSES

Alternative Medicine Foundation Inc.
http://www.amfoundation.org/index.html
5411w Cedar Lane Suite 205-A, Bethesda, MD 20814, USA.
This is a guide for professionals and users of complementary therapies and has good links to other sites and useful information.

The Aromatherapy Organisations Council
http://www.aoc.uk.net
PO Box 19834, London SE25 6WF
Tel: 0208 25 17912
Contact this site for information regarding accredited training schools, professional organisations and AOC registered practitioners.

The British Complementary Medicine Association
http://www.bcma.co.uk
Kensington House, 33 Imperial Square,
Cheltenham, Gloucestershire GL50 1QZ
Tel: 01242 519911, Fax: 01242 227765
This site has a national register and close links with activity related to the government and the European Union.

British Medical Journal http://www.bmj.org/cgi/collection/complementary_medicine
The Editor BMJ, BMA House, Tavistock Square
London, WC1H 9JR. Tel: 0207 387 4499
This link is a valuable resource of up-to-date research and evidence based practice in relation to complementary therapies.

Foundation for Integrated Medicine
http://www.firmed.org/
International House, 59 Compton Road,
London N1 2YT Tel: 0207 588 1881
Formed by HRH the Prince of Wales, the foundation promotes development and delivery of safe, effective and efficient forms of health care.

Institute for Complementary Medicine
http://www.icmedicine.co.uk
PO Box 194, London SE16 1QZ
Tel: 0207 237 5165
This site provides the public with information on complementary therapies.

MEDLINE http://www.ncbi.nlm.nih.gov/PubMed/
This database of clinical research includes complementary medicines with citations and links to relevant journals.

Research Council for Complementary Medicine (RCCM)
http://www.rccm.org.uk/index.htm.
60 Great Ormond Street,
London WCN 13JF.
Tel: 0207 833 8897.
This site provides a comprehensive database (CISCOM) of research information relating to the practice of complementary medicine.

21

Art, drama and music therapies

Richard Manners, Gillian Stevens, Elaine Chaplin

CHAPTER CONTENTS

KEY ISSUES

- Arts therapies are tailored to the individual needs of the clients. Each intervention is different. There is not a standardised process for a standardised ailment, illness or disability.
- Therapy proceeds at the pace of the client and provides natural ways of communicating which have no right or wrong way.
- Arts therapies allow the true voice of a person to be heard by alternative means. A person with learning disabilities may find words or writing intimidating or impossible to use.
- Generally a person with a learning disability can often feel 'done to' rather than 'done with'. Arts therapies can empower the individual: also they facilitate the voice of the person 'within' to be heard without prejudice or judgement and assist the person to have positive relationships and express feelings in a positive way.
- Finally arts therapies promote real choice and offer a flexible way of solving or overcoming problems to facilitate change for people with learning disabilities who have additional needs and/or problems.

INTRODUCTION

In this chapter we deal with three forms of therapy that have their roots in the arts, which have become known collectively as the arts therapies, they are: art therapy, drama therapy and music therapy. The chapter commences with discussion of the common ground and misconceptions to help provide focus and to clarify the role of the arts therapies for the reader. A section devoted to each of these professions follows this.

In general we use the word client to describe the users of the arts therapies. Client does not have the same connotations as patient or resident. It affords the user with learning disabilities a feeling of equity and respect. It is intended to imply that therapy is being developed with them, rather than being done to them.

For the purposes of state registration the newly named Health Professions Council (HPC) recognises art therapy, drama therapy and music therapy as three professions within a single unit. Each profession has a professional association. All vocational training is postgraduate and is university validated. The training of arts therapists qualifies them to practise within various clinical settings and groups of people such as psychiatry, prisons, special and mainstream schools and colleges, and the community as well as with people who have learning disabilities who have additional clinical problems.

These three professions are related, in that they all use an arts medium to offer clients an opportunity for expression, exploration and change. Another link is that they all draw strongly from psychotherapeutic models of intervention. However, one of the strengths of the arts therapies is the diversity of models within each profession that can be offered to this client group.

Historically, within the National Health Service, these professions are employed under Whitely Council regulations, as are occupational therapy, physiotherapy and chiropody. Usually, for the purposes of consultation, they are referred to as Professions Allied to Medicine (PAMs).

The All Wales Network Committee for Arts Therapies Professions describes the arts therapies in this way:

The Arts Therapies offer clients an opportunity for expression, exploration and change. Therapy may be offered to people experiencing specific forms of distress, or who are seeking insight into themselves and their relationships.

The work undertaken addresses emotional and developmental needs, with a view to effecting lasting change. A relationship of trust, built on the needs and wishes of the client, is developed between client and the therapist.

The art becomes a way of communicating within that relationship, and is important for expression, rather than for its purely aesthetic value.

The therapist will act as a witness, carefully attending to what is communicated, whether through words, actions, or the art materials. Therapists will use their considerable understanding of art processes, and of non-verbal and symbolic communications, to work in partnership with the client in recognising and working through areas of difficulty.

Arts therapists may work with individuals and groups. The therapist has an appropriate and respectful relationship with the client. Sessions are usually weekly, and may take place over several months or years (The All Wales Network Committee for Arts Therapies Professions 1997).

Each session takes place in an undisturbed place. Whilst the content of the session is private between client and therapist, care is taken that developments in the session are communicated to other clinicians involved in the care of the client in a sensitive way in order to contribute to the total care plan.

Whilst training, students must take part in their own personal therapy, and whilst practising are supervised on a regular basis. As with any profession, this is not just for personal development, but also as a safe and essential mechanism, to prevent difficulties that may arise from transference, countertransference and related issues that may occur within a session.

Some common misconceptions about the therapies and what they are not

Education

Arts therapists are not teachers. The context of therapy is not generally within an educational process or system. Clients do not undergo therapy in order to gain an educational certificate or reach an acceptable and recognisable level of proficiency. A therapist does not judge a piece of work on its technical merit or aesthetic value. Artwork is not publicly displayed or performed.

Many of these points may often come up in the process of therapy as issues for the therapist to explore with the client. Often, the culture from which a person with a learning difficulty may come can underline or accentuate the individual's feeling of being different. The person may feel it is impossible to attain acceptable levels of educational attainment. This can perpetuate feelings of alienation or inadequacy and result in emotional and psychiatric problems.

The client will often see the therapist as superior, as a person with skills to impart. Often the client will want to learn skills to facilitate the making of a piece of artwork or music, for example a coil pot in pottery, or learning to play notes, or articulating a particular movement. The therapist will, of course, facilitate this but within the context of the therapeutic relationship. The therapist will support the client to feel valued and respected and not judged.

Occupational therapy (OT)

Historically within the NHS the arts therapies have been associated with occupational therapy (OT) because the arts therapists were so small in number and the OT establishment already used the arts as a part of their intervention package. In reality this continues for management purposes rather than because of its appropriateness. This has caused considerable confusion as to the role of the arts therapies and possibly hindered their development.

Art / music / drama with a person with learning disabilities

The arts therapies are often confused with arts activities in a community setting. These days people with learning disabilities can hopefully access the arts in the same way as anyone else. However, some confusion and misplaced criticism for the arts therapies has arisen amongst the proponents of social role valorisation (SRV) and normalisation (see Glossary). They rightly criticise the concept of offering therapy to people solely because they have learning disabilities, but sometimes forget that everyone should have a right to an accessible form of therapy. An arts therapist will not work with clients because they have learning disabilities but because they have extra clinical problems as well as their learning disabilities.

Hospital arts

In recent years many exciting hospital arts projects have been developed in partnership with arts associations and organisations. Artists are commissioned to work within hospitals, sometimes as facilitators and teachers with patients, sometimes as craftsmen and women developing more aesthetic and healthy environments, for example by providing murals in long bleak corridors or setting up studios which patients can visit to participate whilst they are undergoing treatment. These projects are indeed therapeutic, however they are not therapy.

A day service or vocational services

Historically traditional long-stay residential hospitals and institutions provided day services for their residents. These services offered activities to occupy, entertain, educate and rehabilitate. Since the closure of these hospitals day services are now more usually called vocational services. Key to the delivery of these services are the philosophical notions of SRV and normalisation. Clients are supported to access 'normal' activities, education and employment. Individuals are encouraged to advocate for themselves and become integrated into the community. In both the traditional and modern delivery of these services the arts have been used. Indeed, arts therapy services have often grown from these roots. However the distinction is that arts therapists work with the extraordinary problems of those people with learning disabilities. It is a specialist service for those with acute problems. Ideally, nowadays, the services are provided in integrated settings – in those settings that are established to deal with the extraordinary problems that anyone might have.

Therapy solely for those who are good at the arts

Often clients are referred to one of the arts therapies because they are 'good' at it. This is not a reason for referring, nor does it exclude a client.

THE ARTS THERAPIES

The following three sections present each of the arts therapies in some detail, including a brief history, a description of what it is, how it works in practice and case studies.

Art therapy

It is not intended here to linger too long on a theoretical debate or the description and efficacy of the various models of art therapy. Nor is the intention to describe the whole diverse spectrum of models that make up art therapy. It is, however the intention to provide the reader with a 'nuts and bolts' description of art therapy whilst touching on some of the broad debates within the profession. The case studies and description offered here are from a particular perspective, that of the writer as a therapist within the field of learning disabilities over 20 years of practice.

A brief history

The British Association of Art Therapists (BAAT) is the professional organisation that represents art therapists. BAAT's website clearly describes the development of the profession:

BAAT was formed in 1964 from a group of artists and therapists who had been working independently in hospitals, clinics and schools. They realised that in order for Art Therapy to develop and for its value to be more widely appreciated, it was necessary to have a central organisation to which the general public and employing authorities could refer . . . The immediate remit of the association was to pool creative resources, but it quickly became involved in issues of conditions of practice, training and development, emerging as the official voice of the profession of Art Therapy.

BAAT traces its roots to the Second World War and the subsequent requirement for rehabilitation facilities, which included art as a therapeutic tool. Throughout the late 1940s, 1950s and 1960s artists increasingly used their skills in hospitals and clinics, employed mainly on an ad hoc basis and without an umbrella organisation. Despite clear indications of success in its practice, art therapy lacked professional credibility.

In the early 70s, the development of postgraduate training in art therapy heralded a push for appropriate training and a career and salary structure within the profession's chief commissioner, the NHS.

By 1982, the Department of Health recognised the postgraduate Diploma in Art Therapy as the approved qualifying course to work in the NHS.

Currently there are five accredited training courses approved and accredited by the British Association of Art Therapists, the Department of Health and the National Joint Council for Local Authorities and the European Commission. BAAT has a Code of Ethics, Principles of Professional Practice and a Register of Members. In 1997 the Council for the Professions Supplementary to Medicine (CPSM) Act of 1960 was extended to include Art, Drama and Music Therapists, giving State Registration to the profession of Art Therapy and greater protection and confidence to the public in our services (BAAT website).

BAAT currently consists of a governing body, its council of management, and there are 19 regional groups for the members of the Association, plus an international section.

What is art therapy?

It is difficult to define just what art therapy is in a single statement or group of statements. Philosophers and art historians have debated the meaning of art for centuries. If we take art at face value, measuring its meaning and value in aesthetics or skill, it is difficult to see how it might bear any relation to therapy. The notion of psychotherapy is equally difficult to define. It is a generic term for many different approaches. For example, therapists may derive their practice from a Jungian, Freudian, Adlerian, Kleinian or a humanistic or Gestalt perspective, amongst many others. In his book *The Story of Art* Gombrich (1972) writes as his first line, 'There is really no such thing as Art. There are only artists'.

The focus, therefore, is on the person not the product. Art can be seen as an expression of our innermost selves or our feelings in relation to the world around us. Psychotherapy could be described as a group of related techniques to provide insight into and expression of difficult feelings and thoughts that impinge on or cause suffering to an individual, with a view to facilitating healthy change or growth. In the light of these perspectives the link between art and psychotherapy becomes more understandable.

There are as many different therapies as there are therapists. This statement is not just true of art therapy but is also true of all therapies that are rooted in the psychotherapeutic tradition. In addition to a rigorous academic training and practical clinical placements, all postgraduate training of art therapists offers experiential learning such as group and individual art therapy training groups. This facilitates self-knowledge in relation to understanding an individual's internal psychological mechanism, group dynamics, and non-verbal as well as verbal communication. Therapists are therefore prepared to understand and to help their clients by first understanding themselves.

What an art therapist does

Therapists may work with groups or with individuals. They may choose to take a theme orientated directive approach or a client-led non-directive approach. Therapists work in a number of different environments. Client groups and theoretical standpoints vary. Usually art therapists work as part of a multidisciplinary team. Clinical objectives, choice of materials and how much the therapist will become involved in the process depend totally on the individual client. Clients are usually referred because somebody else has identified a need, usually the referrer's need. In other words, the referrer might find it difficult to communicate with the client or there may be a behavioural problem that the social situation from which the client comes cannot cope with. This idea is illustrated in the following quotation:

I believe that for people with learning difficulties, the learning difficulty is not a problem in itself. The real obstacle is other people's often-negative perception of that person and, in turn, the person with a learning difficulty's perception of the way that they are being negatively viewed. I feel that communication, for example, can be as much a challenge to us as it might be to those people with learning difficulties. Some people with learning difficulties exhibit behaviour which we may find strange, but it is actually our inability to recognise these behaviours as valid and acceptable which further alienates the individual with learning difficulties from the community (Manners 1998).

The therapeutic process begins with a period of assessment. Where possible, the objectives are agreed with the client in writing. Where it is not, consent and possible benefit can be gauged by the client response during the assessment. Following the assessment period, an intervention plan and clear objectives can be written, which will include the client's objectives. Objectives are reviewed at regular intervals and changed according to progress.

Typically, the client is encouraged to make an image or an object. The art becomes the central point between client and therapist where strong emotions can be expressed and developed. The therapeutic relationship develops through the medium of art. There is a triangular relationship between the artwork, the client and the therapist. The therapist will observe quietly whilst the client is working. This is usually followed by a period of discussion and reflection. The therapist assists the client to put into words or to make some sense of the images produced. The therapist does not interpret or analyse, rather asks questions in discussion with the client. The danger of interpretation is that therapists will impose their own symbolic assumptions rather than those of the client. Of course an internal dialogue as to the possible meaning and therapeutic potential of the image will be going on in the therapist, based on experience and knowledge; this will help the therapist to formulate appropriately crafted questions to meet the individual needs of the client. Over a period of several sessions the therapist will begin to understand the personal symbolism of the client. Transference will occur, where the client will associate/transfer past experiences and relationships to the therapist. An understanding of the dynamics of transference and countertransference will develop (see Glossary for explanation of these terms). The client may have developed coping strategies that are perceived as behavioural problems or may simply be unhappy because of this pain. Clients may have found it difficult or even impossible to express this. The client can begin to make concrete and tangible those difficult, often traumatic feelings and events that may have been forgotten or avoided because of the emotional pain.

Outlined below are two case illustrations that are intended to illustrate and demonstrate the diversity of an art therapist's caseload. Both case illustrations are of individual clients (because of the nature and intensity of the problems), however much art therapy is delivered in groups. The images used represent fragments of the therapeutic process.

Case illustration 21.1

Janet is a 34-year-old divorced woman living in Wales. When art therapy began she had been detained under Section 3 of the Mental Health Act on and off for two years since 1998 under the categories of mental illness, schizophrenia, and borderline personality disorder. Her IQ rating is 73, which would put her in the category of borderline learning disability. Janet has a 9-year-old daughter Elizabeth who lives with her father and his partner in England. Janet has not seen Elizabeth for 9 years although they have had regular contact by letter and telephone. There is no developmental or psychiatric history prior to Janet having Elizabeth. Janet experienced a difficult labour, which ended with a caesarean delivery. It had been reported that she had had a major psychotic episode in the first year after the birth of Elizabeth. Her past history is a picture of puerperal psychosis, which precipitated her admission to her local NHS psychiatric hospital. Behaviours described, amongst many others, range from attempted suicide, aggression towards property and staff, stripping naked in public, urination and defecation on the floor and smearing. Janet reports feeling depressed inside and has horrible feelings. Janet was referred to art therapy as part of a treatment package within a specialist service provided in the private sector. Other treatments include a women's group, social skills, relaxation, healthy diet, a package of integrated vocational services and a 24-hour nursing environment that is flexible enough to meet her individual needs. Janet is overweight. She is very attractive, always immaculately made up, well manicured and well dressed. Janet always makes sure she is well turned out before attending her therapy session. She presents as a pleasant and articulate woman although quiet and slow in speech; she reports that she has a mild speech impediment. Janet has difficulty in describing her feelings and emotions with appropriate words. Janet attended art therapy for a 1-hour session each week. Janet understood the objectives of art therapy and responded extremely well. In her first art therapy session Janet drew her family. She described how they were all professional and had wonderful families; she felt she let her family down. She said she was embarrassed and ashamed of her behaviour. This was the reason she wanted to present herself as perfect. Her second drawing was of a beautiful vase of flowers (Fig. 21.1). The vase had a chip in the base, which was letting out water; the chip was hardly noticeable. The drawing was perfectly executed – fine line linear drawing. Much of our discussion revolved around the fact that people were not perfect. We all have cracks. We all have emotions and difficulty in our lives. Janet found it difficult to express her emotions because she was frightened of exploding with intensity – she would break the vase. She wanted to control her feelings because she might end up embarrassing herself again.

The third drawing (Fig. 21.2) was of a noticeably cracked and broken vase. Water was pouring out of the vase. Inside she has drawn a picture of herself. She is 'drowning in emotion'. She is very unhappy. This is not what she wants.

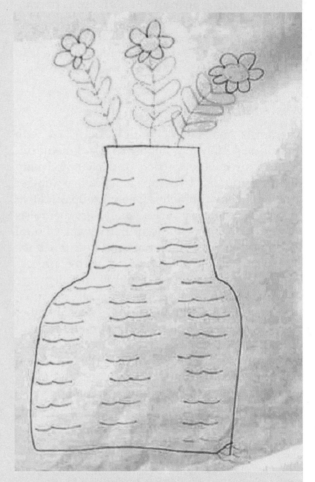

Figure 21.1   Vase.

After a lengthy discussion it occurred to Janet that the figure in the vase might be her daughter Elizabeth. She talked of how her feelings may in fact drown Elizabeth – she was concerned that she wanted to avoid this. She wanted help and guidance on how to approach Elizabeth, should they meet again. Janet's fourth picture followed this theme. She drew two figures standing by a fire. They were both warming their hands. It was herself and Elizabeth. She said this was how she wanted it, a warm and loving glow between her and Elizabeth.

Since these initial drawings Janet continued to articulate her feelings of loss and bereavement. She described how she was so upset that she has not brought up her daughter. Her daughter doesn't know her. She regrets not being able to cope. She wishes she were still married to her husband.

Case illustration 21.1 (*Cont'd*)

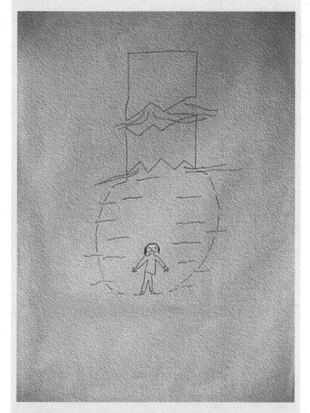

Figure 21.2 Me or my daughter in a vase?

She longs for a 'normal' life. Janet admitted that she wishes she never had Elizabeth sometimes; she feels extremely guilty for this feeling. Much of our discussion talked about the reality of her situation and the needs of her daughter. Janet worries about both her and her daughter's long-term future.

The discussions were extremely moving. Janet used the art therapy as a kind of pressure valve in a similar way to that of a boiling pressure cooker. She didn't want to allow her feelings to explode out. She wanted to talk about them – but in a safe way. She wanted to let her feelings out slowly.

Janet obtained a great deal of benefit from our discussions and expressing her feelings through her drawings. She felt proud of her progress and her growing ability to articulate her feelings in this way. At the time of writing this Janet was released from her Section.

Case illustration 21.2

John was a 21-year-old gentleman who was born in London to parents of Nigerian origin. His IQ rating was 46. This would put him in the category of having moderate learning disabilities. However, the test was administered in English, which may not be his first language. He had a limited vocabulary and had considerable difficulty in understanding language used in an abstract way. He exhibited features related to autism although there is some debate regarding this diagnosis. He has presented with extremely challenging behaviour over a number of years within the family, and in a number of institutional settings. John weighed 17 stones with a muscular frame, which added to both the difficulties, and the perception of his challenging behaviour. His challenging behaviour ranged from kicking, shouting, swearing, and kicking prams with the babies in them to destruction of property. A key feature of his behaviour was his repetitive verbalisation of themes, which included wild animals from Africa mixed with figures from popular cartoons or films such as Popeye.

John left London at the age of 6 due to the divorce of his parents. He lived in Nigeria with his father and grandparents for 7 years before returning to London to his mother and siblings. This whole period was a period of disturbed attachments and, it is speculated, some abusive experiences. It is speculative because there is no evidence other than what John reports amongst his repetitive verbalisations. He reports beatings, being chased out of the village and what seem like ritual exorcisms performed by a witch doctor or shaman. We know there is truth in some of these reports as in one report he described himself surrounded by policemen with batons. Indeed, on one occasion the riot squad were called out when his challenging behaviour was extreme.

At the time of writing this chapter John had been having art therapy for 18 months. He really appreciated his sessions. He was always happy to see the therapist. He greeted the therapist with a hearty handshake and a smile. He made good use of the session, often drawing four to six images.

The primary aim of the session was to facilitate communication and expression of his feelings through the medium of the art materials. The secondary aim was to provide some catharsis and some understanding of John's obsessive repetition of specific events and images from the past that continually 'haunted' him. The approach taken was to listen and to observe carefully the images and stories that John produced in his session. Occasionally he was asked to clarify and expand on some of the subjects. In later sessions there were attempts to lead John away from the subjects he is obsessed by, to subjects currently in his everyday life. He refused to be led. He preferred not to talk about the present or recent past in London. He seemed to be overwhelmed with the need to relate his stories. Often he described them as nightmares; he was extremely distressed and afraid. On his unit the staff were not able to tolerate his obsessive repetition of these images; if ill

Case illustration 21.2 (*cont'd*)

managed this could result in challenging behaviour. He was encouraged to save his images for the art therapy session.

It was difficult for other people in his home environment to take the amount of time to listen that John often demanded. In the art therapy sessions his stories were listened to and explored. He continued to engage in a one-sided monologue. In the early stages his behaviour bordered on becoming extremely disturbed at times, however he was able to control his behaviour and continued to express himself in an acceptable manner. John found it very helpful to have the set time and boundaries that art therapy offered to pour out his stories and images.

It would take too long to describe the rich tapestry of images that were produced. The images were often bizarre and alien to our culture. They came from his native Nigeria mixed with western cultural icons (Fig. 21.3). Often there was a theme that described a real event in the past mixed with an underlying bizarre theme. It was difficult to disentangle what was real from fantasy. For example: did the ritual exorcism happen in Nigeria? Was he describing an actual event? Some research and discussion with a Nigerian psychotherapist confirmed that within Nigeria beliefs still exist where a person with learning disabilities may be considered to be possessed of evil and may have been exorcised; this culture coexists alongside a modern westernised culture.

What evolved were multi-layers of meaning that could only be guessed at, which could not be verified in fact. It would have been very useful to have a family history, which included a history of the cultural environment from which John came. What was certain was that John was genuinely frightened and traumatised in some way. He found it difficult to be understood or even to be heard, partly because of the make-up of his clinical diagnosis and partly because he was a man stuck in his cultural identity, as a Nigerian man who found it difficult to fit in to our culture. The art therapy offered him an opportunity to express his feelings and his identity, to communicate and to be understood.

This is illustrated in Figure 21.4. John drew a caged tiger. The cage was locked and John had the key. He enjoyed the fact that this symbolised him in control of his 'demons'. He was reassured that the image was put in his folder and taken away each session.

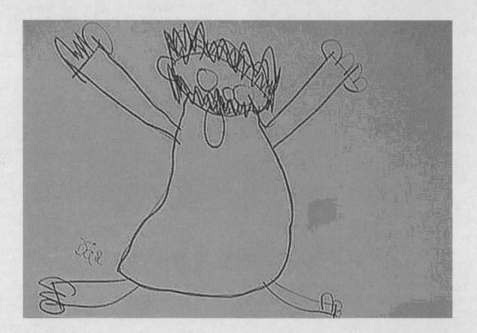

Figure 21.3

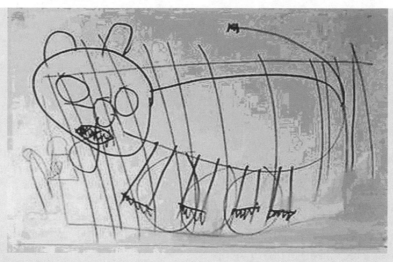

Figure 21.4 Lion locked in a cage.

Reader activity 21.1

The following exercise is used in the context of therapy and as such it is sensitively used to support the individual client. Here the intention is to give the reader an insight into the potential of imagery within therapy. The tone of the exercise should therefore be one of fun and sharing.

Find a partner who is willing to make a drawing or painting and to talk about it and about personal feelings in relation to the image. Both of you should equip yourselves with varied art materials and a reasonable size piece of paper.

The theme of the exercise is to draw or paint the kind of house you would like to live in – your ideal home – and indicate who might live there and where it is, for example the countryside or a city etc. (money and time are no object). Spend 45 minutes completing this. On completion you should return to your partner. Each of you in turn should describe your picture to the other. The listener should strictly encourage the other to use the first person at all times and ask exploratory questions, for example:

Listener: 'Describe what kind of house you are.'
Describer: 'I am large and have big windows.'

The listener should encourage the other to explore each room and to describe each character in the house and what their perception might be.

Each partner should have 30–40 mins to describe his or her house, after which an open discussion should follow. Themes you might want to explore:

- Did you feel there was insight about how you are in the world?
- Did the images afford any personal symbolism?
- Did the images encourage you to explore or expose parts of you that you may not have explored if you used words only?
- Are there some sensitive areas?
- Do you think there was some universal symbolism here – what would be common to others?
- Did you feel there were some insights to your external and internal worlds – private and public? Are there differences or any conflicts?
- How did you feel about the act of drawing?

Please take care of each other. If you do find there are sensitive areas please respect this – don't go in like a bull at a gate. Remember to enjoy the exercise!

Drama therapy

A brief history

The British Association of Drama Therapists' research indicates that drama as a therapy in western culture emerged in Europe in the 19th century. Articles were published identifying drama as a tool for facilitating the experience of catharsis as a healing function. Historically, drama as a therapy holds its roots in anthropological rituals and the mythological wisdom of the collective unconscious. Drama therapy continues to develop and can play a vital part in the construct of the 'real self'. Psychoanalysts such as D W Winnicott and Alice Miller also recognised the importance of play and drama as an integral part of the developing child. Drama therapy has the ability to connect these strands together, which enables individuals to integrate their inner dramas to their true being.

From the emergence of remedial drama in the 1930s in the UK, there have been many pioneers in establishing the profession in this country and abroad. Training needs were identified in the 1960s to validate the unique skills of the drama therapist. Marian Lindkvist, Sue Jennings and Gordon Wiseman established these needs, and from their insight and vision, training became an essential component to the profession. The British Association of Drama Therapists was formed in 1976 and from 1989 Drama Therapists became a recognised professional body under the Whitley Council. As an innovative and dynamic source, drama therapy has had to survive many difficulties, but as it provides healing to others so it did to its profession, and in 1997 it received state registration from the Council for Professions Supplementary to Medicine.

Training courses are now available in England, Scotland, Europe and the USA. Training is at postgraduate level; many colleges offer MA and PhD studies. The qualities required for training as a drama therapist are varied, but range from an involvement in theatre or drama from the student, to experiences of health or education.

What is drama therapy?

The British Association for Drama Therapists has now adopted the following definition for use in its literature and policies:

Drama Therapy has as its main focuses the intentional use of healing aspects of drama and theatre as the therapeutic process. It is a method of working and playing that uses action methods to facilitate creativity, imagination, learning, insight and growth.

In practice, drama therapy can be used within a wide range of clinical settings as well as in education and social/community based environments. Drama therapy, like art therapy, has developed in a number of different directions. Drama therapy can be provided within a multidisciplinary team approach and many institutions and service providers have recognised this. Individuals with learning disabilities respond to a variety of treatments, as we all do. A service with vision and resources can ensure that collaborative planning addresses the individual from a holistic viewpoint. Drama therapists also work with psychologists, psychiatrists, nurses, social workers, teachers and families.

Drama therapists adhere to British Association of Drama Therapists standards as well as those set out by the employing body. Clinical practice and clinical effectiveness are important mediums in which the profession can establish itself. However, a positive therapeutic intervention has its roots in the trust and rapport established between client and therapist. Therefore the therapist is required to have extensive skills and flexibility to ensure that clients within this area fully benefit from the inspiring and cathartic experience of drama as a therapy.

Drama therapy can take a variety of forms suited to the individual, whether that person is able to verbalise or not. It is concerned with the interaction between individuals and their environment or situation or experiences. Drama therapy can become a bridge where different ways of being can occur in a safe therapeutic space. Clients can become empowered to assess their own attitudes and beliefs on their terms whilst having the ability to explore positive interactions of being. It is about an inner drama that can be played within boundaries, which can lead to a more whole person who is able to function more fully in the world. Within learning disabilities this aspect may be especially important to those individuals who have lived in a long-stay hospital or in places that have had levels of high security. As our services change in the provision of support for the client with learning disabilities, so our sensitivity should encompass this expansion of a new person, who feels valued as a member of society.

Drama therapy and learning disabilities

'Ha, ha you can't be a tree they move and you don't.' (Care worker to a client with learning disabilities, taken from the therapist's own work experience.)

Is this true, can we be like a tree, its roots grounded into the soil, or fragile shoots laying half submerged in clay? Does it feel bare and cold with the wind whipping round or a branch full of leaves, ripe with fruit, giving to others? Is its head leaning towards another path, or straight and tall and focused. What could be its destiny?

There are millions of variables, all valued and soaked in symbolism. It may be the client's need to explore, activate, create, ritualise and embody this feeling. This is for the client only, for drama therapy has no right or wrong performance, but allows growth and development to take place.

What a drama therapist does

In the writer's experience of 10 years as a drama therapist within the area of learning disabilities, all clients, regardless of cognitive and/or physical disability, can develop through this creative art

Reader activity 21.2

Drama therapy can't work with people with learning disabilities. Consider this statement. Is it true? Try this exercise and then reflect on the feelings this exercise aroused you.

Sit quietly on your own and reflect on a client you work with.

Then look at how you are sitting.

Make a note of this and then move position.

Do you feel different?

Don't verbalise the feeling.

Now try a larger movement.

What do you feel now? Write or draw or play some music.

Now reflect and write some observations on the client about his posture, and how he may feel if he had an opportunity to explore another way of sitting.

To try even a small change in movement can empower or change your feelings about yourself. If your feelings changed then think about how movement or mime can affect another individual.

Case illustration 21.3 A community based women's group

Aim

To establish a women-only group, to provide opportunities to develop friendships and shared experiences in relation to rites of passage.

This group was identified as a need for those women who experienced rites of passage yet were unable to verbally express their feelings on these changes. Drama therapy and art therapy were recognised as being valuable tools to assist in this process.

7 women were referred with a mean age of 43 years, the youngest being 30 years, the eldest 59 years. The women all had verbal communication skills and independent mobility. 4 women lived with family, 1 woman lived with a foster family, 1 woman lived independently, 1 woman lived in a community home. All women were registered as having learning disabilities.

Method of working

The group was facilitated by a drama therapist and an art therapist and supported by a therapy assistant. The combination of two therapists allowed the women to use media that were suitable to their expressive needs. The assistant provided support to both therapists and clients, through provision of materials, photographic evidence and individual assistance.

The group created their own rules and the therapists provided a contract for the women regarding confidentiality, times, venue and dates. This was to ensure that clear boundaries were set in place, and to validate the importance of the group.

Media used

Photos	Improvisation
Poetry	Role play
Story telling and mythology	Mime
Drawing and painting	Objects of reference

Session content

The sessions ran for 10 weeks and commenced with collective guidelines, boundary setting and media used. The topics listed below were covered:

- Birth
- Early childhood
- Early adolescence
- Maturing women
- Transition
- Here and now (over a two week period)
- Inner peace
- Endings and achievements.

The session content became rich in symbolism and metaphor that was created using different materials. The women especially enjoyed dressing up in different clothes, and taking part in role-play. It enabled them to wear clothes that might have been disapproved of and to change their hair. Essentially the women were able to let go of a mask and be free to discover concepts that they wanted to play with. This promoted a sense of confidence by giving the opportunity to integrate their disabilities within themselves.

Case illustration 21.3 A community based women's group (cont'd)

Evaluation

Evaluation can be perceived as difficult in therapy, as the process can be internal and sometimes subjective. The drama therapist used a standardised culture-free self-esteem inventory (Bartram et al 1991) pre-, during and post-session, to try and establish a more objective perception of the women's self-esteem. The drama therapists also designed an evaluation tool based on a gender-free mannequin and universal symbols. Clients were shown the symbols and their interpretations were recorded, pre-, during and post-session. This allowed the women to be in control of their own self-percep-tions. These two evaluation tools were used to produce manageable data and to correlate the meanings of the sessions to each individual on an internal and external basis. The following areas emerged from the first evalu-ation tool as a defensive approach to needing to be socially acceptable. The concrete standardised test appeared to reveal a protective attitude to their inner vulnerabilities and feelings of inadequacy. However, the central themes from the women over the 10-week peri-od using the second evaluation tool were: sadness, process of change, inner yearning, bereavement, vul-nerability and the conflict of being a woman.

The outcomes of these drama therapy sessions sug-gests that this group of women with learning disabilities share fears over rites of passage, as other women do, yet these expressions appear to become frozen and this may be attributed to:

- perceived emotional development
- a fearfulness of expressing these feelings
- identity confusion (perceived as young girls, yet in fact older women)
- inability to express these thoughts confidently through speech.

It is suggested that the therapy process promoted an open door to explore their attitudes and roles, which was conflicting with their outer selves. This also appeared to reduce behaviours that were seen as chal-lenging in these women.

Reader activity 21.3

As quality services continue to be promoted for this client group, reflect on the following statements from your own viewpoint.

The impact of being socially accepted can be hard for us all at times. We all feel fear and changes in many different forms.

Spend some time on assessing how drama therapy became an 'open door' for the women in Case illustra-tion 21.3.

Case illustration 21.4

This illustration relates to an individual session with a client residing at an assessment and treatment unit. The young man in question is 23 years old and has a history of behaviours that challenge both himself and others, including destruction of his environment. The young man was noted to sabotage and avoid an activ-ity, leading to negative expectations from staff. He also found attachments with others hard to sustain. This may have been due to his inability to trust, as the client had lived in many different settings. The client had a positive relationship with his family and with some staff who had been at the unit for a long period of time.

AIMS

The aim of the sessions was for the client to explore drama therapy as a medium to assist in trusting and in communicating his needs at that time. The sessions were quite chaotic to start with; the client would bite the lycra material and throw equipment away, laughing as he did so. Eye contact would be made and then he would try to hit out or bang an object. Within these sessions the client would verbally advocate that he did not wish for the session to end, yet the situation was created that made it difficult to continue. The client was testing trust to see if the therapist would reject him. The therapist maintained consistency, and although no external props were used, the client began to respond to vocal sounds and story telling. The sounds were used to draw imagi-nation into the story, and the client would mirror these and laugh. Slowly the client created his own sounds to the stories and would then mime them for very short peri-ods. As the therapy process continued a structure was formulated, so that he was able to feel safe in the ses-sion, yet able to create his own choices.

The session was as follows:

- Hello X
- Hello Y
- Vocal sounds
- Story telling
- Enactment of story in client's media (sounds, mime and sound, mime)
- Patting self down as a grounding ritual
- Goodbye X
- Goodbye Y.

The therapy sessions lasted for 3 months, and the tran-sition work into new activities was accepted well. The client appeared more confident and an equal partner-ship was established which the client began to apply to other staff.

form, whether the growth is based on trust, increased confidence, reduction of behaviours that challenge, or a more developed sense of themselves. Drama therapy is a rich medium that

Reader activity 21.4

Select a fairy story or a myth that you like, then think what character you would like to be and why. Ask yourself if this character has qualities that you like or dislike.

Myths and fairy stories are rich in symbolism and can be used as a structure to explore roles, rituals and ideas; they enable you to identify with a given situation in a sensitive, powerful way.

acknowledges a process emerging in an individual, which can take time and patience.

Case illustrations 21.3 and 21.4 are intended to demonstrate the work of drama therapy in practice.

Music therapy

A brief history

The term music therapy is one that has been given to the use of music for therapeutic purposes only in the last 60 years, though examples of the therapeutic use of music can be drawn from numerous historical sources and inferred from anthropological studies and cave paintings. Music and medicine were closely connected in Greek mythology; the god Apollo presided over both fields. The story of the boy David calming King Saul by playing on the lyre is given in I Samuel 16: 14–23. Another frequently cited example is that of Pythagoras, a philosopher from the 6th century BC, who was said to have calmed an angry youth by getting a nearby musician to play calming music.

To return to the 20th century, the increasing use of music in hospital settings probably led to the setting up of various training courses. In the USA, the first full academic course was taught at Kansas University in 1946. Juliet Alvin, one of the pioneers in this field, set up the first British training course at the Guildhall School of Music and Drama, London in 1968. In 1974 another course was started at Goldie Leigh Hospital, London, taught by Paul Nordoff and Clive Robbins, who had gained most of their experience through working with children with learning disabilities. Further courses were set up in Southlands College, London, Bristol University and The Welsh College of Music and Drama, Cardiff. All the courses have common elements of training, which include psychological studies, clinical studies and clinically focused musical training. In addition all trainees have to receive their own personal therapy. The minimum requirement to become a state-registered music therapist is, at present, to have undergone one year of postgraduate training, leading to a diploma in Music Therapy. This may change in future as there is currently a trend towards longer courses, leading to an MA.

What is music therapy?

The power of music All people whatever their age, gender, culture or ability, respond to music. The elements of music (pitch, rhythm, pulse, duration, volume and timbre) are part of our physical being and the raw material of our earliest communications. Few of us pass a day in which we are not in some way affected by music, whether we are aware of it or not. Film-makers and advertisers use it to manipulate our emotions.

Reader activity 21.5

Consider what part music plays in your life. Discuss whether music played during films or in public places affects you.

It is small wonder then that this medium is a powerful means of enabling non-verbal expression and contact between people. 'Music therapists facilitate interaction and development of insight into clients' behaviour through music' (DOH 2000).

Reader activity 21.6

Take some bongo drums or two other small drums (or improvise with, for example, saucepans or books on a desktop) and sit opposite a partner with a drum each. Have a 'conversation' on the drums.

Discuss what happened and what it felt like, for example. Were you nervous? Did you feel silly or childish?

Try not to talk while you are actually playing the drums. Think of all the ways this could be useful to a person with learning disabilities .

Music therapy is a broad field and in the UK alone there are varying approaches. However, it is probably fair to say that the common ground between us is greater than our differences. Most British music therapists have in common that they use mainly improvised music, which can come from the client or therapist or both. Music therapists pay attention, among other things, to the musical elements of their clients' behaviour, whether this is expressed on an instrument or in other actions such as walking, rocking or vocalising. They will usually respond to this with improvised music, either sung or played. The way in which the developing musical and interpersonal relationship is understood may vary according to the therapist's theoretical bias.

Many therapists draw on Winnicott's ideas on play and the parallels between the mother/infant relationship and the therapist/client relationship. He described playing as taking 'place in the potential space between the baby and the mother-figure' (Winnicott 1964). The psychologist and psychotherapist Daniel Stern, who has observed infants' interactive behaviour in great detail, has also had an enormous influence on the way music therapists understand their work. His book *The Interpersonal World of the Infant* (Stern) has been important in this respect.

The concepts of transference and countertransference, introduced by Freud, are also employed as a tool for further understanding. On the other hand some music therapists prefer to look primarily at the musical content of a session. Gary, Ansdell describing the approach known as Creative Music Therapy, says it 'is primarily a practical approach. Most therapists would rather have it seen as a special form of music-making than a musical form of clinical therapy, answerable to another system' (Ansdell 1995).

Who can benefit from music therapy?

Music is a universal means of expression and people at all stages of development are able to respond to and use music. People can be referred to music therapy for any of the same reasons that they would be referred to other forms of therapy or counselling. However, music may be a particularly appropriate medium for those for whom words are not available or easily used.

Reasons for referral could include the following:

- Communication difficulties including autistic spectrum disorder
- Emotional problems, such as anxiety or depression
- Bereavement or other difficult life changes
- Behavioural difficulties
- Concerns over mental health
- Difficulties in relating to others within a group setting.

Many children and adults with autism have been seen to benefit from music therapy. The therapist can tune in to all of the client's behaviours, including stereotypical movements or vocalisations, and by responding to these musically, begin to develop some common ground for further communication and playful interactions. The fact that a music therapist can demonstrate awareness of the client's actions without getting physically too close can be helpful.

Music therapy has been shown to be a useful intervention for those suffering from anxiety (Hooper & Lindsay 1990). The effect of live music made with a therapist was to reduce the pulse rate and behaviour indicative of anxiety.

Music therapists, like the other therapists, usually work as part of a team of various professionals such as community nurses, psychiatrists, psychologists, social workers, occupational therapists, parents and care workers. At times they also collaborate in specific ways. Here are two possible examples:

- Physiotherapy and music: the use of live, specially selected music to support specific therapeutic movements
- Musical interactions: the use of live, mainly improvised music to support play and communication between young autistic children and their parents.

Children and adults with challenging behaviour can sometimes use music as an appropriate and acceptable means of expressing whatever it is that has led to their difficult behaviour. For example, frustration and anger could be expressed in loud or chaotic playing. This could be matched and supported, and through the process of clinical improvisation be led towards becoming more organised. Of course, sometimes things are not straightforward and the therapist has to tolerate and try to contain very disturbed behaviour, which only gradually improves. Ruth Walsh has described 15 half-hour sessions with a 12-year-old girl who initially spent much time overturning instruments and chairs in the therapy room, but who was gradually able to show more of her good feelings as well (Walsh 1997).

People with profound and multiple disabilities are not thereby precluded from experiencing the whole range of human emotions; they can particularly benefit from the non-verbal nature of music therapy. If possible the therapist will try to find a means of enabling the client to play an instrument and will consult a physiotherapist about supported seating. People who have few means of acting on the environment can, through music therapy, be given the opportunity to lead and control another person and to express feelings through the quality of their playing. In some cases clients prefer to vocalise and the therapist can respond to the musical and expressive elements of the vocalisation and use them in improvisation. Where playing an instrument is possible, this can motivate people to use their limited physical skills.

What a music therapist does

When a client has been referred to music therapy, the therapist will usually, after discussion with client and/or carers, arrange for some sessions to assess the suitability of music therapy as an intervention. These will usually take place at the same time each week in a suitable quiet and undisturbed venue. At the end of an assessment period the therapist will formulate some aims and objectives.

Sessions may be with an individual or with a small group. The room will usually be equipped with a keyboard and various tuned and un-tuned percussion instruments, appropriate to the age and abilities of the client, such as xylophone, floor toms, maracas and cymbal. There may also be a guitar or wind instruments. The instruments will be designed to appeal through touch, sound and sight and to be readily accessible to a person with no musical training. When clients come to their first session the therapist will make it clear that this is a time and space for them to use as they wish (though of course appropriate safety boundaries will be maintained).

Some people will immediately start to play one of the instruments. In this case the therapist will pick up on the pulse, volume and mood of their playing and start to improvise alongside them, often on keyboard. Other clients don't use the instruments at first (see Case illustration 21.5 below). Some clients make it clear that they want to play alone. In this case the therapist's task is to listen attentively. Others prefer to listen to the therapist's playing, but will usually give some indication of the kind of music they want to hear. Musical material will develop between client and therapist over a number of sessions (see Case illustration 21.6 below).

The therapist can respond to the client's lead in various ways:

- following
- supporting
- imitating
- initiating
  - leaving gaps to encourage turn taking
  - changing speed or rhythm to see how the client responds.

At the end of the assessment period the therapist may formulate some aims and objectives based on what has occurred during the sessions and on the reasons given for the original referral. These aims are focused on the clients' needs and will therefore vary accordingly. Some possible examples are to:

- support in the expression of feelings of sadness and loss
- assist in the development of pre-verbal communication skills such as turn taking and imitation.

In music therapy an agreement will be reached as to a period of time for the therapy to continue. This will of course be reviewed at intervals by the therapist, the client and other people who are involved, such as parents, carers and teachers.

Case illustration 21.5

Jenny was a young woman in her late 20s, living on the ward of a big hospital. She had been there since she was a child. She was diagnosed as having severe learning disabilities and was thought to be autistic. She was referred to music therapy because she had difficulties in communicating and exhibited demanding behaviour, including smearing feces on herself and the walls. The nurses thought that this often happened when she was bored or frustrated and wondered if music therapy would help her communicate. In her first session she didn't seem to want to play, but continually paced the length of the room, stopping to scratch the wall at each end. The therapist matched the pace and force of her walking with a march-like tune on the piano. Each time she stopped the music was changed to match the tempo of the scratching sound. In this way the therapist hoped to make Jenny aware that attention was being paid to the way in which she chose to communicate. The hope was that she would gain pleasure from controlling her environment in this positive way and would be encouraged to find a more acceptable means of communication than smearing. In the second session the therapist stopped playing for a little while to see what Jenny's reaction would be. Immediately Jenny came over to the piano and replaced the therapist's hands on the keyboard, whereupon the therapist resumed her playing. Over the course of the next few weeks this activity continued and the therapist in return placed Jenny's hands on the keyboard. Soon from this a short musical dialogue developed. She never tried to smear in the sessions and on the ward her smearing decreased. She was always keen to come to the sessions, apparently motivated by her sense of being listened to.

Case illustration 21.6

David was an 8-year-old boy, referred to music therapy because of emotional and behavioural difficulties. He had mild learning disabilities and since he was a baby, had lived in at least 13 different foster homes. His current placement was in danger of breaking down because of his difficult behaviour. It was hoped to give him a non-verbal means of expressing the anxiety and insecurity that had led to this vicious circle of 'bad' behaviour and continual rejection. Over the months a musical theme over a rhythmic repeated bass pattern developed between David and his therapist. To this David sang the words 'Keep on going'. It seemed to express his need for people not to give up on him. Another important theme for David was the oscillating semitone bass from the *Jaws* movie which he discovered for himself on piano. One week he played this and told the therapist she was bitten to pieces. When she said, 'Am I dead now?' he replied, 'Other people can't get better but you can get better.' He seemed to be saying that he knew that the therapist, who in his mind also stood for his foster mother, could survive the worst of his behaviour and not be destroyed. Music therapy continued for 3 years and was probably one of the elements which helped to maintain him at his current foster placement. No other placement had lasted for more than a few months.

Case illustration 21.7

Stuart was a man in his early 40s with Down syndrome and moderate learning disabilities who was suffering from anxiety and depression. He lived in a supported setting with four other people with learning disabilities. He spent a lot of time alone in his room and didn't mix much with the other residents. It was felt he might benefit from group music therapy and he attended weekly sessions for $2\frac{1}{2}$ years. His favourite instrument was the piano. At first he played very tentatively and unrhythmically and didn't like to play alone but as his confidence increased he played more loudly and much more closely in time with the prevailing tempo. He enjoyed the attention given him when he played a solo or duet and became very sensitive to the nuances of the improvised music. When another member of the group annoyed him by disrupting the music, he was able to be assertive and tell this person that he didn't like his actions. He became a particular friend of another member of the group. At home he became more sociable and his antidepressant medication was reduced without ill effect.

Music therapy may continue for several months and occasionally for several years, especially when it is providing a means of emotional support for those who are experiencing continuing difficulties in their life circumstances. Outlined here are three case studies intended to illustrate and demonstrate the diversity of a music therapist's caseload.

CLINICAL EFFECTIVENESS AND EVALUATION

Within the arts therapies there is an abundance of qualitative research whilst there is limited quantitative research (Kliendienst & Frude 1999). Most research in this area is in the form of single case studies, or 'fly on the wall' ethnographic studies which validate the efficacy of these therapies. Appropriate models of research, which reflect the practice of arts therapies and the nature of the clients' problems, are continually sought. Current thought within clinical effectiveness promotes the quantitative tool of randomised control trials (RCTs) as the 'gold standard'. The current political culture promotes only those clinical interventions that can be proven to be clinically effective by the use of the gold standard. A proven standard clinical process or treatment can be applied to a standard illness or ailment to ensure a positive outcome. Any suitably qualified person can then repeat this process. The theory is that the most clinically effective (and cost effective) treatment can be applied with equity to those who need it. It would be impossible to do justice to this debate here. It is worthwhile, however, flagging up some of the issues in this debate from the perspective of the arts therapies (and maybe some other professions?) in learning disabilities.

It would be difficult to find a standard person with learning disabilities with additional problems. Each is unique and very complex. Their problems are not often clear. Each person is treated as a whole person, often by a multidisciplinary team. It would be difficult to isolate a problem or the treatment that was the most effective.

One of the benefits of the arts therapies is their creative and flexible response to meet the individual needs of the client. Therapists will often employ their own personal skills, knowledge and experience as well as proven methods to treat clients. There are as many different therapies as there are therapists. A standard clinical process may not be easily found. Standardisation of treatment plans or processes may invalidate the effectiveness of the treatment!

CONCLUSION

The arts therapies are therapeutic interventions that are ideally suited for people with learning disabilities who have additional problems. Whilst each therapy has its roots in the arts, each has a unique contribution to make. The arts therapies have a number of benefits that include:

- being tailored to the individual needs of the clients
- proceeding at the pace of the client
- providing natural ways of communicating which have no right or wrong way
- allowing the true voice of a person to be heard by alternative means
- empowering the individual
- facilitating the voice of the person 'within' to be heard without prejudice or judgement
- assisting the person to have positive relationships
- expressing feelings in a positive way
- facilitating the person to self-advocate
- promoting real choice
- offering a flexible way of solving or overcoming problems and
- promoting and facilitating change.

GLOSSARY OF TERMS

Social role valorisation (SRV) and normalisation After using the principles of normalisation for a period of time, it was realised that the principles were only being applied to buildings and furnishings, and that service users were still not valued as equal citizens.

In 1983, Wolfensberger proposed a new term for normalisation to overcome this problem; he called this social role valorisation. The emphasis of social role valorisation is to prevent people with learning disabilities being cast in damaging social roles and to establish them in positive or culturally valued social roles in all areas of life (Brown & Smith 1992).

The following actions are required to contribute to social role valorisation:

- improving of situations and living conditions of disadvantaged people
- Creating, supporting and defending valued social status for disadvantaged people
- Developing the experiences and competencies of disadvantaged people
- Minimising differences between disadvantaged people and those viewed as respected citizens
- Presenting disadvantaged people in positive ways.

Symbolism 'What we call a symbol is a term, a name, or even a picture that may be familiar in daily life, yet that possesses specific connotations in addition to its conventional and obvious meaning. It implies something vague, unknown or hidden from us' (Jung 1964). Jung also coined the term archetypal symbolism where symbolic images are common to us all and have a universal meaning. In this context 'individual symbolism' is intended to mean the specific symbols a particular individual has chosen to portray their world.

Transference The client's reaction to the therapist is as if the therapist is an important figure in the client's early development or current life. The client is bringing feelings and beliefs from his or her relationships to the present therapeutic relationship, transferring feelings and beliefs about this person or persons to the therapist. This process can be an important tool in understanding internal or unconscious conflicts.

Countertransference The clinician's reaction to the client is as if the client is an important figure in the clinician's early development or current life. The clinician is bringing feelings and beliefs from his or her relationships to the present therapeutic relation-

ship, transferring feelings and beliefs about this person or persons to the client. This process can be a hindrance to the therapeutic process as it can cloud clinical objective judgement; clinicians guard against this by having external clinical supervision. Countertransference can also be an important tool in understanding internal or unconscious conflicts in the client – therapists can 'listen' to the messages in the feelings they are having towards clients. They may be indicators of how the client has related to individuals in the past, for example does the client engender parental feelings in the therapist?

REFERENCES

Ansdell G 1995 Music for life: aspects of creative music therapy with adult clients. JKP, London

Battle – Culture Free Self-esteem Inventory 1991 NFER-Nelson Publishing

Brown H, Smith H (eds) 1992 Normalisation: a reader for the nineties. Routledge, London

British Association of Art Therapists (BAAT) website. http://www.baat.co.uk/home.htm

British Association of Drama Therapists (BADTH) www.badth.co.uk

Department of Health 2000 Meeting the challenge: a strategy for the allied health professions. The Stationery Office, London

Gombrich E H 1972 The story of art, 12th edn. Phaidon, London

Hooper J, Lindsay B 1990 Music and the mentally handicapped. The effects of music on anxiety. British Journal of Music Therapy (4)2

Jung C 1964 Man and his symbols. Picador, London

Kliendienst M, Frude N 1999 A review of research relevant to outcome measurement in the arts therapies. An unpublished paper commissioned by The All Wales Network Committee for Arts Therapies for the Welsh Office

Manners R S R 1999 A personal journey. In: Rees M (ed) Drawing on difference. Art therapy with people who have learning difficulties. Routledge, London

The All Wales Network Committee for Arts Therapies 1997 Information Leaflet

Wood C 1999 Gathering evidence: expansion of art therapy research strategy. Inscape (The journal of the British Association of Art Therapists) 4 (2): 51–56

Walsh R 1997 When having means losing. Music therapy with a young adolescent with a learning disability and emotional and behavioural difficulties. British Journal of Music Therapy (2)1

Winnicott D W 1971 Playing and reality. Routledge, London

Winnicott D W 1964 The child, the family and the outside world. Penguin, London

USEFUL ADDRESSES

American Music Therapy Association
www.musictherapy.org

The British Association of Art Therapists (BAAT)
Mary Ward House
5 Tavistock Place
London WC1H 9SN
Tel: + 44 (0) 171 383 3774
Fax: +44(0) 171 387 5513

British Association of Drama Therapists
41 Broomhouse Lane
London SW6 3DP

British Society for Music Therapy (BSMT)
Denize Christophers
BSMT Administrator
25 Rosslyn Avenue
East Barnet
Herts, EN4 8DH
Tel/Fax 0208 368 8879

CandoCo Dance Company
Dawn Prentice
2L Leroy House
436 Essesx Road
London N1 2QP

Graeae Theatre Company
Interchange Studios , Dalby Street
London NW5 3NQ,

Heart 'n' Soul
Website: www.heartnsoul.co.uk

Music Therapy Online
www.musictherapyonline.com

Music Therapy for Young Children with Special Needs
www.geocities.com

Nordoff-Robbins Music Therapy UK
www.nordoff-robbins.org.uk

Prism Arts
Carlisle Enterprise Centre
James Street, Carlisle CA2 5BB
Tel: 01228 625700 ext 228

FURTHER READING

Bunt L 1994 Music theraphy. An Art beyond words. Routledge, London

22 Psychological approaches

David Wilberforce

KEY ISSUES

- First this chapter provides an overview of the nature and history of psychology. Next it outlines the main strands of thought that have contributed to a modern definition of this relatively young science. Psychology provides a means of understanding and making sense of human reality, addressing as it does issues of emotion, behaviour, motivation and other internal processes.

- Cognitive, biological, behavioural, psychodynamic and humanistic perspectives are discussed before moving on to look at some specific approaches in more detail. Some of the therapies within these perspectives, for example gestalt, rational, emotive and cognitive analytic therapies, might be regarded as 'talking therapies' and subsequently inappropriate for people with learning disabilities. By way of contrast some suggest that these therapies are appropriate, for example Sinason (1992) has stated that 'emotional intelligence' is not necessarily correlated with cognitive ability. Bates (1993) believes the only differences in working with this population are ones of pace and time scale.

- A large number of these psychological or 'talking' therapies have long been available to the general population, and we are becoming a more 'therapy aware' culture. At the same time there is evidence of an increased demand for such interventions amongst the learning disabled population (Waitman 1993). This may

be due to greater community visibility, growing awareness amongst carers of the emotional needs of people with learning disabilities, or a consequence of the higher than average instances of psychological disorders amongst this population (Bouras et al 1993). Behavioural approaches remain at the heart of much therapeutic work with learning disabled people, but this is well recorded and described elsewhere in the literature and will not be explored at great length here. Instead a basic functional analysis approach will be outlined.

INTRODUCTION

Common to the human experience are emotional and/or psychological problems. Clearly, this will be no less true for people with learning disabilities. Given the devaluing manner in which they are often treated by society with resultant poor self-esteem, allied to other social, psychological and biological factors, one might expect that they are more likely to experience psychological distress. The dramatic shift from institutional care in the recent past means also that people with learning disabilities are now more likely to be exposed to the stresses and demands of life in the community. Recent studies have begun to demonstrate a high incidence of psychological disorders amongst this element of the population (Bouras et al 1993, Crews et al 1994, Patel et al 1993).

The nature and impact of psychological distress in people with learning disabilities is not necessarily well understood by those who care for them. Perhaps the all encompassing concept of 'challenging behaviour' has contributed to a certain element of confusion, particularly in terms of differential diagnosis, with manifestations of psychological distress or mental illness being described as 'challenging behaviour'. Furthermore, services have generally been more focused upon the development of personal life care skills and social skills along with perhaps a general approach to challenging behaviour, whilst the emotional needs of people with learning disabilities have not been so adequately addressed.

Recent health policy documents such as *Valuing People* (DOH 2001), *National Health Service Framework for Mental Health* (DOH 1999) and *Signposts for Success* (DOH 1998) provide guidance and highlight the mental health and behavioural needs of people with learning disabilities. However, there is a sense that it is perhaps still too often the case that needs more specifically related to their learning disabilities tend to dominate others views of their lives, whereas needs associated with their emotional, spiritual or psychological damage are less well understood or acknowledged (Waitman 1993).

As Gates (1998) has suggested, the cause of behavioural difficulties may be multifactorial and may be explained from a variety of theoretical perspectives. However, since this population are generally less verbal and articulate than the general population, unspoken emotional and psychological distress will undoubtedly be a major cause. Clearly there is a need to focus upon helping people who generally have little experience of dealing with the private realm of their emotions, feelings and thoughts. This will entail the development of particular skills amongst professionals in the field and other carers. Too often, direct care staff are being left to rely upon intuition and their own life experiences in their response to the emotional aspects of their work. Whilst this may be potentially helpful, there are clearly drawbacks in this situation. Such an unstructured approach could potentially be professionally abusive (Waitman 1993). Brandon (1990) articulated similar concerns when he wrote 'love is abundant but wisdom rare'. Valerie Sinason (1991), bemoaning the sparse provision with regard to working with emotional disturbance in people with learning disabilities, states that '. . . we cannot love someone out of mental illness'. Professionals and carers need then to develop more skilful and reliable means to facilitate the expression of emotional and spiritual concerns amongst the learning disabled population.

Whereas a large number of psychological therapies have long been available to the general population, we are now seeing an increased demand for such services from the learning disabled. Unfortunately, a great deal of research remains to be done which might show whether psychological approaches or 'talking therapies' are beneficial to this client group. Nor is there much evidence to show which people with what disorder are best suited to which approach. Thornicroft et al (1992) have provided some useful insights for readers who may be interested in this aspect. There is research (Decker 1988, Lambert 1986), however, which shows that there are a number of 'common factors' amongst the therapies which are themselves therapeutic regardless of the techniques used in the therapy (see Box 22.1).

These common factors are relationship based and echo the work of Carl Rogers (1980) who outlined 'core conditions' which needed to be in place within any therapeutic relationship which purported to be helpful. There can be no reason why such findings cannot be applied when working with the learning disabled population, providing a more explicit foundation for the provision of services and support.

This implies a need for practitioners to at least develop an awareness of the range of psychological approaches available, which may enable them to address the emotional needs of the people for whom they care. The scope of their practice can only be broadened and enriched by the general development of such awareness and skills. The origins of psychological thinking and the various strands which, have developed into the modern perspectives that make up psychology today are now briefly outlined.

THE NATURE OF PSYCHOLOGY

With its inception during the latter part of the 19th century, psychology is still a relatively young science. The fundamental idea behind its development is the belief that mind and behaviour could be the subject of scientific study and analysis. Thus psychology can be defined as, 'The scientific study of behaviour and mental processes' (Atkinson et al 1990). Thinking about everyday human reality in order to make sense of it is not new and is, indeed, probably as old as the human ability to reflect. There is ample evidence from ancient history, in the great philosophical works of Socrates, Plato and Aristotle for example, of engagement with fundamental questions related to mental life. These questions have as much relevance and importance now as they ever did.

Up until the late 19th century, these and other academic works of philosophy were the dominant influence in the construction of knowledge, theories and laws about the world. Similarly, many aspects of our lives now are influenced by ideas from psychology, from theories of behaviour and

---

Box 22.1 Common factors amongst the therapies

There are many therapies from various schools of theory, each placing a different emphasis upon different aspects of the helping process and utilising particular techniques and methods. Some research has shown (Lambert 1986, Orlinsky & Howard 1987) that factors common to the various approaches may actually be more important to the success of the therapy than the actual techniques used. These 'common factors' are shown below:

- A *relationship* characterised by trust, genuineness and mutual respect in which the client feels understood and heard, believing the therapist to be concerned about his or her problems.
- A *working alliance* is developed in which the client and therapist feel that they are working in a partnership with shared aims and goals.
- *Support and reassurance* gleaned from the calm and assured presence of another will engender hope in clients that their problems can be resolved. Luborsky et al (1985) showed that therapists who formed such helpful and supporting relationships were the most successful.
- *Insight* is increased within the client with regard to his or her particular problems. How such understanding is developed is perhaps not particularly important; all approaches provide some sort of explanation for human distress and evoke a belief that by engaging in particular activities such distress can be alleviated.
- *Healthy and adaptive responses are reinforced* somehow within the relationship. This may be explicit as in a behavioural approach or implicit in the therapist's behaviour. Therapists may be unaware of their subtle reinforcement of adaptive responses from clients, however all therapies have an aim of producing positive change, which suggests an influence somehow upon clients' behaviour.

mind through to the development of laws and public policy.

Very early psychological thinking would ally philosophical ideas with biological or physiological scientific methodology. These sciences themselves have a long history. Hippocrates, for example, had begun observing how the brain controlled the organs of the body. This type of work paved the way for the development of modern medicine and greater understanding of human physiology. Eventually, these philosophical and physiological strands of thinking would lead to the cognitive and biological perspectives that initially underpinned approaches to the study of psychology itself. Other perspectives, which will be outlined later, have since emerged to make up the modern approach to psychology as a whole (see Fig. 22.1). There are a number of perspectives which contribute to the development of a psychological understanding of the individual. Each brings a different approach and explanation of human behaviour and makes a contribution to the whole.

These various perspectives may appear to conflict in certain areas, however they should not be regarded as being mutually exclusive. Rather, they will each bring a different focus and emphasis to different elements of the same situation or event (see Table 22.1).

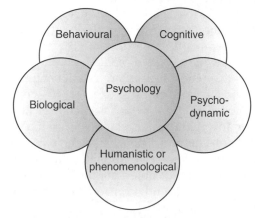

Figure 22.1   Different perspectives of psychology.

Table 22.1   Underlying assumptions and features of behavioural, psychodynamic, cognitive and humanistic models of human behaviour (adapted from Ellis & Gates 1995, with kind permission from Churchill Livingstone)

Issues	Behavioural	Psychodynamic	Cognitive	Humanistic
Philosophical view of the person	All behaviour learned in response to environment	Behaviour originates from our past experiences	Behaviour indicative of a problem-solving organism	Behaviour drives an individual to self-actualise
Internal versus external causes of behaviour	Emphasis placed on external world causing behaviour	Interactive relationship between inner and outer world	Reciprocal relationship between external and internal worlds	Balance is sought between two worlds to create harmony
Self-concept	Self is not central as it is unobservable and therefore unmeasurable	Concept of ego central to understanding self	Important in self-praise, self-criticism and self-regulation	Self a central concept combining thought, feeling and behaviour
State of awareness	Awareness and insight not relevant	Unconscious most important. Interplay between conscious and unconscious behaviour	Behaviour may not be unconscious but automatic and rehearsed	Mostly concerned with the here and now, and existentialism
Feeling, thought and behaviour	Behaviour central; thought and feeling not relevant to (excluding cognitive behaviour therapy)	Feeling, thought and behaviour all understanding behaviour	Cognition thought and understanding important in behaviour	Lived and central to unique experience; feeling and thought and behaviour should be in harmony
Role of past, present and future	Present and future important	The past is most important in understanding the present, and both interact	Cognitive maps and schemata enable expectation	Most importance placed upon present

Carl Rogers (1980) has made a similar point with regard to the integration of different perspectives. He suggested that any understanding of man would need to encompass not only an awareness of 'inner cognitive processes; for example as outlined by Piaget (1952), but also an exploration of what he termed 'inner personal emotionalised meanings'. This represents a humanistic perspective – an understanding of the phenomenological world of man and observations of his external behaviour and reactions.

Developing an awareness of the various ways in which we seek to view our lives and construct knowledge of our world is clearly relevant because these ways influence how we view and thus, ultimately, respond to emotional and behavioural distress (Gates 1995). The broad aim of psychology is that through the development of knowledge about behavioural and mental processes, human beings will be able to lead basically healthier and better lives.

From this perspective and in order to help another person we must clearly develop an understanding of that person; in this respect, our initial position must be one of not knowing. We must acknowledge that at first we do not understand what a person may or may not understand about his or her life. Ultimately, in order to help, we need to know more than the other, but we must not reach too soon for answers. This would be a mistake; using knowledge without an understanding of the other can be handicapping to the helping process and potentially oppressive. The reader should see work by Laing (1982), Szasz (1987) and Masson (1997) regarding the potential for oppressive practice.

Freud (1990) regarded his psychoanalytic approach as essentially an exploration of an individual's life, and although the approach was knowledge based, he did not primarily seek to provide solutions to problems or indeed 'cures' as such. Rather, he sought to enable his patients to develop a richer understanding of their lives thereby helping them to 'work and love more effectively'. Whereas this presents us with particular problems when we look for ways to help people with learning disabilities, it is perhaps nevertheless a useful framework for us when thinking about the uses of psychological approaches in our work with this client group.

The prime focus does not always have to be 'cure' per se – the reduction of aggressive behaviour, for example, enabling a better understanding for both clients and carers, may sometimes be sufficient and therapeutic enough in itself.

The next section briefly outlines five perspectives, which represent the main approaches used by psychology in modern times. Each offers a different framework for understanding why people behave and think as they do and each can contribute something towards our overall understanding of the whole individual.

Biological perspective

As we have stated earlier, the exploration and study of links between the physiological functioning of individuals and their behaviour is not new. All psychological events can be linked to activity in the brain and nervous system. In terms of treatment, for instance, humanity has from the earliest times utilised naturally occurring drugs such as opium and hashish in order to alter mood or to treat anxiety, phobias and so on. However, it was not until the middle of the 19th century that the scientific world began to take an active interest in such remedies (Turkistani 2000).

Biological or physiological psychology is now a huge field of research, which is constantly developing new areas of knowledge, particularly in neurology and genetics. The brain however, with its multitude of nerve cells and infinite number of interconnections, is hugely complex and our knowledge of neural functioning remains, despite modern advances and discoveries, somewhat inadequate.

The biological perspective has made significant progress in a number of areas, which are clearly of use in terms of health care. The search for a neurophysiological basis for learning and memory, for instance, has emphasised the importance of particular brain structures. The hippocampus has been linked with these functions (Gustaffson & Wigstrom 1988) as have various chemical processes within the brain. See work by Green (1987), Atkinson et al (1990) and Thompson (1975) for further information in this area.

The physiological basis of emotions has been explored by William James and Carl Lange. The James–Lange theory suggested that emotion basically consisted of the perception of the physiological changes brought about by an emotional stimulus (Gray 1987). Other areas of success from the biological perspective include work in the area of stress, not only the immediate physiological changes brought about by acute stress but also those from exposure to prolonged stress. Classic work by Hans Selye (1956) provides a good introduction to this work.

The link between eating disorders and the role of the hypothalamus and more peripheral mechanisms, such as the endocrine system, have led to a better integration of treatment regimens, bringing together factors involving personality, social norms and brain physiology. Further exploration of abnormal eating patterns can be found in Logue (1986) or Duker and Slade (1988).

Finally, explorations into the physiological aspects of mental illness have brought about many advances in the treatment of the various illnesses, particularly in the chemotherapeutic treatment of various conditions such as depression, schizophrenia and mania. See Turkistani (2000), Mackay and Iverson (1992) and Weller (1992) for further information.

Freud always believed that there would emerge physiological explanations for many of the psychological disorders that he was exploring and certainly this branch of psychology is producing new data all the time. Many aspects of behaviour and mental functioning can be better understood through knowledge of the biological processes involved and, ultimately, one might expect that the treatment of some disorders will become more successful because of this.

Cognitive perspective

In some respects the cognitive perspective is something of a return to the early philosophical roots of psychology in its focus upon mental processes. However it is more clearly concerned with the study and interpretation of those processes rather than with introspection alone.

It is now regarded as a well-researched approach and is based on the premise that our thoughts and beliefs primarily influence our behaviours and emotions. Hence an individual's appraisal of an event or situation can determine his or her emotional and behavioural response. Helping individuals to change how they view or appraise events can impact positively upon their emotional problems (Beck 1976).

The modern cognitive approach has also developed as a response to the perceived shortcomings and narrowness of behaviourism and, perhaps to a lesser degree, psychoanalysis. Both approaches have been criticised for not distinguishing sufficiently between human behaviour and animal behaviour – psychoanalysis because of its initial emphasis upon the influence of basic instincts and drives and behaviourism for its emphasis on conditioning in respect of learning, neither taking enough account of people's thoughts, beliefs and other internal processes. Tolman (1925) conducted experiments with rats in a maze, which demonstrated that links between an external event and behaviour were not as straightforward as behaviourists suggested. He offered an insight into the interaction of behaviour and mental experience (Gates 1998).

Piaget (1952) and his associates stressed these mentalistic concepts such as 'cognition' – which had fallen from favour with psychologists from the behaviourist tradition – and went on to demonstrate the relationship between cognitive abilities and learning and human development. This chiefly led to the development of modern cognitive psychology.

Generally, a cognitive approach advocates an active role for the therapist in the process of helping and is essentially humanistic in that it emphasises a holistic view of the individual and focuses on personal growth. Turnbull (1998) has outlined the following assumptions underpinning cognitive behavioural interventions:

- Cognitions exist.
- External events are processed by cognitions to create personal meaning for an individual.
- Almost all behaviour is a product of an interaction between external events, cognitions and emotions.

- Cognitions are the primary target for change in therapeutic interventions.

Cognitive behavioural interventions are now seen as the leading psychotherapeutic approach of modern times (Blackburn et al 1981, Hollon et al 1991) enabling people to address and overcome particular emotional difficulties. Matlin (1994) has offered a useful overview of various cognitive approaches for readers who may wish to explore further.

Behavioural perspective

This perspective focuses upon observable behaviour only and is little concerned with mental experience or the brain and nervous system. The American psychologist John B Watson first developed this view in the early 1900s; he believed that only through the study of observable and measurable behaviour could a proper objective science of psychology be developed. He believed essentially that behaviour was largely determined by external, environmental factors. (Watson & Raynor 1920). The offshoot of this approach – stimulus–response psychology – remains influential today. A perhaps better known exponent of behaviourism contemporary to Watson was Pavlov (1902) who identified 'conditioning' and described the relationship between what he called unconditioned responses and unconditional stimuli. Through his famous work with dogs, which has been extensively written about elsewhere (see McCue 1998), he demonstrated how, through a process of association, a conditioned or learned response could be elicited. This notion of how behaviour could be learned was called 'classical conditioning'. This work was developed further by Watson and, amongst others, B F Skinner in the 1950s (Skinner 1953), who extolled the notion that behaviour was mostly functional and stimulated and maintained by external factors. He developed the behavioural definitions of reinforcement contingencies – positive reinforcement, which would strengthen behavioural responses, and negative reinforcement and punishment contingencies, which would weaken behavioural responses. Essentially, Skinner demonstrated that if a particular behaviour was positively reinforced, then the frequency of that behaviour would likely be increased. This work was hugely influential, suggesting that behaviour could be shaped and modified by the use of reinforcement. This aspect of behaviourism, known as operant conditioning or, in an applied form, behaviour modification, has provided an effective technology for helping individuals to change their behaviour. Although much debated and criticised, and with few psychologists today regarding themselves as strict behaviourists, these theories remain important with many modern developments in psychology evolving from them.

Psychodynamic perspective

Sigmund Freud developed the psychoanalytic conception of human behaviour in the early part of the 20th century. The term 'psychodynamic' is a generic term which encompasses Freud's theories along with others concerned with human emotional development. Freud's theories were something of a combination of ideas from contemporary thinking in cognition and physiology, utilising notions of consciousness, perception and memory, with others about biologically based instinctive drives, particularly those related to sexuality and aggression. Freud's basic premise was that much of our mental activity is unconscious and that much of the way we behave stems from that process. Thus, an individual's way of being in the world will be influenced by beliefs, fears and desires of which that person has no awareness. He suggested that these impulses were innate and how they were dealt with within earliest relationships with parents and significant others would influence and shape the nature of an individual's internal world. This internal world, depending upon the nature and quality of our earliest relationships, may be characterised by fears and doubts, anxiety to please or it may, of course, be secure and balanced. Freud believed that these early experiences exerted their impact in powerful ways, shaping and sometimes distorting our experience and behaviour. He believed that all of our behaviour had a cause, usually related to our unconscious, rather than to any rational explanation that we may give. Freud believed that repressed traumatic memories of childhood or other unconscious mechanisms of control caused emotional disorders. He called such methods of control 'defence mechanisms'. These are still referred to commonly as denial, rationalisation, sublimation, repression and projection. His work was to try and help patients recognise and then reconcile these hitherto hidden or forgotten aspects of their psyches into their conscious lives. Freud's work has given us a language which enables us to talk about, and begin to make sense of, our complex internal worlds. Psychodynamic approaches now comprise a wide number of interrelated theories that collectively seek to explain human behaviour and all have roots in Freud's psychoanalytic theories. At the last count there were some 400 different sorts of therapy using such theories. Whilst there is a great deal of overlap between them all, there is no therapy that has been proved definitively to be better than another. 'All have won and all must have prizes' (from *Alice in Wonderland*) is an apposite phrase used by Lambert (1986) in his review of outcome research in this field. This research also shows that it is not, in the end, the theoretical background of the therapist or the techniques used that are the most important factors in successful therapy, but rather the quality of the relationship and the goodness of fit between the therapist and client. Whilst this approach has shortcomings as a scientific theory and plays a less central role in psychological thinking than it did some 50 or 60 years ago, it remains the most comprehensive and influential theory of personality ever created. Many of its ideas have been absorbed into the mainstream of psychological thinking and into the social sciences, the humanities, the arts and society in general. Readers wishing to explore this further are referred to Brown (1993) and Clarkson & Pokorny (1994). Sinason (1991) and Waitman & Conboy-Hill (1992) refer more directly to learning disability.

Phenomenological perspective

A phenomenological approach towards understanding human experience and behaviour developed during the 1950s. Focusing on the subjective experience of human beings, this perspective rejected some of the notions extolled in other perspectives to psychology, believing them to be too mechanistic or based overly upon the behaviour of rats, dogs, pigeons or chimpanzees. The aims and goals of a phenomenological approach would also differ from other perspectives in that they would be focused more upon understanding and describing the inner world of individuals rather than perhaps on developing theories or predicting behaviour. The goal would be to help individuals transfer the gains made through an increased awareness in therapy into everyday life. Carl Rogers (1951) was an early exponent of this approach which became known as 'humanistic psychology', the basic premise of which is that people must be understood in the context of their own unique experience. Although there is no single, clear theoretical focus, two underlying principles to understanding human behaviour were articulated. First, individuals were not simply objects responding passively and unknowingly to forces beyond their control, but they were seen as dynamic and interactive and thus capable of controlling their own destinies. Individuals were the authors of their own unique stories, capable of making choices and setting goals and consequently accountable for their own life choices. This encourages individuals to find the potential for change within themselves. Secondly, people's primary motivation and thus purpose for their behaviour was simply about developing their potential to its fullest. Abraham Maslow (1954), famous for his hierarchy of human needs, suggested that the motivation for all human behaviour is about being alive and moving towards self-actualisation – 'being whatever we can be'. This drive towards self-actualisation is what distinguishes us from animals and it is this emphasis which brings the term 'humanistic' to some phenomenological theories. A phenomenological or humanistic approach would draw from other fields outside of psychology and medicine in order to understand the human condition, believing that psychology alone cannot define what makes a person uniquely human. In this respect it is perhaps more aligned with the arts and humanities than with science. A humanistic approach acknowledges the dangers of 'scientism' and its propensity to view human beings rather too narrowly on occasion, depending on what particular aspects of human behaviour lend themselves to scientific study and analysis. A balanced approach would manage to integrate both scientific and humanistic perspectives to addressing problems of the mind and behaviour. A phenomenological or humanistic approach is essentially an optimistic type of therapy concerned with human potential.

SPECIFIC APPROACHES TO THERAPY

Having outlined the main perspectives that make up the whole that is 'psychology', we will now briefly explore various specific approaches to treatment. There are in fact numerous approaches available, ranging from the purely behavioural which downplays the role of feelings and the nature of self, through to the more humanistic approaches which place the person at the centre and focus more directly upon the individual's unique experience of the world.

Thus far, variations on forms of behaviourism have tended to dominate the field with regard to learning disability. This approach has been extensively reported in the literature and therefore will not be explored in great depth here. We are beginning to see the more widespread application of other more psychodynamically oriented approaches and some of these will be outlined. For a long time, learning disabled people were rarely considered to be appropriate for psychotherapeutic treatment (Bungener & McCormack 1994) due to concerns around IQ and verbal ability. However, we know that communication happens on more than one level and often occurs through processes that we use out of awareness. These may include facial expression and other types of body language, tone of voice and even silence, which may contribute to our awareness of others' mood, meaning or state of mind.

Sinason (1992) has also written about the notion of 'emotional intelligence' which is not necessarily correlated with cognitive ability, wherein an individual can be emotionally aware and knowledgeable despite deficits in cognitive intelligence. Bates (1992) has suggested that working with people with learning disabilities in a psychotherapeutic way is only different from working with non-disabled individuals in terms of the time span and rhythm of the process. Although there is a paucity of research about the suitability of this client group for psychotherapeutic work, Sinason (1988, 1992) and Frankish (1989) have shown that such work is feasible and emphasise that psychotherapy and psychological approaches in general are not necessarily just about speaking.

Cognitive analytic therapy (CAT)

Like all cognitive based interventions, this approach is based on the belief that an individual's thoughts, perceptions and assumptions will have a significant influence over that person's behaviour. The approach focuses upon discovering how problems first arose and how procedures that were originally devised to cope with them may no longer be useful. Thus problems need to be understood in the context of an individual's personal history and life experience. The assumption is that although an individual's actions may seem painful and self-defeating, they began from a positive intention of self-protection and have become too familiar to leave. If the patterns that

Reader activity 22.1

Spend a few minutes looking at a current pattern of behaviour of your own and try to trace it back to its possible origins in how you learned to deal with something earlier in your life. Possible examples might be something that really irritates you, a situation that you have become scared of or how you have overcome a former difficulty. Perhaps you react strongly to something in a way not really warranted by the situation.

- What feeling is associated with this?
- What beliefs/thoughts does it trigger off and how do you act?
- What experience created this pattern in the past?

The most important thing is that you get a sense of just how much past developmental experiences influence your life choices today.

underlie the often chaotic behaviours can be understood and put into words, then perhaps the process can be changed and individuals can be freed from the destructive control of the cycle.

A cognitive analytic approach will focus on recognising how an individual's particular coping procedures originated and on how they might be adapted and improved. The issues that we refer to when talking about 'coping' tend to be emotional ones. Emotions can be generated by events or by our interactions with others. Our ways of coping bring with them beliefs and behaviours which act in the future to constrain our 'ways of being' in response to certain events. Even though a means of survival or way of coping we have developed in the past may no longer serve us very well, we may well continue to use it because it is the path of least resistance. It can be difficult (and scary) to try and change, and will require effort over a period of time. The strengths and resources of the individual are mobilised in the task of ameliorating self-limiting patterns of emotional expression or inhibition. Thus the work is active and shared. The therapist will use diagrams of procedures and written outlines developed with clients in order to help them recognise and revise old patterns that are not working very well. The therapist will try to find the main emotional patterns that clients have in relating both to their selves and to others and then seek to understand their connections to the clients' current problems or distress. Central to this is the identification of 'reciprocal emotional roles' (see Ryle 1990) which are maintained by a variety of old, familiar, established and emotionally driven coping strategies. These coping strategies, as we have seen, may once have provided relief from distressing and damaging early experiences.

Cognitive analytic theory suggests that we all have a repertoire of roles acquired from our earliest interactions with our parents and other significant care givers. We also perceive others as playing reciprocal roles. To understand patterns of interacting now, we need to identify what roles the child was placed in by the parents. This can be done by specifying:

- How the parent was (for example abusive, rejecting, critical)

- How the child responded emotionally (for example frightened, angry, withdrawn).

These reciprocal roles are:

Parent:	Abusive	Rejecting	Over-protective
	↕	↕	↕
Child:	Frightened Hurt	Hurt Worthless Bad	Smothered Taken Over

The number of roles the child develops depends on the number of roles parents (or significant others) assume. For some individuals it is a limited number which then act as the template for all future interaction, as it is all the person knows.

For direct care staff and others, this means that a client with learning disabilities will automatically assign us to one category as well! Individuals learn to play either end of the roles, which are eventually internalised and characterise their own particular internal dialogue. It is this internal dialogue which seeks expression and extension in interaction with others. These processes occur automatically in the form of patterns and routines, which once mobilised remain robust even in the face of contradictory information. Thus, reciprocal roles, in terms of actions and expectations, stick with us (although they may become more integrated and elaborated as we develop). Initial patterns and templates remain even if they are inadequate to our current circumstances.

A cognitive analytic approach is educative in its approach to the helping relationship, giving clients an opportunity to understand and thus collaborate better with both the purposes and methods of helping with their problems. This approach also allows for the development of creative ways of communicating and using the model. This is particularly relevant in working with a person with learning disabilities.

The process has a strong narrative element in the retelling of the client's history and how that person has survived particular difficulties and struggles. There is also a descriptive element in that current damaging or maladaptive procedures are described. Again, these can be presented in creative ways; diagrams are often used.

Reader activity 22.2

This exercise illustrates the way in which each of us has different styles in terms of relating to other people. In a sense, these are all different patterns of reciprocal roles. Find a quiet place and close your eyes. Bring to mind a person with whom you have frequent contact. Have an imaginary conversation with that person. Continue this for about a minute. Now listen to yourself. Notice your tone of voice, the content of your speech, whether or not you are open and relaxed or quiet and defensive. Now imagine another person has joined you. Switch the conversation to that person. Notice the change in your tone, content and status with regard to that person. Continue that conversation for about a minute before switching back to the first person. Notice how you feel at the moment of switching back. Check your thinking, feeling and physical status. Now let yourself imagine a third conversation, this time with the person you feel most comfortable with. Notice how your tone, manner, thoughts, feelings and physical status change again. Explore what it is about this person that makes them so easy to talk to. Notice any similarities between this person and yourself.

Case illustration 22.1

In this case, Adam is a man in his 30s who has a history of self-harming behaviour which has led to many admissions to mental health acute units over the years. The service and Adam seem stuck in a repeating cycle of admissions and discharges; just when things seem to be improving Adam seems to sabotage the progress in some way and ultimately ends up hurting himself. Adam had a mother who switched from being rather needy and somewhat excessively 'motherly' in her relationship with him to being very critical and physically abusive, particularly at times when Adam sought to do his own things without her. Adam learned that in order to get the love he needed from her, he had to stay close and allow his mother to care for him in her way, even if that felt stifling of his own wants in some way. He realised that if he didn't take care of her needs in this way then something bad would inevitably happen and he would not get the love and care that he needed. Adam now lived alone, although he had had a series of relationships which had been characterised by their intensity and volatility. He was unable to hold down jobs for long; despite being relatively intelligent and able he always ended up in arguments with his bosses or would turn up late or not at all.

Cognitive analytic therapy can be a relatively brief process (from 4–24 sessions) which does not lose any depth of psychological engagement and insight with the client and his or her concerns. The overall aim is to help clients and perhaps others involved in their care to develop the capacity to recognise faulty procedures so that they can start to control and replace them. It can help carers to avoid getting stuck in re-enacting and thus colluding with damaging ways of relating. It is this non-collusion and working through of these re-enactments which is at the centre of effective therapy. This approach has been used with couples, in groups and in organisations; it has also been used with adults, adolescents and children and people with learning disabilities.

Case illustration 22.1 shows the insight that can be gained from a cognitive analytic approach.

Adam's reciprocal roles and patterns of behaviour may be shown diagramatically (see Fig. 22.2).

From this it can be seen how Adam switches from one 'self state' (reciprocal role) to another and how he induces others to play their part. This whole process is a re-enactment of early formative relationships and others, including the health

service, unwittingly collude with this pattern. It must be remembered that this is not a conscious process on the part of Adam even though it appears to be manipulative.

Cognitive analytic therapy uses and develops ideas and methods from a number of other traditions. The main sources are:

- **Psychoanalysis** Particularly concepts of object relations, conflict, defence and transference. These are articulated in cognitive terms and therapists are more active within the therapeutic relationship and perhaps also their inteventions are more varied than psychoanalytic therapies.
- **Kelly's personal construct theory** (Kelly 1955) A focus on how people make sense of the world, the concept of 'man as scientist', repertory grids and cooperative, common sense work with clients.
- **Cognitive behavioural approaches** (see Turnbull 2000) The teaching of clients to observe and record their own moods, thoughts and symptoms. The step-by-step planning and management of change. However, the cognitive

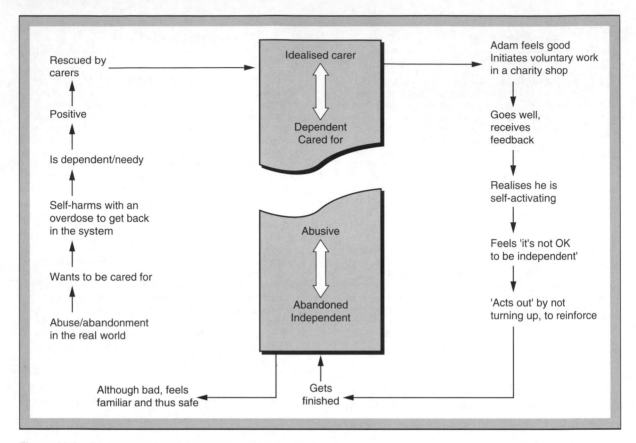

Figure 22.2 Reciprocal roles and patterns of behaviour of Adam.

analytic therapy (CAT) approach is not confined only to visible behaviours and conscious thoughts, however it takes account of transference and unconscious processes too.

Rational emotive therapy (RET)

This approach was developed in the late 1950s/early 1960s by Albert Ellis (1962) and was one of the first therapies to be based primarily on a cognitive model of human behaviour. It is generally considered to be less collaborative and more directive than cognitive behavioural therapy (CBT). The basic premise of RET is that human beings have two basic biological drives:
—a tendency towards irrationality
—the potential to change.

This approach postulates that people perpetuate their psychological distress because of their own theories concerning the cause of their problems. They also tend to attribute the cause of their problems to situations and events rather than to their beliefs about these situations and events. Thus, individuals are less distressed by events themselves than by the way they interpret them. Because people are generally unaware of this process, they continually reindoctrinate themselves with these thinking

Reader activity 22.3

An individual may predict that a social encounter will go wrong, for instance that he or she may become tongue-tied. This belief in itself may well be enough to make the person anxious and thus become tongue-tied! By attributing the cause to the event, the irrational belief is reinforced.

Can you identify similar beliefs in your own thinking? How do such thoughts influence your expectations and thus behaviour, in certain situations?

errors and self-defeating beliefs. Inability or reluctance to change may be due to clients unwillingness to move out of their comfort zone allied to a tendency to be anxious about their own anxiety.

The RET approach focuses on helping people to identify and modify irrational thoughts and beliefs. This may involve helping people to make quite profound philosophical changes to enable them to give up their irrational demands on themselves and others, accepting themselves unconditionally and increasing their tolerance for frustration. Behavioural and educative elements are incorporated into the therapy with the aim of developing and maintaining the client's motivation during the work. The therapy can be offered on a long- or short-term basis and is best suited to treating specific problems that can be clearly identified and articulated.

Cognitive behavioural therapy (CBT)

The terms 'cognitive therapy' and 'cognitive behaviour therapy' can be confusing as they are often used interchangeably. Most types of cognitive therapy incorporate behavioural strategies to some degree. These strategies are an important element of the treatment as they enable clients to experiment with different ways of behaving, which helps them to discern whether certain ways of thinking are either unhelpful or unrealistic. CBT is based upon a model which explains how the relationship between thinking and feeling can evoke and maintain emotional distress and aims to try and change both a person's cognitions (thinking, perceptions, assumptions) and their behaviour. There has been much debate about whether cognitions directly cause behaviour and come before emotional responses to events or whether the relationship between them is less linear and more interactive (Lazarus 1984, Zajonc 1984). Hollin (1990) suggests that cognitions can both shape and be shaped by events. Thus there is a continuous feedback loop between the external event, the cognitions evoked and the emotional and behavioural responses.

Case illustration 22.2

Consider an individual with an obsessive-compulsive disorder, constantly checking that his door is locked when leaving the house for instance, to the extent that the leaving ritual can go on for an hour or more. The external event (leaving the house) triggers anxiety in this person who in turn believes that checking his locks will relieve that anxiety. The act of checking seems to work in this respect and thus the original belief is reinforced. The disorder is sustained by this vicious circle.

As has previously been stated, the assumption of a cognitive approach is that on the basis of experience, people form conclusions about themselves, others and the world. In the presence of appropriate circumstances, these beliefs and assumptions are activated, giving rise to negative automatic thoughts (i.e. specific cognitions). These in turn trigger negative feelings, physiological symptoms and behaviours. The vicious circle is established where negative thoughts lead to painful feelings, changes in physiological arousal and unhelpful behaviour (e.g. avoidance, withdrawal or, as in our example, compulsive behaviour); these in turn act to maintain and reinforce the thoughts. A cognitive model, describing how low self-esteem can be maintained is shown in Figure 22.3.

In this model, adapted from Fennell (1997), it can be seen how the interaction of the individual temperament with early experiences has led to the development of low self-esteem. On this basis the person judges him or herself negatively and expresses this conclusion in various terms (which will differ from person to person). Beck et al (1990) would call these thoughts 'schema'. The person would then develop personal guidelines for living, which will allow him or her to function and avoid the distress emanating from negative self-judgements or schema. These guidelines represent ways of coping although the person remains vulnerable, particularly in circumstances where his or her assumptions cannot or may not be met, for instance when feeling unloved or rejected. Unfortunately, the individual's negative self-judgements or schema remain intact and if a

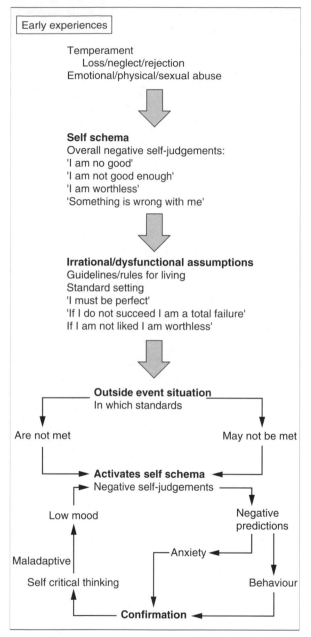

Figure 22.3 depicts:

Early experiences

Temperament
 Loss/neglect/rejection
Emotional/physical/sexual abuse

Self schema
Overall negative self-judgements:
'I am no good'
'I am not good enough'
'I am worthless'
'Something is wrong with me'

Irrational/dysfunctional assumptions
Guidelines/rules for living
Standard setting
'I must be perfect'
'If I do not succeed I am a total failure'
'If I am not liked I am worthless'

Outside event situation
In which standards

Are not met   May not be met

Activates self schema
Negative self-judgements

Low mood   Negative
                             predictions

                 Anxiety

Maladaptive

Self critical thinking   Behaviour

Confirmation

Figure 22.3 A cognitive model depicting how self-esteem can be maintained.

situation arises where the standards set by the dysfunctional assumptions cannot be met, these judgements are activated. This triggers the vicious circle of thinking, feeling and behaviour which ultimately maintains the whole process. It can be seen from this model how a cognitive

behavioural approach can be regarded as interactional. It also illustrates the importance of taking into account both external and internal factors such as early life experiences, significant life events, physiological and psychological factors and the influence of significant others in the life of the individual (Black et al 1997). The central point is that problems are provoked and maintained by faulty or irrational thinking. This is a style of thinking that we all engage in occasionally, however it only becomes problematic when such thoughts begin to have a negative impact upon our lives, on the lives of others or perhaps both.

Reader activity 22.4

Aaron Beck (1976) has categorised errors of thinking. Can you recognise any such errors in your own view of the world?

1. *Arbitrary inference* We draw negative conclusions about an event despite there being no real evidence to support that view. For example, 'my partner no longer cares for me because he/she did not call today'.

2. *Selective abstraction* We focus upon a particular (usually negative) detail and exclude other (usually more positive) evidence. For example, we focus only on the critical content of feedback which also contains good points, and conclude that we are thought to be completely no good.

3. *Over generalisation* We make a broad, generalised conclusion on the basis of one event. For instance, an individual who fails a job interview concludes that he or she will 'never get a job'.

4. *Magnification and minimisation* We overemphasise the importance of a negative event without acknowledging more positive aspects. For example, after one bad day at work an individual may conclude 'I am a terrible nurse/social worker/occupational therapist/psychologist'.

5. *Personalisation* We perceive a situation from a self-centred point of view, relating events to ourselves unrealistically. For example, 'if I had been kinder to my father he would still be alive today'.

6. *Absolutist dichotomous thinking* We can only think things are either all good or all bad with no in between. For example, if the sprouts are under-cooked the whole Christmas meal 'is a disaster'.

Treatment approaches

Treatment is essentially a collaborative process that involves the client and therapist working together on routes to take that feel safe and manageable, seeking to uncover the interpretations and evaluations that might be contributing to a client's distorted view of the world. An initial assessment could include the following:

- Exploration of the client's background, including early experiences
- A functional analysis would identify emotionally arousing situations and other trigger factors
- Arousal levels, patterns of behaviour, current coping strategies could be evaluated
- Psychological questionnaires could be utilised to measure features of anxiety or depression, patterns of relationships and so on
- Cognitions (for example thoughts, expectations and appraisals of events) would be identified
- Motivation to change
- Capacity to follow the treatment plan, which may involve 'homework' and self-report measures.

Treatment could include:

- The provision of information about specific disorders, i.e. agoraphobia, stress, anxiety and so on
- Social skills training. This could involve role play to re-enact troublesome situations and apply new perspectives
- Applied relaxation techniques for situations which evoke distress
- Stress management/anger management techniques
- Problem solving techniques. Castles & Glass (1986) developed a framework for use by people with a learning disability
- Challenging dysfunctional thinking and negative automatic thoughts
- Modelling
- Cognitive distraction – such as imaginary techniques
- In vivo practices of new behaviours and techniques
- Mood monitoring charts and the use of other self-report measures
- Systematic desensitisation, graded exposure to stressful situations.

The aim of therapy is to achieve personal growth through the development of new insights and understandings as well as to acquire new skills. With its focus upon the development of human potential the approach has similarities with humanistic concepts, although most practitioners would not strictly define their approach in this way despite the shared characteristics. CBT has established itself as the treatment of choice for problems such as anxiety and depression (Hollon et al 1991) and other disorders which prevent people from functioning normally, such as obsessive-compulsive disorder, panic disorders, relationship problems and other compulsive behaviours.

There are various accounts that demonstrate how people with a learning disability can be helped. See Stenfert-Kroese et al (1997) and Turnbull (2000) for examples.

Behavioural approaches

There are a variety of therapeutic methods which are rooted in the principles of learning and conditioning emanating from the early work of Watson, Pavlov and Skinner outlined earlier. A strict behavioural approach would focus very much on the behaviour itself and aim to develop fairly circumscribed goals, often relating to the modification of specific behaviours in particular situations.

Early behavioural approaches suggested that behaviour, for the most part, was determined by environmental factors external to the individual. This contrasts with the other perspectives discussed which tend to focus within the individual for causes.

More recently, however, behavioural approaches have broadened their scope and seek to integrate internal factors such as emotion, perception and cognition with biological, social and environmental factors in understanding the causation of behavioural distress (McCue 2000). Interventions are now more likely to reflect this integrative process by being based upon changing systems, culture and environment as well as changing individuals in order to reduce such distress.

Furthermore, the reciprocal influence of carers in the cause and maintenance of behavioural distress, in respect of their personal beliefs, values, attitudes and behaviours, is particularly relevant when developing models which explain the behaviour of people with a learning disability. McGill et al (1996) discuss this process in particular.

Probably the most important beliefs that behaviourists hold are first, that behaviour is functional for the individual in some way and secondly that personal and environmental factors, in particular consequences, will both shape and maintain that behaviour. This process is, to a large extent, dependent upon a process of positive and negative reinforcements, which are presented (or at least anticipated) within that individual's particular context. Reinforcement is defined in Box 22.2.

It must be remembered that what may be experienced as reinforcing for one individual may not evoke the same response in another. Similarly, negative consequences will have variable impacts amongst individuals; what may be punishing to one may actually be rewarding to another and vice versa. Culture, context, personal history and preferences will also play a part in the strength or otherwise of the reinforcement. Thus causal and maintaining factors may vary considerably between individuals. The first stage of a behavioural approach would involve a behaviour assessment.

Box 22.2 The nature of reinforcement (after McCue 2000)

- Positive reinforcement is the presentation of positive consequences and will have the effect of reinforcing the behaviour, making it more likely to be repeated.
- Punishment is the presentation of negative or aversive consequences which will have the effect of weakening behaviour, making it less likely to be repeated.
- Removal of positive reinforcement will also produce a punitive effect through the removal of desirable consequences – this is as opposed to the presentation of a negative consequence. The removal of attention (a desirable consequence) through a process of 'time out' would be an example of this.
- Negative reinforcement is the removal of negative consequences, which has a reinforcing effect also.

Functional analysis

This is the process of seeking to understand the relationship between the various stimuli in the environment and the shaping and maintenance of behaviour through reinforcement. The question to be addressed is: what function or functions does a behaviour serve for an individual in a particular context? This will involve the observation and measurement of behaviours aiming to link reinforcing consequences and behaviour, whilst setting them against an understanding of historical, contextual and cultural factors pertaining to that individual. Emerson (1993) and O'Neill et al (1990) provide good overviews of this process.

The ABC model of functional analysis This is a process of measuring and recording behaviours taking into account the antecedents and consequences of those behaviours.

It is based on the assumption that what occurs just prior to the behaviour (antecedents) and afterwards (consequences) will either partly or fully represent the function of the behaviour. This is represented diagramatically in Figure 22.4 and explained below:

- Antecedents: These are factors that occur immediately before the behaviour in question and could include anything that might seem of significance. This may include location, people nearby, noise, activity, communication and so on.
- Behaviour: This would be as precise and complete a description as possible. Frequency, intensity and duration would be significant along with a clear description of how the behaviour manifested.
- Consequences: Again, a clear description of the consequences of the behaviour is crucial as this will point to the possible function of the behaviour.

This information may be gathered in a structured way using an ABC chart (Antecedent–

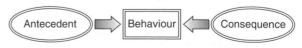

Figure 22.4 The ABC model of functional analysis.

Behaviour–Consequence record). There are a variety of other strategies, which may be used in a behavioural assessment. These could include various interview strategies with the client and/or significant others, structured and semi-structured observational and recording techniques (such as ABC charts) and analysis of and experimentation with setting events (triggers) and other contingencies relating to the behaviour. McCue (2000), Gardner & Graeber (1994), O'Neill et al (1990) already mentioned, and others give examples of various behavioural assessment approaches which the reader may wish to explore further.

A thorough behavioural assessment would not only include a functional analysis of factors serving to precipitate or maintain the behaviour, but also provide a picture of the individual's strengths and skills. In addition one would need to identify reinforcers, which could be used to support the development of new behaviours, and to consider areas of deficit, which could be developed as alternatives to existing behavioural difficulties. Once a reasonable hypothesis has been developed and problems clearly defined, a range of non-aversive interventions can then be considered to effect the desired behavioural change or reduce distress. McCue (2000) has suggested that methodologies can be broadly classified within a framework based upon the ABC model outlined earlier:

- Antecedent based: Focus upon changing the context of the behaviour and modifying setting events or triggers. This is a proactive approach and aims to prevent the behaviour from occurring. This may include: manipulation of the environment, changing how carers approach or relate to an individual, introducing choice and re-scheduling of activities.
- Behaviour based: Focus upon modifying behaviour more directly; ideally alternatives to the behavioural difficulty will be developed. This helps to displace undesirable behaviours. This may include: modelling and behavioural rehearsal of more adaptive behaviours, self-regulation techniques, shaping alternative behaviours and responses through reinforcement, development of behaviours that are physically incompatible with the undesirable behaviour.
- Consequence based: Focus on the contingencies that may be maintaining the behavioural difficulty. This is a more reactive approach, which can produce ethical dilemmas in relation to their sometimes restrictive focus. This may include: positive reinforcement and extinction, time out, punishment, systematic desensitisation, removal of positive consequences and response interruption.

Pyles & Bailey (1990), Matson (1990), Jones and Eayrs (1993) and Day et al (1994) have provided some further reading on these aspects. There are limitations with the process of functional analysis and with a strict behavioural approach. Clearly human beings and their motivations are complex and ever changing; behavioural approaches need to be sensitive to the other factors and processes which contribute towards the cause of behavioural difficulties and distress in order to be effective. Nonetheless this approach still lies at the heart of much work in the field of learning disability, although this is perhaps more true in relation to teaching and instruction with regard to teaching self-care skills, than with addressing behavioural distress and emotional concerns amongst this population.

Gestalt therapy

Gestalt was first developed as a therapy by Friz and Laura Perls in the 1950s (Perls et al 1951) and is now regarded as one of the main humanistic therapies. Gestalt is a German word, the meaning of which embraces a number of concepts which are to do with pattern, form, systems and configurations: a 'gestalt' is a whole pattern or system.

Reader activity 22.5

Considering internal (personal/psychological) and external (socio-environmental) characteristics, list as many variables as you can which may combine and function as setting events for behavioural difficulties. Use the following headings to group the variables:

- Personal (e.g. mental health, stress levels)
- Environmental (e.g. noise)
- Social (e.g. occupation)

Gestaltists believe that human beings have a need to make sense of the world and to create a wholeness or a complete picture of experience and feelings. The aim of this approach is to enable individuals to discover, explore and experience their own form, pattern and wholeness and to integrate disparate parts of themselves. In this way people can reach their potential and experience their lives more fully. Perls believed that one of the best ways of learning about ourselves, each other and the world was by becoming more aware, particularly of what stood out for us from moment to moment, the idea being that the only truth we can know is what is happening in the present moment. The gestalts we form depend on our level of awareness; a completed gestalt creates a whole that is greater than the sum of its parts. A central part of gestalt psychology is the relationship between 'figure and ground'; in other words, every gestalt has a perceived foreground (figure) and a background (ground) that we may only be partly (if at all) aware of. The bringing of background more into our awareness will help us to make a more meaningful whole of our experience. What is 'figure' is that which is most important or meaningful for that individual at any given moment. This may relate to basic needs such as hunger or sleep through to more complex psychological processes. A good figure is one which clearly stands out from the background. As you read this, for instance, your attention is taken up by the words on the page; other elements in the room you are in become background. You may choose to focus upon the other elements and they would then become foreground at that moment. A gestalt approach would suggest that good experience is dependent upon the perception of one clear figure after another. Once one need has been met (or gestalt completed), an individual can focus clearly on the next and move on with full energy. This process can be interrupted by early traumatic experiences. Individuals may have developed ways of acting which at the time may have been adequate coping mechanisms but which now serve mostly to interfere with healthy contact with the world in the present. The natural completion of gestalts is impaired, leading to 'fixed gestalts' or unfinished/unresolved business. Much of the practice of gestalt is focused upon the exploration of how human needs arise, how they are frustrated and how they are satisfied. This process, the cyclic pattern of gestalt formation and destruction, constitutes the gestalt 'cycle of experience' (see Fig. 22.5).

How the healthy cycle of experience is blocked or disturbed is what is of interest. Perhaps past unmet needs have become incomplete gestalten, which now are preventing the formation of new gestalten through becoming the focus of our attention. The cycle can become disturbed or blocked at any point via a variety of psychological defences (see below); bringing these into awareness and experimenting with new ways of being can help people to grow and develop healthier ways of being in the world and getting their needs met. Examples of disturbances or blocks in the healthy cycle of experience, the pattern of gestalt formation and destruction, are shown in Box 22.3. Such disturbances can occur at any stage of the cycle.

There are other examples, which can be seen in Perls et al (1951) or Clarkson (1989). We all use such defences to some degree in order to protect ourselves. However, if they are over-used, we will not endure discomfort long enough to enable us to explore and take constructive action; the defences can become destructive in nature and ultimately self-defeating. A gestalt approach uses a variety of

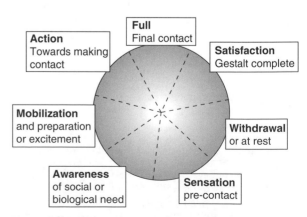

Figure 22.5   The gestalt cycle of experience: After Clarkson (1989).

Box 22.3   Disturbances in the healthy cycle of experience

Desensitisation People avoid experiencing themselves or the world around them. Sensations and feelings become diluted or disregarded and neglected. Pain or discomfort may be ignored and unattended with the ultimate impact upon health unacknowledged.

Deflection People who 'deflect' turn away from contact with others, making their awareness of such contact vague and bland. Feelings will not be shared in their full intensity but are generalised or watered down instead. Such individuals may protect themselves from criticism or hurt but appreciation or love is also kept at bay. This may mean that deep down they continue to feel alienated and abandoned.

Introjection People can be ruled by internalised 'shoulds' taken in or 'swallowed' as children from their families. For example: You're the lazy one, You're the sensible one, Work hard always, Put others first. Perls has suggested that people who introject are always aware of what they should be doing and thus can lack a sense of self-directedness with regard to their own needs. These people can be blocked from taking the appropriate action to get their own needs met.

Projection This is the process of seeing in others what cannot be acknowledged in the self. Thus, traits, attitudes, feelings or ways of behaving that actually belong to our own personality are assigned to others around us and then experienced as being directed towards us. We may be unaware of our own anger or irritation for instance, yet experience someone else as being angry at us. There is often some element of truth in a projection but we may be paying only very selective attention to our environment.

Retroflection This is the process of turning things back against oneself. People can do things to themselves which they really want to do to or with someone else. Instead, perhaps, of expressing anger or aggressive desire towards an abusive parent, individuals harm themselves in some way, perhaps even to the point of suicide. Another kind is when people do to themselves what they want or wanted from someone else. For instance, some people may unconsciously hold or stroke themselves, providing comfort in a way that they wanted a distant or neglectful parent to.

---

techniques and is not entirely confined to being a 'talking therapy'. A gestalt therapist will aim to understand people within their context of race, religion, culture and family and will utilise a holistic frame of reference, which brings together mind and body, action and introspection. Therapists are encouraged to be creative in how they do this, inventing appropriate 'experiments' which may utilise toys, art, role play or actions. The aim is to develop awareness and heighten experiences of contact and relationship with the environment. The patient can address unfinished business through such experiments and through the use of imagination, dreams and fantasies. This approach builds on the idea that the body stores up much of the hurt and pain we experience in our life, particularly in the early stages. It could be fruitful to use such an intervention, acknowledging the possibility of counselling without words, with people who often have a poor sense of self with a limited vocabulary and with limited opportunity to express feelings.

Examples of gestalt experiments

Brainstorming People with learning disabilities are often handicapped in their own emotional and intellectual creativity by the low expectations and judgements of those around them. Engaging in exercises which focus on the generation of ideas about their life without judgement, where what is interesting is more highly valued than what is correct, can provide corrective emotional experiences for such individuals. Brainstorming may involve helping individuals generate as many possible solutions with regard to their problems as they can think of, regardless of how implausible or impractical they may seem. This is done in an atmosphere of playful curiosity where judgement and criticism are set aside. What is possible becomes the focus rather than what is not.

Guided fantasies. People with learning disabilities are often in a position of 'being done to'; using fantasy is a way in which individuals can start to become more active in their lives. New possibilities in terms of feelings, thoughts and actions can be explored and individuals can begin to perceive themselves as being different from the way they are. 'Action' can sometimes start in the head and exercises in imagination encouraged by the therapist can often act as a link between the current reality and the 'conceivable self'.

Dreamwork Perls believed that all dreams have an existential message for the dreamers which they can discover for themselves rather than by relying on the 'interpretations' of others. He regarded all the elements in dreams as projected parts of the self, which could be integrated, owned or at least understood and acknowledged. The intervention involves the dreamer enacting various elements of the dream in the present, as if they were being dreamt now. The possibility is that the dreamer may recognise previously unacknowledged parts of the self in the enactment and thus begin or enhance the process of integration. Freud regarded the dream as the 'royal road to the unconscious'. Perls believed it was the 'royal road to integration'.

Polarisations This is a way in which the different elements of an individual can be explored and experienced. Extremes of personality can be accentuated and acknowledged. Differences between people and within one person can be looked at rather than denied. Individuals who present with an aggressive 'macho' front (perhaps labelled as 'challenging behaviour') may come to recognise a more dependent, passive part of their persona. Through the therapy, via artwork, two-chair work or play perhaps, people can begin to experiment with this less familiar part of themselves. Through this process they may discover new elements and qualities that they can integrate and introduce into their everyday lives. The therapist may encourage or even provoke such polarisations. An obsessive controlling individual may be encouraged to tolerate an element of chaos or uncertainty; a loud, verbose individual could explore silence and wordlessness, a disempowered person could find ways to experience being powerful.

In summary, gestalt is a therapy of awareness which seeks to provide a safe, supportive environment in which individuals can learn about how they relate to themselves and to others, and experiment with new and more satisfying ways of being. It is an approach that has been used with children, adults, individuals, couples and groups.

CONCLUSION

This chapter has suggested that the emotional needs of people with learning disabilities are generally less well understood than their needs associated with independent living skills. However, nurses and other care staff often have to deal with people at their most vulnerable and distressed, addressing difficult and uncomfortable issues from within the context of an intimate caring relationship. Given this, it is perhaps unfortunate that nurses have not always been encouraged to think about feelings, emotions and relationship issues. Although the relationship between psychological and psychodynamic theory and nursing is not clearly defined, these approaches can provide a basis for understanding and working with difficult emotions, both in their clients and in themselves.

This chapter has sought to outline how various perspectives can contribute towards the development of an understanding of human behaviour, and whilst no one perspective can provide all the answers, each contributes something to the whole. Similarly, whilst we have outlined five specific approaches, factors common to each are of equal importance with, if not more important than, particular techniques in bringing about therapeutic change. These common factors are essentially related to the development and maintenance of helping relationships (Lambert 1986). Although behaviour approaches still tend to dominate the field, they have broadened their scope and now seek to integrate internal factors, such as emotion, perception and cognition, with biological, social and environmental factors in understanding and working with behavioural distress. Consequently, practitioners need to develop new skills and awareness in order to be able to work in creative and thoughtful ways in this area.

Whilst it has only been possible here to provide a very brief outline of a few of the myriad approaches available, perhaps readers will be prompted to enquire further in order to develop and expand the boundaries of their practice.

REFERENCES

Atkinson R L, Atkinson R C, Smith E, Bem D, Hilgard E (eds) 1990 Introduction to psychology, 10th edn. Harcourt Brace Jovanovich, Florida

Bates R 1992 Psychotherapy with people with learning difficulties. In: Waitman A, Conboy-Hill S (eds) Psychotherapy and mental handicap. Sage, London

Beck A T 1976 Cognitive therapy and the emotional disorders. International Universities Press, New York

Beck A T, Freeman A et al 1990 Cognitive therapy of personality disorders. Guildford Press, New York

Black L, Cullen C, Novaco R 1997 Anger assessment for people with mild learning disabilities in secure settings. In: Stenfert-Kroese B, Dagnan D, Loumidis K (eds) Cognitive behavioural therapy for people with learning disabilities. Routledge, London

Blackburn I, Bishop S, Glen A, Whalley L, Christie J 1981 The efficacy of cognitive therapy in depression: a treatment trial using cognitive therapy and pharmacotherapy each alone and in combination. British Journal of Psychotherapy 139: 181–189

Bouras N, Kon Y, Drummond C 1993 Medical and psychiatric needs of adults with a mental handicap. Journal of Intellectual Disability Research 37: 177–182

Brandon D 1990 Ordinary magic: a handbook on counselling people with learning disabilities. Tao, Preston

Brown J 1993 Freud and the post-Freudians. Penguin, Middlesex

Bungener J, McCormack B 1994 Psychotherapy and learning disability. In: Clarkson P, Pokorny M (eds) 1994 The handbook of psychotherapy. Routledge, London

Castles E, Glass C 1986 Training in social and interpersonal problem solving skills for mildly and moderately mentally retarded adults. Amercian Journal of Mental Deficiency 91(1): 35–42

Clarkson P 1989 Gestalt counselling in action. Sage, London

Clarkson P, Pokorny M 1994 The handbook of psychotherapy. Routledge, London

Day R, Horner R, Neill R 1994 Multiple functions of problem behaviours: assessment and interventions. Journal of Applied Behaviour Analysis 27: 279–289

Decker R 1988 Effective psychotherapy: the silent dialogue. Hemisphere, New York

Department of Health 1998 Signposts for success in commissioning and providing health services for people with learning disabilities. HMSO, London

Department of Health 1999 A national health service framework for mental health. HMSO, London

Department of Health 2001 Valuing people: a new strategy for learning disability in the 21st century. Cm 5086. HMSO, London

Duker and Slade 1998 Anorexia and bulimia: how to help. Open University Press, London

Ellis A 1962 Reason and emotion in psychotherapy. Lyle Stuart, New York

Ellis R, Gates B 1995 The person in communication. In: Ellis R, Gates R, Kenworthy N (eds) Interpersonal communication in nursing: theory and practice. Churchill Livingstone, Edinburgh

Emerson E 1995 Challenging behaviour: analysis and intervention in people with learning disabilities. Cambridge University Press, Cambridge

Emmerson E 1993 Challenging behaviour and severe learning disability: recent developments in behavioural analysis and interventions. Behavioural and Cognitive Psychology 21: 171–198

Fennell M 1997 Low self-esteem: a cognitive perspective. Journal of the British Association for Behavioural and Cognitive Psychotherapies 25(1): 25

Frankish P 1989 Meeting the emotional needs of handicapped people: a psychodynamic approach. Journal of Mental Deficiency Research 33: 407–414

Freud S 1990 Case histories I. Penguin, London

Gardner W, Graeber J 1994 Use of behavioural therapies to enhance personal competency: a multimodal diagnostic and intervention model. In: Bouras N (ed) Mental health in mental retardation: recent advances and practices. Cambridge University Press, Cambridge

Gates B 1998 Learning disabilities, 3rd edn. Churchill Livingstone, Edinburgh

Green S 1987 Physiological psychology: an introduction. Routledge and Kegan Paul, London

Gustaffson B, Wigstrom H 1988 Physiological mechanisms underlying long term potentiation trends. Neuroscience 11: 156–162

Hollin C 1990 Cognitive behavioural interventions with young offenders. Pergamon, London

Hollon S, Shelton R, Loosen P 1991 Cognitive therapy and pharmacotherapy for depression. Journal of Consulting and Clinical Psychology 59: 88–99

Houston G 1990 The red book of gestalt. Rochester Foundation, London

Kelly G A 1955 The psychology of personal constructs. Norton, New York

Laing R D 1982 The voice of experience. Penguin, Harmondsworth

Lambert M 1986 Implications of psychotherapy outcome for eclectic psychotherapy. In: Norcross J (ed) Handbook of eclectic psychotherapy. Brunner/Mazel, New York

Lazarus R 1984 On the primacy of cognition. American Psychologist 39: 124–129

Logue A 1986 The psychology of eating and drinking. Freeman, New York

McCue M 2000 Behavioural interventions. In: Gates B, Gear J, Wray J (eds) Behavioural distress: concepts and strategies. Baillière Tindall, Edinburgh

McGill P, Clare I, Murphy G 1996 Understanding and responding to challenging behaviour: from theory to practice. Tizard Learning Disability Review 1(1): 9–17

Mackay A, Iverson L 1992 Neurotransmitters and schizophrenia. In: Weller M, Eysenck M (eds) The scientific base of psychiatry. W B Saunders, London

Maslow A H 1954 Motivation and personality. Harper and Row, New York

Masson J 1993 Against therapy. Harper Collins, London

Matlin M 1994 Cognition, 3rd edn. Harcourt Brace, Fort Worth

Matson J 1990 Handbook of behaviour modification with the mentally retarded. Plenum, New York

O'Neill R E, Horner R H, Albin R W, Storey K, Sprague J R 1990 Functional analysis of problem behaviour: a practical assessment guide. Sycamore Publishing, Illinois

Orlinsky D, Howard K 1987 A generic model of psychotherapy. Journal of Integrative and Eclectic Psychotherapy 6: 6–27

Patel P, Goldberg D, Moss S 1993 Psychiatric morbidity in older people with moderate and severe learning disability: the prevalence study. British Journal of Psychiatry 132: 1265–1271

Pavlov I 1902 The work of the digestive glands. Griffin, London

Perls F, Hefferline R, Goodman P 1951 Gestalt therapy: excitement and growth in the human personality. Souvenir Press, London

Piaget J 1952 The origins of intelligence in children. International Universities Press, New York

Pyles D, Bailey J 1990 Diagnosing severe behaviour problems. In: Repp A, Singh N (eds) Perspectives on the use of non-aversive interventions for persons with developmental disabilities. Sycamore Publishing, Illinois

Rogers C 1951 Client centred therapy. Houghton Mifflin, Boston

Rogers C 1980 A way of being. Houghton Mifflin, Boston

Ryle A 1990 Cognitive analytic therapy: active participation in change. Wiley, Chichester

Selye H 1956 The stress of life. McGraw-Hill, New York

Sinason V 1988 Psychoanalytic psychotherapy and its application. Journal of Social Work Practice 4(1)

Sinason V 1991 The sense in stupidity. Psychotherapy and mental handicap. Free Association Books, London

Sinason V, Stokes J 1992 Secondary mental handicap as a defence. In: Waitman A, Conboy-Hill S (eds) Psychotherapy and mental handicap. Sage, London

Skinner B F 1953 Science and human behaviour. Macmillan, New York

Szasz T 1987 Insanity: The idea and its consequences. Wiley, New York

Thompson R 1975 Introduction to physiological psychology. Harper and Row, New York

Thornicroft E, Brewin C, Wing J 1992 Measuring mental health needs. Gaskall, London

Tolman E C 1925 Purpose and cognition: the determinants of animal learning. Psychological Review 32: 285–297

Turkistani I 2000 Chemotherapy and other treatments. In: Gates R, Gear J, Wray J (eds) Behavioural distress: concepts and strategies. Baillière Tindall, Edinburgh

Turnbull J 2000 Cognitive behavioural interventions. In: Gates B, Gear J, Wray J (eds) Behavioural distress: concepts and strategies. Baillière Tindall, Edinburgh

Waitman A 1992 Demystifying traditional therapeutic approaches. In: Waitman A, Conboy-Hill S (eds) Psychotherapy and mental handicap. Sage, London

Waitman A, Conboy-Hill S 1992 Psychotherapy and mental handicap. Sage, London

Watson J, Raynor R 1920 Conditioned emotional reactions. Journal of Experimental Psychiatry 3(1): 14

Weller M 1991 Depressive illness and anti-depressant drugs. In: Weller M, Eysenck M (eds) The scientific base of psychiatry. W B Saunders, London

Zajonc R 1984 On the primacy of affect. American Psychologist 39: 117–123

USEFUL ADDRESSES

American Association of Mental Retardation (AAMR)
444 North Capitol Street
Suite 846
Washington DC 20001–1512
USA
www.aamr.org

Association of Cognitive Analytic Therapists (ACAT)
www.acat.org.uk

British Association for Behavioural and Cognitive Psychotherapies (BABCP)
www.babcp.org.uk

British Confederation of Psychotherapists (BCP)
www.bcp.org.uk

British Institute of Learning Disabilities (BILD)
Wolverhampton Road
Kidderminster
Worcs
www.bild.org.uk

The British Psychological Society
St Andrews House
48 Princess Road East
Leicester
LE1 7DR

The Tizard Centre
Beverley Farm
University of Kent
Canterbury
Kent CT2 7LZ
Tel: 01227 764 000 (ext 7771)
www.speke.ukc.ac.uk/tizard/index.htm/

UK Council for Psychotherapy (UKCP)
www.psychotherapy.org.uk

6

Relationships and learning disabilities

In this section, three chapters are presented that explore areas so very important in the lives of people with learning disabilities. Firstly, Peter Oakes presents a chapter on personal and sexual relationships. This is one area where there is still much misunderstanding and prejudice toward people with learning disabilities. Peter provides a factual but enlightened approach to this area. The recent White Paper has alluded to the importance of the family in learning disabilities. In Chapter 24, Owen Barr presents an excellent overview of contemporary issues concerning families within the context of a member having learning disabilities. As families are acknowledged as being important in the lives of people with learning disabilities, so too is advocacy. In Chapter 25, Steve McNally provides a comprehensive overview of empowerment issues relevant to the field of learning disabilities.

23 Sexual and personal relationships

Peter Oakes

KEY ISSUES

- People with learning disabilities are fully human and in this respect they need to make and maintain close relationships with others.
- Historically people with learning disabilities have been denied this opportunity.
- People with learning disabilities can and do become parents and may need help in this demanding role.
- Direct carers can support people with learning disabilities in their relationships by teaching, advocating and facilitating.

INTRODUCTION

'One could not find a better helper for Human Nature than Love' Plato (Gilmour 1993)

This statement forms part of a symposium on love, written by Plato. The characters who debate the nature, purpose and significance of love include Aristophanes, who tells of a myth which is intended to enlighten the discussion. The myth concerns inhabitants of the earth before people, who were impressive creatures representing both genders and possessing four legs and four arms each. They were mighty creatures, mighty enough indeed to challenge and compete with the gods of ancient mythology. The great god Zeus became unhappy with this state of affairs and decided to split the creatures into people with two arms and two legs. People were from then on enfolded with a longing for unity with others as a symbol of past glory.

In this day and age we would rightly reject the idea of incompleteness without a partner, yet we would also recognise the extent to which many people would identify the loving relationship with another as a call in their lives. The sense of oneness brought about through the faithful union of two people is celebrated in the Christian Bible and has been the subject of poem, novel, picture and song throughout recorded history. Yet where in the literature of learning disability do we find an equal idea of love and intimacy and union?

This chapter is intended to help us understand the need of all people to relate to other people in ways which are special. This is a matter of health for all, when health is understood as wholeness in community with others. It is a matter of policy with the agenda of inclusion, dominating government thinking for the past 4 years (DOH 2001). It has been known as a matter of evidence, not just belief, in the mental health field that isolation and absence of a supportive confiding relationship are serious threats to mental health (Armado 1993); increasingly this is a matter of human rights.

Where people are dependent on other people to meet many of their needs and fulfil many of their desires, issues of love and relationship strike chords which are at once exciting and intimidating. If it is to be useful, then discussion is certain to echo in the personal lives of those who are professionally involved and to range deep in the hopes and anxieties of relatives and carers. At the same time this is known to be a vulnerable group of people for whom the prospect of enduring the sensibilities, needs and emotional pressures of others is appalling.

In the light of these thoughts, discussion in this chapter will range across topics that will carry familiar titles, such as social inclusion, sexuality and abuse. These must not distract us, however, from the essence of our subject. People with learning disabilities, in many instances, will need support to make and maintain relationships which do not exploit and yet which can lead to health in its profoundest sense. This is not intended to be a literary piece, yet it does intend to make real the concerns and longings of the people who receive services.

This chapter has been written to help those who are involved in the care and support of people with learning disabilities to explore some of these issues. It is already clear that this can be challenging and controversial. There will be opportunities to explore the experiences of people who receive services and to relate them to those of people who do not receive support with their sexual and personal relationships. The main body of the chapter will be devoted to looking at the ways in which the social inclusion agenda can address the genuine and personal concerns of people with learning disabilities. This will be put in the context of the history of approaches, before moving to the main dilemmas and opportunities that face modern services. The final section will consider the role of direct carers and other professionals as providers of those services.

SETTING THE SCENE: GROWING UP IN AN EXCLUSIVE WORLD

It is important to begin by considering the experience of children who are identified as having learning disabilities in the modern life of the UK. The experience of both child and family in the early times when the disability has been identified is probably best understood in the tragedy model. Professionals talk of loss and the need to mourn for the child who was not to be. Families are given 'support' to understand 'why' and are cast in the role of heroic victims who must bear the lifelong burden of a disabled child (see Ch. 24). Sometimes the 'tragedy' can be 'blamed' on someone, such as a hospital doctor or a drug company, and the human story is played out in a court of law.

In many ways it is not surprising that these ideas have gone unchallenged from the earliest work on the ways in which parents are first told that their child is disabled. They are, of course, self-perpetuating in that they represent a clear reflection of the genuine ideas and concerns of the wider community. As a community we value the bright, intelligent and successful children who will grow up to hold down important and well rewarded jobs. The loss of such opportunity, if it is the only valued opportunity, is naturally seen as a tragedy. Likewise, parents may harbour many hopes and fears about future relationships for their children. As a community we are reluctant to promote the relationships of people with learning disabilities especially where these might lead to their becoming parents (Booth & Booth 2000). The hopes and fears for future independence, and for the possibilities of long-term partnerships and parenthood are taboo if the child is disabled. It is hardly surprising then if, in later life, people with learning disabilities are not afforded these opportunities and the community held beliefs are maintained.

Childhood and exclusive schooling

The notion of integrated and more recently inclusive education has been accepted in broad principle by governments since the Education Act of 1980. The reality for the majority of people with learning disabilities, especially where those disabilities are more severe, is that access to ordinary schools and hence a peer group in the non-disabled world is denied on a massive scale. It must be said that there may be good social and educational reasons for this and that there are examples where parents, families and other carers would support the notion of special education for their children. The issue here is a specific one and relates to the extent to which a child is enabled to learn about relationships and sexuality. National curriculum subjects are indeed taught in all schools, but the content of personal and social development curricula can vary widely and the extent of successful education in the field of personal relationships is unknown (see Ch. 7). We can, however, make some judgements about the success of such programmes by examining the outcomes. McCabe (1999) undertook a study of the sexual knowledge, experience and feelings of people with disabilities in their 20s. People with learning disabilities were found to demonstrate lower levels of both sexual knowledge and experience than other disabled groups and people without disabilities. In addition to this people with learning disabilities reported more negative attitudes towards sexual relationships than were evident in their peers. It must be noted that this was a study in Australia, but there is good reason to believe that the situation is similar in other countries (McCarthy 1999).

There is a further point about the implications of exclusion in the education system. It seems clear that people with learning disabilities will lack both formal and informal opportunities to learn about and to explore their sexuality and need for intimacy. It can also be argued that young people without disabilities will engage in a poorer social world as a direct result of missing positive contact with people with learning disabilities in the school setting.

Inclusion for all?

Wolfensberger and others have written with great wisdom about the ways in which the community is enriched by the presence of people with learning disabilities (Wolfensberger 1988). This stands in distinct contrast to the notion of disability as tragedy. Where diversity is celebrated, the school community is impoverished by the absence of young people with learning disabilities. Moreover, the roots of prejudice at least in part must be manifest in a school system which fails in its inclusive purpose. People who have grown up without positive contact with people with learning disabilities are then expected to understand the importance of inclusion in adult life. Perhaps this is too much to expect? The wider community is missing out. Indeed many people who do not carry the label of learning disability may be missing out on the opportunity to meet someone with whom they may find love and partnership.

It seems that in modern services, inclusion is not to be sidelined as the concern of purists and radicals. Rather it is to form part of every initiative in the support of people with learning disabilities in relation to both social and health care. Inclusion is clearly more than the use of a post office or leisure centre. Inclusion is about relationship, and we have known for thousands of years now that love and intimacy lie at the foundations of our humanity.

BEING FULLY HUMAN AND THE NEW HUMAN RIGHTS AGENDA

As has been established, the universal view of government policy, and of writing in the field has been to establish, without question or doubt, that people with learning disabilities are fully human. It is simply unacceptable to regard any person as being less human than another person is. Indeed it is seen as a challenge to modern services to recognise and affirm the dignity of people with learning disabilities (DOH 2001).

Despite this important point of progress, it has been the experience of many who work to support people with learning disabilities that there is a considerable amount to do if services are indeed to recognise and affirm the dignity of those for whom they provide support. One of the difficulties in addressing some of these issues has been to establish a frame of reference upon which judgements can be made about the extent to which services fully reflect the fact that those who receive them are fully and completely human.

The notion of establishing that people are fully human finds a curious and somewhat unsettling echo in the history of human rights law. One of the earliest legal cases in the USA concerned a first nation American known as Standing Bear. The case of Standing Bear versus Crook arose because of an attempt to insist that a group of first nation Americans living in Florida should move to North Dakota. Standing Bear did not wish to move and so returned to his home in Florida. The case was brought by US marshall Crook who intended to arrest Standing Bear and return him to North Dakota. The case turned into an argument about the extent to which Standing Bear was a human being. The conclusion, brimming with irony, was that Standing Bear was indeed fully human, and that he was subject to the United States Law, and would have to live where the US marshall directed under the law (Standing Bear v Crook, 18.4.1879).

Since that time, human rights legislation has moved on to establish an international standard for the treatment of all people. In the UK The Human Rights Act (1998) came into force in October of the year 2000. Essentially this involved the UK government adopting all but a small number of the rights contained in the European Convention for the protection of Human Rights and Fundamental Freedoms (Human Rights Act 1998). This is expected to have a number of signifi-cant implications for people with learning disabilities. This is especially so given that actions can be brought under the Act when services or individuals have not taken actions to ensure that an individual's human rights are upheld. It may be that failure to provide opportunities for people with learning disabilities will be the subject of legal challenge under the Human Rights Act.

The implications of this in the field of sexual and personal relationships are untested. However, it is of significance that at least three articles of the Convention may relate to issues of personal relationship:

Article 3   No one shall be subjected to torture or to inhuman or degrading treatment or punishment.

Article 8   Everyone has the right to respect for his private and family life, his home and his correspondence.

Article 12 Men and women of marriageable age have the right to marry and to found a family, according to the national laws governing the exercise of this right. (Human Rights Act 1998, ch. 42 Schedules – articles.)

THE CASE FOR A NEW LOOK AT SEXUALITY AND CLOSE PERSONAL RELATIONSHIPS

The current political and social imperative demands the inclusion of people with learning disabilities in community life, and in the full range of human experience. This is supported by human rights legislation, which gives expression to the fundamental rights and freedoms of all people. Given the pre-eminence of close and personal relationships in the lives of so many of us, it is time to establish work in this area at the centre of professional practice.

It is now possible to move to the historical context, before addressing the main issues for practice in modern services. In moving on however, it is important to reflect on the issues covered thus far. The reader is invited to reflect on and undertake the activity identified in Reader activity 23.1.

A BRIEF HISTORY

It was around 100 years ago that services for people with learning disabilities were set for a

Reader activity 23.1

Consider an individual with learning disabilities who is known to you. How much time and energy is devoted to enabling that person to meet new people, make significant relationships and maintain those relationships. Does this reflect the time and energy which you devote to these issues?

positive move to supportive residential and day services. These would quite possibly have created opportunities to develop close and meaningful relationships, but sadly this was not to be the case and a dramatic change of direction was made. However, the story starts a little before these great events and should be told in its proper order.

There is a detailed account of the history of our response to people with learning disabilities in Chapter 3. This section focuses instead on the main changes that have been related to helping people with learning disabilities to build close personal relationships.

This account begins in the middle of the last century. Literature prior to that time has little or nothing to say about relationships. Rather, it is concerned with people's disposal under law (Gostin 1986), the conditions and regimens of residential services and the process of political change (Skultans 1979). It seems that the mid-19th century brought references to masturbation and the idea that it violated natural law. Indeed, it was seen as both a cause and a result of learning disabilities, with accounts of various attempts to stop the practice in institutions (Rhodes 1993). However, there also developed at this time a sense of benevolence and professional paternalism, which began to influence services. This seemed to arise from the work of a key French pioneer, Sequin. He introduced the idea that a person with learning disabilities can be helped to learn and to develop. Small schools were established and these ideas took hold across Europe and the US. Issues of sexual and personal relationships were ignored, but the conditions were favourable for the introduction of teaching and support in these areas of life.

At the same time, however, Darwin was setting out his theories of evolution, and his cousin Francis Galton was developing the idea of eugenics (from the Greek for 'well born'). Rhodes (1993) tells us that these ideas began to drive a new movement that was particularly important in the US. Other parts of the emerging scientific approach to people and their behaviour were also put to use by the leaders of this movement. Again, in France, Binet had developed the earliest assessments of intelligence. These tests were applied to a series of research projects (Kempton & Kahn 1991) which embarked on major descriptions of extended families. The most notorious of these were the Jukes family and the Kallikaks. Researchers attempted to trace the extent of criminal behaviour in these families and used the new tests to help them in their task. They were attempting to prove a three-point argument: that criminal behaviour was inherited; that learning disability was inherited; and that criminal behaviour was linked to learning disability. Apparently startling results were obtained. The Kallikak family comprised 480 descendants, 143 of whom reportedly had learning disabilities and 75% were said to be 'degenerate'. A remarkable change can be seen in the reporting of data gathered about the Jukes family. In 1877, a study concluded that poor environmental conditions were largely responsible for high levels of criminal behaviour. The study was published again in 1915, this time claiming instead that 50% of the family had a learning disability and that all those who committed crimes came from this half of the family (Rhodes 1993).

These projects had a clear political agenda: they were used to give credibility to a set of ideas called Social Darwinism. It was claimed that the human race depended on a healthy pool of genes, which could be contaminated by learning disabilities and any form of deviant behaviour. These threats were reportedly inherited and were all the more threatening because the people involved were said to be engaging in a good deal of sexual activity. The picture was a frightening one: a group of people were procreating faster than anyone else, and by so doing were spreading the contamination of the human gene pool.

Social Darwinism became the dominant idea in the first 20–30 years of the last century, and effectively contaminated the excellent work that had begun in a range of settings for adults and children with learning disabilities. Services now had a new objective: to halt this frightening decline. The measures taken were fairly predictable, given the understanding of the problem which was to be solved. Men and women with disabilities were taken away to large, separate and usually isolated institutions. The populations of the various institutions increased massively and programmes of enforced sterilisation were begun. It must be said that these programmes were controversial and that they were always secondary to the use of institutions.

The options for people with learning disabilities at this time were extremely limited. Most were to live a life which was celibate and separate. The ultimate expression for these ideas was found in Nazi Germany. Jewish people were not the only group of whom the Nazi Party sought to rid the world: people with learning disabilities also suffered terribly at the hands of those who conducted programmes of experiment and extermination.

The end of the tunnel?

With the defeat and rejection of fascism came the end of Social Darwinism. Programmes of sterilisation were abandoned and some people were released from institutions; although the overall populations remained at a peak until the mid 1960s. It is in the mid to late 1960s that the seeds of change in respect of working to help people with sexual and personal relationships can be found. Learning disabilities were becoming increasingly better understood in terms of adaptive behaviour and community skills, in addition to intellectual ability. The philosophy of normalisation was also introduced, and a small number of workers began to propose help and education for people in these parts of their lives. The 1970s and 1980s saw a proliferation of teaching and support materials available to direct staff, along with a full acceptance of the importance of close personal relationships.

More recently, services have become aware of the implications of attempting to respond to close personal relationships. The acknowledgement of the issue and the development of teaching resources have been significant steps forward. The early ideas and materials have been reasonably straightforward. However, the complexity of the task has begun to challenge service providers in new ways. A range of issues have to be confronted. These include:

- Consent
- Parenthood
- Protection.

What have we learned?

Before moving on it is important to see what can be learnt from this account. Throughout history, if a person has had learning disabilities, other people have taken decisions about many aspects of that person's life. These included everything from when they might have a bath, through to where and with whom they might live. It is this freedom to take decisions that is guarded so jealously by people who do not rely on services. The area of sexual and personal relationships is one of the most treasured parts of a person's life. It is here that some of the most heavy-handed control has, in the past, been exercised, either by failing to acknowledge this part of a person's life or by curtailing the opportunities available to such people. In modern services there remains a reluctance to enable people to take their own decisions and act upon them in respect of sexual and personal relationships. This represents a long history of control and must be understood as such.

The second major point to be drawn from a study of history is the extent to which services are influenced by the wider political scene: people with learning disabilities have always been the object of social policy. This again represents the dependence of individuals who need others for support to cope with the challenges of everyday life. Thus if social policy is concerned with the purity of the gene pool or the economic viability of services, there will be serious consequences for people who are disabled. This remains the case so long as people with learning disabilities are not helped to work together to influence the policies that affect their lives.

Change has come about through the actions of researchers, sociologists, politicians and journalists. This increases the vulnerability of new developments to changes in social and political policy. It may be that those who support people with learning disabilities could usefully spend more time assisting them to exert greater influence on the policies that govern the most personal and intimate parts of their lives. This raises an important dilemma for those who are paid to support people with learning disabilities. The authorities in government are sponsoring this support. It is quite reasonable for those authorities to resist the pursuit of love and personal relationships being seen as a legitimate aim of social and health policy. At the same time it is clear to those in direct contact with people who use services, that matters of personal relationships are central to the concerns of many. It seems important to acknowledge the point of the policy maker, whilst remembering that a definition of health and welfare for the new millennium relates to the whole person and that person's relationships. These include relationships with the wider community and relationships of intimacy. Only by addressing matters of love and closeness can the service make any appropriate claim to be adopting an inclusive approach.

The final lesson that can be learned from the history of services is the ever-present threat to the very existence of people who are learning disabled. David Potter and others have drawn attention to the increasing drive to 'prevent' learning disabilities (Potter 1993). The notion of positive eugenics has significant implications for the sexual and personal freedoms of people with learning disabilities. Women with severe disabilities have undergone sterilisation where consent for such an operation could not be obtained (Campion 1995). The law now distinguishes between the unborn child with learning disabilities, and the unborn child who has no identified disability. There is a time limit after which a child who is not thought to have learning disabilities cannot be aborted. This time limit simply does not apply to the unborn child with a 'serious disability', who can be aborted until the pregnancy is at full term. This procedure is referred to as a 'thera-peutic abortion' and can be seen as further evidence of the drive to cleanse the human race. Our inability to deal with difference shelters the flame of eugenics in the 21st century.

These moves to restrict the population of learning-disabled people strike at the heart of any philosophy that seeks to value such people as being fully human. Without that basic foundation, work to empower people in their close personal relationships is unlikely to succeed. This is so, not least because much of our ability to develop relationships depends on our own sense of security or self-worth. If a person lives in a community which believes that he or she should not exist, or at least should have been prevented from existing, such self-worth will remain a distant hope.

 Reader activity 23.2

Consider again people with learning disabilities. What happens in those people's lives to assure them that they are special and that the world is a better place because they are around?

CURRENT ISSUES
Making decisions

People make hundreds of decisions every day of their lives, ranging from the smallest detail, such as whether to have a cup of tea or a cup of coffee, through to decisions of enormous importance such as a change of job or a move to a new place. Thinking about decisions is not just a matter of the importance of a particular course of action; there are other dimensions. Some decisions affect only the person making them; others may affect lots of people; still others will affect a small number of people in a very significant way. Then there is the quality of the decision that has to be taken: some are practical, others are emotional, and others are moral or spiritual.

A particular decision is likely to involve a number of these dimensions, and the person has to weigh up the different consequences of each option. Important decisions tend to have a whole series of pros and cons. The last confusing piece to this jigsaw is the fact that everybody makes decisions in a different way according to different criteria.

Perhaps the most complex area in which everyone makes decisions is that of close personal relationships. For many people such decisions are the most significant in their lives. People with learning disabilities may need support to reach a decision and to take the resulting action. This raises a series of issues for the people who provide that support.

Service providers are bound by law, and by the demands of good practice, to consider the extent to which a person with a learning disability can make decisions. There are two aspects to this. The first involves deciding to engage in a close relationship and the business of placing boundaries around it. This means that a person must decide whether to become involved with another person and how intimate and/or physical that involvement should be. The second is about the treatment or clinical intervention a person might be receiving. There are a number of options for a person with learning disabilities in this area of life. These include teaching and assistance with personal and intimate matters. Also there may be various forms of contraception available: for example vasectomy or sterilisation, or the use of medication to reduce sexual drive or potency, either deliberately or as a possible side effect.

In considering the ways in which people make these important decisions a number of legal concepts have to be understood. These can then be set alongside the professional issues which are relevant to the making of decisions. Extensive discussions of the legal aspects of these issues can be found elsewhere (Carson 1987, 1991, Gunn 1994). However, some important principles can be set out here.

The main legal issues that surround decision making are known as capacity and consent. Children become able to make decisions in law at different ages for different actions. At 16, a young person can consent to heterosexual sex and to entry into a mental health hospital. Other forms of treatment can also be consented to at 16, although this can be earlier depending on the individual. At 18, a person can decide to vote and to enter into a contract (there are some exceptions to this). At 18 a person can decide to have homosexual sex.

The law is formally concerned with biological age. Once people have reached these ages it is assumed in law that they are capable of making the decisions. However, if people have some form of mental 'disorder', and it can be demonstrated that they are not capable, then different rules apply. Here a person must be able to understand the nature of the action and its consequences to be able to take a legal decision. It is important that the assessment is to be of the person's understanding, not their wisdom (Law Commission 1991).

Allied to the notion of a person's capacity to make a decision is the notion of consent. Issues to consider here are the differences between approval and non-objection, the way a person communicates, and the time at which a person has the opportunity to give consent. It is important to note that fear, force or fraud can undermine consent. Consent can also be undermined when a position of authority is used to ensure submission or acquiescence.

This continues to be an area of debate and consideration by government. The Lord Chancellor's Department is expected to issue further advice about consent in the near future. Given the complexity of decision making and the fact that people with learning disabilities are likely to require support in this area, what are the issues for clinical practice? Some of them are listed below:

- **Legal** It is clear that all practice must be within the law. This is to be achieved by a responsible group of professional people working alongside the person and her or his advocate. These people will require the support of the various organisations involved in the support of that person.
- **Choice** It is essential that work is carried out to understand how a person makes and communicates choices. Following from this, the ways in which a person understands the nature and consequences of a course of action must also be understood. This is certain to involve a consideration of the verbal and non-verbal means of communication the person uses.

- **Personal context** Support in this area is to be given in the context of an understanding of the person as a whole. This is to include issues of development, background and personality.
- **Service context** The philosophies of normalisation and empowerment are widely accepted as a means of helping individuals make decisions when communication and understanding are difficult (Brown & Smith 1992).
- **Assertiveness** A decision usually boils down to saying yes or no to a particular course of action. However, to do this a person must have experience of making decisions, and others must have respected these decisions. To say yes or no, people need to believe that they are of some value, and that it matters if they say yes or no. A person with a learning disability may lack both the experience and the belief. It will be the prime task of carers to help people develop this vital sense of personal value.

 Reader activity 23.3

In considering the life of someone you know who has learning disabilities, how often does that person do things which he or she has not consented to. Is there any work going on to stop this?

Parenthood

It has already been established how the eugenics movement and the setting up of long-stay institutions effectively outlawed the making of close personal relationships and stable partnerships for people with learning disabilities. Reducing the possibility of people with learning disabilities becoming parents has been both a cause and an effect of these ideas and practices. However, recent years have seen a significant increase in the number of people with learning disabilities who have become parents. This is a natural consequence of work to enable such people to live and make choices, like others in the community. Modern practice has given people new opportunities, and they have taken them in increasing numbers.

Clearly the growing numbers of parents who have learning disabilities represent a challenge to services, not least because of the prejudice that they encounter when they interact with children's services. Although research to help understand and meet this challenge has been scarce, a small number of workers have produced work of the highest quality. These include Booth & Booth (1994a,b, 2000) and McGraw (1994) in Britain; Feldman (1994) in Canada; and Tymchuk (1992) in the United States.

Booth & Booth (1994b) reported the first and most consistent finding of research in this area: it is absolutely clear that there is no link between intelligence and the ability to be a parent. There is no point on a scale of intelligence below which a person becomes a bad parent. There is equally no point on a scale of intelligence above which a person becomes a good parent. It follows that treating people with learning disabilities as a homogeneous group is as inappropriate here as it is in every other area of life.

Research does, however, seem to suggest that people with learning disabilities may have difficulties in bringing up children, and may be at greater risk of becoming involved in child protection issues (Feldman 1994, Sheerin 1998). The difficulties reported include being sensitive to the child's development and providing a stimulating environment in which to learn and play. Also noted are problems in expressing love and affection and maintaining good discipline, along with physical safety (Booth & Booth 1994b, Feldman 1994).

However, this work has many weaknesses. The first and most important is an assumption that these difficulties arise from the learning disability. However, the evidence does not warrant the claim that there is a causal link. There are so many other possible reasons why someone can run into difficulties with bringing up a child. Studies seem to be based on small groups of parents, with little attempt to control for key factors such as social and economic circumstances (Campion 1995).

Booth & Booth (1994b) have noted a number of other reasons why research is weak. These include a tendency to study parents who are already in some trouble and known to services.

There is also an enormous conceptual difficulty in defining good, bad or adequate parenthood.

The experience of being parented

In their more recent work, Booth & Booth (2000) have taken an important step forward which reflects more modern and inclusive approaches to research. They spent some time with people who have had the experience of being brought up by parents with learning disabilities to see whether some of the prevailing ideas are helpful. In particular, researchers and participants in research explored what they term the 'damage model' which has dominated work in the field of parenting. This model assumed that the children of parents with learning disabilities are certain to grow up in a deeply impoverished and damaging environment. There is a sense in which the children must survive this the best way they can, and escape to adulthood and independence as soon as possible.

A series of in depth interviews were conducted with people who have grown up with parents with learning disabilities. Individuals talked about problems, but noted that many of them arose from outside the family home. A powerful finding of this work was that many people maintained positive and valued relationships with their parents across the life cycle. This has significant implications for a single model, especially where the model is essentially negative.

In addition to the challenge to the damage model, it is clear from this work and from a wider understanding of people in the context of their relationships with others, that it is not appropriate to regard families in isolation. Not only is it the case that many of the problems for families come from outside of the immediate family; it is also clear that the task of parenting can be better understood as a wider responsibility shared by both family and community. There are positive examples of friends, neighbours and relatives being involved in providing a healthy and stimulating place in which children can grow. It is to be hoped that professionals and other workers will learn to see themselves as part of the range of people who can provide support, an idea central to the concept of person centred planning (see Ch. 19).

What emerges then, is a call to be positive about parents with learning disabilities and to understand parenting as the responsibility of many people who can work in partnership with families in a network of support. This support is beyond that which is available to parents who are not learning disabled, even though the reasons why such support is required may not actually involve the learning disability itself. It is about relationships and emotional support in the first instance. However, it is also about ensuring that the practical responsibilities of parenting are discharged. Four main areas of support can be identified:

- **Making sense of it all** The first kind of support is in the area of practical help and teaching. McGraw (1994) has produced a series of booklets to help people with learning disabilities to learn about the tasks of parenthood. The areas covered are as follows:
  —What's it like to be a parent?
  —Healthy food
  —To be clean, healthy and warm
  —To be safe
  —To be loved
  —To learn right from wrong.

Fundamental to this, and other support, is that it is given in a form that can be understood by many people with learning disabilities. It will be important to use special methods of helping communication, such as Makaton signs and symbols. It is also essential to match the level of information to the ability of the person for whom it is intended.

Another element of communication is the support a person may require to understand the workings of official bodies such as the Departments of Social Services and Social Security. It is possible that parents will fall foul of these bodies, simply because they do not understand what is being asked of them. For example, a social worker may become concerned because a parent does not attend a crucial meeting at school. The reason may be that the parents have been sent a letter about the meeting which they can not read.

- **The answer's no: now, what's the question?**
The second area of support required by parents who have learning disabilities lies in the attitudes of professionals and the services they represent. This involves challenging rather than promoting a 'damage model'.

  In general services, an important movement has fought to ensure that people with a disability are seen as people first, with a consideration of their strengths and abilities next. Only after that should the disability and the support required be looked into. The same is true in the area of parenthood. People with disabilities who have children should be given their full and proper status as parents first (Booth & Booth 1994b). Areas of strength and ability should then be recorded. This can be followed by an assessment of the support needed to maintain the parental relationship, which should not be based on assumptions about people with learning disabilities. It will be unique to the family.

- **Stand up and be counted** The third area of help involves the need of all parents to stand up for themselves and make supportive relationships with friends in the local area. Research suggests that this need is particularly relevant to parents who have a learning disability (Booth & Booth 2000, Campion 1995). At times of stress it is important that parents do not become dependent on services and professionals; rather, workers should be helping people to get together with others in the same situation. Booth & Booth (1994b) make particular mention of the help which can be gained from a 'benefactor' (relative or friend) who does not have a learning disability.

- **First things first** The final area of support which may be needed by parents is environmental. Parents with learning disabilities are susceptible to the same stresses and pressures of modern life as everyone else. It seems that they are also more likely to experience the social conditions of poverty, poor housing and so on. The load is often made heavier by the effects of prejudice and victimisation, which people may experience as a result of their learning disability. Although professionals may be able to do little to lighten these particular loads, it is essential that they understand their impact on a struggling family.

To read the books and articles about parents who have learning disabilities is an encouraging task, and it would seem that the long night of prejudice has passed and a new dawn has begun. Sadly, however, the experiences of many people with learning disabilities who have children suggest that this is a false dawn. Campion (1995) notes that more and more people require the approval of others to bring up a child, and people who have learning disabilities are increasingly under the scrutiny of those who give such approval. Much more work needs to be done to ensure a just outcome for those people and their children.

Reader activity 23.4

What are the most important things for parents to give to their children? How many of these things are dependent on intelligence?

Protection

Perhaps the most significant harm that can be survived by a person is to be abused. Whereas the subject of physical and sexual abuse of children has been taken seriously for some time now, the abuse of people with learning disabilities has been a relatively recent addition to mainstream thinking. Indeed, the early papers tackled the subject as a great taboo, with titles such as *Thinking the Unthinkable* (Brown & Craft 1989), representing one of the earliest treatments of the issue in the UK. Even in 1994 a paper about working with members of staff to help confront issues of sexual abuse needed to be called *Alarming but very necessary* (Brown et al 1994).

However, the issue is now on the agenda and has been extensively reviewed and discussed (Brown et al 1995, Curry 2001, McCarthy & Thompson 1997, Turk & Brown 1993). It has also been encouraging to note the work of the

Association for Residential Care (ARC) and the National Association for the Protection from Sexual Abuse of Children and Adults With Learning Disabilities (NAPSAC) in this important area (ARC/NAPSAC 1997). These initiatives have been brought together by the Department of Health, in its document *No Secrets* (DOH 2000). Here, particular emphasis is given to the need for multi-agency training in responding to vulnerable adults.

Definition

Brown & Turk (1992) have adapted some earlier work in defining sexual abuse. They relied heavily on the ideas of consent that were discussed earlier in this chapter, including the factors that can undermine the person's capacity to give consent. Following this, two main categories of abuse were suggested (see Box 23.1).

Brown et al (1995) have made some minor amendments to this work in a follow-up study. They included the idea that people can be victims to a number of different perpetrators, either in the same incident or over time. Equally, one perpetrator can have more than one victim.

Characteristics

The pattern of abuse seems to have been fairly consistent across studies (Curry 2001). In the UK, Brown et al (1995) carried out a detailed study. Over a 4-year period, 228 reports of sexual abuse were analysed, 169 of which were shown to be proven or highly suspected to be proven. Although it is difficult to work out the national incidence from a regional sample, the study suggested that some 1400 cases of sexual abuse can be expected in the UK each year.

Box 23.1 Types of abuse

Non-contact abuse	Contact abuse
Pornography	Touch
Indecent exposure	Masturbation
Harassment	Penetration/attempted penetration

Men and women are at risk of abuse to an almost equal degree, but the vast majority of perpetrators (96%) were men. It seems that the majority of victims have moderate to severe learning disabilities and have additional difficulties. The victim generally knows the perpetrators, and other people who receive the service made up the largest group of perpetrators. This was followed by members of staff, other known adults and members of the family.

In a different approach to research, Carlson (1998) undertook a qualitative study of 11 people with learning disabilities. During in depth discussion, 6 members of the group reported sexual abuse, and all reported emotional abuse. Indeed the individuals in this study regarded emotional abuse as 'almost universal' in disability services in the US.

Response

Before dealing with the ways of responding to this issue, there is an important warning to heed, sounded by Evans & Rodgers (2000). This reflects concerns that work in this area may be starting from a base of negative assumption. It is assumed, albeit tacitly, that sexual relationships are fraught with danger and in some way to be survived, if indeed they are absolutely necessary. This account seeks to address the issue of protection because it should release people to explore their sexuality in the context of trusting and safe relationships. In the light of this, there is a reasonably simple set of protective measures that could be put together to support a safe and positive approach to sexuality.

Turk & Brown (1993) have stressed the importance of ensuring that sexual abuse is recognised, recorded, responded to, reported and remembered by services. This will increase the likelihood of abuse being taken seriously, and assist in changing the culture of services to one which impedes rather than promotes abuse.

Furey (1989) took up this issue of service culture in a paper about general abuse. It is clear that much can be done to reduce the likelihood of people being abused. Members of staff need support to reduce stress at work and to avoid situations which might lead to abuse, for example late night sessions of one-to-one work. All direct care staff need to be taught to be particularly vigilant, so that perpetrators may expect to be caught. Procedures need to be clear so that perpetrators can expect the most serious outcome following abuse. These issues should fall within a policy which will cover all those who are abused or who are vulnerable to abuse (Fruin 1994).

Baum & Shepperd (2001) have described an interesting contribution to the methods of preventing abuse. In this study, people with learning disabilities were taught to work as 'checkers' of residential services. This was to form part of the wider evaluation of services. Part of the 'checking' role was the 'alerting' role. Here people who were visiting services were taught to be sensitive to signs that the environment might be abusive or that individuals were moving to disclose material. This was seen as a means of bringing information to the authorities, and of extending the idea of openness in services.

Individuals who receive services will continue to need support to say 'yes' and 'no', as mentioned earlier. This will be combined with work to help people who have suffered abuse. Individual and group work with survivors of abuse will be an essential part of the therapeutic work of the future. For example, it has been noted that working with survivors who may be unable to give an account of their abuse will present particular challenges to workers in both the legal and therapeutic services (Pillay & Sargent 2000). There is the genesis of a literature about this (Synason 1994). However, it will be necessary to extend the skills of working in this way to those who have direct contact with people. It will also be necessary to enable people to get together as survivors of abuse. Current research and writing seem very well intentioned, but there is still a sense of the person who is abused as 'subject'. So far the 'subject' has been studied and surveyed. Sometimes

Reader activity 23.5

Are you sure that the people you know with learning disabilities are safe? How do you know?

the 'subject' is given therapy. Maybe the 'subject' could be helped to throw off the role of subject, for that has too many parallels with the role of victim. It may be time for survivors to get together, take control of the services, the writers and the researchers and tell them what should be done about sexual abuse.

ROLE OF DIRECT STAFF

Having considered a range of issues, it remains to pull together the role of direct staff in addressing this area of a person's life. This can begin with the overall requirements of good practice and move to discuss a model of direct work in respect of close personal relationships.

The basics

It is essential that people work within a full legal and policy framework, which means that members of staff will be guided by and accountable to a clear policy. This policy will address specific issues such as sexual intercourse, masturbation, consent and so on. It will ensure that everyone knows exactly how decisions are to be taken within the policy. Nobody will be uncomfortable with actions that they are expected to take. This will all be contained within a legal and philosophical framework. Policies on sexual and personal relationships will include or be related to policies on abuse, risk taking and health and safety.

The second overall requirement concerns the need to maintain general standards of good practice. Members of staff require regular and effective supervision. People who receive services will be active participants in a person centred planning process that addresses their needs, hopes and wishes. Procedures need to be in place which ensure that services have effective means for getting to know the people who receive them; this may include diary work and reliable recording.

There is a well-struck balance in current policy towards people with learning disabilities in the UK. The White Paper *Valuing People* (DOH 2001) builds on earlier guidance in *Signposts to Success* (DOH 1998). Person centred planning and social inclusion are the hallmarks of an approach which might claim to value people and affirm their dignity as people. However, it has also been important to recognise that people with learning disabilities may need support in many areas of their lives, and that accessing positive physical health care has been a difficulty for many years. This will in turn be balanced with the danger of overprotection, but will include specific support in all aspects of sexual health. This may range from the management of menstruation (Rodgers 2001), through to an open approach to HIV and AIDS (Cambridge 1997).

Direct support staff are those who care for people with learning disabilities on a day-to-day basis. This may involve actual social or physical contact. The role of direct staff can be divided into four main areas of activity, each of which can be related to working alongside people to develop close personal relationships (a discussion of some of these issues can be found in Craft & Brown (1994)):

- **Doing** In a number of situations a member of direct staff is required to do something for the person with learning disabilities. Examples of this should be kept to a minimum. However, if people are unable to move their arms and legs someone will need to dress them and place food in their mouths.

  There is a clear imbalance of power in the relationship between staff who are paid by a third party and people receiving the service. Both groups are vulnerable to exploitation and there are enormous dangers inherent in members of staff becoming involved in this intimate part of a person's life. At present this is not regarded as acceptable practice in the UK, but to rule it out leaves open the question of who will provide this support?

- **Advocating** It will often be necessary to speak up on behalf of learning-disabled people. It may be that there are objections and resistance to the idea of such a person becoming close to another. A service may lack the policy framework or the facilities to enable these people to develop close personal relationships. It is also possible that the community at large objects to such people making relationships. Here the member of staff may need to speak up and encourage change. It

is important to remember, however, that it is essential to help people to speak up for themselves and to take control of these issues.

- **Teaching** It is evident from any review of the literature and from contact with people who use services that people with learning disabilities have rarely enjoyed the opportunity to explore, learn about and understand the issues of close personal relationships (Cambridge 2001, McCabe 1999). There are many resources to assist with individual and group teaching. These are of great benefit to people, although it is important that they have the opportunity to learn about relationships at all times (Craft & Brown 1994, McCarthy and Thompson 1994). This will involve members of staff setting appropriate examples and intervening if inappropriate activities are being pursued. Learning is always improved if it takes place in a natural setting. Social settings and gatherings can provide many opportunities for such learning.

- **Facilitating** Loneliness is the landscape through which many people must travel in their lives. It seems that this is the particular experience of many people with learning disabilities (Armado 1993). This has been something of a theme in this chapter, as people need support in so many ways to pursue the dreams which are shared by so many. Building connections between people with learning disabilities and the community and promoting reciprocal relationships between people with learning disabilities and community members would seem to be a foundation of the work of support services. This is about making sure that people who receive the service have the opportunities to meet people, spend time with them and develop close relationships, both inside and outside the home setting. This work has been shown to be successful in the USA (Schwartz 1997), yet seems to lack direction and vigour in the UK. Whatever the reasons for this, 'It is essential to have a support network and a circle of close friends and family to provide strength and assistance. Helping people to develop and maintain relationships . . . allows people to make choices, dream, stay safe and live the way they want' (Pitonyak & Pitonyak 1998).

CONCLUSION

Life without being close to other people is hard to imagine, yet easy to impose on others. This chapter has described the reasons why such an imposition is so devastating for people with learning disabilities, and has charted its history in services for such people. It is now possible to discuss, with reference to all sorts of books and resources, the ways in which this imposition can be lifted. However, the day-to-day experience of a very large number of people with learning disabilities is certainly not one of closeness and intimacy. The ideas, the words and the good intentions need to be turned to action in settings right across the country if they are to prove to be of any real value.

REFERENCES

ARC/NAPSAC 1997 There are no easy answers: service needs of people with learning disabilities who sexually abuse others. ARC/NAPSAC, Chesterfield/Nottingham

Armado R 1993 Friendships and community connections between people with and without developmental disabilities. Paul Brookes Publishing, Baltimore

Baum S, Sheppard N 2001 Recognizing and responding to abuse: training people with learning disabilities to be checkers of residential homes. Clinical Psychology Forum 148: 32–35

Booth T, Booth W 1994a Parenting under pressure: mothers and fathers with learning difficulties. Open University Press, Buckingham

Booth T, Booth W 1994b Working with parents with mental retardation: lessons from research. Journal of Developmental and Physical Disabilities 6: 23–41

Booth T, Booth W 2000 Against the odds: growing up with parents who have learning difficulties. Mental Retardation 38(1): 1–14

Brown H, Craft A (eds) 1989 Thinking the unthinkable: papers on the sexual abuse of people with learning difficulties. Family Planning Association, London

Brown H, Smith H 1992 Normalisation: a reader for the nineties. Routledge, London

Brown H, Turk V 1992 Defining sexual abuse as it affects adults with learning disabilities. Mental Handicap 20: 44–55

Brown H, Hunt N, Stein J 1994 Alarming but necessary: working with staff groups around the sexual abuse of adults with learning disabilities. Journal of Intellectual Disability Research 38: 393–412

Brown H, Stein J, Turk V 1995 The sexual abuse of adults with learning disabilities: report of a second two year incidence survey. Mental Handicap Research 8: 3–24

Cambridge P 1997 How far to gay? The politics of HIV in learning disability. Disability and Society 12(3): 427–453

Campion M J 1995 Who's fit to be a parent? Routledge, London

Carlson B 1998 Domestic violence in adults with mental retardation: reports from victims and key informants. Mental Health Aspects of Developmental Disabilities 1: 102–112

Carson D 1987 (ed) The law and the sexuality of people with a mental handicap. Southampton University Law Faculty, Southampton

Carson D 1991 Clarifying the law on mental responsibility. Health Service Journal 16 May: 14–15

Craft A, Brown H 1994 Personal relationships and sexuality: the staff role. In: Craft A (ed) Practice issues in sexuality and learning disabilities. Routledge, London

Curry M 2001 Abuse of women with disabilities. Violence Against Women 7(1): 60–80

Department of Health 1998 Signposts to success. HMSO, London

Department of Health 2000 No secrets. HMSO, London

Department of Health 2001 Valuing people. HMSO, London

Evans A, Rodgers M 2000 Protection for whom? The right to a sexual or intimate relationship. Journal of Learning Disabilities 4(3): 237–245

Feldman M A 1994 Parenting education for parents with intellectual disabilities: a review of outcome studies. Research in Developmental Disabilities 15: 299–332

Firth H, Rapley M 1990 From acquaintance to friendship. Issues for people with learning disabilities. BIMH Publications, Kidderminster

Fruin D 1994 Almost equal opportunities . . . developing personal relationships: guidelines for social department staff working with people with learning disabilities. In: Craft A (ed) Practice issues in sexuality and learning disabilities. Routledge, London

Furey E M 1989 Abuse of persons with mental retardation: a literature review. Behavioural Residential Treatment 4: 143–154

Galway S 1992 Plato's Symposium. http://cyberpat.com/shirlsite/essays/plato/html

Gostin L 1986 Mental health services – law and practice. Shaw and Sons, London

Gunn M 1994 Competency and consent. In: Craft A (ed) Practice issues in sexuality and learning disabilities. Routledge, London

Human Rights Act 1998. www.hmso.gov.uk/acts/acts1998/19980042

Kempton W, Kahn E 1991 Sexuality and people with intellectual disabilities: a historical perspective. Sexuality and Disability 9: 93–111

Law Commission 1991 Mentally incapacitated adults and decision making: an overview. HMSO, London

McCabe M 1999 Sexual knowledge, experience and feelings among people with disability. Sexuality and Disability: 17(2): 157–170

McCarthy M 1999 Sexuality and women with learning disabilities. Jessica Kingsley Publishers, London

McCarthy M, Thompson D 1994 Sex and staff training. Pavilion Publishing, Brighton

McCarthy M, Thompson D 1997 A prevalence study of sexual abuse of adults with intellectual disabilities referred for sex education. Journal of Applied Research in Intellectual Disabilities 10(2): 105–124

McGraw S 1994 How to be a good parent. BILD, Kidderminster

Orford J 1992 Community psychology: theory and practice. Wiley, Chichester

Pillay A, Sargent 2000 Psycho-legal issues affecting rape survivors with mental retardation. South African Journal of Psychology 30(3): 9–14

Pitonyak D, Pitonyak C 1998 The community journal: building a better Virginia together. Special Issue 4(2): 22

Potter D C 1993 Mental handicap: is anything wrong? Kingsway, London

Rodgers J 2001 The experience and management of menstruation in women with learning disabilities. Tizard Learning Disability Review 6(1): 36–44

Rhodes R 1993 Mental retardation and sexual expression: an historical perspective. Journal of Social Work and Human Sexuality 8: 1–27

Schwartz D 1997 Who cares? Rediscovering community. Westview Press, Philadelphia

Sheerin F 1998 Parents with learning disabilities: a review of the literature. Journal of Advanced Nursing 28: 126–133

Skultans V 1979 English madness: ideas on insanity 1580–1890. Routledge and Kegan Paul, London

Synason V 1994 Working with sexually abused individuals who have a learning disability. In: Craft A (ed) Practice issues in sexuality and learning disabilities. Routledge, London

Turk V, Brown H 1993 The sexual abuse of adults with learning disabilities: results of a two year incidence survey. Mental Handicap Research 6(3): 193–21

Tymchuk A 1992 Predicting adequacy of parenting by people with mental retardation. Child Abuse and Neglect 16: 165–178

United Nations 1983 Human rights: a compilation of international instruments. United Nations, New York

Wolfensberger W 1988 Common assets of mentally retarded people that are not commonly acknowledged. Mental Retardation 26: 63–70

FURTHER READING

Booth T, Booth W 1994 Parenting under pressure: mothers and fathers with learning difficulties. Open University Press, Buckingham

Cooper E, Guillebaud J 1999 Sexuality and disability: a guide for everyday practice. Radcliffe Medical Press, Abingdon *This is an excellent book covering practical issues about health and sexuality for people with all kinds of disabilities. The material concerning people with physical disabilities is of real interest and there are specific chapters relating to people with learning disabilities.*

Craft A (ed) 1994 Practice issues in sexuality and learning disabilities. Routledge, London

Craft A, Members of the Nottinghamshire SLD Sex Education Project 1991 Living your life: a sex education and personal education programme for students with severe learning difficulties. LDA, Cambridge *This is one of the teaching packages available to support people with learning disabilities to explore issues of personal and sexual relationships either individually or in groups.*

McCarthy M 1999 Sexuality and women with learning disabilities. Jessica Kingsley Publishers, London

McCarthy M, Thompson D 1993 Sex and the 3 R's. Rights, responsibilities and risks: a sex education package for working with people with learning difficulties. Hove Pavilion Publishing, Brighton *This is also a package for working with people with learning disabilities in support of their sexual and personal relationships.*

24

Working effectively with families of people with learning disabilities

Owen Barr

CHAPTER CONTENTS

KEY ISSUES

- The majority of people with learning disabilities, perhaps as many as 85% of all people with learning disabilities, up to 60% of adults and a higher percentage of children with learning disabilities live at home with their families.
- Family members often make a major contribution to their care. Parents, brothers and sisters and, at times, members of the extended family provide accommodation, as well as aspects of day care, nursing care, social care, education and social support.
- The need to involve family members in care is not a new idea. Manthorpe (1995) has noted that attention to the needs of families was incorporated into the 1913 Mental Deficiency Act.
- This has been clearly stated in most reviews of legislation and policy documents between 1971 and 2001 (Welsh Office 1971, DOH 2001a).

INTRODUCTION

The importance of involving family members has once again been formally articulated in *Valuing People: A New Strategy for People with Learning Disability in the 21st Century* which stated that 'carers need to be confident that public services will provide reliable support for their family members with learning disabilities' (DOH 2001a, p. 53). Similar views are to be found in the review of services for people with learning disabilities in Scotland and Northern Ireland (Scottish Executive 2000, DHSS NI 1995). Current community care policies rely heavily on the importance of family members in order that people with learning disabilities may live fulfilling lives in their communities, a situation that has been acknowledged by the Government who have stated that the 'support and commitment of carers is critical in enabling people with learning disabilities to achieve independence, choice and commitment' (DOH, 2001a, p. 53). A real challenge remains for professionals to provide effective support to families if the criticism of care in the community being 'a euphemism for care by the family . . . very often with minimal support from health, social services and voluntary agencies' is to be overcome (Udwin et al 1998)

THE NEED TO WORK EFFECTIVELY WITH FAMILIES

The 1990s in particular witnessed increased recognition of the importance of parents and other family members being involved in decisions that affect their children or, when appropriate, their siblings with learning disabilities. It appears to be generally accepted that parents, and at times other family members, have a legal and moral right to be involved in decisions that may affect the life of a person with learning disabilities, and the lives of family members. The opportunities for parents to be involved in the decision making process is evident from early in the child's life; for example under the provisions of the Children Act (1995), and corresponding legislation in Scotland and Northern Ireland, the importance of parental involvement and parental responsibility is highlighted. This is considered to remain important even when children are not living with their parent(s).

It is also evident in the inclusion of parents in the 'statementing process' when plans are being considered for the best way to meet the educational needs of children with learning disabilities (see Ch. 7). Within this process parents have a clear role in contributing to the assessment of their children's abilities and needs, as well as making suggestions about future services for their children.

Their involvement within the area of education is also evident in the discussions that should occur during school leaver conferences when young people with learning disabilities are preparing to leave school. Parents are not intended to be passive participants in these processes and have opportunities to challenge both informally and formally the decisions made by professionals.

Further to being involved in the decision making process, parents and other family members who provide care for people with learning disabilities now have the right to have a comprehensive assessment of their own needs in relation to the care they provide. This can occur through legal rights in legislation such as the NHS and Community Care Act (1990) which introduced comprehensive assessment and care management as one system of care coordination in which the consideration of the abilities, needs and views of the carers is a key requirement. This has been further strengthened within both The Carers (Recognition and Services) Act (1995) and the extended provision within the Carers and Disabled Children Act (2000) that was implemented on 1 April 2001. Within Northern Ireland the need for carers to have independent assessments of their own needs is achieved through the implementation of good practice guidelines within services, which emphasise the need for a separate assessment of carers' needs. In addition to the above legislative and policy guidance many professionals are required by regulations of their own professional bodies to work effectively with families in a manner similar to that outlined within the *Code of Professional Conduct*. This code requires each registered nurse, midwife and health visitor

 Reader activity 24.1

Further to the policy requirements outlined in the preceding paragraphs, write a list of practical reasons that make it important for professionals to work effectively with parents and other family members of people with learning disabilities. What do you believe would be the potential practical outcomes of working effectively with family members? Equally what could be the consequences of failing to work effectively with family members?

to 'cooperate with others in the team... includes the client's family and informal carers' (NMC 2002, p. 6)

Hornby (1995) has pointed out that parents both have needs and can contribute to the care process. All parents have communication needs, most have liaison needs, many require education about their child, and some require the services of counselling and support groups. Despite the developments in the provision of information to family members the difficulties with this continues to be highlighted as a key failing in services (DOH 1999a). Parents can also make valuable contributions to services. All parents can provide information, most are interested and capable of collaboration, and are a resource in the provision of care. Further to this, some may be willing to contribute to the formulation of policies on a local and national level through their involvement in joint planning ventures and support groups. Dale (1996) has provided a comprehensive rationale for parental involvement in relation to children with special needs that can be expanded to include adults with learning disabilities and other family members (Box 24.1).

Box 24.1   The case for parental involvement in the care process (adapted from Dale 1996)

- Professionals need family cooperation to do their own jobs effectively.
- Family members are a potential resource for helping the person with special needs.
- Parents and other family members need support and guidance to help them carry out their parenting and care of the person with learning disabilities.
- Unless professionals work alongside family members supportively, their actions can have a disabling effect on the person with learning disabilities and the family unit.
- The family has a key role in the life of the person with learning disabilities.
- People with learning disabilities are individuals with their own needs, wishes and feelings.
- Families provide continuity for children throughout their childhood, and for many adults with learning disabilities.
- The abilities and needs of the person with learning disabilities cannot be separated from the family process and functioning.
- Carers want to be more involved in activities and decisions on services provided to the family members with learning disabilities.

Much of the literature to date focusing on family involvement in care relates to the role of parents (often more specifically the mother), but it requires more than this and should consider the role of both parents and siblings, and the effect of the impact on the extended family (Burke & Cigno 2000, Carpenter 1997). Active involvement sees the family as valued contributors and not merely as passive recipients of services. Involvement should mean more than the professionals unilaterally collecting data from family members and then deciding priorities, which are then explained to, rather than negotiated with the family.

Recent changes in legislation, professional guidelines and policy statements together with practical considerations mean that the involvement of family members must be an integral part of the assessment, planning, implementation and evaluation of services offered to them. Active family involvement does not require the person with learning disabilities to be living at home (although it is often thought of in this way). Even when an individual lives in a residential facility family members should still be facilitated to have an active part in their life (DOH, 2001b, Dyer 1996).

In order for active family involvement in care to become a reality of service provision, professionals must recognise that there are many different types of family, and how the diagnosis of learning disability in a member will influence this complex structure.

WHAT IS A FAMILY?

As individuals we have a variety of family backgrounds. Often during conversations with friends and colleagues, similarities and differences in our family circumstances may be commented on. These include areas such as the size of the family, the number and gender of children, our ordinal placement and role within the family. Discussions between friends and colleagues about our relationships with our parents and siblings, their abilities and needs and how our parents related to each other provide insight into the differences between families.

Often these differences have their origins in cultural, religious and ethnic beliefs (Diniz 1997).

Consideration will probably have been given to whether our own family members are very close to each other, and whether it is an extended family with grandparents and aunts, uncles and cousins in regular contact, or a much smaller unit consisting only of parent(s) and their children. It is possible that the rules and roles within our family were a topic of discussion and at times debated, both inside and outside the family setting.

During conversations about our families there is an assumption as to what a family is and it is generally recognised as a core unit within society that has a major influence on the development and overall functioning of its individual members as well as on local communities. The possible consequences of the changing composition of families on individuals and on wider society has generated much political debate over the past decade, and this is likely to continue for a considerable time to come. Some 'newer' family structures have been portrayed, often inappropriately, as the origin of many of society's problems whilst almost simultaneously the idea of a stable family whose members are supportive, loving and involved with the interests of their children has been identified as the answer to some of these problems (Giddens 1997, Haralambos & Holburn 2000).

Evidence as to the 'health' of the family in society at present is conflicting. However some trends remain almost constant such as marriage, which continues to be popular, and the majority of children live with both natural parents (ONS 2000). However, as the composition of families within the UK and the demography of people with learning disabilities are changing, some consideration

needs to be given to the increasing diversity of family structures ranging from small nuclear family groups to more extended family structures. Individual professionals and wider service policies should be supportive of an increasing range of family structures that reflect the diversity of social and cultural factors within society (Burke & Cigno 2000). Care must be taken to ensure all families are supported equally and people with learning disabilities are not discriminated against through living in a particular family type.

As noted earlier, the majority of people with learning disabilities live with one or both parents and other family members. At times there can be more than one child with learning disabilities within the family (Tozer 1999). A growing number of parents may have had previous marriages and this may result in an increased number of step-parents and step-siblings. Some people with learning disabilities live with one parent and indeed single parents with dependent children do make up a sizable proportion of the population. The stereotypical image of lone parents being single mothers, who have never been married, is misleading as the majority of lone parents have previously been married and have either become divorced, separated or widowed. It is also important to note that a growing number of people with complex needs and adults with learning disabilities are living at home with older carers who are often alone. Recent estimates for England, Wales and Scotland appear to agree on an estimate that approximately one-third of people with learning disabilities live with carers who are over 70 years old (DOH 2001a, Scottish Executive 2000). Lone parents are often affected by the lack of partner support, unavailability of transport and fears for the future, all of which can increase the degree of isolation felt by the parent (Cigno & Burke 1997).

An increasing number of people with learning disabilities are being cared for either by foster parents or by adoptive parents. The challenges faced by these families may at times be different from those faced by natural parents, but they remain considerable. It is an unwarranted assumption to believe that adoptive or foster parents will cope better than natural parents because they knew the

Reader activity 24.2

Define what the term 'family' means to you; now compare and contrast your definition with that of colleagues, and consider why you have defined a family as you did. Following discussion with colleagues, prepare a list of the components that you feel are necessary for a group of people to be a family.

children had learning disabilities prior to caring for them. In the case of adoptive parents it may be the case that they may have had a child from a very young age when learning disabilities had not been confirmed; but even with advance notice, the same practical difficulties of care arise.

People with learning disabilities who live within extended family networks may receive significant support from grandparents, aunts, uncles and cousins who may be very much part of the 'family'. Some people with learning disabilities may live within a three generational family structure, in which grandparents are active members of the family and may live along with the family in one house. Another possibility is an extended family in which brothers and sisters and their respective families live together, either out of necessity, or as part of a cultural tradition. The impact of support from grandparents and other relatives must be recognised. When they offer practical and psychological support this can be a significant factor in the longer term adjustment of the family to a member with learning disabilities and may increase the coping abilities of the parents and siblings. Grandparents are affected by the birth of a child with learning disabilities: they often feel the pain of their son or daughter. This may be further complicated in situations in which the child with learning disabilities is identified as having a genetic condition that can be traced back to their grandparents either by confirmed tests or by implication of diagnosis (Barr 1999). Grandparents and other relatives may find it difficult to cope with their own emotions, thereby reducing their provision of active support. They may have limited understanding about the care of a child with learning disabilities, or very different views on learning disabilities from those of the child's parent. The views of grandparents may have been informed by limited personal experience or memories of the nature of services for people with learning disabilities some 30–40 years ago. Information about people with learning disabilities should be available to grandparents and, if necessary, other relatives (Mirfin-Veitch & Bray 1997). This should help them talk with the child's parents and reduce the possibility that they will try to cope by not talking about the child's difficul-

ties, by blaming either parent, or holding unrealistic expectations of the person with learning disabilities or their son or daughter.

In contrast to extended family networks living in close proximity, other people with learning disabilities may be in families which have strong family ties, but whose members live a considerable distance apart, for example where there is a need to travel for employment. Some families even move to gain access to what they believe to be better services. Thus a situation can arise where family members are a considerable geographical distance apart. Even so, they can remain actively involved in the decisions and life of the family unit. Equally, because family members live nearby, it must not be assumed that support will be forthcoming as tensions and other barriers to providing support may be present. Some families may regularly move from one location to another for various reasons, such as employment, career prospects, housing, personal interest or as part of a way of life within a specific culture, as, for example, in the 'travelling community' population (now recognised as the largest ethnic group in Northern Ireland under race relations legislation). This can mean that they 'slip through' the net of service provision. They may also not be established in a neighbourhood, and therefore not benefit from the informal community support available because they are unknown in the area.

Families are complex fluid structures and it is reasonable to expect that the nature of family structures will continue to alter over time. This raises as problematic whether it is possible to identify a clear definition that encompasses all families. New family structures will continue to emerge, requiring services to adapt. Family units with partners of the same gender are beginning to be acknowledged in legislation in some European countries. As more people with learning disabilities have children, yet another type of family structure will develop.

From the perspective that families involve structured relationships and stability over time (Carpenter 1997), people with learning disabilities in residential care often view the people they live with as their 'family'. Such people may have lived together in close proximity for 20 years or more and have established close relationships that they value. Unfortunately, this has not always been appreciated in plans for developing new accommodation. Crude measures, which have included original address, level of ability, contracted places and the desires and self-interests of some managers of new services have, on occasions, been applied rather than looking at the importance of the long established relationships between people with learning disabilities. This can result in the destruction of such 'families' and a transitional bereavement type trauma for people with learning disabilities.

It is no longer desirable to have a static definition of the 'family', as this runs the risk of perpetuating the stereotype of what a family should be, a difficulty of this being that when a family fails to match some preconceived idea of what it should be, judgements are placed on its worth. Such judgements could have serious implications for the availability, delivery and evaluation of services for people with learning disabilities and their families, and therefore must be carefully guarded against. Despite variations in definitions it is generally accepted that a family involves the following broad characteristics:

- A defined membership
- Agreed group values
- Relationships between members
- Roles
- Structure
- Functions
- Stability over time.

The emphasis given to each area will be greatly influenced by the values, beliefs and cultural background of the family.

In conclusion, it would be more practical to obtain up-to-date information on the key components that provide an understanding of the individual nature of each family and reflect on its current functioning. Regular revision of any initial information collected must be undertaken to ensure that the changing nature of the family is accommodated in any interventions (DOH 2001a). The importance of the family in person centred planning is pivotal in the recent White Paper on involving the family (DOH 2001b).

FACTORS INFLUENCING FAMILY FUNCTIONING

By the very nature of the interactions between family members' abilities and needs (as individuals and as a family group) within the wider community, families can usefully be viewed as evolving or functioning. 'Family functioning' refers to how the family is structured, its aims, objectives, priorities and purpose, and the strategies used to achieve these. If services are to be effective and family members actively involved, it is important that intervention strategies used by nurses, social workers and other professionals are compatible with the functioning of the family (Burke & Cigno 2000). This will require a clearer understanding of the issues that can impact on family functioning if the regular criticisms that professionals do not fully understand the complexity of family life are to be overcome (Grant et al 1998, Scottish Executive 2000, Shearn & Todd 1997).

People who aim to support families to respond effectively to caring for a family member with learning disabilities need to recognise the wide range of factors that can impact on family functioning. The context of family life is dynamic and has many influences that need to be taken into account. The functioning of families can be viewed on a number of different levels as outlined within family system theory. The main areas for attention within this theoretical perspective are the characteristics of the family, interactions within the family, the stage(s) within the family life-cycle being encountered and the focus of family functioning (Box 24.2).

Reader activity 24.3

List the factors inside and outside the family which you believe influence its functioning and then from the list you have prepared, describe the effects of four factors (two inside and two outside the family) and what implications these may have for professionals working with people who have learning disabilities.

Box 24.2   Components within family systems model of family functioning (adapted from Turnbull & Turnbull 1990)

Family characteristics (Inputs)
Physical, psychological and social characteristics of each individual member.
Physical, psychological and social characteristics of family as a unit.
Special challenges faced by the family and the resources available to meet these

Family interaction
Degree of cohesion and adaptability in interrelationships within the family between parents, siblings, marital rela-

tionship and involvement and relationship of the above groups with the extended family

Family lifecycle (change process)
Developmental stages and transitions (remember possible impact of having family member with learning disabilities).
Change in family characteristics (new members, people leaving, alterations in health, socio-economic status)

Family functions (outputs)
Priorities among functions of economics, daily care, affection, leisure, socialisation, education, reproduction

---

Characteristics of the family

It is generally accepted that although several people may share a similar appearance, the interests or habits that each person has are unique and individual. In considering families, whilst it is possible to group families together on a number of characteristics such as size, income, location, ethnic origin or the presence of a person with learning disabilities, care must be taken not to make the error of viewing families with similarities as the same. Despite similarities, major differences can occur in how individual family members or families as a unit view their circumstances, and the environment in which they live will affect this. Hornby (1994, 1995) has outlined the need to view families within the wider context of an ecological perspective and acknowledge that they are influenced by a number of factors that can affect family functioning, and therefore families require atten-

tion at all stages of the care process. He noted that the factors that may impact on overall family functioning can be grouped within four overlapping domains, namely what he defined as the microsystem, mesosystem, exosystem and macrosystem (Box 24.3).

The nuclear family is at the centre of this model (microsystem). All the personal characteristics of the family members have a direct impact on the family. This makes it necessary to ascertain from family members what they consider their personal characteristics to be, and what impact these have on the functioning of the family. The abilities and needs of a family member with learning disabilities, and that person's carers, should be a major part of this assessment. For example, the presence of communication difficulties or physical illness can result in different sets of challenges in contrast to each other.

Box 24.3   The ecological model of family functioning (adapted from Hornby 1994, 1995)

Microsystem
Parent factors (e.g. age, status, health education, socio-economic status)
Child factors (e.g. age, abilities, needs, cause of disability, prognosis)
Sibling factors (e.g. number, birth order, gender, abilities, needs)

Mesosystem
Impact of extended family, friends, neighbours, colleagues, other parents, nurses, social workers, teachers, psychologists, other therapists. Involves impact as individuals and in relation to professional services, the degree of coordination, cohesiveness and conflict

Exosystem
Images portrayed by local and national television, radio, newspapers.
Voluntary / support groups – availability, resources and response to people as individuals

Macrosystem
Influence of larger social forces and how these affect family unit and individual family members. Involves the influence of community, culture, ethnicity, religion, economics, politics and the legal system

Discussions with family members will invariably point out other influences on the family, such as the extended family, friends, workmates and the professionals involved (mesosystem). Such people can be a critical component in the coping abilities of a family that includes a person with learning disabilities, and their impact should never be underestimated. Practical, emotional and possibly financial support from relations, friends and workmates will reduce the isolation of the family members and assist in maintaining their energy and motivation. On the other hand, a diagnosis of learning disabilities in a family member can also result in the fragmentation of previous relationships, leading to lack of support, increased isolation and further demands. The pain of long-standing friends and colleagues failing to talk about or to a child with learning disabilities, and being reluctant to maintain regular contact with family members, will be remembered by parents and siblings for a long time.

As the move to inclusive services gathers momentum, resources in the wider community (the exosystem) will exert an increasing influence over the abilities of families to care for the person with learning disabilities. Although in most localities services for children have become reasonably comprehensive, frequent difficulties are still reported in relation to flexibility within service provision and the availability of short-term breaks. Adults continue to encounter major problems with access to open employment, choice of accommodation on leaving home (or hospital), inclusive recreational facilities and short-term breaks, which continue to be patchy and often inadequate (DOH 1999a, Simons & Watson 1999).

On the last level (macrosystem), the impact of political decisions and the resourcing of services need to be considered. At a local level professionals should involve family members and people with learning disabilities in project groups to develop new services or policies. At a national level, voluntary organisations should be used to provide valuable insights into policy decisions. The wide consultation process, and the development of partnerships in the development and implementation of the strategies for people with learning disabilities in Scotland as well as in England and Wales, provide some evidence of the recognition of the need for such discussions (DOH 2001a, Scottish Executive 2000).

Recognising the differing levels of factors that may impact on family functioning has the advantage of orientating services to the wider issues affecting the lives of families. In doing so it challenges staff to respond on all levels, not only within the microsystem. However, this must be balanced against ensuring that the family remains central to the whole intervention process whilst acknowledging the importance of external factors. As the different levels clearly impact on each other it is not realistic for individual members of staff or professional groups to take the view that they only deal with one level of influence. Rather they need to realise how their interventions impact on the other levels of influence and develop effective alliances and partnerships for service development, political lobbying and service delivery that maximise the use of their resource.

Interactions within the family

Family systems theory acknowledges both the environment outside the family, and the stage of family development; however, the essential component is considered to be relationships between family members. A series of interactions between two or more family members is considered not only to bring about a change in the members involved, but also in the overall functioning of the family. Equally, a change in the abilities and needs of a family member, such as the development of learning disabilities, illness, leaving home and starting or leaving school or employment, will have an impact on all the other members and the functioning of the family. Any changes in the family life are recognised as potentially having a major impact on family functioning.

Consequently, within this framework any intervention, to be effective, must concentrate on the nature of the interactions within the family, instead of focusing on one particular member. Family systems theory is relevant to the care of people with learning disabilities because a diagnosis of learning disability in a family member will lead to alterations in family characteristics, such as the abilities and needs of child and parents, financial resources, personal energy, as well as the level of commitment and motivation required to maintain previous functioning. Family interaction between the parents as a couple, parents and children, siblings with each other or friends and the impact of the extended family may alter. The increased physical and emotional demands on the family resource (the need to keep appointments, run new programmes of care, changes in working practices) may lead to a change in priorities among family functioning (Hilbert et al 2000). The overall patterns of coping and interaction will also be influenced by the explanation other family members receive about learning disabilities and the rationale for changing roles and expectations with the family.

Family lifecycle

Several authors have attempted to explain how families evolve by outlining the various sequential stages, qualitatively different from each other, that families move through during their 'lifecycle'. Gelles (1995) has highlighted that the number of stages in a developmental framework varies depending on the author of the work (Duvall 1967, 8 stages; Rodgers 1962, 10 stages; Rubins 1976, 4 stages). Despite these variations, each framework follows a remarkably similar path. The age of the eldest child is taken to be an indicator of the developmental stage of the family. However, it is necessary to consider that families may be attempting to achieve a number of goals simultaneously from various stages, depending on the age range of their children.

Viewing the family and its members within a developmental model can provide some insights into the impact of a member with learning disabilities on family development (see Table 24.1). This will differ according to the stage of family development. This approach provides a framework that can assist professionals and family members to understand and put into perspective the goals of the family at any given time during the family lifecycle. However, irrespective of this, families have

to grapple with 'changed expectations for the child, altered perceptions for the future and an acknowledgement of being a different family' (Manthorpe 1995).

There are some limitations to using a framework of stages to coordinate services, as all stages are not directly applicable to all families of people with learning disabilities. The framework is based on the belief that adult sons and daughters leave home, but this may not be the case for many people with learning disabilities. It has been demonstrated that adults with learning disabilities often remain at home with their parents until the parents are old, and can no longer manage (DOH 2001b). This scenario is likely to become more common with the implementation of current government policies aimed at maintaining people at home for as long as possible. Therefore, the final three stages identified in Table 24.1 need to be reconsidered for such families.

Developmental goals have been shown to differ for families that are not 'traditional' in their structure (that is, two healthy heterosexual parents with children). Additional developmental tasks have been reported for adoptive, separated, single-parent, remarried and step-families (Johnson 1992). Revised developmental frameworks have also been reported for divorced, reconstituted, dual-earner and low-income families, and families of people with alcohol dependence (Carter & McGoldrick 1989). Care must be taken in transferring 'norms' developed in the USA to families within the UK, as the structure, function and development of families has been shown to differ across cultures (Giddens 1997).

Focus of family functioning

Issues encountered during the lifecycle and strategies for responding to them will be influenced by the changes noted above. Teaching new skills for physical care or teaching responses to 'challenging behaviour' occur within a family context. Therefore, the best results will be achieved when any intervention acknowledges family functioning. A focus on the person with learning disabilities in isolation from other family members may at best result in inconsistent

Table 24.1   Family developmental tasks and possible impact of having a member with learning disabilities

Stage	Developmental task to be achieved	Considerations when a family member has learning disabilities
1. Setting up home	Establish relationships (Marriage / cohabiting) Integrate with partners relatives and friends Priorities identified (children, career, home) Roles evolve in relationship	
2. First child arrives	Learn about and adjust to new roles Care of the child Keeping time for self and each other Maintaining work plans Readjusting priorities	Increased stress due to care needs. Fears over future children. May be unable to return to work. Blaming partner or oneself if genetic cause is found. Financial pressures. Regular appointments to be kept with increasing number of professionals. Social isolation may evolve due to difficulties with child minding or reluctance to go out socially
3. Out to school	Encourage integration with peers Support child's learning Liaison with teachers Sharing child's care Seek employment (if desired)	Assessment process undertaken. Confirms degree of disability (possibly for first time). Difficulty in nursery and school place. Additional programmes of work and appointments. Child development overtaken by siblings, cousins or children born at same time
4. Living with an adolescent	Readjust boundaries of responsibility Adapt to new peer group Reducing supervision Maintaining educational and vocational progress Facilitating choices and risk taking	Puberty may be delayed. Difficulties in explaining physical and psychological changes. Concerns over sexual expression and risk of exploitation. Unsure about further opportunities. Adult size, possibly with additional physical care needs for parents. Pressure on time due to additional supervision needs of person with learning disabilities. Conflict as person with learning disability realises that some opportunities of adolescence are not open to them
5. A new freedom	Children leave home. Parents readjust to free time and increased living space. Provide financial support in higher education. Pursue new goals and hobbies. Maintain open communication with son / daughter. Possible new role as grandparent. Reappraisal of life. Revise plans for career, possibly consider early retirement. Reinvest time in marital relationship	Person with learning disabilities may leave home for independent living due to increased care needs, possibly limited day-care facilities, or remains at home, imposing new restrictions on parents' time. May be only son / daughter remaining at home. Concerns over further care increasing. Limited time for new interests. May have to explain to other children about risk of learning disabilities in their children. Additional burden of care may fall on siblings (especially older sisters)
6. Together to the end	Leave work, enter retirement, adjust to changes in physical and mental ability. Require support from family members	Alternative care required, separated from son / daughter with learning disabilities. Feeling of failure if residential care is required may be strong for some parents. Expectation that siblings will take over care of person with learning disabilities

progress. At worst, the failure to consider the family context will increase rather than reduce the challenges faced by the family. When an intervention fails to achieve its stated aim, professionals must carefully examine how family centred the care process was. It is not sufficient to attribute the failure to a lack of interest or commitment among family members. Limited resources, lack of explanation, confusion, little or no encouragement, fatigue, and lack of commitment among professionals, as well as inconsistent advice, are only some of the reasons for unsuccessful care programmes.

The context of family life is dynamic, and has many influences that need to be taken into account. Models of family functioning provide some starting points and frameworks to guide intervention. The key task is to make an informed and professional decision in relation to the model that fits best with the family at the time and that can provide a coherent structure within which to coordinate any intervention. Although accepting the individuality of families, research into how families respond to the diagnosis and care of people with learning disabilities provides further insights that are helpful in understanding family functioning.

Reader activity 24.4

Reflect on your involvement with a family of a person with learning disabilities and identify the extent to which you feel services have successfully responded to the range of factors that may influence family functioning. Why do you feel services have been effective and what suggestions would you make for enhancing the services provided?

THE IMPACT OF LEARNING DISABILITIES ON THE FAMILY

Diagnosis

Some mothers with hindsight report having 'a feeling' during pregnancy that things were 'not right', but they had no hard evidence as to what was wrong. However, the vast majority of parents have no evidence that their child will have learning disabilities before the birth. Only a minority of parents have definite advance warning, possibly from screening investigations such as blood tests and ultrasound scans, or diagnostic investigations such as amniocentesis, chorionic villi sampling or other tests undertaken because the parents are perceived as at a high risk of having a child with disabilities (see Ch. 2).

Unless a definite physical abnormality or characteristic signs (as in children with Down syndrome) are present at birth, or a traumatic delivery has taken place, the presence of learning disabilities is often not suspected or diagnosed at birth. Even if clear signs are present it can take several days to confirm test results. The precision of a diagnosis can vary from the confirmation of the presence of a specific condition, for instance Down syndrome, to a much broader 'diagnosis' of developmental delay with no specific condition identified. The more specific the diagnosis the more accurate a prognosis may be, even allowing for the wide variation among individuals with the same diagnosis. A clear indication of likely development and health of the child may reduce uncertainty about the future for family members and give a focus to their interactions with the child, whereas, a broad non-specific definition can leave considerable uncertainty about the future and provides less focus for interventions. It is anticipated that as our understanding of genetics increases, arising from the human genome project (see Ch. 2), more confirmed diagnoses will be provided. While this may provide more specific information for parents and family members it can also lead to added difficulties within parental and family relationships (Barr 1999, Ward 2001). Even then these tests cannot predict the degree of learning disabilities with any accuracy, and for this reason conclusive statements relating to eventual achievement or the possible degree of disability cannot be made. A major determinant of the eventual level of functioning of all people is their environment after birth.

Learning disability is most often diagnosed in early childhood, when the child fails to reach developmental milestones. During the developmental period parents may have concerns over the nature of their child's progress and suspect that a problem exists. It is unprofessional and potentially dangerous of those in contact with the parents at this time (e.g. GP, health visitor, paediatrician or other nurses) to dismiss these concerns and label the parents 'overanxious' or 'overprotective'. Value judgements such as these are prejudicial and negate parents' concerns, and they have no place in family centred services. If it is thought that a parent is unnecessarily anxious professionals involved should record exactly what makes them believe this. In doing so, professionals often realise that parents' concerns make sense. Many parents who have a child with learning disabilities report feeling that they have been 'fobbed off' by professionals (Leonard 1994). Professionals should accept that parents spend a lot of time with their children in daily activities, and therefore see how the child is progressing and become aware of minor fluctuations in progress. Therefore, they must start from the position that parents' concerns usually have some substance.

It is essential that such concerns are taken seriously, are clearly noted, factual information is gathered and that parents are assured that they have been listened to. A regular check should be kept on the child's progress (more often than the usual screening checks) and clear records kept. It is a relief to both parents and professionals to be able, after a period of observation, to show that the child is achieving normal milestones. Parents do not expect professionals to have all the answers, and are heartened by an honest answer that admits limitations in knowledge and an agreement to provide the information when available. Parents are deeply hurt and the prospects for partnership damaged by an illusion of expertise (Vagg 1998). The memory of how a diagnosis was given to parents remains fresh in their minds for many years: some parents state that it will never leave them. The prospects of active family involvement will be damaged in the short term, and possibly for several years, when a diagnosis of learning disabilities is confirmed after repeated concerns have been previously dismissed or received little attention.

The adaptation process

In preparation for the birth of a child prospective parents and other family members often think and talk about their hopes for the child and how things will change in the household. This is the start of an adaptation to a potentially new family composition that commences well before the birth of the child. When the child is born the process continues as parents, any previous siblings and other family members, for example grandparents, have to adapt to changes in family/work routines and changing priorities among other things. As the child grows, new challenges and opportunities arise for parents and other family members as family routines stabilise and become consolidated.

The adaptation process commences in anticipation of the birth of all children and is also underway when a child with learning disabilities is born. However the diagnosis of learning disabilities will have a major impact on the adaptation of the family and while most families adapt successfully to having a member with learning disabilities the nature of the adaptation process is altered. Models have been developed to explain the process; these focus on a series of stages that parents are considered to pass through as they progress from the initial shock and confusion to a state of successful adaptation or adjustment to their new situation (Table 24.2a, b). Progression is not always forward, and family members may find themselves oscillating between different stages at times of difficulty. In addition, adaptation is lifelong, and as the abilities and needs of the person with learning disabilities and the composition of the family in which that person lives alter, family developmental goals evolve.

Table 24.2a Hornby's 1994 model of adaptation to diagnosis of learning disability

Stage	Associated emotion
Shock	Confusion
	Numbness
Denial	Disbelief
	Protest
Anger	Blame
	Guilt
Sadness	Despair
	Grief
Detachment	Emptiness
	Meaninglessness
Reorganisation	Realism
	Hope
Adaptation	Reconciliation
	Coming to terms

Table 24.2b   Miller et al's (1994) model of adaptation to diagnosis of learning disability

Stage	Associated emotion/behaviour
Surviving	Shock, fatigue, physical symptoms, feelings of weakness, fragility and vulnerability. Feelings of grief, helplessness, aloneness, sadness, depression, confusion and chaos, uncertainty and ambiguity, preoccupation with child, worrying, asking questions that appear to have no answers. Guilt, self-absorption, self-pity, self-doubt, shame and embarrassment, resentment and envy, blaming, feelings of betrayal, chosen and unconscious denial (seems to last for ever)
Searching	Begins while you are still surviving. Outer searching: quest for diagnosis, search for a label, contact with other families, new awareness, gaining competence and control. Inner searching: forced self-development, redefining life goals and priorities, asking questions of self, being realistic about child's abilities without giving up hope. Acknowledging that you are not the same person as you would have been if your child did not have special needs and deciding whether this is a disappointment, challenge or a blessing
Settling in	Realisation that there are no quick cures or easy answers, realise that some of your questions do not have answers, you become aware of regular progress in your child's development, sense of urgency, establish new priorities in your life and child's life, you get on with the rest of your life, balancing changes, developing new knowledge and skills, find out what works for you, develop a network of people, increased flexibility and adaptability in responses
Separating	Giving some control over to child and others, admitting you cannot make the disability go away, pride in seeing your child achieve goals, getting 'tough' making decisions and sticking to them.

Similarities have been drawn between the diagnosis of learning disabilities and bereavement following death, in so far as parents, siblings and grandparents mourn the loss of the 'dream child' that they thought about prior to the diagnosis (Allan 1993, Maxwell 1993). While some similarities do exist a key distinction needs to be made, in that on the death of an individual that person is no longer present in the physical sense, whereas the child with learning disabilities remains present, and needs to be looked after. This brings with it challenges and opportunities: the challenge to provide a supportive environment when mourning a loss, and yet the opportunity to work through the adaptation process and facilitate the development of the child and family to achieve whatever is possible. No matter how well parents or individual family members appear to be coping, those people supporting them will do well to remember that 'it never gets easy' (McCormack 1992).

During the 1990s attention shifted from viewing families within a pathological model that emphasised the difficulties they experienced in coping with their situation and highlighted the need for professionals to advise and support families often in a directive manner. Within such a perception of families they were viewed as 'in need' of services rather than striving towards independence (Scorgie et al 1999). The emerging view of families highlights their ability to cope successfully given the necessary opportunities. Patterson (1995) has developed a model known as the Family Adjustment and Adaptation Response (FAAR) model to explain how services can effectively support families.

Within the first phase of this model families work through the process of adjustment during which time demands on the family outweigh their coping resource. The emphasis of intervention is to increase individual, family and community resources in order to facilitate families to develop, establish and maintain successful coping behaviours. The focus is on developing strength and resilience within families and their communities, rather than dealing only with crises that may arise for families. As families increase their range of coping behaviours the demands on the family are successfully dealt with and equilibrium between demands and resources is achieved. The aim of intervention is empowerment of family members and professionals involved; this has been defined as the 'increased ability to meet the needs and goals while maintaining autonomy and integrity'

(Patterson 1995). Such a model is consistent with the requirements of working in partnership with families and to facilitate their development.

Positive and negative impact on family

Depending on family circumstances and the progress of the adaptation process, the impact on individual family members and the family as a unit can vary considerably. The impact on family members is often highlighted as being negative, but positive consequences have also been reported (Grant et al 1998). Some effects will span all family members and others will be specific to one or two members. Although family members may have some common concerns, as individuals mothers, fathers and siblings can also have very different concerns and use differing coping strategies. Siblings may have concerns similar to their parents about the health, abilities, needs, future achievements and care of their brother or sister. Further to this, there may be specific impacts on either parent or individual siblings.

Parents

The main responsibility for providing care and support to a family member with learning disabilities falls on the parents, and often the mother will provide the majority of physical care, while fathers may focus more on supporting their partner and the family in general and focus their involvement with the person with learning disabilities on specific activities such as leisure, recreation, or managing difficult behaviour (Carpenter 1997, Rendall 1997). The range of support provided by parents is multidimensional and has been outlined under eight main headings (see Box 24.4). Through interaction with their son or daughter, parents can gain increased knowledge of the nature of learning disabilities and care skills that will be of assistance in providing support. A sense of confidence and competence can evolve for parents from increased knowledge and skills that can in turn lead to increased life satisfaction and a clear sense of coherence about the things that are important in one's life. A greater clarity about the values, beliefs and possibly religious

---

Box 24.4 Components of day-to-day parental work identified (Sheam & Todd 1997)

Body work
Actions to maintain physical health and comfort including tasks such as washing, feeding, toileting and transporting

Safety work
Action to minimise risk to person with learning disabilities and others

Development work
Action that encourages the person with learning disabilities to acquire new skills and survival competencies

Social and recreational work
Actions to involve and engage the person with learning disability in interaction or leisure

Public work
Action to manage other peoples' views of the family and of learning disability

Service work
Action to manage professionals' and other service providers' views of the family and of learning disability

Articulation work
Action to coordinate a range of disparate activities, prioritising activities, and calculating, arranging and controlling the flow of resources

---

beliefs in one's life may provide a framework, together with the motivation to achieve personal goals (Barr 1996).

Provision of support to a son or daughter with learning disabilities may contribute to a negative outcome for parents. Two key aspects that may generate considerable anxiety relate to the future: first, the possibility of having another child with learning disabilities; secondly, most parents, including those of young children, have concerns about the care needs of their children with learning disabilities when they, the parents, are no longer able to manage. This may include the increased presence of chronic sorrow or depression particularly in mothers, possibly compounded by fragmentation of previous networks of friends at work, and associated with social activities that cannot be maintained due to the needs of the person with learning disabilities.

Fathers also report isolation and difficulty in gaining support from professional services as these are often available only when the father is working, or they are focused on the needs of the person with learning disabilities and the mother, which can have the effect of implicitly downplaying or diminishing the concerns of the father (Carpenter 1997). Similar to the idea that mothers may generate some pressure upon themselves to be the main care givers, fathers may contribute to their isolation by holding self-perceived ideas about the need to remain 'in control' of their emotions and provide support to the rest of the family. This can result in the deeply felt needs of fathers going unnoticed and hence fathers feeling less supported (Rendall 1997).

Siblings

Depending on the age of siblings, their experience of having a brother or sister with learning disabilities may differ accordingly. As with parents, as siblings learn more about learning disabilities and observe the support provided, they will gain more knowledge and skills in providing support to their brother or sister. This in turn may lead to increased confidence and understanding in siblings that can also manifest as increased tolerance of differences, and empathy with other people with disabilities. Burke & Montgomery (2000) have reported that siblings could develop an appreciation of the achievements of their learning-disabled siblings, and be very proud of them. In addition siblings can develop maturity and a strong sense of loyalty, and become effective advocates.

However, siblings may also experience difficulties that can arise from the disruption of their previous pattern of family life resulting from the increased care needs of the family member with learning disabilities. This can have the effect of reducing the amount of time and on occasions money available for other siblings. Furthermore the care and support needs of the individual with learning disabilities may reduce siblings' opportunities for spontaneous activities inside (e.g. bringing friends around) and outside the home (e.g. leisure activities).

There may also be expectations that siblings, both sisters and brothers, will provide practical assistance in caring and supporting, whilst at the same time siblings can feel under pressure from parents who may unknowingly or purposively highlight their increased expectations of siblings to achieve in their schoolwork and other activities.

Siblings can experience difficulties that may arise from mixed emotions towards their brother or sister; as well as pride and loyalty they may experience frustration, guilt, embarrassment and annoyance. Difficulties can also arise from outside the home when siblings are teased or bullied as a result of having a brother or sister with learning disabilities, which can be compounded if siblings do not tell their parents and so the bullying may continue. As siblings become more aware of the presence of learning disabilities they may also experience some confusion about their fears for the future both in relation to having a child with learning disabilities themselves and/or providing support to their sibling; they may be unable to discuss this with their parents (Evans et al 2001).

Other family members

Members of the extended family often increase their knowledge, skills and understanding about people with learning disabilities. For example, they may become more tolerant of people with disabilities or develop an increased awareness of the difficulties they can sometimes face. It is also possible that difficulties may arise for members of the extended family due to feelings of awkwardness about visiting the parents of the child with learning disabilities, because they are not sure what to say or do. They may also be embarrassed and/or have mixed emotions of guilt and frustration about some aspects of the behaviour of the person with learning disabilities. Members of the extended family may also not be aware of the nature of the learning disability, or may deny its presence which can lead to difficulties for parents, for example in visiting the homes of relatives or going to social activities at which they may be present. These uncertain emotions coupled with fears that they may have about a child with learning disabilities (particularly if a genetic origin has been identified) can result in disagreements and conflict within families that can further compound the isolation.

Overall family unit

Overall, in a family unit, the presence of an individual with learning disabilities can have a positive outcome by increasing cohesion within the family and can highlight priorities within the family as a group. Family members may develop an increased sensitivity to the abilities and needs of other members, that could result in an enhanced understanding of difficulties that can arise and the need to resolve these. Thus fewer persistent family problems may be present among family members (Barr 1996). However, consistent with the bullying that some family members may experience, families can sometimes find that they are not well supported or accepted by their local community due to misinterpretation of the behaviour of the person with learning disabilities, which may result from members of the local community lacking information and awareness about people with learning disabilities.

People supporting those with learning disabilities should recognise and reinforce the qualities and abilities that can result from having a family member with learning disabilities. This is an important step toward developing the mutual respect, understanding and trust of family members, which is a prerequisite to an effective partnership. Professionals must also realise that the presence of difficulties is not inevitable, and care must be taken to distinguish difficulties that are part and parcel of normal family life, from those that are a result of having a family member with learning disabilities. The professional carer's awareness of potential negative consequences will help them to recognise these quickly and respond appropriately to reduce the impact.

The impact of having a person with learning disabilities in the family is a combination of positive and negative consequences. The impact on the family spans physical, psychological and social domains, and therefore to be effective family interventions must do the same. It is necessary to take time to obtain a clear understanding of how all family members perceive their situation, and the coping strategies employed by individuals and the family as a functional unit. In doing so a more accurate picture of family interactions and priorities is gained and consequently flexible support may be more successfully targeted to facilitate family adaptation (Hilbert et al 2000, Shearn and Todd 1997).

Variables influencing the impact

Key variables affecting the balance of positive and negative consequences can be grouped under four headings: the characteristics of the child, the parents, the family and the local environment (Box 24.5). There is some debate as to the impact of a child with learning disabilities on the strength of a marriage, and whether the child's presence increases the likelihood of divorce or separation. The strength of a relationship, prior to the birth, is considered an accurate predictor as to whether a relationship will survive the birth of a child with learning disabilities. When a marriage or a cohabiting relationship breaks up, the risk of scapegoating the child is potentially great.

Many other factors can influence the eventual outcome of parental and family relationships, therefore the total picture must be examined and the focus should not simply be on the child with learning disabilities as a causative factor. Parents and siblings who see their circumstances as a challenge, and believe that they have control over their future (internal locus) will manage stress

Reader activity 24.5

Think of a person with learning disabilities with whom you are currently involved, and write down the names and approximate ages of the members of that person's family. Then list the attributes of the family and its members which you feel are as a result of living with the person who has learning disabilities. Following this, select three of the attributes you listed above and outline why you feel they are the result of a person with learning disabilities being in the family. Finally, share your results with colleagues (and family members if possible) and assess the strength of your observations and explanations.

Box 24.5   Variables that impact on the ability of a family to provide care for a member with learning disabilities

The parents
Appraisal of the situation
Perceived locus of control
Perceived life satisfaction of parents
Reported previous coping strategies
individually as parents, and together as a couple
Perceived abilities and needs
Response to other children
Strength of relationship

The child
Communication abilities
Degree of continence
Reduced mobility
Presence of challenging behaviour
Physical health

The family
Family health / vulnerability
Level of disruption to previous family functioning
Level of training and competence of family members in care tasks
Financial stability
Number of children
Reaction of grandparents and other relatives

The environment
Level of social support activity available and used
Values, beliefs, culture
Acceptance of the family
Acceptance of the person with learning disability
Availability and quality of services
Professional response (optimistic / pessimistic)

more effectively than those who perceive a threat and little or no control (external locus). An internal locus of control can be encouraged by asking parents to work in partnership with professionals and by valuing their abilities (Barton 1998). The reaction of professionals in the early days can be critical in determining how each family views its situation. Although at times progress may be painfully slow, there is always something that can be set as a realistic objective. If they are clear, realistic and achievable within a few months, then objectives can provide motivation for family members, professionals and the person with learning disabilities. Pessimistic professionals who do not actively seek to have the person with learning disabilities develop new skills and provide encouragement to the family will probably make a difficult situation worse.

The characteristics of a child with learning disabilities have been associated with the level of stress experienced. In particular, the reduced ability to communicate, incontinence, physical illness or the presence of challenging behaviour have been noted to increase stress levels (Hoare et al 1998, Hodapp et al 1998). The increased needs of a person with learning disability can in turn result in increased hospitalisation, or more frequent medical and other appointments; this results in parents having a greater degree of uncertainty and leads to further difficulties in coordinating activities in the home and maintaining work commitments (Hilbert et al 2000). Therefore, equipping parents and siblings with the knowledge and skills to manage their individual situations is a priority.

Wider issues within the family and extended family will have a bearing on the balance between positive and negative consequences. Maintenance of family cohesion and the successful integration of a person with learning disabilities into a family with limited disruption to lifestyle, together with the perceived fairness of parents in managing siblings, is crucial as this can buffer stress and the perceived need for out-of-home placements (Llewellyn et al 1999). Brothers and sisters must continue to have their own interests and hobbies; their birthdays, clothes, possessions and activities should as much as possible remain individual to them. If the siblings consider that they always take second place to their brother or sister with learning disabilities, then the cohesion of the whole family will be reduced. Siblings may assist in practical tasks when asked but may resent this 'duty' and withdraw from it or the home at the first opportunity.

A local community that takes an interest in people with learning disabilities, and welcomes them into their homes and shops, will help families achieve integration. When this is successful the family can feel valued as well as obtaining support and understanding from the local community. Conversely, when the family feels isolated and unsupported, stress will be increased and maintaining the person within the family home becomes more difficult (Llewellyn et al 1999). This can be a particular difficulty for families who are new to or poorly integrated into an area.

Practical considerations, including accessibility to GPs, nursing, social work, nursery and education provision, are all important. Access to public transport, or a car, will be important if the child has regular appointments to attend. It is not unheard of for families to move house to improve their access to services, although being in a new community can compound the isolation experienced by the family. The provision of flexible short-term care services, and introducing families to support groups in the local area can be very important in reducing their social isolation.

COLLABORATION WITH FAMILY MEMBERS

Active family involvement in care requires collaboration between several groups of people. Family members must assist each other and there must be strong partnerships between family members and staff within both statutory and independent organisations. Staff who work within statutory and independent organisations must be committed to working effectively with each other. Active family involvement does not necessarily require a person with learning disabilities to live at home. People in hospitals, community residences or living independently may desire family involvement. When people with learning disabilities leave home it should not mean that their families have any less significance in their lives (Barton 1998, DOH 2001a, b, Dyer 1996).

Collaboration does not come about simply by putting people together, or because a family 'needs' nursing services. Hennemann et al (1995) have identified the antecedents for collaboration as individual readiness, understanding, acceptance, recognition of the boundaries and confidence in one's own role. These qualities must exist within a culture of trust and respect, and among people who value participation and interdependence. Hennemann et al (1995) outline nine defining variables that are present in the relationships and interactions between people who successfully collaborate and by which collaboration in action can be recognised (see Box 24.6).

The extent to which family members wish to be involved in aspects of care can vary greatly. The

> **Box 24.6** Defining variables of collaboration (adapted from Henneman et al 1995)
>
> - Joint venture
> - Cooperative endeavour
> - Willingness and participation
> - Shared planning and decision making
> - Team approach
> - Contribution of expertise
> - Shared responsibility
> - Non-hierarchical relationships
> - Power sharing based on knowledge and expertise versus role or title

level of interest will be influenced by the abilities and needs of family members (including the person with a learning disability), the time available, urgency of action and the professionals involved. No assumption should be made that family members will rush to be totally involved, and no obligation should be placed on them to take on tasks they do not feel prepared for. Pressure to become involved and exploitation of family members' willingness to assist is just as undesirable as deliberate exclusion. Active involvement is a gradual process, starting with small manageable decisions and proceeding to larger, more complex decisions that may involve challenge and the need to resolve conflict.

Obstacles to active partnership with family members

In attempting to facilitate effective partnership between professionals and family members it is necessary to consider the potential obstacles and barriers that may exist; these can arise due to a combination of views and actions of family members or professionals, as well as wider policies and procedures within services that exclude or fail to involve family members. Whereas the outcome of interactions between individual professionals and family members can be hard to predict with accuracy, several persistent obstacles to partnership have been identified.

Parents and professionals may view the same situation very differently. In identifying family needs professionals have been shown to underestimate the need for parent education and access to services. They have also at times failed to demonstrate an accurate awareness of the changing needs of families and the personal difficulties members may face (Shearn & Todd 1997). Both of the above will result in difficulties in establishing a common understanding of any situation and in developing an agreed basis for action.

Perhaps the most persistent obstacle reported over a number of years is the lack of appropriate information for parents. In response, the most recent strategy for developing services for people with learning disabilities and their families in England has highlighted the need for carers to receive relevant information and to know who to approach for advice and help (DOH 1999a, 2001a,b). A careful assessment of individual parents' and family members' current levels of understanding and identification of the areas in which they feel they require more information is essential. This will increase the probability that information provided is seen as significant. In the absence of accurate information and an awareness of whom to contact, family members may hold unrealistically high or low expectations of individual professionals and overall services. The development of the National Learning Disability Information Centre by Mencap, arising from *Valuing People* (DOH 2001a), is envisaged as having a valuable role to play in providing accurate and relevant information to parents and other family members. Family members may also perceive themselves to be unsupported and more isolated than is in fact the situation, all of which combine to reduce the potential for effective partnership.

All interactions between professionals and family members should demonstrate respect for family members, even if there is disagreement with issues being raised. Professionals should respect the right of family members to have their own views. An interaction with any member of the interdisciplinary team that does not show respect for the opinion of family members can have a detrimental effect, which may last for years. Negative attitudes towards family members, and the stereotypical 'labelling' of family members are often based on information from other professionals and not on direct contact with the family. Such views may prevent any effective partnership developing.

Lack of respect does not necessarily involve the professional being abrupt or unpleasant: failure to listen attentively, dismissing parents' concerns, always offering advice or instructions, inappropriately using jargon to disempower others and exclude family members from decision making, treating parents as 'just another parent', not keeping appointments or not apologising for delays, showing little interest in the person with learning disabilities, and other apparently minor instances of inattention will signal lack of respect (Dale 1996, Maxwell 1993). Family members are not easily fooled, and can quickly recognise when nonverbal behaviour does not match the apparent understanding and empathy of the words being used.

On occasions attitudes of family members toward professionals may not be welcoming. In such circumstances it is useful to attempt to establish why such an attitude exists and work to resolve any understanding/misunderstanding with services. It is also necessary, however, to be clear with family members that professionals need to be treated as valued partners, if effective collaboration is to develop. Unwelcome attitudes on the part of family members are not a reason to keep them out of decision making, but make it imperative to change these attitudes by demonstrating the merits of partnership for all involved (Dale 1996).

Further, the continued presence of rigid inflexible criteria for assessment, service led priorities in care, complex forms to be completed, and no involvement of family members in the evaluation of care can all impede any attempt to develop partnership (DOH 1999a). Also failure to effectively plan and timetable meetings with family members may result in reduced time for discussions or an absence of active family involvement. When negotiating the format of meetings professionals should bear in mind issues such as location, timing and how they fit in with the other commitments of family members.

Many family members need to be taught new skills that can be used when providing care. These can be as diverse as behavioural management strategies (Green & Wray 1999) and the passing of a nasogastric feeding tube. Without skills specific to their situation, family members will be unnecessarily reliant on services. However, caution must be exercised in teaching new skills as professionals who teach these to family members could be held accountable for the quality of their instruction. If family members are poorly instructed or misinformed and their competence is not assessed, the 'teacher' can be held accountable. Therefore, instruction is best provided within a structured yet individualised approach. This makes it necessary for clear records to show how the nurse followed a structured educational programme and was satisfied that family members were competent in the skills. If, after instruction, family members make an error through lack of attention or taking short cuts in safety procedures, the accountability rests with them.

Models of collaboration

The nature of the collaboration entered into with family members can be clarified by considering a continuum of models relating to family involvement in care. Due to variations in family composition, professionals may be working with both parents or single parents, and partnership may develop with some, or all family members. The models may be compared on seven characteristics:

- Role of family member
- Role of professional
- Nature of interactions

 Reader activity 24.6

Think of the family members of two people with learning disabilities whom you have recently worked with, with whom active family involvement in care was limited (despite the wishes of the family). Briefly list the obstacles to active family involvement and describe the impact of these on their involvement in care and relationships with staff. In discussion with colleagues consider what actual or potential solutions to these problems there could be.

- Location of control in decision making
- Identification of the problem
- View of conflict
- Criteria for a successful outcome (see Table 24.3).

Expert

The expert does not provide active partnership for family members. In this model their role is passive and obedient to the instructions of professionals. Such an approach provides a short-term intervention in emergency situations, or at the earliest stages of family involvement. Beyond this, it is limited and does not desire active family involvement in decision making. This model can feel safe for professionals and is visible in services long after initial interventions. This can be damaging to longer-term plans for partnership.

Transplant

The central focus of the transplant model is teaching family members new skills (which are transplanted from professionals) to enable them to care for the person with learning disabilities. As noted earlier, many family members desire new knowledge and skills, and therefore this model has a place in interventions. However, a major limitation is that it is often professionals, and not family members, who decide the skills to be taught. This can result in the specific needs of family members not being addressed, particularly in light of the dichotomy between what professionals view as important to family members and what they view as important to themselves. It is also essential that the risk of family members acquiring new skills and then being left unsupported by services is acknowledged and guarded against (Gibson 1995).

Consumer

The consumer model provides a degree of partnership, recognises the abilities of family members and the changing role of professionals, and in theory the final decision is left with the person

Table 24.3 Comparison of some key characteristics of models for working with parents and family members

Model	Identification of problem	Role of parent	Role of staff	Nature of interactions	Control in decisions	View of conflict	Desired outcome
Expert	Selected by staff based on their expertise	Obeys instructions Passive and accepting of decisions	Make decisions Inform parent. Give instructions	View of parents not valued. Mainly one-way communication from staff to parent. Compliance of parents	Totally with staff	Undesirable Suppressed Expert knows best	Compliance with prescribed care
Transplant	Selected mainly by staff, parents may have some limited involvement	Participates in care, actively learns new skills	Facilitates parent learning, resource person. Retains expert role to a lesser extent	Two-way flow of information. Opinions, knowledge & skills of parents respected, valued to some degree	Staff and parents consult but final decision by staff	May arise in discussion not valued	Family learn new skills & parents become a resource
Consumer (Cunningham & Davis 1985)	Parents and staff	Active in discussions. Full control over decisions	Combination of roles. Consultant, instructor, facilitator	Two way dialogue. Abilities of parents acknowledged	Parents and staff contribute, but final decision is made by parents	Challenge to staff expected & viewed as part of negotiation process	Partners in care. Increased control of resources & decision by parents
Empowerment (Appleton & Minchom 1991)	Selected by parent and professional	Active in decisions, degree of involvement selected by parent	Facilitates parent control. May act as expert, instructor, resource person to help empower parent	Two-way dialogue which includes social network of parents. Aims for partnership	Shared between staff and parents Parents' control promoted but possible need for staff to make decisions to assist parents	Viewed as part empowerment. Valued as creative. Acknowledged & channelled into action	Partners in care. Parents have more control. Social network recognised
Negotiating (Dale 1996)	Problem of mutual concern agreed by parents and staff	Consumer role recognised. Active participation encouraged. Recognises differing levels of involvement desired by parents	Variety of possible roles (expert, instructor, consultant, facilitator). Selected roles agreed with parents. Major listening role	Both parties can learn from each other. Family, community & ethnic differences catered for	Joint control neither party has total control. Both parties may undertake expert, instructor or facilitator roles depending on the decision	Conflict a possibility – part of the process. Dissent & failure to agree common purpose may result in suspension of partnership	Jointly agreed decision on issues of mutual concern

with learning disabilities and the family members. Two issues need to be considered: first, if this results in unilateral decisions by one party it resembles the expert model, with the parent as the expert, and has similar limitations; secondly, if decisions are left to family members it must be clear that the interests of the person with learning disabilities are seen as paramount, and not secondary to the desires of other family members. It is possible that as further opportunities arise for direct care payments, as outlined in *Valuing People* (DOH 2001a), the prominence of this model may increase. This model does not justify professionals abdicating their responsibility by stating that family members made the decision and not them. Partnership between all involved will only result if family members are enabled to implement or see the implementation of the decisions they have made.

Empowerment

The empowerment model seeks to move closer to active partnership. Both family and professionals are recognised as having expert ability and needs, and both are involved in decision making. The implementation of this model requires relevant information to be accessible to family members, and can result in a longer time being necessary for decisions to be reached that will have implications for service resources. It also requires professionals to be open to having their advice questioned, disregarded and not always accepted. Gibson (1991) has highlighted the need for self-determination, a sense of control as well as motivation, to exist within the client for empowerment to evolve. Some of the visible indicators of empowerment in interactions are trust, empathy, mutual goal setting, participation in decision making and overcoming organisational barriers. Braye & Preston-Shoot (1995) emphasise that empowerment must move beyond tokenism. This may require a review of service values, models, policies and procedures, and an investment in staff education and monitoring.

Building on her earlier work, Gibson (1995) has proposed a model for the development of empowerment within mothers of chronically ill children. In this she noted the preconditions of commitment, a bond with the child, love and the influencing factors of beliefs, values, determination, social support and experience. The presence of frustration with the situation was considered to be a driving force in achieving empowerment.

Empowerment is recognised as having both positive and negative outcomes. An increased purpose and meaning in life, self-development, satisfaction and mastery over the challenges are viewed as positive. In contrast, rejection by professionals, becoming overloaded with responsibility, and having reduced support because of managing so well, are negative consequences. In light of this professionals must continue to provide opportunities for empowered family members to ask for help without feeling that they are failing.

Negotiating

Dale (1996) built on the empowerment model (in which she viewed professionals as still having the final decision) to develop the negotiation model. There are crucial differences between the two. The starting point of the empowerment model is the identification of a problem of mutual concern, not a professionally selected problem. The possibility of conflict and temporary suspension, or indeed the breakdown of partnership, is recognised, as are the interchanging roles of both professionals and family members.

Working in partnership with family members and facilitating their involvement in decision making is the stated policy aim of most services. However, it is important to recognise the range of possible levels of collaboration, and their usefulness. The model of involvement must match the abilities and needs of the family members and professionals at any particular time, and may vary with time and with the challenges faced. This flexibility is incorporated into the negotiation model, which accepts the need for expert roles at times, but requires them to be agreed by all involved, and not unilaterally either by professionals or family members. Forcing a negotiating model on a family who are not yet able to respond as required by this model can be just as damaging as adhering to an expert model in a situation where empowerment or negotiation models could be implemented.

PROVIDING FAMILY CENTRED SERVICES

As noted at the commencement of this chapter, and explored throughout, professional, social policy and moral imperatives continue to highlight the need to work in effective partnership with family members. Clear emphasis is given within the reviews of services and corresponding new strategies in Scotland, England and Wales to the crucial support families provide to people with learning disabilities at home and also to those living outside of their family homes in a range of settings. It is not possible to provide a prescriptive and all encompassing list of how to support families, due to their uniqueness and the extent of their changing situations over time.

However, some broad principles that should underpin services that seek to support people with learning disabilities and their families can be identified, and these include the need to communicate openly and honestly, to demonstrate a commitment in words and actions to work in partnership, and to recognise the previous and future contribution family members make. Services must be coordinated across interdisciplinary and inter-agency boundaries, and accountability for services must be evident to family members. Patterson (1995) has further identified a need for professionals to be self-aware and self-respecting, curious about what they can learn from families, genuine and accepting of the person with learning disabilities and the family, and egalitarian rather than paternalistic in their approach. She also identified five principles that professionals should implement in providing family focused services:

- Focus on family competence and strengths
- Acknowledge and validate emotions
- Ask questions rather than provide answers
- Provide information in a clear, timely and sensitive manner
- Work with family members to create solutions.

With the above principles in mind, some practical considerations can be identified in respect of assessing, planning, implementing and evaluating care.

Assessment

The accuracy of an assessment will be influenced by the ability of professionals to develop trusting relationships with family members. In doing so it is important that professionals provide accurate information about the rationale, scope and nature of the assessment, including clarification of the extent of confidentiality, in order that carers can make informed decisions about their participation and the information they provide. Carers should be made aware of their right to an independent assessment of their needs and the purpose this could serve when planning care and allocating resources. Attention should be given to building relationships with all family members with convenient appointments offered to family members who are not usually at home when home visits are made, or for those hard to meet during usual contact. By doing so, a balanced perspective of the family is obtained, and the differing abilities and needs of individual members, be they parents or siblings, are noted. Professionals should recognise the perceived intrusion into personal and family life an assessment can involve and therefore conduct it in a manner sensitive to the personal, social and cultural circumstances of the family unit. At times questions may be difficult to answer if carers have not considered them before, or if they have concerns they are unsure about sharing, for example in relation to future care arrangements. Therefore, families should be given time and quiet encouragement to answer the questions asked.

The instruments used will be influenced by the purpose of the assessment and should be carefully selected so as to provide an accurate picture of the circumstances at that time. The assessment should be 'needs led', seeking to identify what family members believe priorities to be, rather than service driven, in which the purpose is to undertake a limited assessment to ascertain if the individual could benefit from existing services. It is also important to provide opportunities for all family members who may be affected by decisions made at the planning stage to have an input into the assessment process.

The assessment process should acknowledge the contribution of the family in supporting an individual with learning disabilities, and any instrument used should seek to identify family strengths, as well as areas for development (BILD 1998). All interdisciplinary assessments should seek to use instruments that are reliable and valid, and should be comprehensive enough to cover physical, psychological and social aspects of family circumstances. When assessing the circumstances of children in need it is now recommended that the assessment process encompasses the main areas of the child's developmental needs, family and environmental factors and parenting capacity (DOH 1999b). A comprehensive assessment provides a basis from which to make planning decisions as well as providing a baseline from which to measure the impact of any service provided. Assessment must lead to visible action, with information obtained guiding future interventions. Trust, interest and motivation generated by team members will quickly wane if the long discussions, and the sometimes detailed self-disclosure by family members, do not result in tangible progress. People as individuals and families as units are dynamic, and for this reason assessment information must be kept up-to-date if interventions are to be effective.

 Reader activity 24.7

Obtain two information leaflets on services for people with learning disabilities and their families within your locality (leaflets should be obtained from a public place and should not need to be obtained from specialist service offices, or people to whom family members do not have direct access). Evaluate the leaflets in relation to the usefulness of the information they provide that would assist family members in making informed care decisions. If possible, have family members evaluate the leaflets on the above criteria and compare their findings with yours. Explain any differences that exist between the evaluation by family members and your own evaluation. Following this, make recommendations (if required) for any improvements to the leaflets in the light of this exercise.

Planning

The planning process commences with the negotiation of priorities for action that are agreed with family members, people with learning disabilities and professionals. Through negotiation, misperceptions and unrealistic expectations can be worked through until a common understanding of the way forward is reached. This should involve all people identifying what they feel the priorities are and the reasons for this, together with their views on the objectives that should be pursued. The relationship with family members must be based on respect for their right to have views. Central to this is honesty, which means an acceptance that you do not know all the answers. Any pretence or deceit will eventually be uncovered and interpreted as disrespect for family members as well as for the role of professionals.

The planning stage provides an opportunity to review services provided, and consider alternative services if appropriate and real choices are available. This often brings with it challenges and possibly difficult discussions for family members who may have to acknowledge the difficulties they are facing and the need for support. This may be particularly difficult for older carers who realise the possibility of needing out-of-home placements and may perceive this in the context of a failure on their part. Therefore the advice from Vagg (1998) to 'tread carefully, assume nothing and approach each situation with an open mind uncluttered by preconceptions and ill informed ideas' is poignant. Professionals should be careful of pushing for hasty decisions and 'create opportunities for family members to think about possible futures for themselves and their relative over an extended period of time' (BILD 1998).

Any care plan that emerges should respond to physical, psychological and social aspects identified in the assessment and provide opportunities for family members to build on existing strengths and develop coping resources (Grant et al 1998). It should also be realistic and provide practical support, the nature of which will vary, but family members will assess whether it is practical or not. For this reason they should be involved in decisions about priorities of care, and the interventions. Everyone involved must be aware of the expectations, the requirements, the support available, and the advantages as well as possible limitations of undertaking the roles agreed. This agreement should be reviewed regularly to provide opportunities to alter the level of commitment without family members feeling (or being made to feel) that they have let someone down.

Once a care plan has been arrived at and all necessary equipment, education for people with learning disabilities, family members and professionals are in place, the care plan should be implemented. It is essential to keep the progression from assessment through care planning to implementation moving if the services provided are to be consistent with the priorities identified in the care plan. All people affected by the care plan should have a copy of it in a format they can understand and refer to when necessary. Finally a record should be made of any priorities that cannot be met at present and reasons identified why. Evidence of unmet need often indicates the completion of a comprehensive assessment that has not confined itself only to the services available. Conversely, no evidence of unmet need in service planning could either mean that all necessary resources are available to comprehensively meet family needs, or that the assessment was restricted in its coverage so as not to identify gaps in services; often the latter is the case.

Implementation

A crucial aspect of intervention is the ability of individual professionals and overall services to provide a coordinated response to assessed needs. For this reason communication between family members and professionals is of the utmost importance and it should always be possible for family members and the professionals involved to identify and easily contact the person responsible for the coordination of the care package, be it a nurse, care manager, social worker, doctor or another person acting in a key worker role. The target for each family to have an identified 'link person' known and accessible to them has been highlighted as a policy objective (DOH 2001a). Loose partnership structures that result in vague accountability, uncertain management and poor channels of communication are confusing, wasteful and unnecessary.

Family members will vary in their interest and willingness to be involved in care planning and delivery. Although interventions should respect and build upon existing family resources, pressure should not be placed on family members to participate in activities in which they do not feel confident or competent. Procedures that appear straightforward to professionals (because of their education and experience) can appear dangerous, unpleasant or disrespectful to family members. The willingness of family members to be involved in the care process should never be assumed or exploited for any reason (especially to reduce costs, or to overcome service deficiencies), but should be agreed in relation to specific aspects of care.

The majority of direct care and support may be carried out by family members and whilst this is consistent with the development of additional coping resources, professionals must remain alert to the isolation that family members may feel after more frequent contact with services during the assessment and planning stage. Family members continue to benefit from encouragement during this time and professionals should 'show an interest without being patronising, offer a listening ear without feeling under pressure to offer advice and show support without being judgemental' (Vagg 1998).

Professionals should share the ups and downs of caring for an individual with learning disabilities with family members and maintain regular contact as negotiated during the planning stage. Interest in the activities of family members and people with learning disabilities is most often demonstrated through small details of practice, rather than policy statements and glossy pamphlets. Talking and listening attentively, touching, holding (if appropriate), joining in activities and being prepared to learn from the person with learning disabilities and from family members acknowledges their value, whereas an aloof and distant approach will do little to set the scene for understanding the complex dynamics of each family and its members.

Family members often gain tremendous support from contact with other families of people with learning disabilities. Interdisciplinary team members should have up-to-date knowledge of voluntary and private organisations available locally and nationally, which may be of assistance to people with learning disabilities and their family members (see Ch. 4). If an identified need exists for a support group and none exists in the locality, professionals should consider supporting the development of such a group in order to enhance the coping resources within the local community (DOH 2001a).

Evaluation

Evaluation will be both ongoing, as the impact of interventions are monitored, and also summative on an agreed date set during the planning stage and clearly noted on the care plan. All people directly involved in the provision and receipt of services should be given the opportunity to prepare for and attend the review of the care provided. In practical terms this may involve reminding family members that the review is to occur on the date set, providing relevant information about the process and encouraging family members to think about how they may wish to be involved.

A review meeting provides an opportunity to acknowledge the contribution made by all involved and gain insights into which interventions and support were effective in helping the individual with learning disabilities and the person's family members successfully adapt to their circumstances. Equally it is important to learn from the times that did not go as well, and team members must be prepared to acknowledge limitations and mistakes. The accountability · for actions and omissions in service should be transparent to all involved. The review should consider the outcomes achieved for the person with learning disabilities and family members; in addition it should consider both the structure of the way services were provided and the processes involved in making this happen. All of the lessons learned can then be used as a basis from which to further refine the assessment information held in relation to the person with learning disabilities, family members and the family as a unit, and the effectiveness of professional services in that locality. The involvement of family members in project

groups to develop new policies, and in evaluation activities in respect of services they receive, can provide valuable information and suggestions for developing better services, and increasing the needs led approach, yet this continues to a poorly developed aspect of services (DOH, 1999a). The key principles of effective partnership with families are summarised in Box 24.7.

CONCLUSION

Family involvement in care is the stated aim of many services and their policy documents. Although some progress toward this important goal has been achieved, much remains to be done. At times family members wish for greater involvement than seems practical, on other occasions they may want limited or no involvement. Family members may also appear to have expectations that the professional services cannot meet,

---

Box 24.7 Practical considerations for active family involvement in care

C   Collaboration requires two-way communication
A   Assessment of abilities/needs of all family members and the family unit
R   Recognition of +/- aspects of caring
E   Empathy with person with learning disabilities and family members
R   Respect for opinions, concerns and cultural diversity in families
S   Support: physical, psychological, social

I   Individualised approach to interventions and the provision of information
N   Negotiation of roles undertaken by professionals and family members/No abuse of commitment
V   Values and priorities of intervention agreed
O   Organisational policies and procedures may need to be reviewed to facilitate family centred services
L   Link person/liaison known and accessible to family members and professionals
V   Voluntary and private organisations (local and national) known about
E   Existing networks utilised but not exploited
M   Mothers often primary carers. Careful not to overburden
E   Evaluation of structure, process and outcomes involving family members
N   Nurses' and other professionals' accountability for actions and omissions should be transparent
T   Teamwork necessary for coordinated services

and the interaction between the parties can become strained.

Attitudes to professionals can vary from sincere appreciation to distrust, and should be seen as a product of how family members perceive their situation and not as a deliberate unchangeable position. For either party to make value judgements and label each other as overprotective, disinterested, unmotivated, hostile, pushy or uncaring can be the greatest barrier to active family involvement. By noting the facts and discussing individuals' perspectives on situations it is often possible to come closer to understanding their actions and omissions. The life of a person with learning disabilities is of paramount importance in all interventions. There may be differences of opinion between professionals, family members and the person with learning disability about the preferred course of action, but negotiation can normally lead to an agreement about how best to proceed. However, negotiation requires time, openness, honesty, respect, confidence and a willingness to achieve an understanding of all perspectives.

It is the case that people with learning disabilities are members of families, and that caring is a family matter (Hilbert et al 2000), therefore, the role of family members in their lives must be acknowledged, respected and become an integral part of service provision. The development of services which actively involve family members is not easy, but it is well worth the effort.

REFERENCES

Allan I 1993 View of the family. In: Shanley E, Starrs T (eds) Learning disabilities. A handbook of care, 2nd edn. Churchill Livingstone, Edinburgh

Appleton P, Minchom P 1991 Models of parent partnership in child development centres. Child Care, Health and Development 17(1): 27–38

Barr O 1996 Developing services for people with learning disabilities which actively involve family members. A review of recent literature. Health and Social Care in the Community 4(2): 103–112

Barr O 1999 Genetic counselling: a consideration of the potential and key obstacles to assisting parents adapt to a child with learning disabilities. British Journal of Learning Disabilities 27(1): 25–30

Barton R 1998 Family involvement in pre-discharge assessment of long-stay patients with learning disabilities: a qualitative study. Journal of Learning Disabilities for Nursing, Health and Social Care 2(2): 79–88

Braye S, Preston-Shoot M 1995 Empowering practice in social care. Open University Press, Buckingham

BILD 1998 Working with older carers: guidance for service providers in learning disability. British Institute of Learning Disabilities, Kidderminster

Burke P, Cigno K 2000 Learning disabilities in children. Blackwell Science, Oxford

Burke P, Montgomery S 2000 Siblings of children with disabilities: a pilot study. Journal of Learning Disabilities 4(3): 227–236

Carpenter B 1997 Families in context: emerging trends in family support and early intervention. David Fulton Publishers, London

Carter B, McGoldrick M 1989 The changing family life cycle, 2nd edn. Allyn and Bacon, Boston

Cigno K, Burke P 1997 Single mothers of children with learning disabilities: an undervalued group. Journal of Interprofessional Care 11(2): 177–186

Cunningham C C, Davis H 1985 Working with parents. Frameworks for collaboration. Open University Press, Milton Keynes

Dale N 1996 Working with families of children with special needs. Partnership and practice. Routledge, London

Department of Health 1999a Facing the facts. Services for people with learning disabilities: a policy impact study of social care and health services. Department of Health, London

Department of Health 1999b Framework for the assessment of children in need and their families. Department of Health, London

Department of Health 2001a Valuing people: a new strategy for people with learning disability for the 21st century. Cm 5086. Department of Health, London

Department of Health 2001b Family matters: counting families in. Department of Health, London

Department of Health and Social Services Northern Ireland 1995 Review of policy for people with a learning disability. DHSS, Belfast

Diniz F A 1997 Working with families in a multi-ethnic European context: implications for services. In: Carpenter B (ed) 1997 Families in context: emerging trends in family support and early intervention. David Fulton Publishers, London, pp 107–120

Duvall E 1967 Family development, 3rd edn. J B Lippincott, Philadelphia

Dyer B 1996 Seeming parted. New Millennium, London

Evans J, Jones J, Mansell I 2001 Supporting siblings: evaluation of support groups for brothers and sisters of children with learning disabilities and challenging behaviour. Journal of Learning Disabilities 5(1): 69–78

Gelles R J 1995 Contemporary families. A sociological view. Sage, London

Gibson C 1991 A concept analysis of empowerment. Journal of Advanced Nursing 16(3): 354–361

Gibson C 1995 The process of empowerment in mothers of chronically ill children. Journal of Advanced Nursing 21(6): 1201–1210

Giddens A 1997 Sociology, 3rd edn. Polity, Cambridge

Grant G, Ramcharan P, McGrath M et al. 1998 Rewards and gratifications among family caregivers: towards a refined model of caring and coping. Journal of Intellectual Disability Research 42(1): 58–71

Green T, Wray J 1999 Enabling carers to access specialist training in breakaway techniques: a case study. Journal of Learning Disabilities for Nursing, Health and Social Care 3(1): 34–38

Haralambos M, Holburn M 2000 Sociology. Themes and perspectives, 5th edn. Collins Educational, London

Hennemann E A, Lee J L, Cohen J L 1995 Collaboration: a concept analysis. Journal of Advanced Nursing 21(1): 103–109

Hilbert G A, Walker M B, Rinehart J 2000 In for the long haul: response of parents caring for children with Sturge–Weber syndrome. Journal of Family Nursing 6(2): 157–179

Hoare P, Harris M, Jackson P, Kerley S 1998 A community survey of children with severe intellectual disability and their families: psychological adjustment, carer distress and the effect of respite care. Journal of Intellectual Disability Research 42(3): 238–245

Hodapp R M, Fidler D J, Smith A C M 1998 Stress and coping in families of children with Smith–Magenis syndrome. Journal of Intellectual Disability Research 42(5): 331–343

Hornby G 1994 Counselling in child disability. Skills for working with parents. Chapman & Hall, London

Hornby G 1995 Working with parents of children with special needs. Cassell, London

Johnson R 1992 Family development. In: Stanhope M, Lancaster M (eds) Community health nursing, 3rd edn. Mosby Year Book, St Louis

Leonard A 1994 Right from the start. Looking at disclosure and diagnosis. Scope, London

Llewellyn G, Dunn P, Fante M, Turnbull L, Grace R 1999 Family factors influencing out-of-home placement decisions. Journal of Intellectual Disability Research 43(3): 219–233

Manthorpe J 1995 Services to families. In: Malin N (ed) Services for people with learning disabilities. Routledge, London

Maxwell V 1993 Look through the parents' eyes. Helping parents of children with a disability. Professional Nurse 9(3): 200–203

McCormack M 1992 Special children, special needs. Families talk about living with mental handicap. Thorsons, London

Miller N B, Burmester S, Callahan D G, Dieterle J, Niedermeyer S 1994 Nobody's perfect. Paul H Brookes, Baltimore

Mirfin-Veitch B, Bray A 1997 Grandparents: part of the family. In: Carpenter B 1997 Families in context: emerging trends in family support and early intervention. David Fulton Publishers, London, pp 76–89

NMC 2002 Code of professional conduct, 4th edn. NMC, London

Office of National Statistics 2000 Social trends 30. The Stationery Office, London

Patterson J 1995 Promoting resilience in families experiencing stress. Pediatric Clinics of North America 42(1): 47–63

Rendall D 1997 Fatherhood and learning disabilities: a personal account of reaction and resolution. Journal of Learning Disabilities for Nursing, Health and Social Care 1(2): 77–83

Rodgers R 1962 Improvements in the construction and analysis of family lifestyle categories. Western Michigan University Press, Kalamazoo.

Rubins L B 1976 Worlds of pain: life in the working class family. Basic Books, New York.

Scorgie K, Wilgosh L, McDonald L 1999 Transforming partnerships: parent life management issues when a child has mental retardation. Education and Training in Mental Retardation and Developmental Disabilities 34(4): 395–405

Scottish Executive 2000 Same as you: a review of services for people with learning disability. Scottish Executive, Edinburgh

Shearn J, Todd S 1997 Parental work: an account of the day-to-day activities of parents of adults with learning disabilities. Journal of Intellectual Disability Research 41(4): 285–301

Simons K, Watson D, 1999 The view from Arthur's Seat: review of services for people with learning disabilities – a literature review of housing and support options beyond Scotland. Scottish Executive Central Research Unit, Edinburgh

Tozer R 1999 At the double: supporting families with two or more severely disabled children. National Children's Bureau, London

Turnbull A P, Turnbull H R 1990 Families, professionals and exceptionality: a special partnership, 2nd edn. Merrill Publishing Company, New York

Udwin O, Howlin P, Davies M, Mannion E 1998 Community care for adults with Williams syndrome: how families cope and the availability of support networks. Journal of Intellectual Disability Research 42(3): 238–246

Vagg J 1998 A lifetime of caring. In: Thompson T, Mathias P (eds) Standards and learning disabilities, 2nd edn. Baillière Tindall in association with the RCN, London, pp 276–286

Ward L 2001 Considered choices? The new genetics, prenatal testing and people with learning disabilities. BILD, Kidderminster

Welsh Office 1971 Better services for the mentally handicapped. HMSO, London

FURTHER READING

Department of Health 2001b Family matters: counting families in. Department of Health, London (*available free from Department of Health, PO Box 777, London and also available at* www.doh.gov.uk/ukxira.htm)

Dyer B 1996 Seeming parted. New Millennium, London

Miller N B, Burmester S, Callahan D G, Dieterle J, Niedermeyer S 1994 Nobody's perfect. Paul H. Brookes, Baltimore

Vagg J 1998 A lifetime of caring (pp 276–286). In: Thompson T, Mathias P (eds) Standards and learning disabilities, 2nd edn. Baillière Tindall in association with the RCN, London, pp 276–286

USEFUL ADDRESSES

www.autismeurope.arc.be *This site provides clear information about people with autism and coordinates the efforts of 60 national and regional associations of parents of children with autism across 25 countries.*

www.cafamily.org.uk *This is the award winning website of Contact a Family which contains a large online directory of support groups for people with a wide range of conditions. It is an excellent resource for finding local and national support groups and provides additional information related to supporting families.*

www.jrf.org.uk *This is the home site of the Joseph Rowntree Foundation which is a major funder of research in relation to developing services that support people with learning disabilities and their families. A very useful search engine on the site will provide you with a list of relevant research 'findings' that summarise the projects that received funding support from the Foundation.*

www.learningdisabilities.org.uk *This is the site of the Foundation for People with Learning Disabilities. It includes information relevant to wider services for people with learning disabilities and a helpful network of links to other related sites providing further information about people with learning disabilities.*

www.mencap.org.uk *This is the website for Mencap and provides a wealth of information about the activities of Mencap and information relevant to supporting families and people with learning disabilities as indiviauals.*

www.nelh.nhs.uk *This site is contains the National Electronic Library for Health. One of the virtual libraries available is the learning disability library. This site is still in the early stages of development and currently provides access to a wide range of government documents from across the UK. In addition it provides links to a large number of other relevant sites, some reviews of literature on specific topics and is set to develop into a substantial resource for professionals and families.*

25

Helping to empower people

Steve McNally

KEY ISSUES

- Representation is part of citizenship; it is important for all people, including those with learning disabilities.
- Representation is linked with concepts of autonomy and empowerment.
- Self-advocacy and citizen advocacy are approaches which assist representation.
- Carers can support empowerment of clients through advocacy.
- Carers can identify, initiate and support self-advocacy groups in partnership with service users.
- Carers can help clients to develop partnerships with citizen advocates.
- Collective advocacy can be valuable – locally and nationally.
- Professionals must be aware of the dual discrimination which confronts service users from ethnic and cultural minorities, and must ensure that clients have access to services which meet their needs.
- Users have a valuable part to play in research, including service evaluation.
- Users can contribute positively to programmes of training and education: their experiences and thoughts are potent teaching tools.

INTRODUCTION

The principle of representation is fundamental in society. It is connected closely with the concept of citizenship which centres on the relationship between the individual and the state. Marshall (1950) has referred to citizenship as a status bestowed on those who are full members of a community. He described three elements of citizenship: the civil, political and social. The civil element comprises the rights which are necessary for individual freedom. These include personal liberty, freedom of speech, thought and faith, the right to own property and to conclude valid contracts. The right to justice, a significant civil right, is the legal right to defend all of one's rights on an equal basis by means of the legal process. The political element concerns participation in the exercise of political power at local or national level. It may involve participation either as an elector or as a member of an elected body (local government, parliament) which is invested with political authority. Marshall's social element refers to the whole range, from the right to a modicum of economic welfare and security to the right to a full share in the social heritage and the right to live the life of a civilised being according to the standards prevailing in the society. Citizens require access to social resources, including health, education and social services, in order to further their own and other people's civil and political rights (Gould 1988).

Community care legislation in the UK (NHS and Community Care Act 1990) has emphasised the importance of representation of service users. A central policy aim of *Caring for People* (DOH 1989) was to give people more say in the services they use. Local authorities which provide social services are required to consult with service users and user organisations (Monach & Spriggs 1994) The voice of the consumer is crucial (Jowell 1991). This recognition is particularly significant for members of vulnerable groups.

Nevertheless, legislative changes have attracted criticism. Roberts (1997), reviewing the evidence for the effectiveness of community care legislation, has argued that the 'new community care system has contributed little, if at all, to empowering people in their everday lives' (Roberts 1997, p. 156). The NHS and Community Care Act 1990 placed a duty on social service authorities 'to carry out an assessment of need'.

The assessment process has the potential to be empowering for a person with learning disabilities, because it is a statutory duty, which represents a gateway to a package of individually tailored services. Discretion concerning when the duty to assess arises is located with the local authority where it 'appears that a person for whom they may provide or arrange the provision of community care services may be in need of any such services' (NHS and Community Care Act 1990). An excellent opportunity to consolidate and simplify this area of the law was missed (Roberts 1997).

The beginning of a new century seems a suitable time to review developments in policy and practice in the UK relating to the welfare and interests of disadvantaged groups. The 1990s were heralded as the 'decade of the citizen' (Dahrendorf 1990); the incorporation of the European Convention on Human Rights (Human Rights Act 1998, see Box 25.1) sends a clear egalitarian message. Article 14 states that 'the rights and freedoms set forth in this Convention shall be secured without discrimination on any ground' (Human Rights Act 1998, p. 6 Annex). While these rights had existed previously, the advantage of the Human Rights Act is that challenges can now be made in UK courts.

This Convention was originally conceived in the aftermath of the Second World War as a means of helping to prevent a recurrence of the atrocities of that era. The experience of conflicts in the recent past in Europe, and current events in other regions of the world, demonstrate that much is still to be done if these rights are to be secured for all. It has been predicted that the Act will have 'a huge impact on both criminal and civil law' (Edge 2000, p. 18).

 Reader activity 25.1

What are your human rights? These rights seem to be so much a part of our lives that we may take them for granted. What barriers do people with learning disabilities face in asserting their rights? Can you think of situations in which the person's rights could conflict with the wishes of others?

Box 25.1   The Articles of the Human Rights Act (1998)

- Right to life
- Prohibition of torture
- Prohibition of slavery and forced labour
- Right to liberty and security
- Right to a fair trial
- No punishment without law
- Right to respect for private and family life
- Freedom of thought, conscience and religion
- Freedom of expression
- Freedom of assembly and association
- Right to marry
- Prohibition of discrimination
- Restrictions on political activity of aliens
- Prohibition of abuse on rights
- Limitations on use of restrictions on rights

(For a full account of the Act, see government website in references)

WHY IS EMPOWERMENT IMPORTANT?

Freedom of self-determination is considered to be the most fundamental and valuable human right (Gadow 1979). Historically, people with learning disabilities have not had much control in their lives (Wolfensberger 1972). The stigma attached to 'mental retardation' has been powerful; the label denotes a complete lack of basic competence (Edgerton 1967). Hugman (1991) believed that long-term service users are at greater risk of devaluation than those who receive treatment for a curable medical problem.

Empowerment involves the exercise of one's rights as a citizen. Members of disadvantaged minorities have fought back against discrimination, including denial of rights. Strategies such as self-advocacy have played an important role in enabling people to gain control in their lives. Choices which have affected people's lives in a very direct way have been in the hands of others, often family members or service workers. Representation can be seen as a vital tool for members of devalued, disadvantaged groups.

It could be argued that effective representation is more important for a person with a learning disability than for a non-disabled citizen because the former is so far behind in terms of experience of speaking up and making choices, and awareness

of rights. Representation through membership of a self-advocacy group may bring benefits for the person at an individual level, for example developing confidence, improved listening and speaking skills, greater knowledge of rights. It could also have an impact on the services a person receives, so that increasing awareness and assertiveness might lead to paid employment or better housing.

Participation is an important component of representation and an expression of empowerment. Individuals have a right to be involved in decisions which affect their lives. If they are not, there is a danger that the service may meet the needs of staff rather than users (Gathercole 1988). A fundamental principle here is that people with learning disabilities should be involved in the planning, operation and evaluation of services which affect them.

The recent government White Paper *Valuing People: A New Strategy for Learning Disability in the 21st Century* (DOH 2001) is a landmark, 30 years having passed since the previous White Paper concerned exclusively with the needs of people with learning disabilities (*Better Services for the Mentally Handicapped*, DOH 1971). It contains a government objective of promoting more choice and control for people with learning disabilities. The document acknowledges that people currently tend to have little control in their lives: few people receive direct payments; advocacy services are inadequately developed; and service users are often not central to the planning process (DOH 2001, p. 4). *Valuing People* pledges government funding to develop advocacy services. While this initiative is to be welcomed, the amount of money involved (£2.3 million a year for 3 years via the Implementation Support Fund) seems minimal, being devoted to 'key aspects of the new strategy such as the expansion of advocacy services' (NHS Confederation 2001, p. 5).

The Disability Rights Commission was established in April 2000. It has 'a vital role to play in enabling all disabled people, including those with learning disabilities, to gain full access to their legal rights. It will ensure that the needs and views of people with learning disabilities are integral to all the Commission's work' (DOH 2001, p. 24).

This is a laudable objective but we must wait to see how this is to be achieved meaningfully in practice. There is clearly great potential for people with a learning disability to have an influence. A concern might be that the work of the Commission becomes oriented primarily towards other disabled people who, generally, have superior access to knowledge and can articulate their views more readily and effectively in a variety of media.

DEFINING EMPOWERMENT

There is a danger that empowerment, a term which has passed into common usage and is applied in many contexts, could be disregarded as a buzz-word or taken to denote the token involvement of service users. The concept is multifaceted and difficult to define but remains enormously significant. The concepts of empowerment and autonomy are linked closely. Empowerment has several dimensions. There are questions around the extent to which it is about professionals sharing power with users. It has been suggested (Simons 1995) that empowerment is concerned with users actively taking control.

Gibson (1991) has defined empowerment as 'a social process of recognising, promoting and enhancing people's abilities to meet their own problems and mobilise the necessary resources in order to feel in control of their own life'. The concept of empowerment for service users and carers can be characterised both as a process and a goal. It is concerned with people having greater power to express their needs and to decide how these should be met (Parsloe & Stevenson 1993). Empowerment is easy to define in its absence (Rappaport 1984): powerlessness, real or imagined; learned helplessness; alienation; loss of a sense of control over one's life. Individuals may never have achieved power in their lives.

Types of representation

Essentially, there are four types of representation: by self, by an unpaid person (such as a friend, relative or citizen advocate), by a paid person (perhaps a community nurse or social worker) or by an organisation (People First or Mencap, for example). It is important to be aware of the nuance between representation of an individual's interests and collective action by an organisation, which is less pure and direct. The difference here could be characterised as that between advocacy and user representation.

Advocacy

This can be defined as the process of speaking out or acting on behalf of another person who is unable to do so for himself. Upholding the rights and best interests of an individual is a crucial element of the advocate's role. Action should result from this representation. It is important that advocates have a genuine commitment to represent the person's interests as though they were their own (Tyne 1991). Advocacy refers to a process by which service users, individually or in groups, make service providers aware of their views and interests (Monach & Spriggs 1994). It is important to make a distinction between advocacy and user involvement. Advocacy is about service users setting the agenda, not just about being consulted by professionals and organisations. Good practice in user involvement is considered later in this chapter.

Self-advocacy

Self-advocacy is practised by many of us as individuals but groups can provide a good setting for developing self-advocacy skills, particularly for people who are at risk of being devalued in society. Definitions of self-advocacy often include 'speaking up for yourself' but that is only part of the picture. Making decisions, taking action, and *changing* things are significant components which a number of self-advocacy groups have identified. Self-advocacy has great potential to enhance the lives of people with learning disabilities as they become more aware of rights, express needs and concerns and assert interests.

The following self-advocacy skills have been identified (Clare 1990):

- Being able to express thoughts and feelings with assertiveness if necessary

- Being able to make choices and decisions
- Having clear knowledge of rights
- Being able to make changes.

Other important components include: being independent; taking responsibility for yourself; getting things going yourself; being concerned for other people. The Self Advocacy in Action Group have made the point that self-advocacy affects 'the whole of your life the whole of the time' (Self Advocacy in Action Group 1994). Crawley (1988, p. 1) saw self-advocacy as 'the act of making choices and decisions and bringing about desired change for oneself . . . Any activity that involves self-determination can be called self-advocacy'. She makes the vital point that all can be involved. 'Everyone can take part in self-advocacy at some level regardless of the severity of their disabilities' (Crawley 1988, p. 1).

The challenge which faces professionals is to find out how individuals communicate, and to open up pathways, perhaps with augmented communication systems or intensive one-to-one work, which enable them to express their needs and wants. The various types of advocacy are not mutually exclusive. People with severe learning disabilities may be involved in partnerships with citizen advocates, who help them to uphold their rights and represent their views. However, the same people may also be developing their self-advocacy skills at an individual level by making choices and decisions. They might be members of self-advocacy groups, in which their participation is supported by service workers or citizen advocates.

Citizen advocacy

This refers to the supportive partnership which results when a volunteer develops a relationship with a person who is vulnerable to being disadvantaged through illness, age or disability. It is important that advocates are 'valued people', i.e. not themselves disadvantaged. Advocates form a close personal relationship with their partners, helping them to make choices and decisions. They work independently of services to uphold the rights of their partners as citizens.

Citizen advocacy refers to the persuasive and supportive activities of trained, selected volunteers and coordinating staff working on behalf of those who are disabled/disadvantaged and not in a good position to exercise or defend their rights as citizens. Citizen advocates are persons who are independent of those providing direct services to people with disabilities. Working on a one to one basis, they attempt to foster respect for the rights and dignity of those they represent. This may involve helping to express the individual's concerns and aspirations, obtaining day to day social, recreational, health and related services, and providing other practical and emotional support' (Gathercole cited in Butler 1988, p. 2).

The benefits of a partnership with a citizen advocate fall into two broad categories according to the nature of the needs met: expressive (human, emotional and social needs) and instrumental (material needs) (see Box 25.2).

Collective advocacy

This approach is about user representation. There is an important nuance here between advocacy and user representation. Self-advocates represent their own interests; citizen advocates uphold the rights of their partners. User oganisations cannot represent each individual's views but they can promote the cause of minority groups, including people with a learning disability, by raising public awareness and lobbying policy makers on their behalf. Key organisations which help to further

---

Box 25.2   Possible gains from citizen advocacy (Adapted from Sang 1984)

Expressive	Instrumental
Affection	Access to financial benefits
Attention	Access to services
Companionship	Accommodation
Communication	Leisure and recreation
Friendship	Transport
Identity	Training and education
Love	Citizenship rights e.g. voting
developing social	
Networks	Access to facilities e.g. shops, pubs
Warmth	Medical, dental and opthalmic care

the cause of people with a learning disability include: Mencap, People First, BILD (British Institute of Learning Disabilities), Values into Action (formerly Campaign for Mental Handicap) and SCOPE (formerly the Spastics Society).

Opportunities exist for people with learning disabilities to become more involved in the broader disability movement; alliances of disabled people are likely to have greater political and economic power, with concomitant influence on policy makers and service providers. As Napoleon reputedly observed, 'God is on the side of the big battalions'.

HELPING WITH INDIVIDUAL REPRESENTATION

To be in a position to help individuals to represent their rights and interests, one must first build relationships with them. This will involve getting to know, and value the people and to understand their styles of communication. Rogers (1967), considering education, believed that the interpersonal relationship between facilitator and learner is the most significant factor governing the learner's experience.

It is crucial to give people time to say what they want to say and to be aware of one's own communication, keeping vocabulary and pace of delivery at a level which people can follow. Individuality is the key here; knowing the people concerned, their use of language and their range of interests is paramount.

The importance of *knowing* the person cannot be over-emphasised. Goode (1984) has noted the dangers of clinical perspectives which highlight what the service user cannot do and can give rise to a fault-finding approach. The 'etic' perspective is a definition constructed by outsiders (i.e. how professionals believe that the person experiences the world). Goode discusses the desirability of understanding the person's own actual experience of reality. This is the 'emic' perspective. Practitioners need to be aware of the relationship between identity, behaviour and social context. Somebody with a severe learning disability, whose spoken and received vocabulary is limited

in a formal assessment setting such as a clinic, may communicate effectively in the home situation. He may feel more confident and be aware that others – family members or house mates – are better able to understand him. The crucial aspect is that of time spent with the individual.

It is well documented that people who have close, sustained contact with people with severe disabilities tend to have positive, accepting views of them. Four dimensions of the non-disabled person's perspective have been reported (Bogdan & Taylor 1989), and are shown in Box 25.3.

Carers of people with severe intellectual impairment and multiple disabilities maintain a valuing, human perception of those they care for.

A useful approach is to keep conversation relatively simple and as clear and jargon-free as possible. Another important precondition is to find out what the person wants – as opposed to what you think the person should want, although these things may correspond – in terms of achieving life changes.

There is a clear connection between the centrality of service users to the shared action planning process and their actual control of their lives. A key principle here is that people should have the opportunity to participate appropriately in their individual programme planning meetings (Alexander & Hegarty 2001).

Communication

Effective communication is the cornerstone of good practice for caring professionals; it is crucial to have these skills in the learning disability field. Service users need to be confident that staff members are able to understand the points which they are making. A key skill which supporters require

---

Box 25.3   Four dimensions of the non-disabled person's perspective (Bogdan & Taylor 1989)

- attributing thinking to the other
- seeing individuality in the other
- viewing the other as reciprocating
- defining social place for the other.

is the capacity to build a trusting relationship with the client, which creates a context for clear communication. It is imperative that information is provided in a clear and concise way. It should be free of bias because the person may simply acquiesce with the perceived choice of the staff member. An understanding of augmented means of communication which the person may use, for example knowledge of Makaton signs or Rebus symbols (Phoenix NHS Trust 1993) is helpful.

These methods are used along with speech, therefore it is an important ground rule always to use speech as well as signs and to encourage the client to speak. Some clients may use electronic switches and computer generated artificial voices to help communicate. Software programmes produced by companies such as Widgit (www.widgit.com) create text in symbolic form and are designed to help develop literacy skills, and to help in writing minutes for adult non-readers, for example self-advocacy group members.

Pictorial methods of representing text are used increasingly by organisations which are concerned with people with learning disabilities. Photographs can be used to refer to people and activities, and of course they can stimulate thinking and interaction. Photographs can be stimulating in making choices or devising a timetable with a client, who may not be able to read but can see a clear sequence of activities.

Box 25.4 illustrates some of the ways of ensuring that communication is effective.

ASSESSING AND SUPPORTING CLIENT CHOICES

One of the chief ways in which carers can support individual representation is by helping people to

---

Box 25.4   Listening: the Barton Empowerment Group 1994

Listening has been identified by a group of service users in Oxfordshire as vitally important in the lives of clients and staff. They have produced a set of guidelines for new staff, which state clearly the standards which users have a right to expect (Barton Empowerment Group, Oxfordshire Learning Disability NHS Trust, 1994). Here are some the principles of listening which the group highlighted.

Look at the person who is talking to you.
Stand still when somebody is talking to you. It is clear that you are not listening if you keep moving around.
Give people time to get their point over, especially if they have difficulty talking.
Do not walk away – it is very difficult to talk to someone who is always moving around.
Think about what you are doing. Sometimes it may be all right to continue what you are doing while the person speaks.
Think about what the person is saying to you. People will realise if you keep nodding and saying 'yes' in the wrong places. Give them feedback. Let them know if you have not understood them; ask them to repeat it in their own time.
Space for talking and listening is important. People need to be in a place where they feel comfortable. This may be at home, perhaps in their bedroom if they choose, or in another venue away from the house, e.g. a cafe or pub.

People who use wheelchairs sometimes feel left out and not listened to.
Listen to people who are in wheelchairs. Get down and talk to them at the same level.

You have probably heard of the 'Does he take sugar' phenomenon, whereby people tend to address the supporter. Nurses and other workers can use their skills to encourage communication between the wheelchair user and, e.g. the shopkeeper or barman. Ordering or paying for an item presents a very good opportunity for contact for the wheelchair user.
Talking to the right person. Part of listening is talking back and giving the correct information. When people ask questions to which you do not have the answer, you should put them in touch with someone who does know or ask the question on their behalf.
Telephones are an important means of listening and talking. Some people need support to make phone calls and to be listened to on the phone. People need to have the time to speak and listen, and access to a private place for this because calls may be personal.
A staff member might help in getting a number and then leave the room so that the person has the privacy and space required.
Going to house meetings. The group suggested that everyone should have the opportunity to go to a regular house meeting because things come up which people need to discuss. Group members hoped that everybody who lives and works in a house would talk and listen to each other.
Responding. Listening is about what people are saying to you; it is also about acting on the information.

develop their self-advocacy skills. With very few exceptions, people are capable of making choices and decisions at some level. They are able to express individuality and personal freedom by exercising the right to choose. This potential for autonomy can be developed by providing supported opportunities for choice making. There is an onus on organisations providing human services to achieve this 'accomplishment' among others (O'Brien 1987). Choice has been defined as 'The act of an individual's selection of a preferred alternative from among several familiar options' (Shevin & Klein 1984).

For choice making to be meaningful, a number of conditions must be met:

- an awareness that a choice is needed
- an awareness that a choice is being offered
- an understanding of the choice concept
- a self picture
- a choice to be offered
- information about the options
- the capacity and time to respond to the choice offered
- an understanding of the consequences of the choice (Wilson 1992).

It is important to bear in mind that a whole range of factors affect choice making. A person who has had little opportunity to make choices, these always having been made by carers in the past, may take some time to get used to making decisions. The skills will need to be practised and developed. Some people are more assertive than others and may relish the chance to have more say in their lives. Of course, some choices are more significant than others. The consequences of selecting a meal which is not a good choice are less far-reaching than the consequences of deciding on a place to live or work which proves unsuitable. It seems relevant here to say that choice making is not a skill which people suddenly attain as adults. Our parents, teachers and others support us in developing this skill through childhood. For children and young people with a learning disability, opportunities to make choices in a supportive environment are even more crucial because they may be slower in grasping the implications of choice. Therefore choice making and self-advocacy should be a significant part of the school and college curriculum. Environment is an important factor in choice making. A valid, genuine choice may be more likely to be made in the person's home environment (Simons 1990). This is especially pertinent for those with a severe learning disability.

The use of pictorial methods to supplement verbal interaction in research situations is a good practice. Simple faces, usually arranged in a three point scale – ranging from happy to indifferent to unhappy – can be very effective in ascertaining clients' feelings about an issue (Conroy & Bradley 1985).

In order to support choice making effectively, carers need to have a positive approach towards their clients' autonomy. This involves:

1. being prepared to accept that a choice made by a person with a learning disability is as valid as our own
2. being prepared to accept and support choices made by a person with a learning disability
3. being prepared to look for imaginative and challenging ways of encouraging people with a learning disability to make choices in their own environment
4. being prepared to support bad choices (CMH 1987).

To the above could be added:

5. being prepared for new, different choices to be made
6. being prepared to support developing knowledge and social networks.

Partnership with a citizen advocate could prove most valuable in enhancing the capacity to self-determine, particularly for someone with a severe learning disability who is developing assertiveness skills. It is important for nurses working in NHS Trusts and other practice settings to be aware of local advocacy initiatives. There may be an independent advocacy organisation locally. This could be an Advocacy Alliance or Advocacy Development Group (or other scheme) which is involved in the recruitment, training and support of citizen advocates. Such schemes provide advocates for various user groups, including older people, mental health service users and people with a physical disability. A suitable citizen advocate can play a crucial role in strengthening a client's identity and developing the person's social networks. The relationship would usually begin with a sensitively managed introduction and develop through time spent together. Friendship is distinct from advocacy but advocacy can occur as a progression. For various reasons, not everyone will want to join a self-advocacy group (some people may feel that they manage well on their own) but this is also an avenue for support of the individual.

Group representation

Another key aspect of representation is the potential of the group to nurture individual development. Self-advocacy groups for adults with a learning disability are becoming increasingly influential. Recent years have seen an upsurge in their growth. The person whom you support may benefit from membership of a self-advocacy group. Confidence, growth, trust and information are some of the gains reported for members (Williams & Shoultz 1982). There is evidence of growth in the numbers self-advocacy groups but do increasing numbers necessarily mean increasing influence?

Some writers have seen self-advocacy as the form to be attained ('Self-advocacy rather than advocacy should be seen as the goal') because speaking out independently increases the recognition of the person's citizenship (Walmsley 1993; p. 264). Parallels have been drawn between the practice of self-advocacy skills and establishing an identity as an adult (Mitchell 1997).

What do self-advocacy group members themselves think about their self-advocacy work? Dawson (1995), in a project supported by the Department of Health, interviewed seven groups across England. He found that across the groups there was a commitment to being in the group. This characteristic does seem to come over strongly from advocates, as does an interest in supporting people seen as less able to assert their rights and wishes. The groups generally perceived themselves as meeting to 'speak up for themselves and for other people with learning difficulties who could not speak up for themselves and to "sort things out"' (Dawson 1995). One group came together to give each other help and advice; a lot of discussion took place around problems at work and feelings members had about situations they faced. Another of the groups met to 'have more say to the authorities' (Dawson 1995). A group working through course materials felt they helped each other to learn and gained much from 'seeing people progress' (Dawson 1995, p. 3). Things that members felt were important about meeting as a group included:

- 'having opportunities to get used to speaking in groups'
- 'speaking up to MPs and directors of services'
- 'getting involved in staff training'
- 'protesting about cuts in services'
- 'gaining confidence from meeting together'
- 'learning from each other' (Dawson 1995).

The brief excerpts above do convey something of the range of activities of groups, and the benefits identified by individual members. Increasingly, individual self-advocates are taking opportunities to disseminate their ideas and share their experiences.

Self-advocacy groups

Four types of self-advocacy group are described in the literature (Crawley 1988). This typology has been used in various studies (Dowson & Whittaker 1993, Simons 1992). Each model is thought to have advantages and disadvantages.

The 'autonomous' or 'ideal' model

Such groups are independent from professional services or parent bodies in terms of time, organisation and finance. This independence is advantageous, as is the independence of an adviser. Essentially, group members are free from conflicts of interest with professionals or parents and are free to voice opinions without fear of embarrassment or recrimination. The main disadvantages are that groups have to support themselves from the beginning and gaining finances and other resources can be problematic. (It is interesting to note that a small number of established, autonomous groups have gained funding from the National Lottery Commission.)

The 'divisional' model

This type of group is formed as a section of an existing parent or professional organisation concerned with people who have a learning disability. Mencap and various advocacy organisations are examples. The chief advantages here are that the group probably has easy access to a range of resources including venues, finances and administrative support (with access to telephone and photocopying). It is also likely that the adviser is well-versed in advocacy skills. Disadvantages centre on the aspect of conflict of interests between self-advocates' demands and those of parents and professionals. The other potential negative is the issue that the group is subservient to the organisation, the needs of which will take precedence.

The 'coalition' model

This involves bringing together people with different types of disabilities to form a self-advocacy group. Crawley (1988, p. 3) gives an example from the USA – the Massachussetts Coalition of Citizens with Disabilities. Another example would be organisations like the Council of Disabled People or Independent Living initiatives. Within the overall structure, members with learning disabilities have their own section but meet with other sections for certain events and to determine policy. The strengths of this model include the increased political power and power to attract funding that alignment with other disabled people brings. Being part of the wider disability movement can help to nurture a positive identity as a disabled person. The possible downside of this model is that people with a learning disability may be in a position of being overpowered by other interest groups and indeed by more articulate, politically aware members, who may be taking their agenda forward. (However, it may be said that this phenomenon – of more articulate, aware, forceful individuals having an undue influence – can also occur in the setting of a group exclusively for people with a learning disability.)

The 'service-system' model In this the self-advocacy group is based in a service setting, such as a committee at a day centre (adult training centre/social education centre), or residents' or users' groups within a residential service operated by an NHS Tust, social service department or independent sector organisation. Crawley (1988) observes that there are no difficulties in relation to transport or access to the group, as it uses the same set of resources as the service (as in the 'divisional' model). Recruitment of members tends not to be problematic and focusing on service issues is facilitated. There are several potential disadvantages. There exists a constant threat of conflict of interests between self-advocates and personnel if the members challenge the service system; accounts of groups being stopped by day centre staff have been recorded (Shearer 1986). Conflict arising within the group may be continued in the service setting. The group may be seen simply as an extension of existing activities and so become token rather than real self-advocacy (the 'if it's Friday morning it must be self-advocacy' syndrome).

The autonomous type of group tends to be seen as the most empowering (Dowson & Whittaker 1993). The 'service-system' type has been the form most susceptible to criticism, particularly because the embrace of self-advocacy by the system can be seen as limiting and subverting it. Downer & Ferns (1993) try to overcome the apparent tension between self-advocacy initiatives and services by proposing that although it is important that self-advocacy happens in day and residential services, people should be assisted by services in setting up groups without the services taking these over and allowing them to be merged into sevices (Downer & Ferns 1993, pp 145–146).

The above typology reflects the literature, but it is not necessarily exhaustive. It should be pointed out that there is a considerable crossover between the divisional and coalition models.

Getting started

It may be that you are aware of service users whom you believe would benefit from a self-advocacy group but no such group is running in the area. In these circumstances, you may wish, along with potential group members and supporters, to think about getting an initiative going. You may well find that your employer, whether a statutory or independent sector provider (for example Mencap), will support the development. The establishment of a users' forum locally will fit the objectives of a forward-looking organisation.

The process of considering a new group, discussions with potential members and the search for an appropriate venue are part of an interesting and rewarding (though time-consuming) process. Planning the group and negotiating with staff and venues can be an enriching learning experience for prospective group members and supporters. The foundations of a successful, active self-advocacy group are to be found with a small nucleus of people who are concerned about their rights and wish to achieve changes in their lives, including in local services.

Potential members will know some other members, probably through the services that they use in the area. They will have an interest in, and commitment to, meeting regularly for about 2 hours. Meetings might range from weekly to monthly. At this stage, the emphasis is on spending time together and enjoying one another's company. From social beginnings, and the discussion of common interests and concerns, the group takes shape. Major points to consider at this stage include: finding a suitable venue, identifying members and advisers, investigating the possibility of obtaining funding, organising transport if needed.

Developing valued roles

A central tenet of self-advocacy is that the agenda is constructed by service users. Another is that service users occupy the official roles in the group and have the opporunity to practise and develop the skills of meetings, e.g. chairing a meeting. Typically, a self-advocacy group would have elected officers in the roles of Chair, Deputy Chair, Secretary and Treasurer. Advisers to groups are in a position to support service users in these roles. A new chairperson might need help in asserting order in a meeting; a recently-elected secretary may need assistance in taking minutes (tape recording a summary of discussions and decisions is a very useful strategy).

Gains include:

- Growth and confidence
- Trust
- Self-valuing
- Identity
- Determination
- Responsibility
- Ability and knowledge
- Sensitivity to others
- Finding a voice (Williams & Shoultz 1982).

Advising a group

Members tend to value the support of an adviser greatly; if there is more than one adviser in a group, one has to be wary of interaction between or by advisers dominating the meeting. A self-advocacy group of eight or nine members should have only one adviser present, unless an individual requires one-to-one support in order to participate in a meeting. Advisers should have knowledge of local services and of learning disability issues. It could be argued that it is more appropriate to have an adviser who has no professional care background or links, because the person is less likely to have a perception of disability which is steeped in the individual or medical model. In order to promote the empowerment of users effectively, advisers should not hold negative stereotypes of service users as 'victims' but have beliefs which are congruent with the social model. For an account of the social model of disability see Oliver (1990,1996). This does not exclude professionals of course, nor is it the case that an adviser would necessarily have a more positive perception of service users simply by being independent of services. Another view is that the person who is in an ideal position to be an adviser is another self-advocate: 'the most well-meaning, helpful, sensitive and committed advisor will never be able to do the job of self-determination as effectively as a well-prepared, well-trained self-advocate' (Worrel 1988, p. 13).

An effective adviser concentrates on helping group members to acquire the skills which are needed to run meetings properly. Helping members to generate agenda items and supporting the discussion of issues and possible courses of action is crucial: 'In our groups we have support. That helps us make decisions' (user's view, Dawson 1995, p. 8).

The adviser should be responsible to the group. The person may have been interviewed by service users for this position. Essentially, the adviser should be at the group's disposal. Group members might ask the adviser to leave the meeting at times.

Commitment is crucial. The adviser should want to be at the meeting, not have to be there (Dowson & Whittaker 1993) While there is an argument which suggests that advisers should be completely independent of services (because of a potential for conflict between the role of adviser and the service role), suitable people are not necessarily always available. This misses the point and does not address the question of the motivation of an independent adviser. Why is the person taking on the role? The characteristics and skills of the adviser are much more important than whether the adviser is independent. In some situations, the link with services can be an advantage. People do value the support of advisers who know about their lives, providing that this contact is not too close. Tension could be present if, for example, a member of a group who lives in a staffed group home has a member of the house staff acting as adviser. This may inhibit the member's freedom to talk in the group. The member may wish to comment to members of staff on the service received, but this belongs in a different type of group, namely a users' committee.

People in the group will need help in finding out who to contact and what to do in order to answer their queries. An adviser who is part of a network will be in a strong position to enable group members to become more independent. The practical aspect of this is that service users may not have access to a telephone during office hours, possibly on account of their own timetables at work experience, day centre or college. A key skill for the adviser is the capacity to demonstrate how to do things, rather than actually doing them for the group, but there may be times when it is the only practical solution because of time or resource constraints.

Listening is crucially important. In the group context, including less assertive members is important. There are strategies for achieving this, e.g. doing a 'round' of the group. Complex issues and impenetrable, jargon-laden documents need to be 'translated' into an accessible form which retains the essence of the original meaning. Raising awareness of possible options in a situation, including the strengths and weaknesses of each, is a process which the adviser can facilitate. Ultimately, the group is responsible for its decisions, including mistakes. The adviser will have helped to explore consequences, particularly on major issues.

Box 25.5 Supporting a self-advocacy group: features of support (Brechin & Swain 1987)

Enhancing mastery and control for self-advocates
Learning to be on their side (e.g. people with a learning disability) in seeing problems
Commitment
Belief in people
Knowing, and enjoying the company of group members
Emphasising positive qualities
Sharing skills and information
Monitoring own communication
Learning to assist without control or power

An interesting insight into the perception of professionals of someone labelled as mentally retarded comes from the work of Bogdan & Taylor (1982, p. 67) who have quoted 'Ed Murphy', one of two people who told the authors their life stories in a series of unstructured, tape-recorded interviews.

I was picked up when I arrived in Central City. My social worker came to pick me up. I had only been in that city when I came in for the state fair once. There are two different kinds of social workers as people. There was the kind that came to find out what your situation for the week was. Then there was the kind like the guy who took me to Central City. He had what I would call a young attitude. He was nice and didn't want to restrict you. He wasn't formal – he hung in there. It was tiring – all the moving and talking to all the new people (Bogdan & Taylor 1982).

COLLECTIVE REPRESENTATION
Involving service users

In recent years there has been increasing acknowledgement that users have valid views about their lives, including the type and quality of services they receive and how these should be provided. People with a learning disability have always been a rich source of information about their own lives and aspirations (Atkinson 1988). The growth of the self-advocacy movement has brought new opportunites for people to express themselves and to listen to the concerns of others. Many self-advocacy groups are willing to discuss their work and to participate in research (McNally 1999).

 Reader activity 25.3

Are there clients whom you support who would like to participate in a self-advocacy group?

How do you think they might benefit?

Do self-advocacy groups exist in the local area? Are these based at social service department day centres, or within NHS Trusts? Are there any independent groups or People First groups in the area?

If groups do not function locally, would you or a colleague be prepared to help set up a new initiative with users?

Commissioners and providers of services, including NHS Trusts, social service departments and independent organisations, have an onus on them to involve users in an appropriate way. It is clear that service users have a very positive contribution to make. They must, however, be supported through the process and have access to information that is presented in a comprehensible way and have enough time to understand and form a view on it. A potential trap here is for planners to think that user involvement is a 'good idea' and to 'consult' a token client about a *fait accompli*.

A good approach would be for service planners to elicit users' views by meeting them in an advocacy group context. In this way, a wider range of views would be gathered and service users would be less daunted in a familiar setting. There are significant differences between consumer participation and advocacy. While common concerns undoubtedly do exist, for example housing, support, work, transport, we must not lose sight of the individuality and diversity of needs and wishes of people with a learning disability.

Service users in the West Midlands have drawn up a useful list entitled 'Things That Will Help Us To Get Involved':

- 'Being clear about what we can do'
- 'Involving us from the start'
- 'Go at our pace'
- 'Make us an important part of the organisation'
- 'Keep our involvement going'
- 'Give us choice about how we are involved'
- 'Use places we know and which are easy to get to'
- 'Make sure that we feel relaxed'
- 'We are the best judges of our wants and needs' (Service User Groups in the West Midlands 1995).

Meeting ethnic and cultural needs

Historically, people with learning disabilities have been regarded as an homogeneous group, having uniform needs predicated on their intellectual impairment, but this is not the case.

A discussion of representation must address the needs of people with learning disabilities from ethnic and cultural minorities. They may be vulnerable to 'dual discrimination' (Baxter et al 1990), a phenomenon which refers to the doubling effect of being a member of a disadvantaged minority twice over.

The evidence indicates that ethnicity and culture have significant implications for the provision of services to people with a learning disability (Baxter 1998). Concern exists regarding the under-use of services by families from black and ethnic minority communities. Gunaratnam has reported that the most significant stereotype applied to Asian carers is that all families live within an extended family, where clearly defined roles and responsibilities exist and 'caring for ill or disabled family members is a natural function' (Gunaratnam 1993, p. 115) In setting out to provide flexible, individualised services for all clients with learning disabilities, it is important that service planners have an accurate profile of the local community (the 2001 Census should provide a basis for this). By establishing a demographic profile of the community and monitoring the use of services, it is possible to estimate the level of unmet need (Baxter et al 1990). Consultation with black professionals and other members of, for example, the Afro-Caribbean community would be invaluable for this purpose. Existing services must develop to meet the needs of ethnic minority clients. These services must be accessible physically and in terms of communication. The key questions here for the service user might be expressed as:

- Is the resource (e.g. day centre) within a reasonable distance of my home?
- Is there a worker whom I can see at home or at the centre who speaks my first language?
- Do the staff understand the cultural implications for my needs? There are several dimensions here: physical care, e.g. personal hygiene, hair care, food and drink; social and emotional care; access to users of one's first language; presentation of self; spiritual care.

Services have tended to be based on the needs of clients from the white British population. Also, the label of learning disability has tended to mask issues like ethnicity and culture, as though every-

Reader activity 25.4

Does your organisation have a forum in which users can express their views?

Do people with a learning disability have the opportunity to contribute to the locality Strategy for People with a Learning Disability or Community Care Plan?

How would you ensure that users' views could be represented, e.g. in the local strategy for meeting the needs of people with a learning disability?

What links exist for clients whom you support, e.g. with People First or BILD?

one with a learning disability had the same set of needs. Action is necessary to ensure that the needs of people from black and ethnic minorities who have a learning disability are met. Black People First groups can be influential in this. There are some successful local developments but the national approach needs to be more unitary, with financial support from central government.

CONCLUSION

What is the future for empowerment? Professionals and carers have an influential role to play in supporting empowerment through self-advocacy for people with learning disabilities. Support comprises the encouragement of choice making and expression of views. It may involve assistance in forming a partnership with an independent citizen advocate or in becoming a member of a self-advocacy group. Citizen advocacy is a valuable approach which can do much to promote the identity and dignity of the individual. Unfortunately, it seems that there are far fewer citizen advocates than people who, carers feel, could benefit from their input.

Because citizen advocacy is a voluntary, unpaid activity for which an advocate could expect only to receive expenses, it requires a level of financial security and commitment of time and energy which many would find too demanding. The indications seem to be that the self-advocacy movement is growing rapidly. This can be seen not only in the increasing numbers of self-advocacy groups in the country (Crawley 1988) but also in the development of independent groups, as well as those which are based within services (Whittaker 1991).

The potential of service users to participate in the development and delivery of the local services and policies that affect their lives so profoundly will increasingly be recognised and utilised, e.g. through the consultation process involved in formulating Community Care Plans. The future should also see a greater utilisation of users' skills and experiences in conducting service evalu-ations and acting as trainers, and being paid for operating in these roles.

Valuing People (DOH 2001) has set out the government's vision for the empowerment of people with learning disabilities. Implementation of the policy, as it translates into practice, will be reviewed closely by service users, their families and professionals. It is encouraging that the needs of a marginalised section of society have secured a place on the political agenda.

REFERENCES

Alexander M, Hegarty J 2001 Measuring client participation in individual programme planning meetings. British Journal of Learning Disabilities 29: 17–21

Atkinson D 1988 Research interviews with people with mental handicaps. Mental Handicap Research BIMH 1(1): 75–90

Atkinson D 1999 Advocacy: a review. Pavilion/Joseph Rowntree Foundation, Brighton

Barton Empowerment Group 1994 The empowerment group guide- lines part 1: listening. Oxfordshire Learning Disability NHS Trust, Oxford

Baxter C 1998 Learning difficulties. In: Rawaf S, Bahl V (eds) Assessing health needs of people from minority ethnic groups. Royal College of Physicians, London, pp 231–241

Baxter C, Poonia K, Nadirshaw Z 1990 Double discrimination. King's Fund, London

Bogdan R, Taylor S 1982 Inside out: the social meaning of mental retardation. University of Toronto Press, Toronto

Bogdan R, Taylor S 1989 Relationships with severely disabled people: the social construction of humanness. Social Problems 36(2): 135–148

Brechin A, Swain J 1987 Changing relationships: shared action planning with people with a mental handicap. Harper and Row, London

Campaign for People with Mental Handicaps (CMH) 1987 Values into action. Talking points 5. CMH, London

Caring for People 1989 Government White Paper. HMSO, London

Clare M 1990 Developing self advocacy skills. Further Education Unit, London

Conroy J, Bradley U 1985 A five-year longitudinal study of the court-ordered deinstitutionalization of Penhurst. Temple University, Philadelphia

Crawley B 1988 The growing voice: a survey of self-advocacy groups in adult training centres and hospitals. CMH, London

Dahrendorf R 1990 Decade of the citizen. Guardian, 1 August

Dawson P 1995 Report on visit to self-advocacy groups for Department of Health. EMFEC, Nottingham

Department of Health 1971 Better services for the mentally handicapped. HMSO, London

Department of Health 1989 Caring for people. HMSO, London

Department of Health 2001 Valuing people: a new strategy for learning disability for the 21st century. The Stationery Office, London. Available online www.doh.gov.uk/learningdisabilities/strategy.htm

Downer J, Ferns P 1993 Self-advocacy by black people with learning difficulties. In: Beresford P, Harding T (eds) A challenge to change: practical experiences of building user-led services. National Institute for Social Work, London

Dowson S, Whittaker A 1993 On one side – the role of the adviser in supporting people with learning difficulties in self-advocacy groups. Values into Action/King's Fund Centre, London

Edge J 2000 Human Rights – an Act with teeth. Community Living, July/August

Edgerton R 1967 The cloak of competence: stigma in the lives of the mentally retarded. University of California Press, Berkeley

Gadow S 1979 Adcocacy, nursing and new meanings of aging. Nursing Clinics of North American 14(1): 81–91

Gathercole C 1986 cited in Butler K, Carr S, Sullivan F 1988 Citizen advocacy: a powerful partnership. National Citizen Advocacy, London, p. 2

Gathercole C 1988 Involving people with learning disabilities. In: Towell D (ed) An ordinary life in practice. King's Fund Centre, London, pp32–42

Gibson C 1991 A concept analysis of empowerment. Journal of Advanced Nursing 16(3): 354–361

Goode D 1984 Socially produced identities, intimacy and the problem of competence among the retarded. In: Tomlinson G, Barton L (eds) Special education and social interests. Croom Helm, London

Gould C C 1988 Rethinking democracy: freedom and social cooperation in politics, economy and society. Cambridge University Press, Cambridge

Gunaratnam Y 1993 Breaking the silence: Asian carers in Britain. In: Bornat J, Pereira C, Pilgrim D, Williams F (eds) Community care: a reader. Macmillan/Open University, London

Hugman R 1991 Power in caring professions. Macmillan, London

Human Rights Act 1998 The Stationery Office, London Available online www. doh.gov.uk/ human rights

Jack R 1995 Empowerment in community care. Chapman & Hall, London

Jowell T 1991 Community care: a prospectus for the task. Joseph Rowntree Foundation, York

McNally S 1999 Professionals and user self advocacy. In: Malin N (ed) Professionalism, boundaries and the workplace. Routledge, London, pp 47–64

Marshall T H 1950 Citizenship and social class. In: Turner B (ed) 1991 Citizenship and social class and other essays. Pluto Press, London

Mitchell P 1997 The impact of self-advocacy on families. Disability and Society 12(1): 43–56

Monach J, Spriggs L 1994 The consumer role. In: Malin N (ed) Implementing community care. Open University Press, Buckingham, pp 138–153

NHS and Community Care Act 1990 HMSO, London

NHS Confederation 2001 Briefing (May). The NHS Confederation, London

O'Brien J 1987 A guide to personal futures planning. In: Bellamy G, Wilcox B (eds) A comprehensive guide to the activities catalog: an alternative curriculum for youth and adults with severe disabilities. Paul Brookes, Baltimore

Oliver M 1990 The politics of disablement. Macmillan, Basingstoke

Oliver M 1996 Understanding disability: from theory to practice. Macmillan, London

Parsloe P, Stevenson O 1992 Community care and empowerment. Joseph Rowntree Foundation, York

Phoenix NHS Trust 1993 A guide to using symbols. Connect, Bristol

Rappaport J 1984 Studies in empowerment. Prevention in Human Services 3: 1–7

Roberts G 1997 Empowerment and community care some of the legal issues. In: Ramcharan P, Roberts G, Grant G, Borland J (eds) (1997) Empowerment in everyday life. Jessica Kingsley, London, pp 156–171

Rogers C 1967 The interpersonal relationship in the facilitation of learning. In: Kirschenbaum H, Henderson V (eds) The Carl Rogers reader. Constable, London

Self Advocacy in Action Group – working together and helping others to speak out 1994 Speak up for yourself: some ideas about self advocacy groups. Fairdeal, Leicester

Service User Groups in the West Midlands 1995 Together we can get what we want. BILD, Kidderminster

Shearer A 1986 Building community with people with mental handicaps, their families and friends. CMH/King's Fund Centre, London

Shevin M, Klein N 1984 The importance of choice-making skills for students with severe disabilities. Association for Persons with Severe Handicaps 9(3): 159–166

Simons K 1990 Learning to listen. In: Booth T, Simons K, Booth W (eds) Outward bound: relocation of community care for people with learning difficulties. Open University Press, London

Simons K 1992 Sticking up for yourself – self advocacy and people with learning difficulties. Joseph Rowntree Foundation, York

Simons K 1995 Empowerment and advocacy. In: Malin N (ed) Services for people with learning disabilities. Routledge, London, pp 170–188

Tyne A 1991 A report on an evaluation of Sheffield citizen advocacy. Sheffield Citizen Advocacy/National Development Team, Manchester

Walmsley J 1993 'Talking to top people': some issues relating to the citizenship of people with learning difficulties. In: Swain J, Finkelstein V, French S, Oliver M (eds) Disabling barriers – enabling environments. Sage, London, pp 257–266

West Midlands Learning Disability Forum 1994 Planning for change. BILD, Kidderminster

Whittaker A 1991 How are self-advocacy groups developing? King's Fund, London

Williams P, Shoultz B 1982 We can speak for ourselves. Souvenir Press, London

Wilson E 1992 Contemporary issues in choice making for people with a learning disability: part 1. Underlying issues in choice making. Mental Handicap 20(1): 31–33

Wolfensberger W 1972 The principle of normalization in human services. National Institute of Mental Retardation, Toronto

Worrell B 1988 People First: advice for advisors. National People First Project, Ontario

FURTHER READING

Atkinson D 1999 Advocacy: a review. Pavilion/Joseph Rowntree Foundation, Brighton

Braye S, Preston-Shoot M 1995 Empowering practice in social care. Open University Press, Buckingham

Dawson P, Palmer W/East Midlands Further Education Council 1991 Self-advocacy at work. Training materials. EMFEC, Nottingham

Jack R 1995 Empowerment in community care. Chapman and Hall, London

Shakespeare T (ed) 1998 The disability reader: social science perspectives. Cassell, London

USEFUL ADDRESSES

The following websites and addresses may be useful to the reader:
British Institute of Learning Disabilities www.bild.org.uk

Center on Human Policy, Syracuse University, New York
www.soeweb.syr.edu/

Joseph Rowntree Foundation www.jrf.org.uk
People First www. peoplefirst.org.uk

Royal College of Nursing www.rcn.org.uk

'New Ideas' Project
c/o Community House
Coleshill Road
Atherstone
Warwickshire

7

European dimension

This section explores the nature of learning disability services in three European countries. Firstly, Truce Soeter outlines the nature of learning disability services in the Netherlands. Next, in Chapter 27, Barbro Blomberg presents a chapter on the construction of services in Sweden, and finally, in Chapter 28, Sabine Rothe presents a chapter on the nature and configuration of services in Germany. In each of these chapters, the various histories and future direction of services is discussed. This section has been added to the new edition to assist readers in making comparisons between the ways in which services are configured and managed in different member states of the European Community.

26

The Netherlands

Truce Soeter

KEY ISSUES

- The Netherlands has a different history of care for people with learning disabilities, compared to other leading countries such as the USA, the UK or Sweden.
- Community care was introduced a number of years ago, the process to reach it has been a difficult one.
- The brief history presented in this chapter shows how care for people with learning disabilities has gradually changed from institutional orientated medical care.
- Changing ideas about people with learning disabilities have affected the models for the provision of care during the last four decades.
- Currently, a broad spectrum of services is available for clients and their parents, who decide themselves how to meet their own needs within the available resources.

INTRODUCTION

The country

The capital of the Netherlands is Amsterdam, but historically the government and the parliament resided in The Hague. Other major towns are Rotterdam, important because of its harbour, and Utrecht, in the middle of the country, important because all railways are connected from there.

The Netherlands has a land mass of 36 174 km^2 (13 967 square miles). In 2000 the number of citizens was estimated to be 16 million, with roughly equal numbers of men and women. Demographic data demonstrates an increase in the number of older people, particularly those over 80. Immigrants are, as in many other countries, an influencing factor in the increasing number of the population. Two-thirds of the population increase consists of people with a foreign background. About 30% of the population of the three large municipalities (Amsterdam, Rotterdam and The Hague) have an immigration background. About 89% of the population live in urban areas, 11% in rural areas. The population density is 463 people per km^2 (1199 per square mile). In the Netherlands Dutch people speak the Dutch language, with regional varieties of dialects; in the province of Friesland, the Frysk language is spoken. Most Dutch people can speak other languages: English, French and German are usually learned at school. It is often said that it is necessary to learn another language because the country is so small, but the other reason is that Dutch people seem to like it, and because many are travelling so much they can use it regularly.

The population

Looking at the ethnic make-up of the citizens of the Netherlands, we find that 96% of the population are Dutch, 1% are Turkish, 1% Moroccan, and 2% belong to other nationalities. These figures are reflected in the religions of the country. Although only a small percentage of the population are active members of a church, formally 27% are Protestants, and 36% Catholic; 3% are Muslim. Islam is the most common religion among immigrants from Turkey, Morocco and Surinam. 34% of the people have another or no religion.

Politics and economics

The Netherlands is a wealthy country, which is mainly explained by the country's policy. This policy, known as 'the Poldermodel', means that in a positive atmosphere, negotiation meetings between the government, the employer's organisations, and Trade Unions, lead to wage restraint, a kind of voluntary pay cut that will be used to increase the total employment. Due to this policy,

industrial actions are limited and wage restraint is common. Unemployment is rather low, 5% of the working population, and the number of vacancies is high and stable (Ministry of Economic Affairs 2001).

System of government

The Netherlands has a constitutional monarchy. Legislative power is vested in parliament, with two Chambers of the States General. The monarch (Queen Beatrix) has only nominal power. The First Chamber (75 seats) is indirectly elected, the Second Chamber (150 seats) is directly elected. It is a democratic system with the Social Democratic Labour Party, the Liberal Party, the Democrats, Christian Democratic Party, other christian parties, the Socialist Party, the Green Party and other smaller parties. Coalitions and a high degree of consensus characterise Dutch politics. Most Dutch people agree on a social function of government and readily accept relatively high taxes and a generous social security system (World Desk 2001). The Netherlands is a member of the European Union and NATO. The national currency of the Netherlands was the Dutch guilder of florin; from January 2002 the currency is the Euro.

HISTORY OF CARE FOR PEOPLE WITH LEARNING DISABILITIES
The 50s: the medical model

Although some large institutions for people with learning disabilities did exist in the Netherlands at the end of the nineteenth century, most institutions for over a thousand people were built in the twentieth century, in the 50s and 60s, after the Second World War. Before that time care for people with learning disabilities was given either at home or in psychiatric hospitals. The first institutions offered only custodial care without special treatment, therapy or activities during the day. Residents had no privacy in their rooms, no individual property or clothes. They lived in large groups of up to thirty or more persons, spending their days in communal areas instead of their own rooms, sleeping in dormitories with several rows of beds.

Food looked like an unidentifiable mix of potatoes, vegetables and meat, without any necessity to chew. Hospital clothes were shared with other residents and they all looked alike. In this model the 'feeble-minded' were seen as patients with an irreversible disease that could not be cured, so only physical care was given. It was mostly delivered by religious institutions, nuns and brothers caring for them in cloister-like institutions with a strict division between male and female. Only in children's residences were the groups mixed, up until the age of 12. This type of care in the 50s was later labelled as the 'medical model'. After 1960 care of people with learning disabilities changed quickly toward a more humane and personal care system. The living conditions changed first; modern buildings with windows gave the residents a view of the outside world. The rooms were better furnished and decorated. Around the pavilions playgrounds and sufficient recreational devices were available, and a swimming pool could be used daily by each group. Visitors from the USA and from other European countries came to see these much-improved environmental settings. Arguably at that time the Netherlands maintained far better living conditions for people with learning disabilities than anywhere else in the world.

The 70s: the developmental model

At the end of the 60s a developmental model was introduced and people were no longer called feeble-minded; the new name was 'mentally handicapped'. The first clinical psychological and orthopedagogical scientists entered clinics to help nursing staff to shape and change the behaviour of the residents; play therapy and speech therapy were also introduced. Work and activities were available for groups with mildly and moderately handicapped people. The numbers of residents in a group decreased from 30 to about 12 persons or less; however, this did not immediately change the fact that it was still an institutional group treatment: everything was done by everybody in the same place and at the time. Group walking, group swimming, and group singing were normal; there was no individual distinction.

After the publication of *Asylums* by Goffman (1961), it was clear that institutions were responsible for the lack of personality development, due to a highly controlled situation with strict rules and regulations, block treatment and group living, and a great social distance between staff and residents. The improved physical environment had not really changed this aspect of the institutions, unlike when the psychiatric hospitals were closed down in Italy, during the anti-psychiatric movement; nothing happened so dramatically in the Netherlands.

No revolutionary change had taken place; nevertheless there was an impact on the care of people with learning disabilities in the Netherlands. Some action groups – mainly group leaders and psychologists – occupied buildings and wrote 'black books' about the degrading conditions in the institutions. One important affair known as the Dennendal affair attracted political interest, and it turned the whole care system in another direction. The Dennendal staff protested against the separation of people with learning disabilities in institutions far from their communities. They argued that 'normal' and 'handicapped' people should live together and that they should learn from each other. The Dennendal affair and other actions were in fact not only aimed at improving care of people with learning disabilities; they were also a battle against conservative hierarchical administrators who did not want to change the concept of the old-fashioned institutions. There was a conflict between group leaders and management, as there had been at the Universities, between students and professors. It was mainly a protest against hierarchical systems, and it marked a new period of more democratic relationships in organisations.

Wolfensberger (1972) made a critical analysis of the situation of mentally handicapped people in society. He stated that institutions should either be improved or eliminated. Although Van Gennep (1978) suggested ideas for the decentralisation of institutions, and changing to another type of living, nothing changed dramatically. In the Netherlands all the institutions still existed and were even better equipped. New ideas were being brought into the country again, and slightly new approaches to the residents' care situation. The concept of normalisation was introduced from the Scandinavian countries in the 70s. The normalisation principle (Nirje 1986) stated that people with learning disabilities had the same rights as any other citizens: the right, for instance, to live in a normal house, the right to learn and work, to earn money; the right to have normal living conditions with a structured day like other people had; the right to a normal life cycle, being a child, an adolescent, an adult and then ageing; having a normal life rhythm with the experience of a year divided into months, weeks, days and nights, birthdays and holy days; also the right to live in a sexually inclusive world with men and women together.

Unfortunately many direct care workers, managers and even scientists did not have a clear understanding of the principle and it was seen as trying 'to force people with learning disabilities to be normal'. It did not really work as an instrument for transformation, but some alternatives were born from this concept that were to be revitalised some 10 years later. The so-called 'socio-houses' were a first alternative for residents who were able to live in the community, but needed a place near the institution in a sheltered situation. Outside the institutions other services were providing care through group homes and day centres. The group homes each had about 25 people with learning disabilities, and were built in the cities and villages instead of far away in the woods like the large institutions before. People had their own rooms, and more freedom of movement, but actually the care approach in these group homes was still very much the same as in the institutions. It was time for renewal.

After the 70s: the interaction model

In the following years a new model was used and referred to as the interaction model, or social model, because it stated that people with learning disabilities could grow personally and intellectually through interactions with other people. It was evident that the monotonous institutional environment was causing speech and language delay and behavioural problems. In the interaction model the physical and social–emotional environment was given more attention. It was seen as an important tool for interaction; the daily life of the group was seen as a major variable in a person's living, wellbeing and happiness. Structure and affection in the daily situation and the living climate were the leading principles in this approach. The relationship and communication between nurse and client were the most important conditions. The clients received more attention from the staff, who were very close to them. This initial idea of client-orientated care was better than before, but it was highly dependent on the state of the relationship with the nurse or group leader. This type of relationship was rich in intimacy and communication, but also dependent on sympathy towards clients. This changed when the 'mentor' was introduced. Every resident was allocated to a personal staff member, called the mentor. This person, who was usually a registered nurse (RMN) but could also be a social educational worker, was responsible for personal care, clothes and money and contact with the resident's family. The mentor was the forerunner of the case manager who evolved much later. This was an important step because it took into account that every resident needed personal attention, not only the nice ones or the sympathetic ones or the ones with challenging behaviour. It was evolving towards a more professional way of acting in practice.

Scientific and professional knowledge had turned care for persons with learning disability in a new direction; but in the Netherlands it was the Federation of Parents' Associations who played an even more important role in the living conditions of their sons and daughters.

PEOPLE WITH ABILITIES

The Netherlands has an extensive network of patient and consumer organisations. Over three hundred foundations, associations and working groups are engaged in protecting the interests of health care consumers. Collectively they represent the patients' movement. Patient and consumer organisations play an important role in the Dutch health care system. The patients' movement proceeds from various social developments, especially the growing discontent with the health care system's inability to offer care adjusted to the exclusive needs of patients.

Government has encouraged this development in order to promote a third force in health care. Collaboration with health providers and health insurers not only offers the potential to enhance services but can also help to reinforce the movement's position in the health care system (Blaauwbroek, 1997).

One of these consumer groups is the Federation of Parents' Associations (FvO). In their report *People with abilities* (FvO 1989) the new adage was: 'normal if possible, only special when necessary'. It is still heard and used in institutional and other care concepts. This gave way for more community orientated care and living for people with learning disabilities. For the Dutch government and the health insurance companies this concept was corresponding with their ideas about 'tailor made care'. The Federation's attempt to change the name of people with learning disabilities into 'people with abilities' or 'people with chances' was not adopted. It was considered too broad, including everybody. The terminology has changed over the years from feeble-minded, to mentally handicapped, toward intellectually handicapped. This is how people with learning disabilities are still referred to in the Netherlands. As in other countries, it is a qualification that is neither correct nor adequate, but it is an attempt to treat these people with the proper respect.

The Federation of Parents' Associations had argued in their report that in the process of formulating care needs through to delivery of care the emphasis should be on the client, and the client's parents or other family members. Formulating the client's care needs was seen as a negotiation between client, health insurance agencies and providers. Negotiation is a common Dutch issue in all aspects of life and usually it is a successful process. The parents can get help from the Federation, or the Association, or from social services to formulate their needs. The needs of the client are discussed within an indication committee in the client's region, consisting of a GP or a specialist, a psychologist, a social worker, and a nurse. The Regional Indication Committee will screen the client to determine the amount of social support, nursing care, treatment and daily activities needed and they decide whether the living situation should be substituted or not. The committee will indicate to these services how they can support the client's needs. The committee is not responsible for the immediate and direct delivery of a placement or support. This is the client's task. After the indication procedure the client can, in collaboration with the health insurance agency, with or without help from social services, ask the service providing organisation for delivery of the indicated service at a day care centre, an institution or in supported living. This does not mean that clients can get whatever they want and whenever they want it. There are still waiting lists and personnel problems that can delay or extend the support they need. Currently several parents have taken legal action to get the care they want, and in some cases the insurance companies have been forced to fulfil their wishes immediately.

The more emancipated and demanding the parents are, the better care the clients get. The strong Federation and each individual Association of Parents support them with professional offices, and a wide range of services. Their website is impressive. In addition, social services provide clients with all kinds of information and help.

In this way the concept of normalisation, the leading concept since the 70s, has transformed services into the concept of inclusion. Real inclusion in society, in all respects, is the main goal of the Federation of Parents' Associations. The government is not against it, nor the insurance companies. Their ideas seem to complement one another.

THE NEW APPROACH: SUPPORTED LIVING

The support model is the last model explored in this chapter. It has the potential of autonomy for people with learning disability built on the paradigm of normal citizenship. Almost 30 years after the normalisation principle (Nirje 1985) was published, some of the very same principles can be recognised in the model of supported living

(Steman & Van Gennep 1996); every person with a handicap – the name changed from resident to client – has a right to the same living conditions in society as every other citizen. That means a normal living situation within a social network, education, work or daily activities and their own financial budget to get the special care they need. Support and empowerment have taken over from old care concepts.

Currently individuality is a widespread value in our country (and the rest of the western world) and therefore the new way of support is now seen as a civil right. It is included in the individual future plan, or individual care plan for each client.

Living in a normal house in a normal street and being treated with all the ordinary rights of all other citizens is the most important change; but support in employment is another. Job coaches are available for people with learning disabilities who want to work. They function as intermediaries between client and employer; they support the client in all the aspects involved in getting and keeping work and training.

Supported living means that children with learning disabilities – whatever their level of understanding – do not have to live in institutions any more, if they or their parents would like otherwise. Social services support parents to find accommodation for their sons and daughters. Severely disabled children nowadays live in ordinary houses as well. Supported living has meant that the number of 'normal' houses in a normal street has increased. Although it is normal right now, not all clients warmly welcome it. A difference can be seen between two groups of clients: the new ones who are starters on the market of care and education; and the older clients, who are used to a system of institutionalised care.

It has to be said that in the last group, not all parents are happy with this general decision, and some prefer their son or daughter to stay in the safe environment of an institution; some clients feel the same way, and they are not forced to move. But within 10 years the whole situation in the Netherlands will have been transformed towards community orientated care.

CURRENT SERVICES

Approximately 110 000 people in the Netherlands have learning disabilities, or 7.4 per thousand persons, and approximately 57 700 of them have a severe handicap (Ministry of Economic Affairs 2000). All people with learning disabilities get some form of care from care providers: in institutions, in the community or in group homes. They receive education in primary schools, or in special schools; they have their daily care and activities in day care centres for children or adults; they have employed work, sheltered work or work in a company; or another form of support (see Table 26.1).

More than 40 000 people with learning disabilities live in institutions and are provided with 24 hour service (ten Horn 1997). Compared to countries like Britain, Sweden and some American states, this is a very high rate. The author does not wish to defend this, but it is important to explain developments in care, and it must be said that these institutions can no longer be compared with the ones of earlier days, as described in Chapter 3. Institutions are now communities in themselves, with an open terrain and with many contacts with

Table 26.1 Current services in the Netherlands for people with learning disabilities

Type of Service	Number	Days of Care	Number of clients
Institutions	151	12 651	30 270
Group homes	690	6674	12 500
Day centres	385	4984	13 570
Sheltered work			23 700
Primary special schools			24 000

These figures are a compilation of two resources: Ministry of Economic Affairs 2000 and Schrijvers 1997.

the outside community. Institutions are collaborating, and they have reorganised themselves into 'care groups'. From these merged institutions there has arisen a broad and strong network of services throughout all care providers. An increased distinction of service was the claim of the Federation of Parents' Associations, to serve any client with any imaginable kind of support, and that is possible nowadays, within or outside the institutions. Institutions offer support through nursing care, medical care, speech therapy, physiotherapy, sensory activities (snoezelen), recreation and holidays, special treatment or therapy for challenging behaviour, and in many other ways. There are generic and special institutions for multiply handicapped people.

Four concepts from government and from professional groups underlie this process of care provision: the concept of tailor-made care, the Quality of Care Act, the personal contract and the individual care plan, along with the coordinating role of the case manager.

Tailor-made care

The strategy for care is totally different from what it was in the past. Instead of fixed services for certain levels of disabilities, it has changed to a flexible system where generally everything is possible for any client. The indication procedure, discussed earlier, should enable a person with learning disabilities to obtain 24 hours care; or only a few hours a week in an institution or group home; or a placement in a day centre for an entire week or for some days; a few hours a week home care, weekend care, pedagogical help or support in an independent living situation; employment support, or whatever a person needs. This, however, is only possible within the limitations of each person's personal financial budget. Every person can obtain a personal budget from the insurance company. For clients who do not apply for it, the costs are paid by the AWBZ-Fund (General Act for Exceptional Medical Expenses). This flexible system is available, however, this does not mean that everybody is served in this way. Many people with learning disabilities still live in an institution 24 hours a day.

Quality of Care Act

Much attention is currently placed on quality of care. Quality is a common issue in all organisations in the Netherlands, and the law regulates this for the care sector. Since April 1996 the Quality Act for Care Institutions commands institutions to deliver an annual report to the Public Health Inspector. In this report the organisation is required to describe and provide figures for all dedications, activities and the effect or progress of client care, organisational structures (decentralisation), personnel policy (applying, training, treating), inclusion of clients and personnel in decision making procedures, the treatment of complaints and the financial situation.

These annual reports are published and sent to other organisations and related groups. Organisations learn from each other by reading each other's quality reports. Quality of care is also a general issue for discussion at every level of care provided. Every team will set goals and will try to implement the direction of the organisation to achieve quality of care. One example of quality improvement is the daily activities for severely handicapped clients. Every institution now offers this service. For a number of years all clients have been able to visit an institutional day centre for creative activities. Quality of life is improved by a change in environment for 4, 6 or 8 hours a day; being in contact with and having experiences of different people is as important as the activities themselves.

Individual care plan: a contract

The call for individual care plans came from the nursing profession from 1980 (Soeter 1989), mainly in education. It was tried in practice but was not very popular, because it was seen as an extra component of workload. This has changed since in April 1995 the issue of the contractual relationship between the care giver or care provider and client was regulated by law in the Medical Treatment Agreement Act (WGBO). It states:

- the client's right to be informed about examinations and treatment
- the client's consent for every treatment or action

- the client's right to have access to reports and files
- the right of strict confidentiality by caregivers
- the right of privacy in case of data collection for research (Verbeek 1999).

This applies to all clients and patients in the national health care system. For clients with learning disabilities and/or their parents, this means that their contract with the care provider or care giver determines what kind of care they will receive and how this will be delivered. An individual care plan should be written for every client. This care plan is not only a tool for the case manager and staff; it also represents a kind of informed consent.

Each year the plan will be adjusted to meet the changing needs of clients. Clients are present at meetings and express their desires, wishes and expectations. If not the client, the family (representing by law) is present. The individual plan contains all aspects of multidisciplinary care. The nurse, social worker, doctor, psychologist, physiotherapist and others may participate. Not every discipline, however, is present at every meeting; this will depend on the client's and the case manager's decision. Psychologists who had a leading position in the former years may now be more in the background; they only become involved when there is a problem, or a difficult situation, and their expertise is required. If necessary they provide support workers with knowledge and expertise about assessment, special issues like autism or multiple handicap, sexuality, education, etc.

The clients' needs play a central role in the formulation of the goals for the future. Personal Future Planning (PTP) is a procedure used to formulate goals for housing, work and the social network (Steman & van Gennep 1996, Kröber 1997).

The case manager

Every client has a personal case manager; a nurse or a social worker, also called a personal guide, or care coordinator. The main role of the case manager is to act as the client's advocate, giving the client support in all aspects of life. The case manager is responsible for the formulation of goals in the individual care plan and must discuss this with the client and the family, other disciplines and other colleagues in the team. The case manager must ensure that the client is treated in a respectful way, that the goals have been set, and that they are reached. The case manager can discuss a client's further abilities or can adjust the plan if goals are not attainable. The case manager is the coordinating person, and as such might be thought of as the spider in the web beside their client.

Social services

People with learning disabilities can access a variety of services within or related to institutions and day care centres. Social services or social pedagogical services provide all kinds of care and support for children and their families, for adult clients who are living at home with their parents, or for clients who live independently. Some of these services are shown in Box 26.1.

Box 26.1 Services provided by social service departments (SPD Gelderse Poort 2000)

Adult clients

Social support for all kind of problems
Work integration: supported employment, job coaching
Guided independent living
Care constancy
Group training
Leisure home projects
Support for parents with learning disabilities
Crisis interventions
Intensive care: trauma, sexual abuse

Children at home

Early interventions 0–4 years
Home assistance to relieve parents
Educational helps and support
Playrooms and toys
Crisis intervention
Group training

Other Services

Case management
Foster parents for clients
Social network for clients
Support in multiple problem families
Support for autistic people with learning disabilities
Families first projects

The number of houses in the community for people with learning disabilities (individuals or small groups) is increasing very rapidly. The 50 social services (SPD) support these clients with all kinds of consultation and assistance. The social services have also adopted a support model, but this was a natural consequence of their already existing 'as normal as possible' approach towards their clients. In contrast with the institutional approach, social services were always more client orientated and community orientated, obviously to the benefit of their clients. Social services now collaborate with the institutions and group homes to promote shared new projects in the region. Their ideas are increasingly growing toward each other. Every client who wants to use this service gets a personal case manager or support worker. A client is free to use the service or not, and clients can always disconnect their relationship with social services.

Education and activities in school and day centres

Children with learning disabilities attend a special school, depending on their level of performance. Schools are separated for non-handicapped, mildly handicapped and moderately handicapped children. Special schools are based in every city or region. More and more parents however, especially of children with Down syndrome, dislike the system of non-integration, and prefer a normal primary school education for their disabled child. It is not always easy to find a place, but it is an increasing demand. Central government's plans are developing in the same direction. However, as in the UK, discussion still continues. After primary school people with mild learning disabilities can attend further education in secondary vocational schools.

Many clients attend day centres where they spend their time on activities that are useful and pleasing; they can choose from a variety of tasks, according to their desires and needs and their level of abilities. Most day centres offer programmes such as training in communication skills, cooking, computers, working in a farm house, gardening or technical work, but also producing art objects such as jewellery, wooden tools, postcards, clothing, candle lights, or paintings. The paintings and other art products made by people with learning disabilities are sold in many shops and Art Galleries.

Leisure time

It is not only the professionals in institutional care, community care, day centres and schools who support people with learning disabilities. In their leisure time, people with learning disabilities can benefit from the availability of a large group of volunteers who offer a range of interesting and enjoyable programmes such as wheel chair dancing, truck driving, swimming, football and other sports, theatre and making music.

CONCLUSION

The Dutch situation for people with learning disabilities is client centred, based on clients' needs. History shows how care for people with learning disabilities has changed gradually, influenced by ideas that have affected the models for the provision of care, towards the current situation. Quite a large number of clients still live in institutions. However, institutions have changed their care providing strategies from custodial care, through to client centred care, and on towards community care. Community care is also provided by social services. Social services support adult clients and parents of young clients or severely disabled clients at home. In the current situation a wide variety of services are provided to clients. Institutions and social services are more flexible now, and they collaborate together in order to provide care that meets the individual needs of people with learning disabilities. Clients are supported, according to their status as normal citizens in all respects. Central government, health insurance companies, parents' associations, institutions and social services are complementary in their ideas. Although ideas and practice are not yet synchronised in every service, any client can benefit from the new system.

REFERENCES

Blaauwbroek H G 1997 Patient organizations and patient's rights. In: Schrijvers A J P (ed) Health and health care in the Netherlands. de Tijdstroom, Utrecht, pp 223–236

FvO 1994 Nota Gewoon doen. Federatie van Ouderverenigingen, Utrecht

FvO 1989 Nota Mensen met mogelijkheden. Federatie van Ouderverenigingen, Utrecht

Goffmann E 1961 Asylums, essays on the social situation of mental patients and other inmates. Doubleday Books Anchor Books, New York

Kröber R Th, van Dongen H J 1997 Mensen met een handicap en hun omgeving: bouwstenen voor anders denken. Nelissen, Baarn

Medical Treatment Agreement Act (WGBO) April 1995

Ministry of Economic Affairs 2000 Centraal Bureau voor de statistiek

Ministry of Economic Affairs 2001 Statistics Netherlands. Public internet site

Nirje B 1985 The basic and the logic of the normalization principle. Australia and New Zealand Journal of Developmental Disabilities 11(2)

Nirje B 1986 Het normalisatieprincipe. Samenvatting van de publicatie voor het Congres in Berchem, België: Normalisatie: hebben we het wel begrepen? Vertaling Eddy Bonte, WVI, St Amandsberg

Quality Act for Care Institutions 1996 Ministry of Health

Social Pedagogische Dienst Gelderse Poort 2000 Jaarverslag. Arnhem

Soeter T 1989 Een verantwoorde zorg voor zwakzinnige mensen. Tijdschrift voor Ziekenverpleging 43(5): 144–149

Steman C, van Gennep A 1996 Supported living, een handreiking voor begeleiders. Nederlands Instituut voor zorg en Welzijn / Vereniging Gehandicaptenzorg Nederland, Utrecht

Ten Horn G H M M 1997 Care for people with a mental handicap. In: Schrijvers A J P (ed) Health and health care in the Netherlands. de Tijdstroom, Utrecht, pp 132–138

Times Atlas 1995

Van Gennep A 1978 Het recht van de zwakste. Meppel

Van Gennep A 1997 Paradigmaverschuiving in de visie op zorg voor mensen met een verstandelijke handicap. Oratie, Universiteit van Maastricht

Verbeek G 1999 Zorg in Samenspel, Samenwerking tussen clienten en hun zorgverleners in vraaggerichte of vraaggestuurde zorg. NIZW, Utrecht, pp 19–22

Wolfensberger W 1972 Normalisation. Institute on Mental Retardation, Toronto

World desk 2001 Internet site

Schrijvers A J P 1997 Health and healthcare in the Netherlands. de Tijdstroom, Utrecht

USEFUL ADDRESSES

Arduin, a community	www.arduin.nl
Communication platform	www.zetnet.nl
Dreamhouse	www.svgw.diva.nl/driestroom
Federation of Parents' Associations	www.FvO.nl
Gallery Herenplaats	www.herenplaats.nl
Gentle teaching	www.gentleteaching.nl
Inclusion Europe	www.inclusion-europe.org
Inclusion International	www.inclusion-international.org
The Jostiband (orchestra)	www.josti.band.nl
Journal for Intellectual Disabilities	www.klik.org
Ministry of Health (VWS)	www.minvws.nl
National Centre for Information and Documentation	www.nizw.nl
Professional Centre for Nursing	www.lcvv.nl
Very Special Arts	www.vsan.nl/

27 Sweden

Barbro Blomberg

KEY ISSUES

- Sweden is a large, sparsely populated country that has a universal welfare system.
- Historically Sweden has moved from institutionalised forms of care that were segregated.
- A range of services is provided to children, adults and older people with learning disabilities that are developing into community based services located in the community.
- Sweden has recently published a White Paper that deals with all issues of disability, and that seeks to promote a community based on diversity, a society that enables full participation of all its citizens and equal opportunities for all.

INTRODUCTION

Sweden is a relatively large country in terms of area, 450 000 km² (174 000 square miles) but is sparsely populated with only 8.9 million inhabitants. Stockholm is the capital, and other major towns include Malmö and Göteborg (Gothenburg). The official language is Swedish, but all children study English and some other languages at school. Most of the Swedes are Lutheran, but there are several other faiths, including Roman Catholic, Muslim and Jewish. The currency is the Swedish krona (crown). It is abbreviated Kr or SEK. Sweden has a monarchy, and is a member of the EU.

Sweden is governed and administrated at three different levels: central, regional and local. The central public bodies include the single chamber parliament, Riksdag, the highest representative of the Swedish people, the government and central agencies. There are parliamentary elections every 4 years and from the age of 18 citizens have the right to vote. About 44% of the parliamentarians, 349 members, are women. The government governs the country but is answerable to parliament. The ministries prepare government decisions and the organs of public administration execute the decisions.

At the regional level Sweden is divided in 18 county councils (landsting), with two health care regions and the municipality of Gotland as regional units. Their main areas of responsibility are medical and health care services, including primary care and hospitals, public dental services and psychiatric care. At the local level Sweden is divided in 289 local municipalities (kommun) with responsibility for education from pre-school age to adult age, as well as all forms of social services, physical planning and building, environmental tasks and rescue services.

A universal welfare system covers the whole of the population, and the social insurance system, health care and schools, amongst others, are financed mainly through taxes and employer payroll fees (Swedish Institute 2001).

BRIEF HISTORY

This section describes and analyses the development of welfare services for people with disabilities in Sweden, especially with regard to people with learning disabilities.

In 1866 Emanuella Carlbeck, a teacher and daughter of a priest, established the first special school for pupils with learning disabilities in Sweden. In 1944 the first special law for people with learning disabilities came into force; it was followed by another law in 1954. The first law primarily provided education for children and young people with mild learning disabilities. From 1954 the counties got the responsibility of providing care for all children and adults with learning disabilities. Different perspectives have influenced the development of services, begin-

ning with a medical approach, then an educational approach and now a social policy perspective. Earlier trends considered how to protect society from a person with disability; this later changed to how to protect the person with disability from society. Sweden also had legislation about sterilisation, including non-voluntary sterilisation from 1935 to 1975. The 1934 Sterilisation Act had a limited range of application. It applied solely to certain legally incompetent persons who were incapable of giving consent to sterilisation. Many women with learning disabilities were sterilised during this period (Qvarsell 1996).

The 1950s and 1960s saw Sweden develop more large residential homes for people with learning disabilities, as was the case in many countries. By 1968 they housed more than 50% of all adult persons with learning disabilities. Since then there has been a reduction in the number of homes and people in this type of care. As time moved on more and more of the residential homes were closed down, and converted into different kinds of units, such as group homes. A new law came into force in 1967, Omsorgslagen, that promoted the principles of normalisation and integration. This law was formulated and passed during a time of great ideological debate in Sweden. Democratic issues were high on the agenda in many areas, not only in the disability field. After 1967 a major development of services took place that included group homes, day care centres, leisure activities and multidisciplinary teams staffed by social workers, psychologists, speech therapists, occupational therapists, staff for leisure activities and physicians, offering services and support for families. The roots and ideas of normalisation have their origin in the creation of the welfare state in the late 1940s. The systematic presentation of the normalisation principle originated in Denmark and in the late 1960s in Sweden, and also developed in the UK and the USA. Nirje, in Sweden, outlined the normalisation principle as follows: 'The normalisation principle means making available to all mentally retarded people patterns of life and conditions of everyday living which are close to the regular circumstances and ways of life of society' (Nirje 1980, p. 33).

Theoreticians, such as Goffman (1973), had pointed out the negative consequences of living in institutions in general. In *Åke's Book* (Lundgren

1993) Åke, a man with 32 years of experience of institutions, has given a true inside description of the brutal life in such institutions and his way back to society. He often lectures, as a spokesman for self-advocacy, and has done much work within the National Society for Persons with Mental Handicap (FUB) in Sweden. He has actively participated in many national and international conferences.

In 1985 a new law was passed in Sweden, the Special Services Act, that required all residential or nursing homes for adults with learning disabilities to close down. Those for children and young people had already been closed. This law emphasised the importance and influence of empowerment of users. Giving information and providing transparency were highlighted, and the rights of the individual, rather than the duties of the service providers and other public organisations were emphasised (Lewin 1998).

Bringing about the closure has been a very long process, but by the year 2000 all these homes will be closed. Most of the people now have moved to group homes, each with their own contract for their own flat, consisting of a kitchen, bedroom, bathroom and living room. Four or five persons can live in the same house sharing some communal areas such as rooms for laundry, a large living room and a staff room. Staffing is provided on different levels in order to enable each person to live as independently as possible. There are various kinds of group housing solutions, with a greater or lesser dependence on staff support. New research studies (Färm 1999, Mallander 1999) have shown that the closure of the nursing homes has given people with learning disabilities more opportunities to make their own decisions, and that staff support needs to be given in a more personal and individualistic way. People with learning disabilities also have access to their communities, just like any other citizen, for example using ordinary primary health care facilities.

CURRENT RANGE AND EXTENT OF SERVICES

In *Åke's Book* (Lundgren 1993) Åke described his vision of the future like this:

That all mentally retarded people should feel – just as I do – that we are members of a society and that a disability should not be looked upon as something strange; that all people should regard it quite natural that also mentally retarded persons have the same rights and obligations as all other human beings (Lundgren 1993, pp 135–136).

All citizens have the basic rights of service and support according to the Social Services Act (Socialtjänstlagen 1982) and the Health and Medical Services Act (Hälso och sjukvårdslagen 1983). Since 1994, when the Act concerning Support and Service for Persons with Certain Functional Impairments (Disability Act) was passed, local authorities have taken over responsibility for the support and provision of services for persons with learning disabilities, autism and other severe disabilities. The main principle behind this law was that people with severe disabilities have the right to live their lives as any other citizen in society. The law concerns rights of support and service, and is based on the United Nations Standard Rules on the Equalisation of Opportunities for Persons with Disabilities (1993), with declaration of full participation in society and equality in life conditions for persons with disabilities as the main goals. Governments were urged to work for achieving these goals. 'With equalisation of opportunities' means the process through which services are made available to people with disabilities. The Disability Act also emphasised the idea that people with disabilities should actively demand their rights (Lewin 1998). Those who would benefit from using their rights according to the Disability Act are:

- people with learning disabilities
- people with autism
- people who have impaired mental ability as a result of brain damage in adulthood
- people with other permanent and severe physical or mental disabilities, if in need of constant care and attention.

There is a legal right to 10 different kinds of support and service, which are:

- Advice and personal support from someone with expert knowledge such as a social worker, psychologist, speech therapist etc.

- Personal assistance for those with severe disabilities who need help with personal hygiene, dressing, eating and communicating with others.
- Guidance service for people who need someone with them when they go out, to work or to leisure activities.
- Contact person who should be like a friend, helping the person to take part in leisure activities, visiting each other, phoning each other etc. The local authority pays a small remuneration to the contact person.
- Relief service in the home especially for parents of children with disabilities.
- Short-term breaks away from home. There are special units for short-term breaks for children and others for adults available 24 hours a day all the year round.
- Short-time minding of schoolchildren over 12.
- Foster homes complementary to the parental home.
- Special housing for adults in group homes.
- Daily activities: this right is only for people with learning disabilities and/or autism and those who have suffered brain damage in adulthood (Sjöberg 1994).

How successfully has the law been implemented? Are people with learning disabilities included in society? Do people with learning disabilities have rights to make their own decisions? A survey of knowledge about attitudes to persons with disabilities has been conducted by the Committee of Inquiry into Attitudes to Persons with Disabilities (SOU 1999:21). Research material from Sweden, other Scandinavian countries, the USA, UK and Canada has been included. The main results are that there are still many negative attitudes to people with disabilities among both professionals and people in general (SOU 1999:21).

Bengt Lindkvist, who was charged by the government to review and analyse the issue of attitudes to people with disabilities, has written about many aspects of the gap between the ideal and reality. In interviews, seminars, letters and discussions with people with disabilities he got this picture of attitudes: 'Unfortunately I have to draw the conclusion that there are considerable deficiencies in attitudes to persons with disabilities. Many feel violated, controlled and called in question' (SOU 1999:21, p. 15). In the study Lindkvist recommended nine ways to make living conditions better for people with disabilities. These ways are to:

- establish a statutory right to participate in society
- put a stop to contempt of court
- make the legislation clear
- expand the right to access to public information
- introduce a new function for handling points of view and criticism of attitudes
- develop user support centres
- increase competence
- strengthen research on disability
- reveal prejudices (SOU 1999:21).

All these suggestions have been intensely debated by political parties, within disability organisations, local authorities and county councils. Some results in disability politics are local handicap plans, employment of information officers to give accessible information and the generation of a broad discussion about disability issues in Swedish society. The Social Services Act (Socialtjänstlagen 1982) stipulates the basic rights for all people in society, and the Disability Act stipulates specific rights for disabled groups. The overall goals for social services for people with learning disabilities, including that of democracy, should also be maintained at an individual level. People with learning disabilities and their families often have difficulties in using the opportunities and possibilities presented to them.

Children and the family

Children with learning disabilities generally live with their parents and siblings, and the families have support, and are offered services in many different ways to make it possible for them to take care of their child at home. The Disability Act gives parents the right to support and services from a multidisciplinary team, child care, health care, short-time care, special schools, training and allowances from the National Social Insurance Office. Young people have contact persons, guidance services and can have a disability pension from an early age. All families in Sweden have parental allowances for 480 days in order to stay at home from work to look after the child. Parents together are entitled to a temporary parental allowance of 60 days off work per child per year for children up to 12 years of age and up to 16 years of age if the child is in special need of care and supervision or if the child is sick. Parents can also have childcare allowance if they care for a sick child, or a child with disabilities in the home. They can obtain this child care allowance as soon as the child is born, and until the child reaches the age of 16 (National Social Insurance Office 1999).

All children and young people in Sweden have to attend a comprehensive basic school for 9 years from the age of six or seven. Before starting school, children have an opportunity to attend a pre-school; the pre-school has its own curriculum. The local authorities are responsible for planning and organising the schools. There are also independent schools and about 3.5% of all pupils in compulsory basic schools and upper secondary schools attend these. Since 1994, Särskola (special school) has had the same curriculum as the other comprehensive schools and offers the right to an extra year of schooling. The same basic subjects are covered by all pupils regardless of their level of development, but särskolan have their own syllabuses, adapted to meet the various needs of each pupil. Särskolan are divided in compulsory basic schools and training schools for those with more severe learning difficulties (National Agency for Education 2000). In the training schools the subjects are focused on, among other things, communication, social interaction and everyday skills.

Families can choose if their child should attend an ordinary school or go to a special school. After compulsory school, there is the right to take part in upper secondary school for 4 years, until the person is 21 years old. The number of children in special schools has increased during the last 10 years. Some research explains this as the result of cutbacks in economy in ordinary comprehensive schools, which has led to a reduction of resources. The principle and framework of high quality inclusive education is not always realised in the practical field (UNESCO Salamanca declaration 1994).

Parents are interested in working together with the professionals; they are experts on their own children. In order to decrease the number of professionals every family has to deal with, the multidisciplinary team tries to identify one team member who is responsible for contact with each family. The family and the child have the opportunity to meet different experts from the child and youth multidisciplinary team when they need to.

Adults

Support and services for adults with learning disabilities cover several areas such as housing, daytime activities, work, finance, education and technical aids. Today 17 500 adults with learning disabilities/autism or acquired brain damage live in group homes, about 4000 in their own apartments with or without support from home help services, and others live together with their parents. Only a few people with learning disabilities live together with a partner and a few have children.

21 100 adults with learning disabilities/autism or acquired brain damage have daytime activities in day care centres. According to the Disability Act (1994) all adults with learning disabilities have the legal right to have daytime activities. People with learning disabilities also work in the ordinary labour market, and in different kinds of supported employment. The special state-owned company The Samhall Group, which is located throughout the country, offers employment for 29 000 people, most of them with one or more forms of occupational disability. The Samhall Group produces a broad range of goods and services in about 800 workplaces. One target is that after a period people will be able to leave Samhall to work elsewhere in society.

Adult education for people with learning disabilities is a form of education for adults wishing to supplement their education. There is a greater interest in adult education today although available resources are limited. In multidisciplinary teams there are specially designated staff responsible for leisure activities, and they work in many different ways together with adults to find opportunities for leisure activities in the community, where people with learning disabilities can also be active.

Adults with learning disabilities can get a disability pension if they require it, and they are also entitled to housing allowances. One important task is to ensure access to high quality technical aids in order to make it possible for them to live more independently, to improve their quality of life, and to be able to participate more in society. These products are mostly free of charge for all users. However the possibility of obtaining computer-based technical aids varies between the county councils.

Older people with learning disabilities

In the past ageing of people with learning disabilities has been either little understood, or hidden. Those with severe learning disabilities had relatively short life spans, and those who survived into late adulthood were likely to be invisible, either in institutions or in the protective care of their families. The existence of a growing number of older people with learning disabilities moving into the community, as well as those already established in it, poses new challenges for all service providers. There is a dilemma of institutional ageism and service fragmentation, which means that older people with learning disabilities often face double jeopardy (Walker et al 1994). Today many project teams are working with the aim of finding good housing and meaningful daytime activities for older people with learning disabilities in Sweden. An interest in questions about older people with learning disabilities is growing, and both research and conferences have featured this topic on the agenda in the Scandinavian countries.

The Disability Act

The Disability Act is based on the principles of full participation in society and equality in living conditions, as in the 22 United Nations Standard Rules (United Nations 1993). The rules are divided in three parts: the first is concerned with preconditions for equal participation, the second about target areas for equal participation and the third about implementation measures and actions to reach the goals of full participation in society and equality in living conditions.

In order to reach these goals quality aspects such as influence, accessibility, participation, continuity and a holistic perspective have to be paid attention to. Fundamental to the Disability Act is that people with disabilities will actively demand their rights, while responsible authorities will actively seek out those needing assistance, as well as cooperating with one another and with organisations representing disabled people. Some of these rights concern personal assistance, group home living, daytime activities or occupation, contact person, short-term care and support and services from the multidisciplinary teams. The law guarantees all citizens who fulfil certain criteria special rights, without having to pay for them. In group homes the residents pay for rent, food, and medicines but not for staff costs and common areas such as staff and living rooms. Users have a right of appeal to a court of law against decisions made by social service employees that affect their lives.

People with learning disabilities and/or other disabilities and their organisations have argued that the right to personal assistance is the most important way of achieving independence and participation in society. This right is the newest and perhaps most valuable for many people; it should thus be described more fully. Those with severe disabilities are entitled to personal assistance. This applies to people who need help with personal hygiene, dressing, eating or communicating with others. An assistant should also be able to give professional help to people who want to go out, work or study. Where assistance is required for less than 20 hours a week it is paid for by the local authority. If assistance is required for more than 20 hours a week, an allowance can be obtained from the National Social Insurance Office. This allowance can be used either to pay for assistants employed by the local authority, or directly to employ one or more assistants of one's own choice.

Another right is to have a contact person who should be like a friend, preferably someone about the same age and with similar interests. A contact person should, for instance, be able to give advice on everyday situations, and help people take part in leisure activities. Work as a contact person is not a full time job, but a spare time activity for which the local authority pays a small remuneration. In Sweden there are about 12 000 contact persons, in accordance with the Disability Act. In 1994 the government entrusted the task of monitoring the rights and interests of people with disabilities to the office of the disability ombudsman, which is a national authority. Other government appointed ombudsmen are the consumer ombudsman, the equal opportunities ombudsman, ombudsmen against ethnic discrimination and discrimination because of sexual orientation, and the children's ombudsman. The disability ombudsman has responsibility for and supervises the implementation of the Disability Act. Important tasks include ensuring that deficiencies in laws and regulations are rectified, providing guidance, counselling and information and the formation of opinion.

Today new ideas are on the agenda in Sweden. The concepts of social inclusion and social exclusion are useful in looking at conditions for people with learning disabilities. Inclusion is a term which expresses a commitment to people with learning disabilities to enable them to live in their communities and to provide support and services in those communities, instead of, and rather than, excluding these people and providing special services in special settings.

The concept of citizenship is widely used in literature in many countries to analyse different kinds of difficulties in society related to ethnicity, gender and poverty but it can also be used to analyse citizenship and disability (Gynnerstedt & Blomberg 2001). Citizenship is also concerned with relationships between people and between people and institutions (Twine 1994). Marshall (1950) has analysed citizenship and divided it into three components: political, civil and social. The political citizenship of a person with learning disabilities in Sweden includes the right to vote, marry, build a family and have children. Civil citizenship includes freedom, rights and equal opportunities, but people with learning disabilities do not have all these rights in reality. Social citizenship is the most critical one and includes housing, employment, leisure activities, support and service and full participation in society, and it is in this area that there is still a lot to do.

The concepts of inclusion and exclusion are relatively new; social exclusion has its roots in a political context and was first described in France. There is a union, Inclusion International /ILSMH, which represents the field of learning disabilities. Looking at citizenship and learning disability is a relatively new way of analysing the social and political issues for people with learning disabilities.

The World Health Organization (WHO) has defined learning disabilities at four levels. But a new publication to describe, understand and measure health and disability, The International Classification of Functioning, Disability and Health (ICF), was accepted by 191 countries and published during 2001 (WHO 2001). A discussion about the concept of disability is represented in the new classification system. By focusing on concepts such as activity, participation and accessibility, people are perceived as actors, subjects, and part of society; this contrasts with a focus on concepts of disease, impairment, disability and handicap, which all express individual characteristics and encourage perception of persons as objects.

The concepts of the Swedish welfare state, and a Nordic welfare state model have enjoyed broad support. All countries, however, are unique. It is always difficult to compare the welfare systems of different countries, but there are many similarities between the Nordic countries. Examples of this are that basic needs in social security, social and health services, education and housing are met through public measures, and the government's involvement has been, and still is, strong. All people are entitled to basic social benefits and services and the levels of benefits appear fairly high compared to other industrialised nations (SOU 2000:83, p. 11).

FUTURE DIRECTIONS FOR LEARNING DISABILITY

The objective of all disability policy should be a society that enables people with disabilities to participate fully in the life of their communities. The goals are full participation in the society and equality in life conditions for all people with disabilities. A Swedish White Paper (Ministry of Health and Social Affairs 2000) *From Patient to Citizen – a National Action Plan for Disability Policy* has stated that obstacles that prevent the disabled from participating in society must be removed. Both the environment and activities in our society affect people with disabilities, and therefore disability policy must permeate all spheres and all sectors of society.

The Swedish Minister for Health and Social Affairs, Lars Engqvist, has written in the preface of this proposal: 'We still do not have a society where people with disabilities have the same opportunities as other citizens. The national action plan for disability policy that the Riksdag has adopted represents a great step forwards for modern disability policy' (Government Bill 1999/2000, p. 3). There are many issues that remain to be addressed, and in the White Paper (Government Bill 1999/2000) they are highlighted and divided into three parts: national objectives, special tasks to pay attention to, and special areas to prioritise.

The national objectives of disability policy are:

- a social community based on diversity
- a society designed to allow people with disabilities of all ages full participation in the life of the community
- equal opportunities in life for girls and boys, women and men with disabilities.

Work on disability policy is to pay particular attention to the following tasks:

- identifying and removing obstacles to full participation in society for people with disabilities
- preventing and fighting discrimination
- making it possible for children, young people and adults with disabilities to lead independent lives and to make decisions that affect their own lives.

Special areas to be given priority in the coming years are:

- ensuring that a disability perspective permeates all sectors of society
- creating a more accessible society
- improving the way the disabled are treated.

In more than 50% of the 289 local authorities there are local action plans for disability policy based on the UN Standard Rules, The Disability Act and the National Action Plan.

CONCLUSION

If we look back in time people have been excluded from citizenship or citizens' rights due to class, gender, ethnicity, age or disability in many countries and we can still see traces of this today.

The most critical issues seem to be about citizenship and the possibilities for full participation in society. Are people with learning disabilities included or excluded in society? Citizenship is closely connected to human rights, and there are a lot of obstacles at different levels: legislation, the professional discourse, theories and methods and the practical field. All these areas interact with each other (Lundström 1993). People with disabilities in general are less represented in political parties, have a higher rate of unemployment, lower incomes, less power and less influence in social services.

In the future issues of empowerment will be more in focus. There are also changing patterns in the research and evaluation programmes. People with learning disabilities, and their relatives, are interested in more active roles. Participatory research is one way forward and another is to be active evaluators of the services provided in group homes and day care centres. Citizenship is about empowerment and influence. In June 1999 the first research conference with people with learning disabilities was held in Sweden. This conference was arranged by the interest group FUB, the association for children, young people and adults with learning disabilities. People with learning disabilities were very pleased with the conference and felt that they were really listened to. Disabled researchers have offered a lot of criticism of research based on official definitions.

The disability perspective must be a natural, integrated element of every public authority's regular operations. When people with learning disabilities have access to products, activities, the labour market, information, culture and the media, control of services and education and the accessible society are a reality, and the concept of citizenship can be fulfilled. When people with learning disabilities learn to speak for themselves the possibility of them being recognised as active citizens becomes apparent. There is an ongoing change in attitudes in Sweden from needs to rights.

REFERENCES

Färm K 1999 'Socialt problem' eller 'Som andra och i gemenskap med andra'. Föreställningar om människor med utvecklingsstörning. Tema kommunikation, Linköpings universitet

Goffman E 1973 Totala institutioner. Fyra essäer om anstaltslivets sociala villkor. Rabén & Sjögren, Stockholm

Gynnerstedt K, Blomberg B 2001 Medborgarskap i brytningstid. (In press)

Lewin B 1998 Funktionshinder och medborgarskap. Institutionen för folkhälsovetenskap, Socialmedicinska sektionen, Akademiska sjukhuset, Uppsala

Lundgren K 1993 Åke's Book. Riksförbundet FUB, Stockholm

Lundström T 1993 Tvångsomhädertagande av barn: en studie av lagarna, professionerna och praktiken under 1900-talet. Rapport i socialt arbete;61, Stockholm

Mallander O 1999 De hjälper oss tillrätta; normaliseringsarbete, självbestämmande och människor med psykisk utvecklingsstörning. Meddelanden från Socialhögskolan/Lunds universitet; 1999:2, Lund

Marshall T H 1950 Citizenship and social class. In: Marshall T H (ed) Citizenship and social class and other essays. Cambridge University Press, Cambridge

Ministry of Health and Social Affairs (Sweden) 2000 From patient to citizen – a national action plan for disability policy 1999/2000: 79. Ministry of Health and Social Affairs, Stockholm

National Agency for Education (Skolverket) 2000 The Swedish school system. http://www.skolverket.se/

National Social Insurance Office 1999 Social insurance. Försäkringskasseförbundet, Stockholm

Nirje B 1980 The normalization principle. In: Flynn R J, Nitsch K E (eds) Normalization, social integration and community services. University Park Press, Baltimore

Qvarsell R 1996 Vårdens idéhistoria. Carlsson, Stockholm

SFS 1993:387 Lag om stöd och service till vissa funktionshindrade. (The Disability Act)

Sjöberg M 1994 New rights for persons with functional impairments. Swedish Institute, Stockholm

SOU 1999:21 Lindkvists nia Utredningen om bemötande av personer med funktionshinder. Stockholm

SOU 2000:83 Two of a kind. Mikko Kautto, Stockholm

Swedish Institute 2001 Facts about Sweden. http://www.si.se/

Twine F 1994 Citizenship and social rights. The independence of self and society. Sage Publications, London

Walker A, Walker C, Ryan T 1994 The de-institutionalisation of older people with learning difficulties. A new challenge to service providers. Sheffield Hallam University, Sheffield

UNESCO 1994 Salamanca declaration. http://www.unesco.org/education/educprog/sne/

United Nations 1993 Standard rules on the equalization of opportunities for persons with disabilities. http://www.independentliving.org/STANDARDRULES/

World Health Organisation 2001 International classification of functioning, disability and health. WHO, Geneva

USEFUL ADDRESS

http://www.who.int/

Germany

Sabine Rothe

KEY ISSUES

- The term 'people with mental disabilities' is used throughout this chapter. This is because it is the most commonly used term in Germany by service users and organisations; professionals also use it in both research and literature.
- Government statistics of severely disabled only include those eligible, and having applied for a 'severely disabled card' that proves a degree of disability between 50% and 100%, measuring the extent of limitation and additional handicaps (Statistisches Bundesamt 1999). According to these statistics some 406 297 people with mental disability live in Germany.
- Increasingly another approach of defining 'mental disability' is being adopted by service providers through identifying different target groups of people with varying needs of support, so that their abilities can be built upon. Discussion amongst service users and professionals is ongoing as to how definitions and terminology should be changed to focus on an individual's 'chances and possibilities and personal development' instead of their weaknesses and/or perceived deficiencies (Wernicke 1996).

INTRODUCTION

In Germany the history of people with mental disabilities over the centuries is very similar to developments in other European countries. However, when it comes to the 20th century we have to deal with the darkest period of history concerning people with mental disability in Germany. Between 1933 and 1945 170 000 mentally ill, mentally disabled and physically disabled people are thought to have been murdered on the order of Adolf Hitler. This was perpetrated by medical doctors, professors, nurses and other professionals in hospitals and nursing homes both in Germany and Austria. Because of limited space this chapter will necessarily leave gaps concerning this period but some comprehensive texts in English that deal with these issues can be found in the further reading section at the end of the chapter. Box 28.1 gives up-to-date information on demographic details on Germany today.

The eugenic debate in Germany and Europe

After the First World War several European countries, as well as the USA, were engaged in a eugenic debate (see Ch. 3 for a full discussion of this). Friedrich v Bodelschwingh who was director of Bethel (Germany's largest institution for the care of people with epilepsy and mental disabilities) wrote: 'It is the case that this war called the capable and physically useful individuals to the front line and let them die on the battle fields, whereas physically and mentally useless people stayed at home' (Kühl 1997, pp 54–67).

Medical and other professionals were also calling for the sterilisation of 'inferior' people in order to prevent them from reproducing. By 1920 two scientists, K Binding, a lawyer, and A Hoche, a psychiatrist, had published a book *The Problem of Lifting Control over Extinction of Life Not Worth Living* (*Das Problem der Freigabe der Vernichtung unwerten Lebens*). In this book 'sympathy with people suffering from non-remedial conditions' was expressed but simultaneously they noted how those people were a burden both for their relatives and society: 'There are people whose death means release for them, at the same time enabling society to "get rid" of them and releasing the state from a burden . . .' (Binding & Hoche 1922, p. 28).

As a result of these ideas, that incidentally were shared quite widely by European doctors, churches and politicians, laws of sterilisation were passed in the Scandinavian countries and even earlier in the USA (Kühl 1997, p. 59; Peter 1934, pp 187–191). In the United Kingdom and the Netherlands such laws only narrowly failed to materialise. When the Nazis seized power in 1933; in Germany, Hitler passed a law of 'Prevention of hereditary ill offspring' in July 1933; this was supported both for 'racial hygiene' and economic reasons (Pörksen 1997).

This law applied to the following conditions:

- Congenital mental deficiency
- Schizophrenia
- Manic depression
- Hereditary epilepsy
- Huntington's chorea
- Hereditary blindness and deafness
- Profound hereditary physical disabilities.

Box 28.1   Demographic details on Germany

Status	Federal Republic
Area	357 000 square kilometres
Population	82 163 500 (female: 42 072 700, male: 40 090 800) (includes 7 336 100 foreigners)
Capital	Berlin (approximately 3.3 million inhabitants)
Other major towns	Hamburg, München, Köln, Frankfurt/M, Stuttgart
Languages	German
Religions	Protestant, Catholic, Muslim, Jewish communities etc.
Currency	EURO
Membership	EU, NATO, European Council
System of Government	Federation of 16 states that includes: Bavaria, Baden Württemberg, Berlin, Saarland, Rheinland Pfalz, Hessen, Thuringia, Saxony, Brandenburg, Saxony Anhalt, Lower Saxony, Mecklenburg-West Pomerania, Schleswig Holstein, Hamburg and Bremen (Stadtstaaten = towns as autonomous states)

On the one hand this law reflected the spirit of the time, whilst on the other it deliberately engineered the extinction of mentally ill and mentally disabled people. An application for sterilisation could be made by people affected, relatives, carers, guardians, the doctor at the health authority or a residential institution. A decision to sterilise could even be made against the will of the patient by the 'Court of Hereditary Health' (Erbgesundheitsgericht), involving a judge and two doctors (Pörksen 1997). From 1933 to 1939 it is estimated that some 400 000 men and women were sterilised, and of these approximately 5000 women and 4000 men died. At the same time hospital and nursing budgets in psychiatric hospitals and nursing homes were being continuously reduced, with an acknowledgement that this would lead to starvation of patients and ultimately their deaths (Steppe 1996, p. 143). From 1 August 1939 all newborn children with mental disabilities and/or serious physical disabilities had to be registered. During this period, known as 'the time of children euthanasia' it is estimated that some 5000 disabled children died on 'special children wards' at 30 hospitals and nursing homes all over Germany. Their deaths were brought about by the application of overdoses of luminal and also the withdrawal of food (Steppe 1996, pp 143–144). This paved the way for 'euthanasia', which resulted in the systematic murder of people with mental diseases and disabilities. Because of high priority secrecy a villa in Berlin, 'Tiergartenstraße 4', was chosen as the operational centre for the 'euthanasia' programme, hence the codename 'Aktion T4'. By using this anonymous suburban base those responsible intended to mask the administrative connection with Hitler's Chancellory. Immense pains were taken to keep T4 operations (killing of patients) covert (Burleigh 1994, pp 122, 162). A central working group of hospitals and nursing homes was established to undertake this work.

Euthanasia

After the beginning of the war in September 1939 all mental nursing homes and psychiatric hospitals were obliged to register their patients and inmates. From 1940–1941 six nursing homes and psychiatric hospitals in different areas of Germany and Austria were identified as 'killing institutions'. The patients were transferred to these institutions from other hospitals. Many leading doctors took part in selecting patients who should be killed by gas, injections and/or food withdrawal. Between 1939 and 1941 approximately 70 000 inmates of hospitals were killed (Steppe 1996, p. 144). Relatives were 'notified' by post of their family member's death, but were given another disease as the cause of death; they would never see their relative again. On 3 August 1941 the Catholic bishop Graf von Galen preached a sermon against this criminal extinction of children and adults. As a result the 'Aktion T4' was stopped officially for political (internal and external) reasons, but it later proceeded on to the so-called 'wild euthanasia' from 1942 to 1945. During these years another 100 000 people were murdered by injection and/or starvation. These atrocities were grounded in financial reasons on the one hand, and supposed practical reasons on the other; beds were needed because of war casualties (Steppe 1996, pp 138–165). During the Nuremberg Medical Trial (1945), and at other trials of doctors and nurses who were involved in Hadamar (1947), Obrawalde and other locations, many, but not all were sentenced. Sentences included death penalties, and longer or shorter imprisonment for doctors and nurses. Several defendants committed suicide, others received a 'not guilty' verdict and continued to work as doctors after the war in qualified positions (Hohmann & Wieland 1996, p. 130).

Resistance

Resistance among doctors and nurses was rare but it did take place. Some psychiatrists, for example, tried to conceal the diagnoses mentioned in the law. Others transferred patients into smaller hospitals; they realised that such practices had no scientific basis and contradicted humanistic ideals (Hohmann & Wieland 1996, pp 33–35).

As previously mentioned, some officials of the Catholic Church also protested. Some parents and relatives protested by writing letters to hospitals and tried to take their relatives out; some actually succeeded and some relatives were saved. Several doctors, nurses and also directors of institutions and hospitals advised relatives to take away inmates, and some left their positions because they did not want to take part in this crime. In fact passive resistance was far more commonly found; however, at no time was there a collective ground swell opposition by way of protest by the German population as a whole.

CURRENT RANGE AND EXTENT OF SERVICES

The Federal Republic of Germany's welfare system is based on cooperation between the public sector and non-statutory agencies (charities). These agencies perform on behalf of the whole community; the non-statutory welfare services are recognised as a vital part of the welfare state. Six central voluntary welfare organisations currently providing services in Germany are shown in Box 28.2.

These organisations have provided services for many years and in some cases for over a century. The social network of care service provision in Germany would tear apart if it were not for their contribution. The overall aim of such public and private partnerships, which incidentally are beginning to emerge in the UK, is to provide effective and complementary welfare services for the benefit of people needing help and/or care.

Box 28.2 Six central voluntary organisations who work with the public sector

- Diakonisches Werk der EKD (Protestant Churches 1848)
- Deutscher Caritas Verband (Catholic Church 1895)
- Paritätischer Wohlfahrtsverband (an umbrella for over hundred provider organisations keeping their independence from state and churches 1924)
- Arbeiterwohlfahrt AWO (Workers Welfare Organisation 1919) provide single services for people with mental disability
- Deutsches Rotes Kreuz DRK (1869 German Branch of the Red Cross, re-established 1950)
- Zentrale Wohlfahrtsstelle der Juden in Deutschland (Jewish community welfare organisation 1917) re-established after 1952

Whereas this cooperation involves the effort of public and non-statutory agencies, it is guided by a 'subsidiary principle', which in simple terms means that whatever the individual, family, group or organisational body can do for themselves must not be turned into the responsibility of the state. It should therefore be ensured that the competence and responsibility of the respective social group is recognised and made use of. However, this also places a responsibility on the state to strengthen smaller units where necessary thereby providing the means to deliver a service. The recognition of social initiatives expressed in the subsidiary principle grants citizens in need of assistance the right to choose according their religion or political attitude. The cooperation between public and non-statutory welfare agencies is governed by the Social Code and the special legal arrangements for the area of child and youth welfare (Children's Assistance Code).

For some 70 years these welfare associations have worked closely together at the federal, state (Länder), district and community level. They have developed a strong position by slowly building up their role as the primary partners of service provision, alongside social services at local level. The implementation of the 'subsidiary principle' (1961) has granted these voluntary organisations a special public status: they have to be contracted in the first place whenever a publicly funded new social service or institution is to be established. The public sector provides the money at all levels of administration. Another financial source is long-term care insurance (Pflegeversicherung) which covers the cost of home care services through fees paid into it by all citizens (Federal Association of Non-statutory Welfare/Bundesarbeitsgemeinschaft der Freien Wohlfahrtspflege 1995).

Residential facilities for service users

Box 28.3 shows the number of people with mental disabilities and also the composition of this population accounted for by age. There is a range of residential care and other housing facilities available for people with mental disabilities and these are identified by Wacker (1999, pp 65–66) and shown in Box 28.4, the reader might like to

---

Box 28.3 Number of people with mental disability in Germany and where they live (Lebenshilfe 2000)

- Total number (approximately)   420 000   including those who have no 'Disability Card'
- Children   185 000   85% (160 000) live with their families
- Adults   235 000   60% (140 000) live with their families

Box 28.4 Residential alternatives for people with mental disabilities in the FRG

Nursing homes	24%
External base of a home	6%
Hostels linked with sheltered workshops and day care training groups	53%
Shared flats	5%
Supervised flat (for single or couple)	4%
Village communities	5%
Large psychiatric institutions including mentally disabled residents	3%

compare these with residential options identified in Chapters 5, 26 and 27.

Day facilities

Work

The Bundesministerium für Arbeit (BMA) currently provides 131 372 places of employment in sheltered workshops for those people with mental disabilities who, because of their profound disability, cannot be integrated into working schemes or the first step of the labour market. A two-year introductory training programme is provided to those who need it and this qualifies people to perform at their best. Personal and productive development training encourages workers to develop personal efficiency. People who work are entitled to paid employment dependent upon their results. Sheltered workshops are also provided by welfare organisations; these are usually smaller private or community based facilities. They are the most frequently used and the best available facility, providing employment for 52% of people with mental disabilities, and having a high priority in their lives. Working hours vary considerably according to the individual situation of the person attending; for example, some only work 2 hours per week whereas others will work up to 35 hours.

Provision of services to relieve the strain on families caring for relatives with mental disabilities

As shown in Box 28.3 85% of children (7–18 years) and 60% of adults (19–40 years) live with their families, who undertake the main responsibility of care. Services to relieve the strain on families were mainly developed in the 1980s by the largest self-help association for people with mental disabilities, 'Lebenshilfe', as a mobile service for families with mentally disabled relatives. Approximately 350 agencies with some 300 professionals as managers and 4000 voluntary helpers provide support for approximately 12 000 families. The kinds of support available to families are shown in Box 28.5.

There is additional demand for services where the main carer goes out to work. Special support is sometimes needed for non-disabled siblings who may sometimes be neglected. Spending time away from home and parents, especially from mothers, is crucial for children and young people as service users. Counselling regarding relationships and sexuality, help with behaviour problems, and training in social and cultural skills and living activities are also available. The goals of such a service for the main carer are recreation opportunities and the chance to participate in social, cultural and political life; also the child can be positively influenced through short-term care towards growing autonomy and independence from the mother and father. In addition counselling concerning financial

---

Box 28.5 The FED services to relieve family strain

Relief and support for informal carers
Care may take place in and out of the family:

- Organisation of and company during leisure time
- Nursing care and home help
- Psychosocial support (counselling, conversation)

matters and initiating self-help support groups is another service provided (Lebenshilfe 1999).

Children and young people with mental disabilities

Residential care for children and young people

There are some 169 residential homes providing places for 5407 children and young people with mental disabilities. The largest group of children in residential care are those between 6 and 15 years whose families cannot cope with caring for them at home because of the severity of the disability, social background and/or social problems; this is if no foster family can be found. Most of the residential homes have integrated schools allocated to them. Approximately 3% of younger children will be found in residential care (Wacker 1999, pp 69–70).

Kindergarten

Special kindergarten for children with mental disabilities is provided for 11 300 children by voluntary organisations caring for children with mental and multiple disabilities. Currently there are a few integrative groups (mainstream institutions) where children with and without disabilities learn together; this supports the development of more positive social attitudes, as well as developing personal and cognitive abilities. Kindergarten teachers will have special qualifications, and if necessary therapeutic and nursing staff will be available (Dittrich 1998).

School and day care facilities for children and young people

School

In Germany generally attendance at school is compulsory school for 9 years; this is followed by 3 years vocational education. For children with mental disability there are at least two ways of attending school:

- Special schools and special educational programmes in mainstream classrooms

- Joint (integrative) education of children with mental disability in mainstream schools.

Education is orientated towards cognitive, linguistic, sensory, psychomotor, emotional and social development. As well as classes in the morning, a programme in the afternoon is available that fosters social competence and independence. Since 1994 integrative classes have taken children with all kinds of disabilities and support needs. Some 4% children with mental disability receive special integration support in mainstream schools, of which 60% was at primary, 15% at secondary, 1% at grammar and 22% at comprehensive levels. These figures demonstrate that children with mental disabilities rarely go in to mainstream education, whereas 16% receive special educational support in special schools for children with mental disability.

Integration classes

These are designed to enable children and young people to attend mainstream schools instead of special schools. This is regarded as beneficial for both the disabled and the able-bodied children. The highly gifted child will learn from the child with mental disabilities and vice versa. Integration classes are person- and needs-orientated and have at their disposal a flexible range of equipment and provisions for different types of schools. Instead of the single track of special education, it is thought that the children should be part of mainstream education. Children receive support from specially qualified teachers, together with their regular teacher in their regular classroom, or they are separated for a few hours of the week. Joint education for disabled children takes place only in schools where facilities for staff can be adapted to the requirements of children with special needs. In practice children with mental disabilities will still have limited choices. This is because mainstream schools will only take children into integration classes if facilities are adequate, and if they have the appropriate number of qualified teachers. Also, the size of the class needs to be appropriate before the child can be integrated in the classroom (2–4 children with special needs in a classroom) (Kultusministerkonferenz 2001, pp 3–64).

Integration schools

These are provided by welfare organisations such as churches or special self-help organisations such as the 'Lebenshilfe'; they work as 'model schools' offering joint (integrative) classes of 20 children of which five will have a disability. A typical schedule for such a school would be as follows. Between 7.30 and 8.00 a.m. children would work on their weekly tasks. This would be followed by breakfast and outdoor games. Classes would commence at 10.00 a.m. and would include mathematics, German or another subject. Lunch, games, supervised homework in groups and projects would follow this. Children would then leave at approximately 4.00 p.m. These schools provide common ground and a sense of community with others; arguably this is a basic human right. There are 6 years of joint classes with team teaching, day care and integration of therapies into class. Such schools are open to all children, including those with all kinds of impairments, disabilities and handicaps (Lebenshilfe Gießen 2001).

Early detection and early intervention

Each new-born child is entitled to medical screening in order to find possible metabolic diseases which may lead to mental disabilities. From birth to 6 years (and again at the age of 10 years) children are entitled to receive ten precautionary medical check-ups in case of a disability, or impending disability. Germany has some 700 multidisciplinary centres for early diagnosis and early intervention measures, providing services for children (0–6 years) with disabilities or impending disabilities and their families. Neighbourhood interdisciplinary teams are available which include educational, psychological, medical, therapeutic and social work specialists, and adopt a holistic approach.

Early intervention services and procedure

Mobile services will work with the child at home, in the kindergarten or nursery school. Alternatively mothers will bring their children to the centre. In the former East Germany services take place in schools or day centres. Social paediatric centres with specialists and therapists, will in some cases identify the need for medical and/or therapeutic treatment.

Parents and their child will see the agency with a referral from their family doctor or because of their own concerns. Waiting lists are increasing, as is demand. Tests, diagnosis and if necessary the support needed to identify resources and overcome problems for the family are available. This is followed by a rehabilitation plan that includes weekly treatment over 2 years. Group therapy sessions will be offered where a single child needs support in groups. The current approach adopted is to see the parents, the child, siblings and early intervention workers as systems that influence each other. Development of standards of excellence, quality assurance and transparency of costs are crucial aims for the purchaser to buy only services that provide best value for money.

Special support and advice centres support children with special needs working in mainstream schools. Such centres provide a pool of specially educated teachers that aim to keep children at their regular schools. This link supports the child in the mainstream school with special services and also provides a bridge to other health and social services.

Young persons in vocational training programmes (Federal Institution for Labour 1997)

Vocational training institutes are national facilities providing vocational training especially for young people with mental disabilities for occupations that require recognised training courses. These young people, who are not able to follow regular vocational education in a company, will be offered training courses tailored to their needs. This training will take place in a residential setting where all facilities can be found under the same roof: for example training workshops and vocational courses adapted to the special needs of respective disabilities. An integrated hostel and sport and leisure facility is also available. Germany has around 50 vocational training institutes with just under 14 000 places covering some 170 different occupations. In these training centres a team of doctors, psychologists and social workers will help these young people to develop. Where necessary the services of the vocational support centre are provided by the Federal Institution of Labour, and financed by the Employment Exchange. This centre offers rehabilitation and training courses for people who have already had a job but cannot carry on because of medical problems; they will receive training for a new job.

Services for elderly people with mental disabilities

In Germany the ageing of people with mental disability has only relatively recently received attention. This is as a result of the history of this particular group of people (see earlier in this chapter). The number of elderly persons continues to increase gradually, and therefore research studies on this group are beginning to be published (Gusset-Bährer 1991). Service requirements are changing as the needs of the elderly change rapidly. Though the rate of employment (in sheltered workplaces) is high the inability to continue working commences earlier compared to people with other disabilities; however the wish to stay at the workplace in familiar surroundings is strong. Working hours can be reduced and a new structure of day care in residential homes or in supervised flats will be offered. It should be noted that the housing situation for people with mental disability, especially for the elderly, is still quite poor. Although it was stated earlier that 65% of people with mental disabilities live with their parents, this does not apply to elderly people. Many moved to residential care in large institutions when their parents died and those who had lived independently in supervised flats had often to move because of their increasing dependency when growing older. Only 15% live in facilities where a more independent life is possible. For the majority ageing means living in residential care; 25% live in smaller institutions (of approximately 50 people), and approximately 60% live in larger institutions and often have to share a room with others. Only 38% live in a single room compared to 60% of people with other disabilities. Some of them even share a room with three or four other people. Fortunately in the former East Germany (Neue Bundesländer) the situation has improved a lot, since efforts were made to build new housing facilities for people with mental disability. But also in the western states (Länder) of the FRG continued efforts are being made to improve the situation for residents who experience considerable variation in the quality of services.

Several services for elderly people with mental disability are available in different institutions. Special areas are provided for senior citizens in sheltered workplaces to ensure a gradual transition from work to retirement. At day centres and clubs for elderly residents group activities are planned according to the needs of the people. These events may include cultural events and organising meeting places where the disabled and non-disabled can socialise.

At the moment there is an ongoing debate about the financial responsibilities of the long-term care insurance scheme (Pflegeversicherung) and the provider of services according to Federal social assistance. Normally, the long-term care insurance scheme will only pay for care in the home of the client, but in residential institutions a flat rate of DM 500 per month will be paid for each resident, regardless of each person's real nursing care needs. If a person's care needs result in higher costs then either the client or social assistance will make good the difference. There is also an ongoing reform in that the social assistance provider is interested in transforming as many institutions as possible into pure nursing homes, where only the long-term care insurance scheme would have to provide the financial contribution.

New legislation

A new law, the Seriously Handicapped Persons Act (Schwerbehindertengesetz) was enacted by the government of the Federal Republic of Germany in October 2000. The ninth book of the Social Code (Sozialgesetzbuch IX) states: 'The focus of the new legislation is less on care and provision of people with disabilities than on self determined participation in society and removal of obstacles preventing equal opportunities' (Sozialgesetzbuch 2001, p.2).

In this legislation rehabilitation and the integration of people with disabilities into the labour market is an important issue. Promoting participation in the labour market is crucial. All employers, public or private, have to fulfil a quota of 5% of employees with severe disabilities, otherwise they have to pay a rate per person for not fulfilling their obligation. If by 2003 the number of unemployed disabled people is not reduced by 25%, then the government will take measures, yet to be specified, against both private and public employers. The representatives of disabled employees (Schwerbehindertenvertretung) now have more rights to participate in employment planning, in order to enhance the employment opportunities of applicants with disabilities. Where applicants with disabilities have equal qualifications compared to other applicants, and need possible necessary adaptation of the work place, which may also include a personal assistant, they must be considered equally otherwise the post would have to be disposed of.

Following this legislation a new service was introduced. Special integration services help possible applicants by consulting, and by giving advice and support in finding a job. They should evaluate applicants' strengths and abilities and produce a profile of abilities, interests and achievements, in order to prepare them for their first entry into the labour market. This should be done in close cooperation with the disabled person and with any potential employer, along with the person's former school or workshop. Possible tasks for this new service include: finding the right job, accompanying the person on the job, informing future colleagues about the disability, and possible consequences, intervening in case of crisis, giving psychological support and being available for ongoing support.

CONCLUSION

This chapter has provided a brief overview of services for people with mental disabilities in Germany. A brief history has been provided that has alluded to a very dark part of Germany's past during the 20th century. Now Germany provides a range of services for people with mental disabilities and their families, which are comparable in many ways to services in other countries in the European Union. The unification of Germany has brought about positive developments in former Eastern Germany. Recent legislation has concentrated upon the importance of work as a mediator of self-worth and one's role within one's community and in society at large.

REFERENCES

Arbeitsgemeinschaft der Deutschen Hauptfürsorgestellen Ed 2000 Schwerbehindertengesetz LV Druck, Münster

Bundesarbeitsgemeinschaft der Freien Wohlfahrtspflege 1993 Bonn

Binding K, Hoche A 1922 Die Freigabe der Vernichtung lebensunwerten Lebens, 2nd edn. Meuner, Leipzig.

Bundesministerium für Arbeit und Soziales Ed 1998 Die Lage der Behinderten und die Entwicklung der Rehabilitation. Vierter Bericht der Bundesregierung. Bonn

Burleigh M 1994 Death and deliverance. 'Euthanasia' in Germany, 1900–1945. Cambridge University Press, Cambridge

Dittrich, G 2001 Behinderte Kinder in Kindertagesstätten. (Disabled Children in Daycare facilities) http://bidok.uibk.ac.at/texte/g13-98-kinder.html (4 Oct. 2001)

Glass J 1997 Life unworthy of life. Racial phobia and mass murder in Hitler's Germany. Basic Books, New York.

Gesamtstatistik der Einrichtungen der Freien Wohlfahrtspflege 1997 Bonn

Gusset Bährer S 1999 Alte und älter werdende Menschen mit geistiger Behinderung. Institut für Gerontologie, Heidelberg (hekt.manuscript)

Hohmann J, Wieland G 1996 MfS Operativvorgang "Teufel". Euthanasiearzt Otto Hebold vor Gericht. Metropolverlag, Berlin

Kühl S 1977 Eugenik und 'Vernichtung lebensunwerten Lebens' der Fall Bethel aus einer internationalen Perspektive. In: Benad M (ed) Friedrich von Bodelschwingh d.J. und die Betheler Anstalten. Kohlhammer, Stuttgart, pp 54–67

Kultusministerkonferenz 2001 http://www.kultusministerkonferenz.de/schul/blick.htm (30 Aug. 2001)

Kultusministerkonferenz Ed 2001 Schule in Deutschland Zahlen Fakten, Analysen Nr. 155 – Sekretariat, Bonn

Lebenshilfe 2000 Gießen (personal communication)
Lebenshilfe 2001 Familien entlastende und unterstützende Dienste www.lebenshilfe.de/fachfragen/OHFED_FUD/FED_FUD_home.htm-5k (21 Oct. 2001)
Lebenshilfe Gießen 2001 Sophie-Scholl-Schule ist irgendwie anders. http://www.sophie-scholl-schule-giessen.de (1 Sept 2001)
Peter, W.W. 1934 'Germany's Sterilisation Program' American Journal of Public Health and Nations Health 24, quoted in Glass J 1997 Life Unworthy of Life. Basic Books, New York
Pörksen N 1997 Zwangssterilisation in Bethel In: Benad M (ed) Friedrich von Bodelschwingh d.J. und die Betheler Anstalten. Kohlhammer, Stuttgart, pp 270–274
Sozialgesetzbuch IX 2001 Rehabilitation und Teilhabe behinderter Menschen. Luchterhand Neuwied

Statistik der Bundesanstalt für Arbeit 1997 Berufliche Rehabilitation. St 37, Nürnberg
Statistisches Bundesamt 1999 Metzler-Poeschel Verlag, Wiesbaden
Steppe H (ed) 1996 Krankenpflege im Nationalsozialismus, 8th edn. Mabuse Verlag, Frankfurt/M
Wacker E 1998 Leben im Heim. BMFG. Nomos Verlag, Baden-Baden.
Wacker E 2001 Wohn-Fürder-und Versorgungskonzepte für ältere Menschen. In:Deutsches Zentrum für Alltersfragen Expertisen zum Altenbericht der Bundesregierung. Band 5 Leske Budrich, Opladen
Wernicke C Aspekte der Abgrenzung und Definition "Geistige Behinderung" email:bv fachfragen@t-online

FURTHER READING

Burleigh M 1994 Death and deliverance. 'Euthanasia' in Germany 1900–1945. Cambridge University Press, Cambridge

Glass J 1997 Life unworthy of life. Racial phobia and mass murder in Hitler's Germany. Basic Books, New York

USEFUL ADDRESSES

http://bidok.uibk.ac.at/texte/g13-98-kinder.html
http://www.kultusministerkonferenz.de/schul/blick.htm
fachfragen@t-online

Education and leadership

In this section, two chapters are presented that outline some of the important education and training issue initiatives, as well as challenges, for leadership in the field of learning disability. Both of these areas received considerable attention in the new White Paper. Firstly, Cathy Renouf and Rob Parry trace the complexities surrounding educational and training issues in the field of learning disabilities. Finally, in Chapter 30, Mark Jukes presents a detailed chapter on a range of management and leadership issues that future practitioners will need to address. There is considerable scope in the field for development of new leaders able to carry forward new agendas in pursuit of the best possible chances for people with learning disabilities.

Education and training

Rob Parry, Cathy Renouf

KEY ISSUES

- This chapter focuses on education and training issues. It acknowledges that while the policy documents cited are from England many of the issues presented can be transferred to any other country within the UK.
- There is a very large workforce employed to support and care for people with learning disabilities in widely dispersed settings.
- Some of this workforce hold professional qualifications, some have had training but have no qualifications, whilst others have had no training, and this has implications for the configuration of future services.
- Services for those with learning disabilities will require people who are able to work in partnerships between various agencies and professionals, with users/patients and carers, in order to meet changing expectations.

INTRODUCTION

The first part of the chapter identifies the political drivers influencing the requirements of training and education. The second part addresses various education and training frameworks from a historical perspective through to the current and contemporary preparation for the future learning disability workforce to the benefit of service users/patients and their carers. The chapter also considers the implications of the most recent publication from the Department of Health *Valuing People* (DOH 2001) and its likely impact on education and training for the health and social care workforce.

POLICY AGENDA: THE DRIVERS OF EDUCATION AND TRAINING

In recent years a plethora of reports, policy documents and pseudo political commentaries have been published in an attempt to shape the future worker within learning disability services. Countless government departments under the umbrella of health or social care have produced the policy agendas. Many governments have not looked for radical departures from existing policy, but quite often have considered that the problem with learning disability services does not stem from policy framework itself, but from difficulties with implementation. The requirement is for services to be responsive to client need and to ensure, through leadership and commitment at local levels, that policy can be delivered. The latest policy driver from the Department of Health *Valuing People: A New Strategy for Learning Disability for the 21st Century* (DOH 2001) sets new national objectives for services for people with learning disabilities, supported by new targets and performance indicators, to provide clear direction for local agencies.

The National Health Service Executive (NHSE) in England is responsible for assessing the workforce development implications of national policy developments. It is accountable for the planning processes and investment made nationally in education and training for health professionals. Workforce Development Confederations in England will be responsible for integrated workforce planning for health communities based on Health Improvement Plans and National Service Frameworks, and for supporting individual employers with the planning process. Furthermore, they are required to secure the involvement of non-NHS providers of health care (e.g. local authorities, social service departments and the independent sector) and will commission and manage education and training for all clinical staff. The confederations will negotiate and manage contracts with local education and training providers to ensure quality, appropriateness of

the programmes and value for money. They will also develop strategic partnerships with higher education institutions to assist in the construction of programmes that understand and respond to the developing needs of health and social care providers. Local employers will review skill mix, workforce planning and the development needs of staff to address the policy. Local authorities and service providers in the independent sector are responsible for determining and meeting their own workforce needs. The Training Organisation for Personal Social Services (TOPSS) has a central role in the development of workforce analysis, and in providing a national training strategy for those employed in the social care sector. The participation of local authorities and the independent sector in the Workforce Development Confederations enables their needs for health staff to be taken into account when the overall health workforce is planned.

QUALITY STRATEGY FOR SOCIAL CARE

The government report *Modernising Social Services* (DOH 1998a) focused on the need to change systems and structures in a way that will put people who use social services at the centre of care. This quality strategy will consult on the reforms needed in working practices, local management and training in order to enhance the quality of social services in England. Although the mechanisms for achieving the right workforce in social care vary from those of the NHS, the same precepts apply to all services engaged in the delivery of health and social care. It is the responsibility of individual organisations to meet these challenges and to build supportive, family-friendly organisations that are able to reconcile the needs and aspirations of patients, service users, carers and staff.

As identified in *Modernising Social Services* (DOH 1998a) frontline managers play a key role in maintaining standards of practice by supervising, supporting and developing staff. Training is seen to be a priority, with skills and competencies in managing practice and delivery, and working in partnership with agencies and professional and occupational groups all requiring particular development. Given broader workforce planning, in relation to social care policies which are aimed at combating poverty and social exclusion, new roles are being created for workers. The social care workforce will need to be geared to this new environment. Many staff already working in social care will be capable, with the right training, of doing more skilled work.

The creation of the Social Care Institute for Excellence (SCIE) makes available information on systems that improve quality and that actually make a difference. It will become a major lever for creating a culture within social services that prioritises quality based on evidence based knowledge and a commitment to continuous service improvement. Key points within the new quality framework include a full commitment to staff development and training through the introduction of lifelong learning. A clearer focus on the establishment of local partnerships with users and carers and the local health services is required. Through this it is anticipated that the local community will develop new ways of delivering services in response to identified user need.

Modern social care will require a workforce that is better trained and able to work across service boundaries, in partnership with users. This workforce will be required to update its knowledge and skills continuously, and to link training and development clearly to career progression. The primary responsibilities for training will lay with employers, who should take the lead responsibility for training and development for staff at all levels. This investment is a crucial component in delivering quality through an informed, responsive and stable workforce. The changes planned for learning disability services outlined in *Valuing People* (DOH 2001) will have significant implications for staff in terms of both working practices and educational requirements. The relationship between service providers, educational establishments and practitioners must be strengthened in order to improve practice and ensure good quality care.

The integration of health and social care organisations has become a core component of government policy in recent years. *The New NHS: Modern and Dependable* (DOH 1997), stressed the need to integrate across health and social care in order to

deal with people with multiple needs, who have previously fallen between care agencies. This is legislated within the Health Act (2000) Partnership Section 28–31.

In the Government's policy document *Modernising Health and Social Services: Developing the Workforce* (DOH 1999b) and in the NHS(E) document *A Health Service of all the Talents: Developing the NHS Workforce* (DOH 2000a), the consultation document on the review of workforce planning, it was noted that some £2 billion a year is spent on supporting training and education for clinical staff. In addition to this local staff development and training is also undertaken. The recommendations of *A Health Service of all the Talents* are summarised in Box 29.1; it can be seen that these are wide ranging and radical.

The NHS(E) document (DOH 2000a) identifies that there is a requirement to improve the current arrangements and its recommendations cover four key areas. First, greater integration and the need for more flexibility, where it is recognised that current workforce planning and development arrangements inhibit the development of multiprofessional planning and have not supported the creative use of staff skills. Secondly, better management ownership, and clearer roles and responsibilities. Thirdly, improved training, education and regulation builds on, and further

---

Box 29.1   Proposals and recommendations (DOH 2000a)

1. Team working across professional and organisational boundaries.
2. Flexible working to make the best use of the range of skills and knowledge which people have.
3. Streamlined workforce planning and development which stems from the needs of patients not of professionals.
4. Maximising the contribution of all staff to patient care, doing away with barriers which say only doctors and nurses can provide particular types of care.
5. Modernising education and training to ensure that staff are equipped with the skills they need to work in a complex, changing NHS.
6. Developing new, more flexible, careers for staff of all professions and none.
7. Expanding the workforce to meet future demands.

develops, partnership with those providing training and education for the NHS workforce and with the relevant regulatory bodies. Educational providers should be fully involved in developing workforce plans and in return it is expected that the NHS will work with higher education providers and regulatory bodies to improve the flexibility of pre-qualifying and post-qualifying education programmes. Importantly, emphasis will be placed on the development of training and education arrangements for staff which are genuinely multiprofessional and provide greater scope for switching training pathways without staff having to start their training afresh, by accrediting prior learning. Fourthly, the focus is placed on staff numbers, career pathways and the need to enhance the efficiency and effectiveness of the workforce. The need to provide a flexible career structure and progressive pathways for staff, which reflect the changing ways in which staff will wish and will need to work in the future is also recognised. This is addressed in part by *Improving Working Lives Standard* (DOH 2000c), committing NHS employers to improving the lives of people who work in the NHS.

In *The NHS Plan: A Plan for Investment, A Plan for Reform* (DOH 2000b) the overall direction and priorities for the next 4 years and beyond are established. It provides a comprehensive plan of action against the major challenges for health and identifies 10 core principles which underpin the National Health Service, as detailed in Box 29.2.

Within the context of the *NHS Plan* (DOH 2000b) politicians have framed a policy and assertively outlined the principles for those that deliver the services on how they should plan to deliver health services and how this should be taken forward. The process of creating this Plan has seen the establishment of a Modernisation Action Team comprising NHS staff and patient representatives. Their findings, which informed the NHS Plan, will continue to influence the way future health services are delivered in a quest to raise performance standards across the whole of the NHS.

With regard to the care and management of people with learning disabilities the government has focused upon 'partnership' to determine how all

---

Box 29.2   The NHS core principles

1. The NHS will provide a universal service for all based on clinical need, not ability to pay.
2. The NHS will provide a comprehensive range of services.
3. The NHS will shape its services around the needs and preferences of individual patients, their families and their carers.
4. The NHS will respond to different needs of different populations.
5. The NHS will work continuously to improve quality service and to minimise errors.
6. The NHS will support and value its staff.
7. Public funds for health care will be devoted solely to NHS patients.
8. The NHS will work together with others to ensure a seamless service for patients.
9. The NHS will keep people healthy and work to reduce health inequalities.
10. The NHS will respect the confidentiality of individual patients and provide open access to information about services, treatment and performance.

---

parts of the health and social care sector systems could work better together in order to ensure that the right emphasis is placed at each level of care with the aim of improving clinical performance and health service productivity. The health care professions, and the wider NHS workforce, should experience increasing flexibility in training and working practices with the ultimate aim of removing rigid boundaries between services and care providers.

For learning disabilities the core principles of the *NHS Plan* (DOH 2000b) outlined in Box 29.2 are supported and should be accompanied by a commitment to provide extra resources. Closer links between health and social care are proposed, underpinned by better coordination in training clinicians, be they doctors, nurses or other professions allied to medicine, alongside those within the social care and independent sectors. The NHS Health Act 2000 enables local councils and the NHS to work closely together. The Act swept away the legal obstacles to joint working by allowing the use of 'pooled' budgets; this involves local health and social services putting money into a dedicated budget to fund a wide range of care services. This will enable the provision of 'lead commissioning' either by the local authority or health authority/Primary Care Trust to coordinate the commissioning of services on behalf of both health and social care bodies. Integrated providers, local authorities and health authorities will increasingly merge their services to deliver a one-stop package of care for service users and their families.

Within the *NHS Plan* (DOH 2000b) proposals to modernise education and training are set out. The Plan sets out a radical reform agenda that is planned to reshape care around the patient with new training across professions in communication skills and NHS principles and organisations. Interprofessional learning will be put in place to enable health care students and staff to switch careers and training paths more easily.

Specific policy reports in relation to services for people with a learning disability include *Signposts for Success in Commissioning and Providing Health Services for People with Learning Disabilities* (DOH 1998b). This document attempted to provide direction in commissioning and providing health services for people with learning disabilities and identified foundations of good practice. These are listed in Box 29.3.

In *Signposts for Success* the Department of Health identified that 'there is a very large workforce employed to support and to care for people with learning disabilities in widely dispersed settings, some of this workforce have professional qualifications some have had training but do not have a qualification and others have had no training' (DOH 1998b, pp 22–23). They reiterate this further in the statement 'there is widespread concern about the need for an adequate supply of suitably trained staff. There is a tendency for the relevant skills to be held by health care profession-

als, whilst the majority of care is carried out by unqualified staff.' The Department of Health endorsed this in *Valuing People: A New Strategy for Learning Disability for the 21st Century* (DOH 2001, p. 96) by estimating that of the 83 000 people in the learning disability workforce, 75% of staff are unqualified, and few have recognised accredited training qualifications.

These are major issues that require to be addressed in order to deliver this latest government learning disability strategy which is shared across the social care, health, education and employment sectors. This strategy clearly identifies what might be achieved and is supported by clear objectives and a range of targets and performance indicators that will be closely monitored in the future. A 3-year modernisation programme is proposed for learning disability services that will involve identifying models of good service provision, addressing management and leadership issues and involving users and carers in designing and evaluating services.

Facing the Facts: Services for People with Learning Disabilities: A Policy Impact Study of Social Care and Health Services (DOH 1999a) was carried out by a joint group including the social services inspectorate, NHS(E) and social care group, plus an independent consultant. This report highlighted that little progress had been made since the 1990s in transforming services. It proposed that detailed work on the development of a strategy should address five key areas: health issues, supporting independence, building partnerships, children, and workforce and leadership issues. These themes formed the focus of the Government's White Paper *Valuing People* (DOH 2001).

The idea of partnership runs through the entire range of the Government's modernising agenda for health and social services. Partnership and its corollary, 'joined up services' are not solely concerned with the interface between social care and health services, but also with a range of public services that includes housing, education, employment, social security, the police and transport and the voluntary and private sectors. It is against this backcloth that future education and training strategies should strive to prepare the workforce for the future.

Box 29.3 Foundations of good practice (DOH 1998b)

Shared values
Partnership and cooperation
Shared responsibilities
Availability of information about needs
Using guidance, documents and reports
Training development and workforce planning

The attainment of higher levels of qualifications is a further key government objective for the workforce. Qualifications are seen as a measure of the outcome of training, by which competence can be demonstrated in order to determine that the workforce and its members are 'fit for purpose'.

DEFINING THE WORKFORCE

Historically, the approach to education and training in the care fields was undertaken by two dominant professional groups, i.e. nursing and social work. Since service delivery has integrated, a greater movement to a more 'joined up' approach to education and training has developed which has challenged our understanding of the way in which professionals work. The origins of some of the challenges to how professionals work in learning disability can be traced to policy proposals arising in the 1970s. Briggs (DHSS 1972) proposed that a new caring profession for the mentally handicapped would gradually emerge. The Jay Report (DHSS 1979) concerning the future of mental handicap nursing favoured a unified training for nursing and social work staff. Both Briggs (DHSS 1972) and Jay (DHSS 1979) concluded there was little need for a speciality of nursing for the mentally handicapped. The question rather polarised whether learning disability nursing is a health (therefore nursing) or a social (therefore social work) occupation. Nurses forcefully opposed the recommendations from these two reports. The Government was unwilling to implement the changes proposed, albeit they had a clear desire to promote shared training. An important argument was that there would be a danger of losing an effective tried and tested workforce education and training programme, and therefore a commitment to and focus on learning disability itself. Because the recommendations of the Jay Report in particular were not fully harnessed, the legacy today is that we have continued to segregate nursing and social work education and training programmes.

For nursing, following the rejection of Briggs (DHSS 1972) and the Jay Report (DHSS 1979), the General Nursing Council critically examined the content of the mental handicap nurse training programme, since at that time it reflected a curriculum that had strong links to general nursing and a specialist training with particular reference to the physical needs of service users. The English National Board (ENB) introduced a new syllabus that departed radically from previous training, with an emphasis on the principles of normalisation and on working in community and domiciliary settings rather than in hospitals (ENB 1982). By 1984, the United Kingdom Central Council for Nursing, Midwifery and Health Visiting (UKCC) had initiated a review to determine the education and training required for nurses, midwives and health visitors in relation to the projected health care needs in the 1990s and beyond (Elkan & Robinson 1994). This review culminated in *Project 2000: A New Preparation for Practice* (UKCC 1986). *Project 2000* envisaged a new nurse practitioner who would be flexible, knowledgeable and able to work within a variety of settings both in the hospital and in the community. *Project 2000* was designed to enable students to achieve the required level of role competence – as defined in (15) Rule 18A (UKCC 1989) – in their chosen branch of nursing, namely working with adults, with children, in mental health or with learning disabled people. Elliott-Cannon & Harbinson (1995) commented that this new form of preparation moved all nurses into an 18-month common foundation and an 18-month specialist branch programme, thus moving away from a 3-year specialist programme. Debate occurred as to whether this helped or hindered preparation of learning disability nurses.

At the same time as the Government accepted the *Project 2000* proposals for the far-reaching reform of nurse education, *Working Paper 10* (DOH 1989a) was also published. This report precipitated the integration of nursing and midwifery education into higher education and has extensively reshaped the current nurse and midwifery education programmes in the UK. Another difference to previous training was that nurses would now undertake a 3-year diploma in higher education training. These changes were accompanied by the physical move of schools/colleges of nursing and midwifery out of Trusts and into higher education institutions which in turn created its own difficulties because some have advised that this has separated education from service provision. Other difficulties have included securing adequate student placements in a range of different care settings outwith the old long-stay hospitals.

In spite of the radical changes to nurse training the debate regarding health and social care continued following the publication of the White Paper *Caring for People: Community Care in the Next Decade and Beyond: Mental Handicap Nursing (The Cullen Report)* (DOH 1991). It acknowledged the need for specialist training so those practitioners could advise other workers. However, uncertainty continued within the profession regarding the present and future role of mental handicap nurses despite guidance from the DOH (Sines 1993). Then in 1993 the Department of Health organised a one day conference known as the 'Consensus Conference' to consider the future direction for the specialist nurse practitioner in learning disabilities (RNMH). Five options were outlined in a paper entitled *Opportunities for Change: A New Direction for Nursing People with a Learning Disability* (Sines 1993). The option proposed by the panel for the profession rejected a 'specialist training only at post-registration level'. Brown (1994) noted that amongst the other options support was strongest for training and practice to be linked to National Vocational Qualifications (NVQ) competencies. This was often presented in combination with two other options regarding the development of interdisciplinary training and widening the application of the skill base. The outcome was the retention of the specialism within the 'family of nursing' (e.g. Project 2000) albeit with renewed recognition of the value of shared learning and inter-professional working.

In endorsing the value of pre-registration specialist learning disability nursing education a Department of Health Learning Disability Nursing Project was commissioned in 1994 by the Chief Nursing Officer for England. The project was in response to concerns expressed by nurses and employers regarding the evolving field of learning disability nursing and the decreasing number of students undertaking pre-registration nursing programmes. The project resulted in the publication of a report *'Continuing the*

Box 29.4 Eight key areas for the learning disability nurse (Kay et al 1995, pp 18–35)

Assessment of need
Health surveillance and health promotion
Developing personal competence
Using enhanced therapeutic skills
Managing and leading teams of staff
Enhancing the quality of support
Enabling and empowerment and
Coordinating services

Commitment' Learning Disability Nursing Project (DOH 1995a) which emphasised the work of the learning disability nurse in eight key areas. Box 29.4 lists these areas.

The salient points in relation to education were 'to continue to explore opportunities for shared learning at pre- and post-registration levels' and 'to review the content of pre-registration training to ensure that appropriate emphasis was given to leadership and management skills development' (DOH 1995a).

Meanwhile, Brown (1994) had identified that in the early 1980s the promotion of joint training approaches by the nursing and social work validating bodies did not meet with a receptive audience in either profession. The climate of the time meant that when two reports on qualifying and post-qualifying training were published, in 1982 and 1983 respectively, they were greeted with antipathy at best, and hostility at worst, both from some nurses and from some social workers (GNC/CCETSW 1982, 1983), since this could be considered to be a joint position statement and could be a new framework for education and training. It was not until the announcement late in 1986 of a new initiative between the ENB and CCETSW that it was possible to take the debate and tentative schemes forward (ENB/CCETSW 1986). Although the proposals proved unsustainable, they provided a basis on which others came to build. In 1988, for example, two 3-year joint training courses (two years for the Certificate in Social Service (CSS) followed by a further year to cover the requirements of the Registered Mental Handicap Nurse qualification) were launched between the ENB and CCETSW. These ventures did not survive because major policy changes were already taking place in both the education and service sectors, and by the time the students completed the programme the qualification and skills were not considered to be contemporary to meet the needs of service providers since both the Certificate in Social Services (CSS) and the RNMH (Part 5, UKCC Professional Register) were being reviewed with a view to being replaced.

Further social care training developments followed, including the introduction of the Diploma in Social Work (Dip SW) providing a single UK professional generic qualification for social work. This generic qualification enabled students to apply social work skills in particular settings (CCETSW 1989). Such changes coincided with the implementation of *Project 2000* nursing preparation programmes. As CCETSW (Central Council for the Education and Training of Social Workers) noted in 1984, it is important 'not to develop separate training schemes', consequently encouraging affiliation to health or social services when clients would be moving between facilities. It was stated that flexibility must be the keynote of this provision.

The importance of continuing collaboration between nursing and social work was endorsed in 1989 in the White Paper *Caring for People: Community Care in the Next Decade and Beyond* (DOH, 1989b). This stated that 'It will be important to develop multi-disciplinary training for staff in all caring professions, including the provision of joint training at both qualifying and post-qualifying stages'.

The interface between the professions of learning disability nursing and social work has frequently been questioned both by individual practitioners working together and by their employers, their managers and teaching staff. Tolerance of overlap, duplication, inflexible work patterns, isolated training courses and over-protectiveness by the professions are seen as being unacceptable.

The establishment of vehicles for the generation of ideas and the management of education and training initiatives has, in some areas, been slow and time-consuming. Nevertheless, CCETSW and the National Board have demonstrated their commitment to making progress, despite the many difficulties and differences that they have experienced. In the case of the ENB shared learning has been steadily pursued in relation to learning disability. With the joint publication of *Shared Learning: A Good Practice Guide* (ENB & CCETSW 1995), it was noted that health and social services are now delivered within a highly complex multi-professional organisational framework, with the focus having moved from institution based care to the community. The resultant framework is reproduced in Box 29.5. In order that vulnerable groups are not disadvantaged and to ensure that good

---

Box 29.5 Framework for good practice in shared learning (ENB & CCETSW 1995)

1. Increase practitioners' understanding and develop the skills required to work in multidisciplinary teams, across professional boundaries and in extended networks.
2. Provide practitioners with an understanding of the roles, cultures and values of different professions leading to benefits for service users as a result of increased cooperation and collaboration.
3. Help to address the perceptions and stereotypes that impede interprofessional work.
4. Aid the development of a common language between health and social care professionals which is also easier for service users to understand.
5. Lead to greater confidence for individuals in performing their roles by addressing 'professional protectionism' and identifying the usefulness of the overlap in roles which is different from wasteful duplication.

6. Ensure a more comprehensive knowledge of current practice, research and theoretical developments, which is more likely to lead to collaborative research and development. Such collaboration enhances interprofessional and inter-agency understanding and facilitates common knowledge.
7. Secure a more cost effective way of providing education and training.
8. Facilitate a more effective response to government policy and local service needs.
9. Facilitate changes to career pathways.
10. Facilitate flexibility, creative thinking and the development of leadership skills, essential for collaborative working across complex professional and agency boundaries.
11. Contribute to a learning culture, which fosters reflection, analysis and evaluation by focusing on interactive learning.

quality care is provided, the coordination and integration of services were considered to be essential. Successful shared learning and joint education and training provide a model for effective collaborative working and an integrated approach to practice in order to ensure that the care provided is focused on meeting the needs of those using services.

Against this background, services, practitioners and educationalists had striven to balance their independent professional identities with a desire to review, update and share their particular areas of expertise with colleagues serving similar client groups, thus providing people with learning disabilities with a seamless service. Weinstein (1994) has stressed the need for joint training to achieve this end. The situation that has been highlighted by May (1997) found that most learning disability nurses working within four case-study sites, were employed at the point of qualification in a variety of service settings, namely hospital, private sector and voluntary sector. Half the students from one college gained employment at the point of registration as support workers and the rest as nurses. According to Kay et al (1995) the skills of learning disability nurses had now been deployed in a range of settings: community, day centres and respite homes, specialist hospitals, secure facilities, in social services departments, independent sector providers, the voluntary sector and the new commissioning agencies. They were also part of new specialist service developments, such as challenging behaviour and support services for parents of children with learning disabilities. Kay et al (1995) found that staff employed in residential care homes consistently complained that they were not permitted to practise as nurses and, in some cases, learning disability nurses themselves had questioned the value of continuing their registration with the UKCC.

QUALIFIED WORKER VERSUS UNQUALIFIED WORKER

The English National Board (1996) conducted extensive interviews in selected learning disability case-study sites throughout England. Interviews were held with Trust managers, purchasers, nurses, unqualified workers, other professionals, service users, carers, lecturers and some students. Respondents to this English National Board for Nursing, Midwifery & Health Visiting (ENB) funded study noted that, although undervalued by care managers, support workers were the mainstay of many learning disability services. Employers did not always seem to regard staff with nursing qualifications as necessary even though research evidence demonstrated a direct positive relationship between quality of care and grade of nurse (Carr-Hill et al 1992). Employers determined that they wanted health care workers who were trained to deal with any situation, and able to meet the needs of any service user (Norman et al 1996). The nursing profession, however, has consistently rejected the notion of a generic learning disability worker and regarded the knowledge and skill base of the learning disability nurse as often being the most appropriate for supporting the complex needs of some people with learning disabilities (Brown 1994).

Since that time efforts have been made to familiarise commissioners, managers and practitioners with the role and function of learning disability nurses in care provision (Sines 1993). Kay et al (1995) for example, have described in more detail the knowledge and skills of learning disability nurses, and the contribution they make to the support of this client group. Their report concluded that learning disability nurses are required to make key contributions in the assessment of need, in health surveillance and health promotion, developing clients' competence and feelings of control, the use of enhanced therapeutic skills (specialist roles), managing and leading teams of staff, enhancing the quality of support, enabling and empowering clients and coordinating services. Norman et al (1996) have also reported that learning disability nurses need these qualities to function effectively in the current health and social care environment. These role requirements are very different to those expected of previous generations of learning disability nurses who were primarily hospital based.

There is general recognition that people with learning disabilities need specialist support. For example, having undertaken a comprehensive review of epidemiological data concerning the health status of this client group, Moss & Turner (1995) identified a range of health conditions associated with learning disability: problems with physical health (central nervous system and gastrointestinal functioning, obesity, incontinence, infections, respiratory conditions, epilepsy), dental health and mental health (particularly in older clients). More significantly, this review also found a tendency for these health problems to remain undetected until conditions become severe due to the inability of clients and carers to identify these problems and secure appropriate help (see Ch. 16). Learning disability nurses do have the knowledge base and skills to identify, manage and prevent these health problems (Kay et al 1996, Norman et al 1996). Kay et al (1995) have also reported that there is overwhelming support for retention of a specialist practitioner for people with learning disabilities. The Department of Health (1996) *Guidebook for Purchasers and Providers of Learning Disability Services* identifies a range of areas where learning disability nurses can contribute to maintaining and promoting of the lifestyle of people with learning disabilities. Despite these efforts there still seems to be a reluctance, amongst some service providers, to fully acknowledge the learning disability nursing qualification or, indeed, the need for specialist skills to care for people with learning disabilities (Norman et al 1996). This is perhaps due to some continuing lack of understanding of the role of the modern learning disability nurse and residual suspicion that such nurses label and exclude people with learning disabilities. Learning disability nurses would disagree and in practice the reverse can be demonstrated.

In the last few years, as a result of ongoing debate and emerging evidence, a consensus has been reached that the *Project 2000* model has not fully met the requirements of service providers. The UKCC has recently published the report *Fitness for Practice: The UKCC Commission for Nursing and Midwifery Education (Peach Report)* (UKCC 1999), a clear imperative of which was to address the perceived deficits of the *Project 2000* programmes. Key recommendations included producing a 1-year common foundation pro-

gramme followed by a 2-year learning disability branch programme, strengthening links with NHS Trusts and private and voluntary providers of care, and the establishment of a competency based framework with outcomes for the end of years one and three. This document was published alongside a key government report, *Making a Difference: Strengthening the Nursing, Midwifery and Health Visiting Contribution to Health and Health Care* (DOH 1999c). The latter requires the implementation of an education and training strategy that is both flexible and receptive to service needs and which is patient focused. In meeting these requirements programmes of nurse education are now designed to facilitate the notion of 'stepping off' whereby students can leave a programme, having clearly achieved a defined level of competence, which would have been mapped against National Vocational Qualifications for Care at the end of year one. Thus any students 'stepping off' at the end of year one will have to demonstrate evidence which can be used either to step back on to their programme of nurse education at a later date or to apply for accreditation towards a National Vocational Qualification, without having completed their 3-year initial nurse education programme.

The overall aim of current pre-registration nursing programmes is to ensure that students are fit for practice at the point of registration, and flexible and skilled in meeting changing health care needs by working in partnership with others across professional boundaries. This is not particularly different from the previous aim, certainly in learning disability, but the emphasis in employer-led education is on competencies which are defined much more by the employing purchasers.

Current nursing programmes have involved a refocusing of emphasis on practice so that students are prepared to function effectively and with confidence as registered practitioners. The programmes aim to ensure that nurses will be receptive to their changing roles and responsibilities. Factors such as those listed below have all had a major impact on the health and social care arenas:

- demographic changes
- the growth of information and medical technology

- increasing expectations from users of health services
- the increasing complexity of primary/secondary interface in nursing health care
- the blurring of roles between health and social care professions
- the growth of self-help/health care interest.

As these radical changes to learning disability nurse education are implemented, a major overhaul of social care standards and training in England is taking place through the Training Organisation for Personal Social Services (TOPSS). The TOPSS strategy (TOPSS 2000) is identified in Box 29.6.

The ultimate aim of this strategy is to improve standards of care throughout the learning disability services. TOPSS's mission statement (TOPSS 2000) is to improve employers' confidence in the competence of their workforce, employees' confidence in their own knowledge and skills, and service users' confidence in the quality of services that they will receive. Modernising the social care workforce will provide a comprehensive national training strategy to analyse the skill needs of people working in the social care sector, and to propose an action plan to improve both the qualification base and the quality of training over the coming 5 years. It is a response both to the White Paper *Modernising Social Services* (DOH 1998a) and to the restructuring of further and higher education arrangements.

For the first time the learning disability sector has the opportunity through TOPSS (England) to bring together, under a single training and workforce strategy, all strands of human resource development. This presents a unique opportunity to address long standing and deep-rooted problems arising from under-investment in education and training for a significant number of staff employed in the social care sector.

All these changes are now firmly rooted within the latest White Paper *Valuing People: A New Strategy for Learning Disability for the 21st Century* (DOH 2001). One of the first tasks identified in it is the commitment to create a national framework of qualifications matched to posts and career pathways which make sense to service users, carers, employers and their staff and promote lifelong learning. However, no links to professional training are intimated within the White Paper.

The idea of a partnership between health, social, voluntary and private care, with users and carers, runs through the entire range of the Government's modernising agenda which frames the developments driving this training strategy. In addition the TOPSS learning disability strategy in social care has advised that social care workers will have a training framework that integrates and accumulates study days and in-service training into a qualification of Related Vocational Qualifications (RVQ). This initiative refers to the accreditation and development of competencies specific to an area of work, for example learning

---

Box 29.6   Training Organisation for Personal Social Services (TOPSS) strategy

1. Strategy is placed within a vision of:
   a. a fully skilled and qualified workforce to meet
   b. the performance culture
   c. national service standards
   d. individual registration with the General Social Care Council
2. A national qualification framework matched to competencies and posts and underpinned by a comprehensive map of national occupational standards.
3. Career pathways promoting lifelong learning through flexible training opportunities and accreditation of prior experience and learning.

4. Modern partnerships between service users, carers, employers and training providers to ensure all training and assessment meets skill requirements of responsive and high quality services.
5. A tripartite approach between employers, employees and government to fund the necessary training to fill the knowledge, skills and qualifications gap outlined in the strategy.
6. A workforce which reflects the ethnic communities and diversity of background and perspectives in society as a whole.

disability and the National Vocational Qualifications framework (NVQ).

As a result of the White Paper two new qualifications have emerged to improve standards of care throughout the learning disability sector. For example, staff could be trained within the context of the TOPSS guideline, which includes an 'induction' for staff in their first 6 weeks in a learning disability service complemented by a foundation programme for staff during their first 6 months in a learning disability service. More experienced staff can either take National Vocational Qualifications or two new qualifications, the Certificate in Working with People who have Learning Disabilities at NVQ level 2 and an Advanced Certificate in Working with People who have Learning Disabilities at level 3. The two courses will be known as the Learning Disability Award Framework (LDAF) and will be a key feature of the training framework; LDAF registration will be required for all future entrants to the workforce and credits will be given for training that meets standards. *Valuing People: A New Strategy for Learning Disability for the 21st Century* (DOH 2001) also advises that the next phase of work to be planned will bring NVQ levels 4 and 5 within the Framework for more experienced and advanced practitioners.

The health and social care workforce strategies detailed in *Valuing People* (DOH 2001) will be implemented via the NHS Workforce Confederations in England who will involve all service providers, namely the health, social care, independent and voluntary sectors. As a group they will form new Learning Disability Partnership Boards who will develop a workforce and training plan. The plan will detail how service users and carers are being involved in training and workforce matters, the content and quality of health professional training and define how best to provide and resource training and development needs across all organisations in the field. In delivering the strategy consideration will be given to the education and training requirements for carers who work with those people who not only have learning disabilities but also have additional and complex needs. Such needs are detailed in Box 29.7.

Box 29.7 People with additional and complex needs (DOH 2001)

Those people who:

- have severe and profound disabilities (including those with sensory impairment)
- have epilepsy
- have autistic spectrum disorder, and also learning disabilities
- present with a behaviour that challenges their carers and service providers
- develop conditions associated with old age

Modernising Health and Social Services: Developing the Workforce (DOH 1999b) stated that 'all health and social care employers will be looking to the same limited pool of professionals'. In practice this will mean that collaborative approaches are likely to be the most effective in order to meet workforce demands. The Government gave a clear signal that, although they would not be merged, social services and health should work collaboratively with each other and in the White Paper *Valuing People* (DOH 2001) the Government again spelt out that services should meet the requirements of users and carers.

One way that education and training commissioners are addressing this issue is by developing dually qualified practitioners in learning disability, i.e. learning disability nurse and social worker. The benefits of producing a jointly trained worker are detailed within Box 29.8.

Box 29.8 The benefits of producing a jointly trained worker (reproduced with permission from University of Teesside)

- Ability to conduct holistic assessments and adopt a holistic approach to practice.
- More likely to work effectively in multi-disciplinary teams.
- More likely to adopt balance and compromise when applying professional knowledge to practice.
- Complementary awareness of both social work and nursing needs when working with service users.
- Trained specifically for joint working.

It could be argued that the value of joint training also encapsulates the notion that it produces a more 'needs led' service and thereby:

- reduces the likelihood of carers having to deliver a service themselves due to disputes between the professionals involved in the care planning process
- takes care managers out of the central focus of balancing professional, political and public agendas and sets them in a service user-led model of practice.

Joint training also benefits health and social services in the following ways:

- Shared philosophy and values
- Better understanding of each other's issues
- Improved service to users and carers.

There are further benefits to health care in that joint programmes have an enriched understanding of:

- Community care issues
- Social care assessment
- Social care infrastructure
- Care management.

Benefits for social services include:

- Increased expertise to plan, develop and manage services
- Specialist social workers
- Managers in specialist residential/day care services
- Improved care management
- Recognition of health issues and interventions (reproduced by permission from University of Teesside).

The ability of joint practitioners to meet outcomes across health and social care boundaries may result in joint educational programmes shifting their position from the margins to the mainstream.

The benefits of training and providing qualification frameworks have been highlighted in order to ensure the provision of a skilled workforce with transferable skills that is fit for purpose. The National Vocational Qualifications framework has further defined set occupational standards representing agreed benchmarks that specify staff competence and performance outcomes. Such an approach complements earlier work undertaken. Enhanced links between professional, academic and vocational qualification systems and education supported by the use of occupational standards to underpin existing professional curricula have therefore been evolving. Such changes have been based upon the adoption of an outcomes/competency approach to education and training in health and social care. The nursing profession, for example, has gone some way to responding to this agenda by mapping professional qualifications against NVQ competencies, with the introduction of the new preparation for nursing programmes (UKCC 2000). The promotion of an increased awareness and understanding of occupational standards, their conceptual origins, structure and language and acceptability and applicability to future practice appears to have much to offer the health and social care professions.

THE FUTURE PREPARATION OF THE WORKFORCE

A number of options are proposed for the future workforce in learning disability service provision:

- Learning disability nurse
- Social worker
- Joint trained worker – learning disability nurse and social worker
- Learning disability worker.

Whichever option is selected, that is assuming that anyone single model or option is desirable or possible, it is clear that the linking of professional education with the complex arena of service planning and delivery should be at the heart of all education and training for the workforce. Where employer-led education and training determines and shapes the workforce skill mix, it may be likely that the majority of the care and support will be provided by those holding vocational qualifications, whilst the leaders and managers of the service may come from a range of occupational and professional backgrounds. However, whilst some students completing such programmes may be restricted in their employment choices to a specific profession, their responsibilities may well cross the boundaries of health and social care, opening up new career pathways.

It is clearly the responsibility not only of validating professional bodies but also of the employing authorities to ensure that workers undertaking education programmes in the future have a distinct and valued role in service provision.

Education and training in the field of learning disability has a proven track record of innovation. Such developments have been successfully led both by the profession of learning disability nursing, and by that of social work where the need for a jointly trained worker has emerged from a number of sources. However, the real impetus for change can be traced as the result of Section 47 of the National Health Service and Community Care Act 1990 (NHSCCA) which has provided for the individual assessment of need from a multidisciplinary perspective. Guidance issued by the Department of Health on the implementation of the NHSCCA 1990 commended this process by stressing the need for collaborative working. Since 1 April 1993, when the new statutory arrangements for community care fully came into force, local authority social services departments have had lead responsibility at a local level for developing new patterns of services. They work in close partnership with statutory health and housing agencies, with the independent, voluntary and private sectors and with service users and carers.

Additionally, reports such as *Partners in Caring* (DOH 1995b) have encouraged us to think about providing people with learning disabilities with a 'seamless service'. Weinstein (1994) stressed the need for joint training to achieve this end. CCETSW published *Building a Partnership to Promote Shared Learning in the Field of Learning Disability* (Elliott-Cannon & Harbinson 1995) and confirmed that fundamentally each professional discipline should seek to make its own distinctive contribution to the 'jigsaw puzzle' of continuing professional development. When all the pieces come together it could be said that interagency and interdisciplinary cooperation have been achieved.

CONCLUSION

Throughout this chapter it has been recognised that statutory professional and vocational awarding bodies and the further and higher education sectors need to work together in partnership to ensure that education and training will support the Government's agendas. In meeting these agendas the education and training debate will need to focus on 'professional versus vocational' preparation for people working with people with a learning disability. The debate will also need to consider the role and place that 'work based learning' (which is employer driven) will play in the future as opposed to the retention of predominately small professionally determined education programmes such as those designed to train learning disability nurses and social workers.

The future will demand that a continuous review of skills and of education and interprofessional training provision is undertaken in order to achieve the re-engineering of care delivery that is required in order to deliver the *national strategy for learning disability service* within the context of contemporary government policy imperatives.

REFERENCES

Brown J 1994 Analysis of responses to the consensus statement on the future of the specialist nurse practitioner in learning disabilities. Department of Social Policy, University of York, York

Carr-Hill R, Dixon P, Gibbs I 1992 Skill mix and the effectiveness of nursing care. Centre for Health Economics, University of York, York

Central Council for the Education and Training of Social Workers 1989 Social work training for the 1990's. CCETSW, London

Department of Health 1989a Working for patients: education and training. Working Paper 10. HMSO, London

Department of Health 1989b Caring for people: community care in the next decade and beyond. Cm 849, HMSO, London

Department of Health 1991 Caring for people: community care in the next decade and beyond: mental handicap nursing (The Cullen Report). HMSO, London

Department of Health 1993 Consensus conference, 12 March

Department of Health 1995a 'Continuing the commitment' learning disability nursing project. HMSO, London

Department of Health 1995b Partners in caring. HMSO, London

Department of Health 1996 Guidebook for purchasers and providers of learning disability services. HMSO, London

Department of Health 1997 The new NHS: modern and dependable. HMSO, London

Department of Health 1998a Modernising social services. HMSO, London

Department of Health 1998b Signposts for success in commissioning and providing health services for people with learning disabilities. HMSO, London

Department of Health 1999a Facing the facts: services for people with learning disabilities: a policy impact study of social care and health services. HMSO, London

Department of Health 1999b Modernising health and social services: developing the workforce. HMSO, London

Department of Health 1999c Making a difference: strengthening the nursing, midwifery and health visiting contribution to health and health care. HMSO, London

Department of Health 2000a A health service of all the talents: developing the NHS workforce. Consultation document on the review of workforce planning. NHSE, London

Department of Health 2000b The NHS plan: a plan for investment, a plan for reform. HMSO, London

Department of Health 2000c Improving working lives standard NHS employers committed to improving the working lives of people who work in the NHS. Department of Health, Leeds

Department of Health 2001 Valuing people: a new strategy for learning disability for the 21st century. Cm 5086. HMSO, London

Department of Health and Social Services 1972 Report of the committee on nursing (Briggs report). Cmnd 5115. HMSO, London

Department of Health and Social Services 1979 Report of the committee of enquiry into mental handicap nursing and care (Jay report). Cmnd 7468. HMSO, London

Elkan R, Robinson J 1994 Project 2000: a review of the published research. Department of Nursing and Midwifery Studies, Faculty of Medicine, University of Nottingham, Nottingham

Elliott-Cannon C, Harbinson S 1995 Building a partnership: cooperation to promote shared learning in the field of learning disability. ENB and CCETSW, London

English National Board for Nursing, Midwifery & Health Visiting 1982 Syllabus of training: professional register – part 5 registered nurse for the mentally handicapped. English and Welsh National Boards for Nursing, Midwifery and Health Visiting, London

English National Board for Nursing, Midwifery & Health Visiting 1996 The changing educational needs of mental health and learning disability nurses. ENB, London

English National Board for Nursing, Midwifery & Health Visiting/Central Council for the Education and Training of Social Workers 1986 Co-operation in qualifying and post qualifying training: mental handicap. Report of the ENB/CCETSW joint working group. Circular 1986/89/EDG. ENB and CCETSW, London

English National Board for Nursing, Midwifery & Health Visiting and Central Council for the Education and Training of Social Workers 1995 Shared learning: a good practice guide. ENB and CCETSW, London

General Nursing Council/Central Council for the Education and Training of Social Workers 1982 Report of the joint working group on training for staff working with mentally handicapped people; co-operation in training. Part I Qualifying training. GNC and CCETSW, London

General Nursing Council/Central Council for the Education and Training of Social Workers 1983 Report of the joint working group on training for staff working with mentally handicapped people; co-operation in training. Part II In service training. GNC and CCETSW, London

Kay B, Rose S, Turnbull J 1995 Continuing the commitment: the report of the learning disability nursing project. Department of Health, London

May N 1997 Evaluation of nurse and midwife education in Scotland: 1992 programmes. National Board for Nursing, Midwifery and Health Visiting for Scotland, Edinburgh

Moss S, Turner S 1995 The health of people with learning disabilities. Hester Adrian Research Centre, University of Manchester, Manchester

NHS and Community Care Act 1990 HMSO, London

NHS Health Act 2000 HMSO, London

NHS (EL(95)84) Building on the benefits of occupational standards and NVQs in the NHS. NHS, London

Sines D 1993 Opportunities for change: a new direction for nursing people with a learning disability. Department of Health, London

Training Organisation for Personal Social Services (TOPSS) 2000 Strategies for quality: improving services for people with learning disability through training. TOPSS, Leeds

United Kingdom Central Council for Nursing, Midwifery & Health Visiting 1986 Project 2000: a new preparation for practice. UKCC, London

United Kingdom Central Council for Nursing, Midwifery & Health Visiting 1989 PS.D/89/04 Legislation enabling project 2000 programmes. UKCC, London

United Kingdom Central Council for Nursing, Midwifery & Health Visiting 1999 Fitness for practice: the UKCC commission for nursing and midwifery education (Peach report). UKCC, London

United Kingdom Central Council for Nursing, Midwifery & Health Visiting 2000 Requirements for pre registration nursing programmes. UKCC, London

Weinstein J 1994 Sewing the seams for a seamless service: a review of developments in interprofessional education and training. CCETSW, London

USEFUL ADDRESSES

The following are useful web addresses for any reader who wishes to explore ongoing issues of education and training in the field of learning disabilities.

www.arc.org.uk

www.ccetsw.org.uk
www.doh.gov.uk
www.enb.org.uk
www.tees.ac.uk
www.ukcc.org.uk

30 Management and leadership in learning disabilities

Mark Jukes

KEY ISSUES

- This chapter focuses on the process of managing change within the current context of service provision for people with learning disabilities.
- Theories of management and leadership are explored to assist practitioners to apply contemporary theories to enhance the management of the change process through effective strategies.
- The chapter explores the need to empower individual staff to assist them to acknowledge changes in service delivery, which require a new kind of leadership with the creation of flexible networks within services and professions that have replaced traditional hierarchies of care provision.

INTRODUCTION

For many practitioners in learning disability the role of management and leadership is seen as the responsibility and assumed role of the few, whilst for those at the face of direct service provision their role is about fundamentally getting on with the job in hand. In the past management within learning disability has focused upon the macro picture of managing services (Sines 1988,1992, Thompson & Mathias 1998) within the context of the NHS & Community Care Act (DOH 1990), and therefore emphasis has been upon broad quality, audit and organisational service related issues.

However, it has been identified that the key managerial competence of the 1990s has been the ability to handle change (Buchanan & Huczynski 1997). Recent reform, research and policy documents such as *Making a Difference* (DOH 1999), *Health care Futures 2010* (UKCC 1998) and *Valuing People* (DOH 2001) emphasise both leadership and change management skills as essential for nurses. The leadership role of health service managers amidst turbulent change, has been explored by Davis (1997) and she identifies that an attempt to address change without a vision of how to manage, is to invite chaos, and further adds that we need to have some idea of how to cope with the uncertainties and questions caused by change, and how to shape the consequences of change on our path to our preferred outcome. Changes in the services for people with a learning disability, have not only been the subject of continual debate but have continually been reconfigured in accordance with how politicians and society have viewed what needs to be done. Change has also been a predominant feature within learning disability nursing, and particularly over the last 30 years when major reconfigurations and role fluctuations have acted upon its field of practice. Alaszewski et al (2000), in an English National Board report on learning disability nurse education, have also found that nurses have presented a picture of sustained fighting to gain recognition of the value of their skills in relation to people with a learning disability. Parrish & Birchenall (1997) have also suggested that change is a permanent feature of learning disability nursing.

There are, of course, many other different professionals working at the heart of providing a service for people with a learning disability, whether in the home, in acute settings, in dispersed housing schemes, or through specialist support teams across the interface of primary and secondary care, and within health and social care teams. They have also had to adjust as reforms have impacted on and influenced the way they work, and Loxley (1997) has identified 25 different Acts and government documents published between 1970 and 1990, with 10 national professional coordinating bodies, concerned in some way with cooperation issues between health and social services. Professionals have often become frustrated by the incessant cycles of continual change and reform which have often resulted in feelings of anxiety and uncertainty, coupled with a loss of control, and fears about whether these changes will further enhance services or leave people with a learning disability more vulnerable, and about whether key human service professionals will be out of a job. Such changes have been referred to as being particularly present within such large organisations as the NHS (Walton 1984), but can equally be applied within and across those various voluntary and social care sectors which provide a service to people with a learning disability. Walton (1984) has maintained that the clearer one is as a manager about how decisions are taken within a locality, the more informed and appropriate the resultant actions will be. He identified politics, power, anxiety, uncertainty and change as constant factors that need to be faced and managed effectively by practitioners, rather than denying that such forces are in play. For leadership, Davis (1997) has proposed that managers can draw upon six core competencies (Box 30.1), which can be adopted in assisting them to navigate the difficult waters of current health care restructuring and reform.

Practitioners are accountable and responsible for providing quality direct care; the core competencies are useful to adopt as a means of gaining a more coherent understanding about where we have been, where we are, and where we are likely to be going. They provide a personal and professional barometer for gaining further insight into and awareness of our position and purpose within the learning disability service.

Box 30.1   Six core competencies (Davis 1997)

Know who is involved
Know where we are
Know where we want to go
Knowing the certainties
Knowing the uncertainties
Deciding how we must be on our way

Know who is involved

Since the 1960s policies and providers of services to people with a learning disability have clearly illustrated that there is no monopoly over who provides what. Key practitioners of direct services and key players need to be identified so they can work in partnership to make the overall health and social care system work. An emphasis on joint working, interdisciplinary and inter-professional working, changing roles of practitioners along with the concept of lifelong learning is promoted. As a consequence of professional roots and of dissimilarities among practitioners, which have originated from separate training, the professional socialisation process has stirred up professional barriers against and jealousies towards inter-professional working (Weinstein 1998), coupled with a parochial view of practice and of the world. This is now being challenged. This is an era where strategic partnership groups embody the wider involvement of housing, employment and leisure services, which in turn warrants new working approaches from health personnel who are not used to integrated systems of this nature. The culture today is very much advocating a cross-functional expertise from professionals where the role boundaries are less rigid and defined. In coping with such changes to meet success we must engage more readily with service users, the general public, social agencies, government, the media and the private sector. We cannot ignore others in this process of change, and more importantly we must have a clear understanding relative to our own domains of professional practice.

Know where we are

It is 30 years since the last White Paper was published for people with learning disabilities. The new White Paper (DOH 2001) specifically outlines an ambitious strategy which will attempt to tackle such issues as: poor coordination and planning of services; insufficient support for carers; a deficit in health care needs being met; choices in housing; day services; leisure; employment; meeting the needs of people from ethnic minorities; a general inconsistency in expenditure and service delivery; and further real evidence of partnerships between health and social care.

Valuing People: A New Strategy for Learning Disability for the 21st Century (DOH 2001) embodies the principles of rights, independence, choice and inclusion and as such demands that a further look be taken at the impact of those issues in the context in which current and future learning disability services are developed. This means looking at the wider picture, for example the political view and societal stance on community care and primary health care, amidst those priorities identified through various policy papers such as *Valuing People* (DOH 2001). There is a need to acknowledge and understand the media's and the public's expectations regarding learning disability, the implications of the NHS Plan (DOH 2000a) for long-term care, and the impact of Emerson et al's (1999) evaluation of different service models, which from its representation of the best provides a daunting picture of the overall present situation in terms of quality and poor management outcomes (see Ch. 5). Recent abuse inquiries such as Longcare (1998) and *Lost in Care* (DOH 2000b) along with documentaries like *Perfect Victims* (Panorama 1995) and *MacIntyre Undercover* (MacIntyre 1999) reveal that there is a long way to go in ensuring practices are of high quality and not inappropriate or negligent. The evidence underlining our interventions is the main ethos behind Clinical Governance (DOH 1998), where evidence based practice, clinical effectiveness and risk-assessment and management have never been higher on the quality agenda. Social Care also has a similar emphasis in its quality framework (DOH 2000c).

Know where we want to go

Coping with so many competing demands, coupled with the myriad of policies, guidance documents and providers, makes it difficult to have a vision of where we want the service to go, what it should look like and what our role is within that service. Having such a vision of course promotes a sense of ownership of learning disability provision in those who deliver it, and in those people who use services, i.e. a close collaborative sense of need and direction. Visionary change requires practitioners to appraise models of practice and service provision that have gone before, and not to discard wholesale past values and practices by throwing out everything from the past. Examples could include reviewing past and present approaches to case and care management; moving from individual programme planning and shared action planning to person centred planning within a socio-political context of ordinary living (King's Fund 1980); looking at the purpose of specialist teams and resources; reviewing the use of behavioural technologies within the context of an ethical and human rights framework; and further developing one's own professional knowledge and appraising the evidence in terms of what works in the context of present challenges.

Knowing the certainties

Change is a reality of modern living. What appear to be constant, however, are those values which underpin service delivery, which include respect and choice, the attitude of pursuing empowerment for the individual coupled with accountability, competence, encouragement of lifelong learning and the participation of one's colleagues and other stakeholders, and the ability to work in the community with others. The respect and value of a shared vision of all professionals within the health and social care system is one that is promoting quality, equality and independence for service users. If practitioners are guided by these convictions then they need not fear the fluctuations, disturbances and imbalances created by changes and transitions, or by systems that may leave us with a sense of disenchantment and may create a sense of personal professional paranoia. We therefore must be instrumental in making and contributing to change rather than responding to change negatively and with anticipated pessimism.

Knowing the uncertainties

We need to understand that new developments, services and roles are not set hard and fast in stone and should be allowed to evolve rather than being imposed. Involvement of all staff in engendering

commitment should be appropriate to the situation rather than imposed by a heirarchical structure. Risk assessment and management, innovation through the change process and clinical interventions are made using professional reflective practice within the context of clinical supervision and should direct us to where we want to go. Knowledge of self combined with an accurate understanding and appraisal of ideologies, policies and roles people play from a range of professionals and agencies is therefore vital.

Deciding how we must be on our way

Vision is an important guide for practitioners within learning disability services as they address change or reform. Nevertheless, within learning disability services, strategies, theories and frameworks also need to be in place so as to evaluate the results of change, that is the continuum of process and outcome of change. Practitioners need to select and adopt strategies in methods of change – turning what might be seen as a threat into an opportunity, since change is always present. Therefore it is important to have the ability to manage change by taking a step-by-step and conceptual approach to leading and managing the change process, along with the adoption of appropriate management and leadership theories and styles. Managing change is not only confined to individual practitioners and singular services, but is also perceived as a multidisciplinary and agency activity, and those practitioners responsible for change must possess or have access to a wide range of skills, resources, support and knowledge, in order to activate the change process. The following recommendations serve as an aid to this process:

- Communication skills are essential and must be applied both within and outside the managing team.
- Maintaining motivation and providing leadership to all concerned is necessary.
- The ability to facilitate and orchestrate group and individual activities is crucial.
- Negotiation and influencing skills are invaluable.
- It is essential that both planning and control procedures are employed.

Reader activity 30.1

Discuss and reflect with a colleague on the six core competencies as they relate to your personal knowledge, and how your service provider is responding to current change requirements. Assess to what degree you need to enhance your personal knowledge and development in preparation as a change agent.

- The ability to manage on all planes, upward, downward and within the peer group, must be acquired.
- Knowledge of, and the facility to influence, the rationale for change is essential (Paton & McCalman 2000, pp 36–37).

Leadership is the predominant ethos and focus within today's health and social care sectors where leaders will require special attributes to guide both the professions and the services into the 21st century (Sofarelli & Brown 1998). Leadership is paramount today, due to the Department of Health's modernisation agenda (DOH 1999), which has reinforced the need for more effective clinical leadership. In application terms, this means that more nurses require better leadership skills, which is considered to be a major factor for improving direct person centred interventions and decision making for quality care provision. This era of radical reform, where the profession requires strong leadership, empowers nurses to lead and assist in reshaping learning disability services in the future. Within learning disability services across the country diverse service models and practices exist, where risk-taking and innovation mean challenging the status quo and being creative in response to managing change; to manage change therefore means being an effective leader.

Before entering into a discussion of management, leadership and managing change, it is important to consider the nature of who we are as individuals, since having a clear awareness and analysis of who we are is vital in our own understanding and knowledge of self, and this can be further enhanced and made more available and productive by considering the responses and reactions of others. As practitioners not only do we need to find out more about ourselves, we also need to make use of and relate more effectively to other people. We therefore need their feedback and perspectives on who we are. The whole art of managing effectively and intervening appropriately with people is about forming and developing relationships and networks, not only within our own profession but also with others. The Johari window (Fig. 30.1), as formulated by Luft (1963), is one model which offers a perspective from which individuals can be seen by themselves and by others.

Figure 30.1 illustrates how two dimensions – things that are known to me, and things that are known to others about me – can be put together to give four panes of a window. The complete window is me and the four panes represent areas of knowledge about me. There is an area of information known to all, called the open pane. This is information about me which I am clear about and which is also quite visible to other people: for example, I am male, five foot nine, wear a beard and ride a motorcycle etc. In direct contrast, there

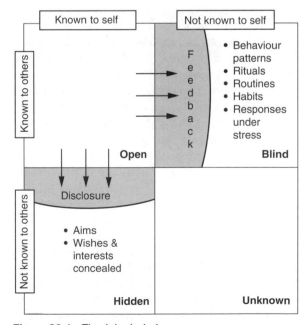

Figure 30.1 The Johari window.

is part of me about which I know nothing and which is a totally inaccessible area as far as other people are concerned. We call this area the unknown pane. The area of which I have knowledge but which I choose not to disclose to others is the hidden pane. Examples here would be some of my personal aims and objectives which I have chosen to keep to myself, or perhaps some interest areas that I have not talked about. There is another pane yet to consider – it is concerned with information about me of which I am unaware, but which is occasionally seen by others. Examples could be the way in which I react in certain situations, or some 'unconscious' habits or ways of doing things. This is the blind pane. Even by looking at ourselves in this simple manner we do not have all the information about ourselves at our disposal. Payne (2000) applies the Johari window in teamwork as a technique for looking at group dynamics, used simply for sharing information about the team or its work, or about more complex problem situations and conflicts.

To be an effective leader and manager it is essential to know about your specialist field of practice, the boundaries, policies and philosophies underpinning that area, and to have a strong sense of who you are with a continual striving for further self-knowledge and awareness. A more contemporary theory and extension of the Johari window idea is that provided by Crow (2000) who has developed the theoretical model for leadership and knowing illustrated in Figure 30.2. Effective leaders, according to Crow, are in tune with what they know, not only in the professional domain but also in having a strong sense of who they are within this social-political world. The model has been the result of his reflective experience as a nurse and as an emergent, developing person. Its properties involve five factors used to describe an individual's system of wholeness, but include a sixth factor which relates to the idea in gestalt psychology that the system is found to be greater than the sum of its parts; this sixth factor is the meaning or culmination of the knowledge, experiences, values and beliefs that are derived from both our professional and our personal lives and which makes us more than the sum of our parts. Figure 30.2 illustrates a summarisation of

Crow's model where each factor is broken down into a brief review of its properties as they relate to a professional working within a learning disability service. The model is meant to be flexible and continuous, not static and therefore non-linear, so practitioners can study and review their 'selves' in the wider context of the environment in which they are located.

THE INFLUENCE OF ORGANISATIONAL MANAGEMENT THEORIES

Moving from a position where we have developed a more accurate understanding and appraisal of contemporary service developments, coupled with a review of self-knowledge and awareness leads us towards the development of a more structured, theoretical and informed basis on how to approach and manage people. It is at this point that a review of the influence of organisational management and leadership theories can be of benefit. This chapter does not intend to provide a comprehensive review of theories of management and leadership, as a plethora of textbooks already exists which do justice to this vast subject area. There is, however, the intention to review the development and influence of some of the major theories. This can be achieved by briefly summarising the key movements as identified by Marriner-Tomey (1996), ranging from scientific management (or Taylorism), through to the classic organisation movement, human relations management and the behavioural theorists. A more comprehensive account of these movements can be found in Marriner-Tomey (1996) (see Further reading).

Taylorism (scientific management)

Frederick Winslow Taylor (1856–1915) developed one of the first models of organisational and management behaviour in the early part of the 20th century. He conducted time and motion studies to determine the most efficient means of production in workers and noted managers' responsibilities for planning, separating them from the function of workers. The basis of Taylor's work was that in

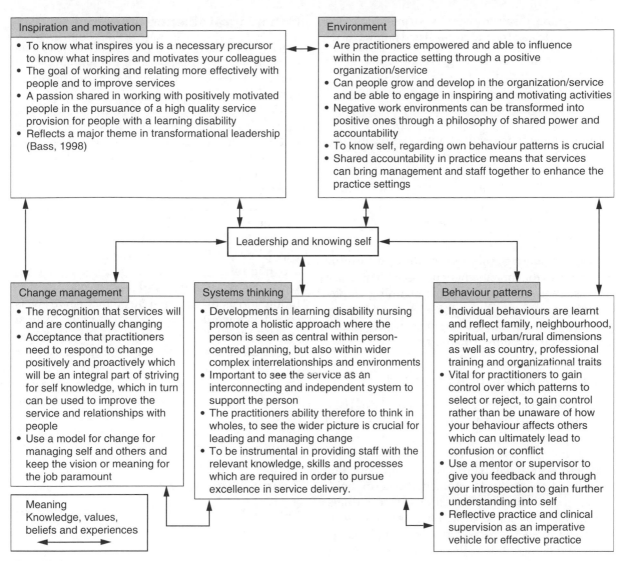

Figure 30.2

applying the principles of observation, measurement and scientific comparison he could determine the most efficient way of completing a task. His studies also encouraged specialisation and emphasised that the selection of qualified workers could be developed for a particular role and purpose.

Classic organisation

Henri Fayol (1841–1925) is identified as being the originator in defining management functions.

Fayol studied the functions of managers, and concluded that management is a universal activity and that managers fundamentally have the same tasks which are broadly categorised into planning, organisation, command, coordination and control. Marquis & Huston (2000) have identified that Fayol's management function is similar in many ways to the nursing process and that both processes are cyclical and many different functions may occur simultaneously as the following example illustrates.

A learning disability service manager carried out in one day all the functions listed below:

- reviewed the annual budget (planning)
- met with staff to discuss meeting the changed needs of one of the service users (organising)
- altered staffing rotas to include waking night staff (staffing)
- held a meeting to resolve conflict between care staff, GPs and hospital staff over not having any guidelines for assisting people with a learning disability in an acute hospital setting (directing)
- and gave a service worker a job performance appraisal (controlling).

The service manager here is seen to be performing all phases of the management process, but it is also the case that each function has a planning, implementing and controlling phase. Just as nursing practice requires that all nursing care has a plan, so does each function of management.

Human relations management

Here, theorists such as Elton Mayo (1880–1949) and Kurt Lewin (1890–1947) can be acknowledged for their studies of group dynamics. Lewin maintained that groups have personalities of their own and demonstrated that group forces can overcome individual interests. He coined the term field-forces to describe group pressures on individuals. Lewin will be looked at again when managing change strategies is reviewed later on in the chapter. Mayo demonstrated through the 'Hawthorne effect', named after his research studies at the Chicago Hawthorne Plant of Western Electric (Mayo 1945), that effective performance was associated with understanding the linkages between the individual, that person's social role among other members of the group within the workplace, and the degree of independence given within the group. Group norms were shown to have significantly more influence than financial incentives. This movement was therefore interested primarily in the nature of job design, where to achieve successful results in managing an organisation managers must be concerned for the motivation, aspirations and personal needs of employees.

Behavioural science movement

Abraham Maslow (1908–1970) is identified as the chief architect and initiator of the human behavioural school with his development of a hierarchy of needs (Fig. 30.3).

Maslow's work can be identified and found most appropriate when relating to human needs in the application of direct individualised client care. Individuals have varying needs at different levels, and it may be more appropriate to think of Maslow's contribution as a model which recognises the different and variable types of needs we each have and which demand attention, the focus on each level being variable within our own and clients' personal situations, with individual and separate future goals and aspirations. Maslow's work has very much influenced management thought in its progression through the five levels, commencing with ensuring that our own security in our activities at the lower levels is ensured, before moving on to higher order needs such as autonomy and independent thought and action, leading to a further development of our capabilities and aspirations towards self-actualisation. Maslow's model promotes the human as a positive, creative and innovatory individual who also acts in a self-determined manner.

Theory X and theory Y

McGregor (1960) has suggested that the style of management adopted by managers was a func-

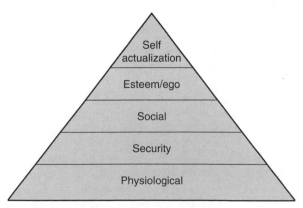

Figure 30.3   Maslow's Hierarchy of Needs.

tion of their assumptions about people and how they go about their working practices and relationships. In fact McGregor further followed through the implications of Maslow's theory for management approaches. Dependent upon one's personal philosophy and view of the person, according to McGregor if one perceives an individual as having characteristics of theory X, one assumes that the person needs to be directed and controlled and has little capacity for either self-motivation or problem solving. The motivation of these individuals is seen as being limited to Maslow's lower physiological and security levels. If, however, one perceives an individual as having theory Y characteristics, one assumes that the person is self-directed, motivated, and creative in thinking and problem solving, and for these individuals motivation occurs at all levels of the hierarchy. Payne (2000) suggests that employees like theory Y management and that most senior managers like to think that their organisations operate like that. However, to retain financial and procedural control, middle managers are forced to use theory X procedures.

Two-factor theory of motivation

Hertzberg's theory (Hertzberg et al 1959) identifies differences associated with job satisfaction. The satisfiers or motivators were achievement, recognition, the work itself, responsibility, advancement and the potential for growth. The dissatisfiers or hygiene factors identified were supervision, company policy, working conditions, interpersonal relations with superiors, peers and subordinates, status, job security and effect on one's personal life. Hertzberg's theory complements Maslow's where the satisfiers and dissatisfiers can be related to Maslow's maintenance levels and motivational factors for achievement (see Fig. 30.4). Nevertheless, Hertzberg has attracted criticism due to his narrow and limited research covering the occupations of engineering and accountancy.

Table 30.1 summarises the contributions made by different authors to management theories.

From reviewing these theorists we can see that both the scientific management and classic organisation movements emphasise the physical environment, and distance the manager and worker functions in not recognising or appraising the human dimension. The human relations and behavioural movements, however, focus upon individuals, group processes, interpersonal relationships and the manager's role in leadership of individuals and groups. It is here that practitioners who are managers can assist workers to develop their potential and can help them in meeting their needs and goals for recognition, accomplishment and a valued sense of belonging within a service or organisational culture. There are of course other models and theories representative of organisational management thought, but those

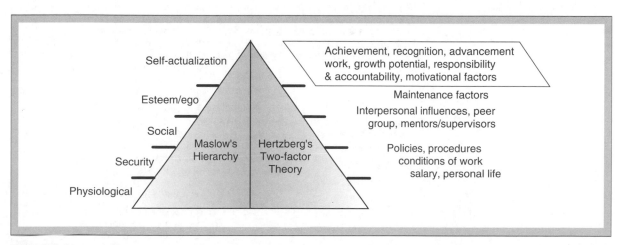

Figure 30.4

Table 30.1 Review of contributors to management theory

Theorist	Movement	Contribution to management theory	Relevance to practice
Taylor	Scientific management	• Division of labour – everyone has a place • Task specialisation • Perpetuates status – prevents contribution and maintains managerial control	• Limitations are that it fails to recognise the full potential of the individual • Perpetuates status and separates managers from Human Service workers • Benefits are that practitioners can study the complexity of care through a task analysis to predict staffing needs and study the efficiency and effectiveness of nursing care, e.g. a functional analysis of a client's behaviour can determine the level of expertise a member of staff requires i.e. the establishment of an appropriate staff team and skill mix • Setting of standards and protocols
Fayol	Classic organisation	Defines management functions • Planning • Organisation • Command • Coordination • Control	Stages similar to the nursing process. Nurse practitioners being aware of their managerial tasks and functions. NURSING PROCESS / MANAGEMENT PROCESS Assessing ———— Planning Planning — Planning / Staffing / Organizing Implementing — Organizing / Directing Evaluating ———— Controlling Source: Marquis & Huston (2000)
Mayo	Human relations	• Hawthorne studies • Work patterns and quality of work achieved are influenced by the individual's acceptability within the work team • Social needs are a major motivator above financial incentives	• Development of team work • Importance of developing learning disability service workers to their potential
Lewin	Human relations	• Study of group dynamics, groups which are democratic and solve own problems and have access to consult with the team leader are most effective • Group forces can overcome individual interests	• Meeting needs for recognition • Accomplishment whilst having a sense of belonging • Mindful of the environment and setting for staff i.e. stress factors, isolation, lack of effective support mechanisms, example through supervision
Maslow	Behavioural science	• Development of a hierarchy of needs theory • Central tenet is that each of us has a range of capacities & skills that we will use if given the right opportunities	• Theory embraces the concept that each member of staff is viewed positively • Is capable of mature and creative behaviour • A degree of autonomy and interdependence in setting mutually agreed standards and protocols for practice • Acts in a self-determined manner
McGregor	Behavioural science	• Two-factor model	• The importance of achievement, recognition, responsibility and advancement as satisfiers

Table 30.1   Review of contributors to management theory—cont'd

• Based upon workers' satisfiers and dissatisfiers within the work environment	• A crucial consideration for developing individual potential within services that do not have an obvious career structure • Emphasis on lifelong learning and continuing professional development • Learning Disability Awards Framework should enhance and support these satisfiers for achievement (DOH 2001)

Box 30.2   Factors to be considered for an effective team

- How practitioners as managers perceive the learning disability worker
- How individual staff relate to one another
- How we can achieve the maximum cooperation and contribution and
- How we go about changing from a situation which is dysfunctional or ineffective to one which is promoting higher standards.

---

presented above, albeit briefly, have had a significant influence on the development of management style. What is acknowledged and emphasised through these theories is that management in services and organisations today is largely about managing people. As identified in *Valuing People* (DOH 2001) 75% of the workforce is unqualified which means that qualified practitioners need to harness their management skills and recognise that the workforce within learning disability services is an important asset, and that the effectiveness of workers within a team is related to several factors, which are shown in Box 30.2.

THE INFLUENCE AND DEVELOPMENT OF LEADERSHIP THEORIES

Just as there are numerous management theories, so there are numerous theories of leadership, and current research demonstrates that there is certainly not just one style of leadership that will be successful in all situations (Margerison 1979).

Nevertheless nurses can select and familiarise themselves with various theories and adapt the most suitable approach for dealing with each different situation. A brief review of theories will be given, followed by what are seen as the more appropriate and contemporary theories for leadership within the context of managing change in learning disability services.

First, we need to distinguish between leadership theory and style. Theory is a term used to explain and to offer general principles that attempt to represent the real world, and style is the way in which a practitioner performs within a particular situation and offers the leader alternative ways to enact a theory of leadership. Many leadership theories exist but they can be broadly categorised under three main approaches: traitist, behavioural and contingency–situational.

- Traitist. Traitist theory attempts to determine what characteristics a successful leader possesses by examining the leader's personality. The assumption behind this approach was that leaders were in possession of special qualities which made them stand out and students of the traitist theory hoped that once the qualities were identified, these could be studied and acquired through experience. According to Stogdill (1974) cited in Rumbold (1995), studies were found to be ambiguous; some leaders were found to have many characteristics, such as intelligence, scholarship, acceptance of responsibility, participation and socio-economic status, whereas others only had perhaps one. Ghiselli (1971) showed that certain traits do seem to be important, i.e. supervisory ability, need for occupational achievement, intelligence, decisiveness, self-assurance and initiative.

- The behavioural approach. This theoretical approach moves away from the idea that leaders are born. Instead it promotes the view that leaders can be developed and the focus is shifted away from what leaders are like in terms of characteristics, and instead towards what tasks they can achieve and to the process of social relationships with individuals or groups of people. Key contributors in this field are Blake & Mouton (1964, 1985) who created the 'managerial grid', which focused on task and employee orientations of managers. Figure 30.5 is an adaptation of the original grid by Blake & Mouton (1964), from which Blake, Mouton & Tapper's (1981) nurse administrator grid was developed. The grid, as in the original formulation, is essentially divided into two axes;

concern for task orientation is shown on the horizontal axis and concern for people on the vertical axis. The grid offers a range of combinations of the two concerns. Someone in the position 1,1 has scored low on both task and people orientation, indicating an abdicator, and at the other extreme someone in the 9,9 position is the ideal type of leader to function as an effective manager.

Blake & Mouton (1964, 1985) insisted that a high concern for both employees and production was the most effective type of leadership behaviour, and sought not a balance (5,5 management) but leaders who attempted to achieve both the best task performance and the best social relations (9,9 management) who would then support each other to the greatest possible extent. In essence, to achieve effective team work it is important to achieve a high degree of attention

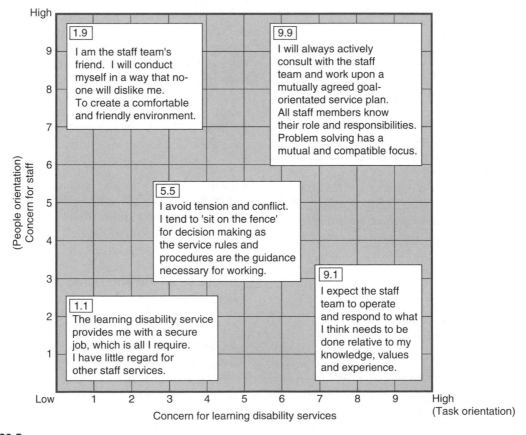

Figure 30.5

to both; it is also suggested that this is an ideal leadership style in all situations.

- Contingency–situational approach. During the 1960s Fred Fiedler introduced the contingency model of leadership. He argued that a leadership style is dependent on the situation as to whether it will be successful or not, and he played down the assumption that there will be an ideal leader for all situations. Within the context of learning disability there are many variables to consider when managing and leading a team of practitioners. Such variables include individual and group behaviours, knowledge and experience, dynamics, the environment, the history and culture of the service along with the background and personality of the team leader. Two prominent theorists in this field are Hersey & Blanchard (1977) who developed the

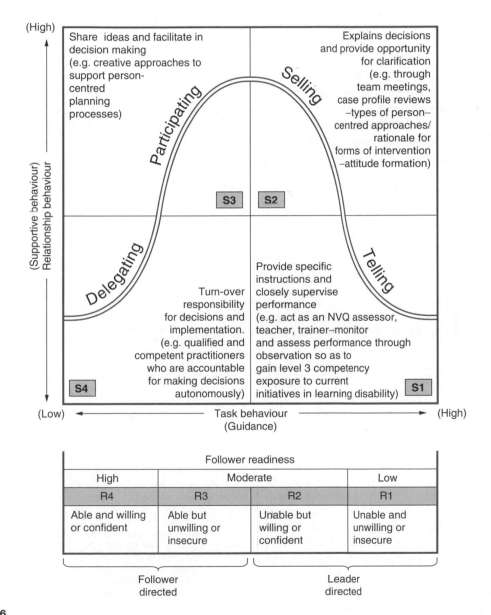

Figure 30.6

situational leadership theory based upon the maturity level of the individual or group. The theory advocates an assessment of the group or individual on a continuum from a low-level maturity to a high-level maturity and is illustrated in Figure 30.6 in a four quadrant model.

At the bottom of the diagram four classifications are represented where the staff member(s)' (or followers') motivation or readiness is assessed. In R1 the team member is neither willing nor able to accept responsibility. In R2 the team member is willing but unable to accept responsibility. In R3 the team member is able but unwilling to accept responsibility and in R4 the team member is both able and willing to accept responsibility. On deciding which level of readiness is best represented by the team an appropriate style may be selected by the leader. According to Hersey & Blanchard, a curvilinear relationship exists within each of the quadrants and through their research they have determined, within each quadrant, a relational style which can be adopted. The high task, low relational style is called 'telling', where the leader has total control. The high task, high relationship style is called 'selling', where the leader has more control than the team group members. The low task, high relationship quadrant style is 'participating', where the leader has equal control with the team. The low task, low relationship style is called 'delegating', where the leader is seen as having very little control. In effect, team members with the lowest level of readiness can be led by adopting the 'telling' style, and those with the second lowest level respond better to the 'selling' style. For team players in the R3 state of readiness, 'participation' is most effective and for those in the highest level of readiness, R4, 'delegation' is seen as appropriate. To determine the most appropriate leadership style, one must assess the maturity level of the individual or group, plot it on the maturity continuum, and project a line at a right angle from that point until it intersects with the curvilinear line. The quadrant in which intersection occurs depicts the most appropriate leadership style. With increased maturity, less structure and emotional support

are needed. In contrast, high task and low relationship style is considered best for below average maturity. Leadership styles in quadrants two and three are recommended for the average group or individual.

Case illustration 30.1 gives an example of how situational leadership theory could be used to analyse and improve teamwork.

Transactional and transformational leadership

Burns (1978) identifies that for managing change, there are two types of leadership styles, transactional and transformational. Transactional leaders, who organise groups around their personal goals and who believe that others are also motivated by personal goals, are likely to use coercion

Case illustration 30.1

Over the years the media have produced documentaries which have not only illustrated the need for more resources for people with learning disabilities, but have also heightened awareness in the public domain that in some service provision poor quality and inappropriate care practices, which include negligence and abuse, unfortunately exist. Documentaries such as *Perfect Victims* (Panorama 1995) and more recently *MacIntyre Undercover* (MacIntyre 1999), which through secret filming gave an account of Donal MacIntyre's first hand experience of abusive practices within Brompton Care Home. This documentary observed and recognised a dysfunctional team of staff who quite clearly required leading and managing in terms of appropriate individual attitudes to working care and team practices. Using Hersey & Blanchard's (1977) situational leadership model, a newly appointed home leader would assess in this instance that the staff were at the lowest level of readiness and would require to be effectively led by using the 'telling' and 'selling' styles which are leader directed and controlled. Eventually the staff team could reach a level of maturity and competency through training, education and supervisory support. With attitudinal change from the outset, staff members could reach a stage of skills development and maturity where a more collaborative and negotiated style of participation could emerge and develop which would lead to an acceptable level of competent practice. Although perhaps a rather extreme example is portrayed here, the emphasis on providing an accurate assessment of team members' readiness to be led through an appropriate style is quite clear.

and rewards. Transactional managers are more conforming, explicit and orderly in achieving their tasks. Turrell (1986) has suggested that the orderly breaking down of tasks by transactional managers often leads to a loss of vision and energy, whereas the transformational leader can keep a distance, and a strategic or a helicopter view of the whole, to motivate others through values, vision and empowerment. As Broome (1998) has stressed, 'The Transformational leader is more effective at large visionary changes of a new or renewing organisation', and 'The Transactional leader is best at the systematic work of a leader at the consolidation stage'. Box 30.3 illustrates the qualities of the two leadership styles.

Reader activity 30.2

Think of the most influential role-model and leader you have had. It can be anyone inside or outside of your professional education or practice experience, anyone that particularly stands out in your mind as a leader. Write down and discuss with a colleague what it is that this person did that made them an 'effective' leader. Don't explain how they made you feel, instead focus on what behaviour they demonstrated to make you feel that way.

Transformational leadership

More than likely your responses will fall into four dimensions that comprise the central tenets of transformational leadership:

Box 30.3 Core factors of transactional and transformational leadership

Transactional	Transformational
Bargains	Empowers
Is task-centred	Inspires vision, ideals
Separates home from work	Mixes home and work
Has a short-term/ medium-term focus	Has a long-term focus
Coaches sheltered learning	Challenges
Rewards formally	Rewards informally, and personally
Is comfortable, orderly	Is emotional, turbulent
Complicates	Simplifies

- Idealised influence. Leaders engender trust and respect from their followers, ensuring they are doing the right thing rather than ensuring they do things right.
- Inspirational motivation. Leaders raise the 'bar' for their employees, encouraging them to achieve levels of performance beyond their own expectations.
- Intellectual stimulation. Leaders engage the rationality of colleagues, getting them to challenge their assumptions and think about old problems in new ways. They help employees to answer their own questions.
- Individualised consideration. Leaders treat employees as individuals, being compassionate, recognising and celebrating their achievements (Bass 1998).

Transformational leadership is now well established with most authors having a consensus on key elements, placing interpersonal communication, mutuality, affiliation and empowerment at the heart of leadership – but how do we do it? According to Kellaway & Barling (2000) the payoff in promoting transformational leaders is making small consistent changes in behaviour. These authors say that this form of leadership can be taught, and they make the point that although many books on leadership strategies are available, sadly most of such works are bought but not read or read but not implemented. They make a number of recommendations that are reproduced in Box 30.4

Leadership qualities

In terms of learning disability services Boulter & Cook (1997) have rejected transactional leadership due to its emphasis on systems rather than cultures, whilst Moore (1999) has promoted transformational leadership with a number of recommendations:

- Clarification of the 'vision' of providing high quality health care and encouragement of networking and best practice initiatives.
- Identification of charismatic, emergent leaders and provision of a structure that creates

---

Box 30.4 Recommendations for effective transformational leadership

Idealised influence

- Leaders do what is right, rather than what is expedient or the most cost-effective
- Leaders take some time to make their decision making more transparent and to be consistent in their reasoning across people
- Consistently making decisions using the same criteria builds respect and trust
- Leaders who are seen by their colleagues/employees as people who can be counted on to 'do the right thing' epitomise idealised influence.

Inspirational motivation

- Leaders who display enthusiasm and optimism, communicating the message 'I know you can do it' raise the employees' sense of self-efficacy and inspire individuals to try harder to carry out a broader and more proactive role beyond traditional prescribed requirements
- Ability of the leader to communicate optimism and enhance role breadth self-efficacy is critical to enhanced organizational outcomes.

Intellectual stimulation

- Is enhanced by a leader's ability to get employees to think about work related problems in new ways
- Responding to questions by asking 'What do you think we should do?' or 'What would you advise if you were me?'. This engages employees' minds in the work place
- This encapsulates the concept of lifelong learning and partnerships within a workplace which is resource or career pathway limited
- Leaders enhance intellectual stimulation by providing colleagues and employees with opportunities for development that are permanent.

Individualised consideration

- Ability of the leader to respond to individual needs by acting as a coach, mentor, supervisor and confidant
- Making time to pay attention to individual concerns is one of the key behaviours
- Scheduling time to talk to staff
- Personally thanking colleagues for their efforts.

Kellaway & Barling (2000)

---

opportunities for them to maximise their contribution and development.

- Ensuring that there is as equal an emphasis on values and ethics as there is on objectives and goals and paying attention to the compatibility of organisational and service philosophy.
- Involvement of service users in service planning where transformational emphasis on individual needs should prove a good vehicle for assisting them in their contribution.
- Strengthening links with professional organisations and academia to improve political awareness by contribution to and attendance at conferences, steering groups and focus groups (Moore 1999).

Klakovich (1994) has promoted a more connective style of leadership and maintains that transformational leadership is seen as competitive rather than fostering an interdependency through networking, which lends support for Moore's (1999) recommendations. Bowles & Bowles (2000) have found that leadership within Nursing Development Units had more of a transformational nature than the leadership of their counterparts working within more conventional clinical settings. This, they suggest, may be due to Nursing Development Units providing a workplace that is more conducive to transformational leadership through, for example, enhanced staff participation and empowerment and new forms of clinical leadership. Certainly the broad spectrum of learning disability work environments would also share this propensity towards a transformational style of leadership. Moore (1999) has suggested, that this arises through working within multi-agency teams and in community settings where the adoption of an empowering, non-paternalistic philosophy, coupled with creativity, reflection, commitment and consistency are also advocated concepts in transformational leadership familiar to learning disability practitioners.

MANAGING CHANGE

Change agents

So far we have been concerned with those theories of management style and leadership which can aid practitioners to promote positive effective change within individuals and staff teams. Practitioners within learning disability services are purposefully positioned within services to bring about best practices, not only in positive client behaviours, but also in immediate service provision as well as in the context of the wider community. As explored previously, practitioners within learning disability services are in a position of influence to act as essential change agents, not only in personal care and development strategies with individuals, but also in the wider provision of service delivery, since there are no longer strict boundaries or role demarcations. It is vital that practitioners reach across the various stakeholders and contribute to the change process, not only for their own professional survival but to ensure positive developments within services. There are many terms used to describe individuals charged with effective implementation of change, examples being problem solvers, facilitators, project managers or task groups. The focal point of a change need not necessarily be a specific individual – a specialist working party or group could just as easily be designated as responsible for managing the change process – nevertheless, the practitioner who manages and leads a local service or team is ultimately responsible and accountable as an 'agent of change'.

There are principally two types of change agents. The first type is usually identified as a consultant who has specialist knowledge or is seen as an expert appointed to the service to assist them in the process of change for a specific project; this type of change agent is outside the service or organisation and is known as an external change agent. A service may look to an external change agent to review the quality of that service following a poor internal review, so as to make recommendations and commence a change strategy to improve the delivery and level of that service for people with a learning disability. These areas of change, in this instance for a global improvement in individuals and a corporate approach to service delivery, may be described under four targets of change defined by Hersey & Blanchard (1977): a need for a change in knowledge, a need for a change in attitude, a need for a change in individual behaviour and a need for a change in group

behaviours. The advantages of an external change agent are that such a person can be completely objective in making any recommendations. Drawbacks to external agents of change are that the process of assessment is usually lengthy and that because the external change agent will not benefit from or need to adjust personally to the change, members of the target group may not fully cooperate.

The second type of change agent comes from within a service or organisation and is called an internal change agent. The advantages are that such a change agent has first hand experience of and familiarity with the organisation's philosophy, culture, policies and procedures and internal politics. In contrast with the external change agent, the internal change agent may already be recognised as trustworthy, and the target group will recognise that the internal change agent will also be part of the adjustment to change and will therefore be more willing to support this individual. Internal change agents can also come from any level within the service and can be identified as formal change agents where an official appointment to be in charge of change is made due to recognition of the person's level of skill and experience. However, informal change agents can also evolve as a result of the support and sanction of a staff group who are dependent on that person's degree of skill in engendering a cohesive working team.

Change theories

Now that change agents have been identified, change theories which can support change agents' approaches will be reviewed, commencing with Lewin (1951) whose origins were in social psychology within the human relations movement. His legacy is in the acknowledgement that a true understanding of behaviour requires not only an in-depth knowledge of the person, but also a knowledge of what surrounds the person. It was from this basis that the 'force-field' model was conceived, using psychological terms as a basis for helping us to understand what keeps an individual, service or organisation in equilibrium. Lewin described behaviour within an organisation as a dynamic balance between driving and restraining forces. Driving forces are forces that facilitate change – they lead members of an organisation in new directions, towards a new goal. Restraining forces are forces that impede change and work towards maintaining the status quo. A manager has to analyse these forces and shift the balance between the two sets of forces. Lewin has suggested that this change is brought about through a three-step process of unfreezing, moving and refreezing.

Unfreezing

The goal here is to clarify what is and make the staff team aware of the need for change. Unfreezing attempts to bring about readiness for change by creating dissatisfaction with the present.

The nurse leader assists the group to raise questions and explore attitudes and feelings about the present scenario. When the team acknowledges dissatisfaction they have committed themselves to change.

Moving

This is dependent on the outcome and results of the unfreezing stage. To bring about change, driving forces must exceed restraining forces.

Refreezing

The goal of the refreezing phase is to stabilise change with new knowledge. Attitudes and behaviour are learned during the moving phase which must continue to be practised until they have become as familiar as the preceding attitudes and behaviour. This is achieved either by increasing the driving forces or reducing the restraining forces, or a combination of both. While the two sets of forces remain in balance, or to use Lewin's terminology frozen, there will be no change. According to Rumbold (1995) this can be compared to Orem's nursing theory in that the need to change results from an imbalance. In Lewin's theory there is a need to create an imbalance in which the driving forces are greater than the restraining forces, and then move towards a new goal and

state of equilibrium. Rumbold (1995) also identifies Lippitt et al (1958) who expanded Lewin's theory into a seven-step process and focused more on the behaviour of the change agent. This is shown in Box 30.5.

Boddy & Buchanan (1992) have identified that change agents face core tasks which aim to reduce the uncertainty associated with the change situation and then encourage positive action. In this challenge they suggest a five point plan to be pursued by the change agent:

Box 30.5 Seven step process for change

1. Diagnosis of the problem

   - Involve key personnel in collecting data and problem solving.
   - What are the problems?
   - What opportunities are there for development and change?
   - What do we have to offer?

   Collects external data, for example through government reports/Trust policies/demographic and epidemiological data on learning disability through profiling. This data supports the need for change.

2. Assessing the motivation and capacity for change

   - How motivated are team members to effect proposed change?
   - Are resources sufficient to help change?

3. Self-assessment

   - How committed are you, as the change agent, to proposed change?

   (This might be more appropriate as a first step to pursue.)

4. Selection of progressive change agents

   - Involves development of an action plan.
   - How is it to be carried out?
   - How will it be evaluated.

5. Identifying a role as a change agent

   - How are you going to act? As an expert, as a consultant or as a group facilitator?

6. Maintaining the change

   - This is the same as Lewin's refreezing stage.
   - Involves both communication and feedback.

7. Ending the helping relationship

   - As change becomes implemented within the service, part of how things are done, the team leader gradually drops the role adopted as change agent and resumes her/his usual role. (Lippett et al 1958)

1. Identify and manage stakeholders, thereby gaining visible commitment.
2. Work on objectives, making them clear, concise and understandable.
3. Set a full agenda. Take a holistic helicopter view and highlight potential difficulties.
4. Build appropriate control systems. Communication is a two way process, feedback is required.
5. Plan the process of change. Pay attention to:
   a. Establishing roles – clarity of purpose
   b. Building a team – do not leave it to chance
   c. Nurturing coalitions of support – fight apathy and resistance
   d. Communicating relentlessly – manage the process
   e. Recognising power – make the best use of supporting power bases
   f. Handing over – ensure that the change is maintained.

According to Paton & McCalman (2000) an effective change agent must be capable of orchestrating events, socialising within the network of stakeholders, and managing the communication process.

Strategies for changing

Chin & Benne (1985) have proposed three well known strategies for changing, i.e. empirical-rational, normative-re-educative and power-coercive:

- *Empirical-rational* This is most frequently the strategy adopted by practitioners within health and social care. Human beings are seen as rational and as following a pattern of self interest, i.e. people will change when they are shown that the proposed change can be justified rationally and that they will ultimately benefit from such a change.
- *Normative-re-educative* Here, what people do is determined by the norms to which they subscribe and the degree of commitment they have to these norms. Norms come from one's society, culture, religion, family and other sources. Change occurs when commitment to some present norms decreases to a point where new norms can be adopted. It is more than an

increased knowledge, it is a modification of values and attitudes, as well as of behaviour. It requires direct intervention by a change agent to aid in the learning and relearning process.
- *Power-coercive* This is the use of legitimate political and economic power to force compliance with change. It may be used by a person who is in a high hierarchical position within an organisation to effect change that he or she personally feels is desirable or necessary. The group affected by the change is forced to comply, without having any input. When selecting a strategy, nurse leaders as change agents must take into account both their relationship with the group and the target of change. Such nurse leaders will be most effective when the strategy adopted has consistency with the overall goals of the planned change and does not sabotage their relationship with the group.

Putting it all together

Theory on change agents, change theories and change strategies can be rather daunting and so the following case studies should assist in relating theory to practice. The recently published White Paper *Valuing People* (DOH 2001, Ch. 6) identifies that the community learning disability team is well placed to undertake the role of health facilitators and proceeds to indicate that learning disability nurses are appropriate practitioners to pursue such a role in improving health care links between the primary health care team and secondary care providers.

Bollard (1999) has provided an example of a change strategy which adopted Boddy & Buchanan's (1992) framework. This first case study (30.2) identifies how, as an internal change agent, he applies change theory and it also illustrates how Lewin's 'unfreezing, moving and refreezing' model can be applied. As a change agent it is clear that Bollard adopts both an empirical-rational and normative-re-educative approach appropriate both to individuals and to the practice setting.

The second case illustration (30.3) is a hypothetical scenario relating to dispersed housing schemes which are not achieving their potential because of a weakness in management, training and monitoring (Mansell 2000).

Bennis & Nanus (1985) have suggested that good leaders should contribute the following:

- a clear vision for the future
- a culture of change
- dynamic management of the boundaries and
- development of an organisation as a learning community where skills are actively developed in tune with the emerging issues.

This case illustration also demonstrates Lewin's 'unfreezing, moving and refreezing' model of change and reflects what may be a typical service organisational issue and dilemma for staff working within managed dispersed housing schemes for people who have a learning disability, within the context of an independent provider. As many providers are involved in the delivery of a service to people with a learning disability, whether it is provided by the independent or the statutory sector, the service that is being delivered is dependent upon the qualifications, skills, motivation, attitudes and experience of its workforce. The qualities expressed in the management of change are dependent upon the quality of the skills engendered within those practitioners charged with the responsibility of leading and managing that service.

The service manager, by virtue of her position, predominantly works with individuals, groups and systems, and is continually involved in management of change within the service she manages, which is a group of six homes that are located in a rural county and are part of an independent company.

Conclusions to be drawn from both these case studies are that change, when planned strategi-

---

Case illustration 30.2 Improving access and health screening in primary health care

Identify and manage stakeholders
Bollard (1999) provided evidence from a locally conducted survey. He was proactive across stakeholders within the Trust and ensured involvement in the project bid. He met and maintained contact with commissioners, gave progress reports coupled with the submission of formal reports and communicated with the funding agency on a regular basis. (**Unfreezing stage**.)

Work objectives concise and understandable
He clarified and discussed whilst continuing to raise awareness of the project objectives from the outset. He engaged primary health care teams in the project through initial meetings and presentations. He ensured a mutual understanding of the project aims and allowed time to do this. Clear and reader friendly documentation was used at all times. He communicated widely, from practice receptionist and practice nurse to the senior GP partner. (**Unfreezing stage**.)

Set a full agenda
He set the project plan, with times and dates to achieve, but was prepared to change it. Outcome measures were set, and problems met head on, through being visible in practices. He listened and changed the health screening tool. The tool is an evolving concept; despite the benefits of standardisation it needs to suit the way each practice works; this allows ownership. Engaging with service users and carers, getting feedback wherever possible and keeping a diary throughout, which assisted at report writing time, were all important. (**Moving**).

Build appropriate control systems
It was important to communicate widely, establish health screening protocols and ensure these were in place and understood. Leaders need to make themselves available. Projects deserve and demand ongoing evaluation and formal and informal systems were included to achieve this. A database was set up in specialist services mirroring information on health check tools kept in GP notes. Practice nurses were allowed to conduct health checks, in order to value and recognise others' expertise. Leaders' own expertise should be recognised, valued and shared. Bollard linked in with specialist services and checked the project demands with them, and GP practice ownership was fostered. (**Moving to refreezing**.)

Plan process of change
Information was disseminated widely during and after the project through conferences and keynote speeches, publications and a project report. Opportunities to influence were sought.

Board presentations on local, regional and national forums were given. Being political and identifying and using people with influence were important as was ensuring good hand-over at project completion. Giving support and advice on similar projects, and making themselves available to others ensured that leaders shared experiences so others could learn. (**Refreezing.**)

(Bollard 1999)

cally can work to great effect once an overall vision is communicated and realised with all concerned, and change can be both painless and exciting, with a renewed sense of ownership shared by all involved in the change process.

THE INFLUENCE AND RELATIONSHIP BETWEEN THEORY AND PRACTICE

If nurses are to be seen to manage people and services effectively as well as providing appropriate leadership, these qualities and principles need to be grounded upon a knowledge base which ultimately informs assessment and intervention strategies. We have seen how by adopting theories of management and leadership we can effect change through strong personal and interpersonal attributes, strategies and styles. Nevertheless this can all be to no avail if we have no sense of direction; we need a fundamental knowledge base in which we can usefully apply these theories to that which underpins health and social care practice – the

Case illustration 30.3 Strategic development of a staff team within a dispersed housing scheme

The case illustration is based on 3 Turngate Drive, a fictitious home for six people with a severe learning disability. It is located in a town approximately 25 miles from its nearest managed home, where other staff work, and is part of a group of six managed homes which come under the auspices of the same provider. Up until the present time the homes have gained a favourable evaluation both from within the service and from the local authority funding and inspection agency. Nevertheless, due to impending changes within the service, bringing new and improved systems and a review of management functions into place, there is a necessity to improve in areas of collaboration and partnership with other stakeholders and interested parties.

The service manager is aware and concerned that a small number of heads of homes have become resistant to change, and that areas such as communication, attitudes and taking on of new roles are perceived as problematic. There is a feeling of 'why does the present culture and way of doing things have to change?' The overall service is also in the process of having its 'Investor in People' award reviewed. The following procedure is based upon and adapted from Broome (1998), who provides a more in-depth discussion on change processes (see Further reading).

Defining the current state
As with any service for people with a learning disability, environmental mapping with key people demonstrates a complex system with many boundary issues, which would need addressing in any change process. The demands on the service in this case had recently changed, in that service managers needed to relinquish more of the operational home management responsibilities to heads of homes in favour of a more strategic, quality monitoring and research role. Service managers would therefore need to have faith in and reliance on heads of home to perform well and rise to the expectations of effective management and leadership within each of the homes. A first stage could be to employ a force-field analysis to get a feel for the nature of change.

The service manager could conduct individual and structured objective interviews so as to engender an attitude of desire for change in the workforce within 3 Turngate Drive, in those involved in the total organisation supporting the home, as well as in the boundaries, i.e. all those people who have formal or informal contacts with the home (see Fig. 30.7).

Individuals from different levels in the structure were selected to represent the widest range of roles and responsibilities from the bottom to the top. The analysis of the interviews and a subsequent force-field analysis revealed the following issues:

- A low level of internal cohesion – information and communication was not being widely shared, but potentially there were good informal social relationships between staff.
- A dysfunctional relationship with specialist teams, for example when called upon initially staff comply the with assessment proposed, but subject programmes to sabotage when left to implement them with clients.
- Specialist team attitudes are also an issue when visiting the home, i.e. evidence of arrogance and 'we know best' – health versus social care staff.
- The home has a low level of creative thinking and problem solving, and a lack of consistency in approach to care practices.
- Although the home staff team had a company philosophy and mission statement, this was not adhered to.
- Involvement/engagement of people who lived at the home was minimal.
- Although staff development was evident, it didn't appear to logically fit in with the developmental needs of the people who lived at the home.
- Company initiatives appeared to be imposed rather than owned or discussed with staff teams.
- Poor image and relationship with social service contract and purchasing representatives.

Case illustration 30.3 (Cont'd)

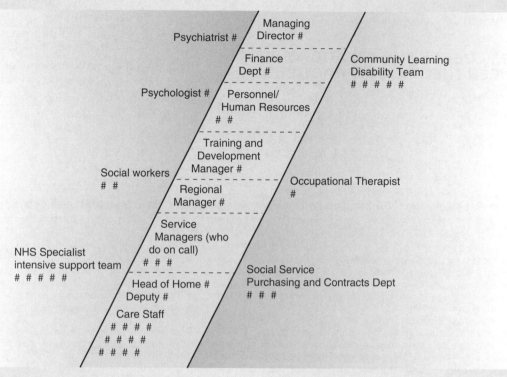

Figure 30.7 Transverse section illustrating boundaries.

- Poor image and relationship with the community learning disability team – especially the community nurse.

From reviewing the broad picture both within and outside the home, it could be seen that overall there were some good staff who were receptive to new ideas and would welcome a cultural change which contained a more structured and supportive approach to their work. As identified by Øvretveit (1994), the dynamics of the existing team members might be to do with power differences and conflict, and could as a consequence overflow on to service users, and therefore lead to a dysfunctional approach which impedes the purpose and delivery of effective care strategies, and the need for change. Maslach (1982) has also observed the process of 'burnout', particularly within the human services, where without appropriate support and professional development, practitioners can become both frustrated and exhausted. Nevertheless, to commence the change process the above information needed to be shared first with those staff who contributed and then with other key people, both within and on the boundaries of 3 Turngate Drive. It was agreed that those with ideas about change (the staff team) should be given assistance to bring their ideas to fruition (*The unfreezing stage*).

Describe future/desired state
It was agreed that the service manager would form a project group (internal change agents) consisting of the six heads of home. The purpose of this group was to define the future running of the homes, creating a vision so as to drive the changes through, as well as supporting each head of home with a personal development and action plan. The service manager during this stage would assess the readiness and capability of people to *move* and would spend time with those individuals who would help in the moving stages. As a transformational leader she would empower people and encourage them through mutual support and vision.

Force-field analysis
This was compiled from an analysis of the key people who, as well as being insiders of the organisation, had a feel for some of the critical issues from informal discussions, observations and visits to the home and partaking of meetings. The analysis showed where some of the difficulties were: for instance, some individuals were pushing for change, but they were not very good at formulating ways of making those changes happen (e.g. top down directives to be interpreted and implemented at a local level in the homes).

Case illustration 30.3 (*Cont'd*)

Change equation
These are the areas which require specific pressure and cumulatively these areas are greater than the actual cost of change:

- Building up a vision of the future that the staff team desires
- Allowing them to become dissatisfied with the present situation and level of performance

- Demonstrating through target setting that it is easy to change by designing the initial programme.

In the beginning of any change process it perhaps feels far easier to continue to do things the same way. Egan (1986, p. 334) identified that within the problem management process there is a fear of starting a change programme (inertia). This is followed by a fear of things falling apart once change has started (entropy). The management

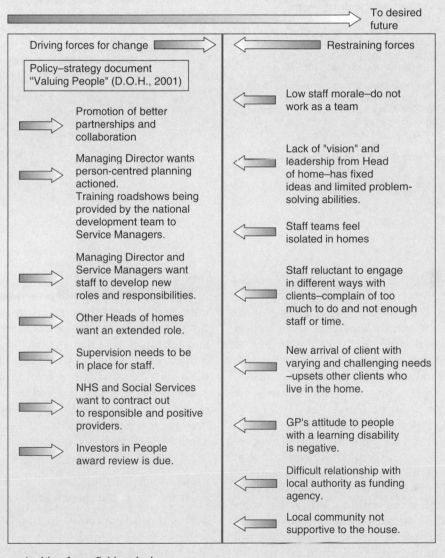

Figure 30.8 Turngate drive: force-field analysis.

Case illustration 30.3 (Cont'd)

of change process is a magnification of Egan's problem management model; problem management is individually applied, whereas change management is organisationally applied. Nevertheless, for change to occur in this case the service manager as an internal change agent needs to be skilled in using leverage to motivate and assist staff to realise that changes are preferable to standing still. The change equation outlines the areas of focus that can cause dissonance and upset the current status quo, and pushes staff towards feeling that change is less threatening and more desirable than standing still.

Summary of leverage (*moving and refreezing*)
This is where staff teams recognise that the future can be different. The force-field analysis (Fig. 30.8) had shown that many forces were working for change, which became more obvious during staff and project team meetings; a five stage process was developed as a result of this:

- *Stage 1* Staff team members brainstormed and defined each of the driving and restraining forces.
- *Stage 2* For each driving and restraining force they allocated each problem to an appropriate staff team.
- *Stage 3* Each team weighted the factors for their power and influence.
- *Stage 4* Each team and overall staff group collectively decided on which forces promoted or constrained an action plan.

- *Stage 5* The collective team identified those forces which they could do something about and planned what to do.

The how, who, where and when approach
This strategy, coordinated by the service manager, culminated in a staff team being able to foster:

- An increasing interest in working towards a better, more cohesive and strategic future with those people identified on the boundaries
- Use of their strong informal friendships to gather support and extend it to others
- A need to develop further working staff groups and develop more informal change agents to take forward initiatives such as person centred planning and supervision.

Other outcomes were as follows:
- Heads of homes viewed the future as more strategic, objective and with a renewed sense of value and purpose.
- Individual staff members had a personal development plan with specific targets to pursue.
- Positive relations were pursued with specialist teams, the GP/primary health care team and with carers.

foundation of a hands on approach with people with a learning disability. Many practitioners find it difficult to link theory and practice or to acknowledge the importance of any theoretical framework (Dalrymple & Burke 1995), but as Turnbull (1999) has emphasised, the construction of learning disability-specific models for practice, such as examples provided by Baldwin & Birchenall (1993), Turner & Coles (1997) and Bollard & Jukes (1999), will be an essential and dominant feature in giving leadership to the profession in the future and will be a key milestone in the empowerment of nurses within the learning disability field. For one of the recognised hallmarks of practitioners within a profession is an underlying knowledge base, a body of specialist knowledge which acts as the basis of professional expertise (Thompson 1995). Within services for people with a learning disability no one particular

professional group has a monopoly over providing a service. Therefore all practitioners, within or outside the nursing profession, must examine and reflect on their individual sets of beliefs, values and assumptions which in turn have been and are influenced by the various theories to which they have been exposed during their training and education. Sibeon (1990) has outlined a three level classification system of theory, which is adapted here for learning disability nursing practice (see Table 30.2) and is based on theories of:

- What learning disability nursing practice is
- How to do learning disability nursing
- The nature of the client world.

This classification is further subdivided in terms of 'Formal' and 'Informal' theory, the former being representative of what is found in the academic literature, whereas the latter constitutes 'the practice wisdom' of a profession, or the assumptions which are transmitted and formulated through actual practice with colleagues within diverse service models.

Within the myriad of learning disability services the ratio of professionally qualified nurses to unqualified staff is relatively small, and therefore the influence of informal theory as a means of direct application to practice is significant as it addresses more directly the day-to-day practice issues. Therefore the likelihood of unqualified or 'inexperienced' practitioners adopting ambiguous forms of practice which are based upon observations from more or less experienced role models within the service will not necessarily lead to an objective and informed approach to nursing practice. Formal theory, however, is subject to more open debate and critical examination and is explicitly expressed and located in the literature. Learning disability needs more theory and practice experience and application (Jukes 2001), since there exists at present in some services an attitude of anti-intellectualism and opposition to a specialist qualified workforce.

Therefore it is vital for professionally qualified practitioners to understand, differentiate between and articulate what constitutes 'formal' and 'informal' theory, and for management and leadership purposes, to distinguish between an informed and an ill-informed approach to practice and service delivery, as well as embracing and promoting anti-discriminatory and anti-oppressive practices.

ANTI-DISCRIMINATORY AND ANTI-OPPRESSIVE PRACTICE

These are important, indeed crucial concepts to be considered and operationalised in today's services for people with a learning disability. It is vital that within human services we continually question the nature of the work in which we are engaged.

Learning disability affects all members of our society, and so practitioners, managers, academics and researchers cannot afford to be seen as discriminatory or oppressive in their practices, values and assumptions across different cultures. One

Table 30.2 Classification system of theory adapted for learning disability nursing practice (after Sibeon 1990)

	Formal theory	Informal theory
Theories of what learning disability practice is	Formal written paradigms/theories which define the nature and purpose of nursing practice. Grand and middle range theories defining 'what is' health, the human, nursing and the environment. Theories on SRV, empowerment, humanism, behaviourism, psychology, sociology, health promotion and education	Individually influenced moral, political, psychological, socio-cultural values of viewing the work as internalised by practitioners. Defining individual nature and purposes of learning disability practice within society and the community
Theories of how to do learning disability nursing	Formal written theories and frameworks for practice, e.g. nursing models, transcultural models, crisis theory, behaviour theory, person centred planning, case work, family centred care, individual and group work, advocacy and empowerment	Unwritten informal practice. Theories constructed experientially from the practical experience of doing learning disability practice, e.g. how to approach and relate to people
Theories of the client world	Formal written theory, e.g. social science and psychological theories on disability, deviance, oppression, personality, relationships, marriage, family, gender, race and the community	Practitioners' use of and exposure to experientially acquired general cultural meanings and definitions, e.g. nature of the person, social behaviour, norms, good and bad parenting. Role of the person in society and the community

predominant philosophy that has significantly impacted upon learning disability is that of normalisation. Chappell (1992) has suggested that normalisation serves a functional model, whereas empowerment has an opposite dimension in that political power is redirected to the person, so that normalisation and empowerment become opposing ideologies in what they are designed to achieve.

In terms of definition of difference, anti-oppressive practice is about minimising the power differential within society and this potentially works best with a model of empowerment (Dalrymple & Burke 1995). This liberating position demands a rethink of existing values, services and relationships between learning disability nurses and people with a learning disability. Anti-discriminatory practice, however, is more about using specific legislation to challenge the discrimination faced by particular groups of people within our society, for example equal opportunities and employment law.

Anti-discriminatory practice and anti-oppressive practice can complement each other, but to adopt a purely anti-discriminatory stance would not confront the power differentials which exist within structured organisations such as the NHS and the social care sector in the provision of services from both resources and professionals. This perspective can be illustrated by looking at a specialist community learning disability team operating within a multicultural population (Case illustration 30.4).

What is interesting about this case illustration is that it shows how we need to have a clear perspective on what informs what we do: we need to examine the power relationship with others, and subsequently generate explanations of why things should be the way they are, both from an individual and a service perspective. This involves a clear identification of what represents our personal political ideology, our professional experiences, theoretical knowledge, self-image and experience from practice and training. That means examining our practice ideologies from a service perspective and translating these into service mission statements which in turn translate into a truly multicultural and anti-discriminatory service.

CONCLUSION

This chapter has focused upon the relationship between management and leadership within the context and ethos of developing learning disability services. In this chapter emphasis has been placed not only on styles and theories of management and leadership, but also on the process of managing change by informed and knowledgeable practitioners. Self-awareness is a critical starting point within the current climate, where many stakeholders are involved in service provision, and where managing change is perceived as a multi-agency and inter-professional activity in

Case illustration 30.4

A white community learning disability nurse (CLDN) is working with a young Asian man. Communication and understanding of cultural issues is a concern to the community nurse who feels inadequate and therefore unable to address fully the needs of this young man. The community learning disability nurse utilises services and legislation to ensure the services of an interpreter. From an anti-discriminatory perspective, the CLDN quite rightly adopts the resources to address the issue. From an anti-oppressive perspective the CLDN would use the legislation to ensure that the needs of the family were being addressed, but would also promote further enquiry within the service and team to consider wider issues beyond what is immediately obvious as a service requirement, such as:

- Why are only white CLDNs available within a multicultural population?
- What existing resources and interventions/treatments apply appropriately across different communities?
- How many Asian nurses are employed or attracted to work and train within learning disability nursing and health care?
- What local strategies are in place to promote access to professional training and which reflect equal opportunities?
- What education and training exists for multicultural working amongst health and social care teams?
- It is important that white CLDNs do not abdicate their responsibility in furthering knowledge and expertise within multicultural communities.
- CLDNs could become instrumental in developing a community profile.
- There is a need to further acknowledge strengths and expertise of individual practitioners as a resource.

which collaborative and appropriate team working practices can be fostered. A number of issues have emerged which suggest that in providing quality services for people with a learning disability, practitioners are the keystone in such partnership endeavours, and it is they who can develop appropriate management and leadership strategies to effect positive and visionary innovations within a consistent resource-limited climate. Practitioners who manage change, and who can provide effective leadership, also recognise that change needs to be responded to positively; the need to evaluate the results of change following a strategic process can assist in narrowing the theory–practice gap. It is important that foundations are laid that lead to effective strategies, which promote anti-oppressive and anti-discriminatory practice. This practice must be based on the principles of rights, independence, choice and inclusion and will need to be placed within the context of fully inclusive service provision, as promoted in *Valuing People* (DOH 2001).

REFERENCES

Alaszewski A, Gates B, Ayer S et al 2000 Education for diversity and change: final report of the ENB-funded project on educational preparation for learning disability nursing. The University of Hull, UK

Baldwin S, Birchenall M 1993 The nurse's role in caring for people with learning disabilities. British Journal of Nursing 2(17): 850–855

Bass B M 1998 Transformational leadership: industry, military and educational impact. Lawrence Erlbaum, Mahwah, NJ

Bennis W, Nanus B 1985 Leaders: the strategies for taking charge. Harper & Row, New York

Blake R R, Mouton JS 1964 The managerial grid. Gulf Publishing Co, Houston

Blake R R, Mouton J S 1985 The managerial grid III: the key to leadership excellence. Gulf Publishing Co, Houston

Blake R R, Mouton J S, Tapper M 1981 Grid approaches for managerial leadership in nursing. Mosby, St Louis

Boddy D, Buchanan D A 1992 Take the lead: interpersonal skills for project managers. Prentice-Hall, London

Bollard M 1999 Improving primary health care for people with learning disabilities. British Journal of Nursing 8(18): 1216–1221

Bollard M, Jukes M J D 1999 Specialist practitioner within community learning disability nursing and the primary health care team. Journal of Learning Disabilities for Nursing, Health and Social Care 3(1): 11–19

Boulter P, Cooke H 1997 Leadership in learning disability nursing. Nursing Management 4(1): 12–13

Bowles A, Bowles N B 2000 A comparative study of transformational leadership in nursing development units and conventional clinical settings. Journal of Nursing Management 8: 69–76

Broome A 1998 Managing change, 2nd edn. Essentials of nursing management. Managing change, 2nd edn. Macmillan Press, London

Buchanan D A, Huczynski A A 1997 Organizational behaviour: an introductory text, 3rd edn. Prentice-Hall, London

Burns J M 1978 Leadership. Harper & Row, London

Chappell A 1992 Towards a sociological critique of the normalisation principle. Disability, Handicap and Society 7(1): 35–52

Chin R, Benne K D 1985 General strategies for effecting changes in human systems. In: Bennis W G, Benne K D, Chin R (eds) The planning of change, 4th edn. Holt, Rinehart & Winston, New York, pp 22–45

Crow G L 2000 Knowing self. Chapter 2, pp 15–31. In: Bower F L (ed) Nurses taking the lead, personal qualities of effective leadership. W B Saunders, Philadelphia

Dalrymple J, Burke B 1995 Anti-oppressive practice social care and the law. Open University Press, Buckingham

Davis E 1997 The leadership role of health services managers. International Journal of Health Care Quality Assurance incorporating Leadership in Health Services. 10(4): 1–4

Department of Health 1990 The NHS and Community Care Act

Department of Health 1998 A first class service – quality in the new NHS. HMSO, London

Department of Health 1999 Making a difference: strengthening the nursing, midwifery and health visiting contribution to health and healthcare. HMSO, London

Department of Health 2000a The NHS plan. HMSO, London

Department of Health 2000b Lost in care. HMSO, London

Department of Health 2000c A quality strategy for social care. HMSO, London

Department of Health 2001 Valuing people: a new strategy for learning disability for the 21st century. HMSO, London

Emerson E, Robertson J, Gregory N et al 1999 Quality and costs of residential supports for people with learning disabilities: an observational study of supports provided to people with severe and complex learning disabilities in residential campuses and dispersed housing schemes. Hester Adrian Research Centre, Manchester

Egan G 1986 The skilled helper: a systematic approach to helping, 3rd edn. Brooks/Cole, Monterey, California

Ghiselli E 1971 Explorations in managerial talent. Pacific Palisades, Goodyear, California. In: Megginson LC et al 1986 Management: concepts and applications, 2nd edn. Harper & Row, New York

Hersey P, Blanchard K H 1977 Management of organizational behaviour, 3rd edn. Prentice-Hall, Englewood Cliffs, New Jersey

Hersey P, Blanchard K H 1988 Management of organizational behaviour: utilizing human resources, 5th edn. Prentice-Hall, Englewood Cliffs, New Jersey

Hertzberg F, Mausner B, Snyderman B B 1959 The motivation to work, 2nd edn. John Wiley & Sons, New York

Jukes M 2001 Learning disability nursing needs theory practice experience. British Journal of Nursing 10(3): 164

Kellaway E K, Barling J 2000 What we have learned about developing transformational leaders. Leadership and Organization Development Journal 21(7): 355–362

Kings Fund 1980 An ordinary life. Project Paper No.24. Kings Fund, London

Klakovich M D 1994 Connective leadership for the 21st century: a historical perspective and future directions. Advanced Nursing Science 16(4): 42–54

Lewin K 1951 Field theory in social science. Harper & Row, New York

Lippitt R, Watson J, Westley B 1958 The dynamics of planned change. Harcourt Brace & World, New York

Longcare 1998 Independent Longcare inquiry. Buckinghamshire County Council Press Statement, 22 June 1998

Loxley A 1997 Collaboration in health and welfare: working with difference. Jessica Kingsley, London

Luft H 1963 Group process. The National Press, USA

McGregor D 1960 The human side of enterprise. McGraw-Hill,

MacIntyre D 1999 MacIntyre Undercover. 16 November, BBC1

Mansell J 2000 Commentary. The quality & costs of village communities, residential campuses and community-based residential supports for people with learning disabilities. Tizard Learning Disability Review 5(1)(Jan): 17–19

Margerison C 1979 How to assess your managerial style. University MCB Press, Bradford

Marquis B L, Huston C J 2000 Leadership roles and management functions in Nursing. Theory and application, 3rd edn. Lippincott, Philadelphia

Marriner-Tomey A 1996 Nursing management and leadership, 5th edn. Mosby, St Louis

Maslach C 1982 Burnout: the cost of caring. Prentice-Hall (Spectrum), Englewood Cliffs, New Jersey

Maslow A H 1970 Motivation and personality. Harper & Row, New York

Mayo E 1945 The social problems of an industrial civilization. Andover Press, New York

Moore D 1999 A force to be reckoned with. Learning Disability Practice 2(3): 25–28

ovretveit J 1994 Coordinating community care, multidisciplinary teams and care management. Open University Press, Buckingham

Panorama 1995 Perfect victims. BBC

Parrish A, Birchenall P 1997 Learning disability nursing and primary healthcare. British Journal of Nursing 6(2): 92–98

Paton R A, McCalman J 2000 Change management. A Guide to effective implementation, 2nd edn. Sage, London

Payne M 2000 Teamwork in multiprofessional care. Macmillan, London

Rumbold G C 1995 Management skills for community nurses. Quay Books, Mark Allen Publishing, Salisbury

Sibeon R 1990 Comments on the structure and forms of social work knowledge. Social Work and Social Sciences Review 1(1):

Sines D 1988 Management of the mental handicap nursing services. Senior Nurse 8(2): 27–29

Sines D 1992 Managing services to assure quality. Chapter 5, pp. 61–73. In: Thompson T, Mathias P (eds) Standards and mental handicap: Keys to competence. Baillière Tindall, London

Sofarelli D, Brown D 1998 The need for nursing leadership in uncertain times. Journal of Nursing Management. 6: 201–207

Thompson N 1995 Theory and practice in health and social welfare. Open University Press, Buckingham

Thompson T, Mathias P 1998 Standards and learning disability, 2nd edn. Baillière Tindall/RCN, London

Turnbull J 1999 Who will lead the way? Learning Disability Practice. 2(2): 12–16 (July)

Turner M, Coles J 1997 Meeting the needs of people with learning disabilities: developing an interactive model of care. Journal of Learning Disabilities for Nursing, Health and Social Care 1(4): 162–170

Turrell E A 1986 Change and innovation: a challenge for the NHS (IHSM), London

United Kingdom Central Council for Nursing, Midwifery and Health Visiting 1998 Healthcare futures 2010. UKCC, London

Walton M 1984 Management and managing: a dynamic approach. Harper & Row, London

Weinstein J 1998 The professions and their interrelationships. In: Thompson T, Mathias P (eds) Standards and learning disability. Baillière Tindall/RCN, London, Ch 20, pp 324–343

FURTHER READING

Bernhard L A, Walsh M 1995 Leadership. The key to the professionalization of nursing, 3rd edn. Mosby, St Louis

Broome A 1998 Managing change. Essentials of nursing management, 2nd edn. Macmillan Press. London

Marriner-Tomey A 1996 Guide to nursing management and leadership, 5th edn. Mosby, St Louis

Paton R A, McCalman J 2000 Change management – a guide to effective implementation, 2nd edn. Sage, London

Payne M 2000 Teamwork in multiprofessional care. Macmillan, Basingstoke

USEFUL ADDRESSES

www.kingsfund.org.uk
www.doh.gov.uk/london
For both websites click on leadership development.

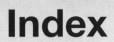

Index

Note: page numbers in italics refer to figures, tables and boxed material; Acts of Parliament refer to British Acts unless stated otherwise.